Library of Congress Cataloging-in-Publication Data

Names: French, Duncan N., editor. | Torres Ronda, Lorena, editor. |
  National Strength & Conditioning Association (U.S.), sponsoring body.
Title: NSCA's essentials of sport science / Duncan N. French and Lorena
  Torres Ronda, editors.
Other titles: National Strength & Conditioning Association's essential of
  sport science.
Description: First. | Champaign, IL : Human Kinetics, Inc., 2022. |
  Includes bibliographical references and index.
Identifiers: LCCN 2020043103 | ISBN 9781492593355 (hardback) | ISBN
  9781492593362 (epub) | ISBN 9781492593379 (pdf)
Subjects: LCSH: Sports sciences. | Sports--Physiological aspects. |
  Exercise--Physiological aspects.
Classification: LCC GV558 .N83 2022 | DDC 796.01--dc23
LC record available at https://lccn.loc.gov/2020043103

ISBN: 978-1-4925-9335-5 (print)

The web addresses cited in this text were current as of August 2020.

Senior Acquisitions Editor: Roger W. Earle; **Developmental Editor:** Laura Pulliam; **Managing Editor:** Miranda K. Baur; **Copyeditor:** Joyce Sexton; **Indexer:** Nan Badgett; **Permissions Manager:** Dalene Reeder; **Senior Graphic Designer:** Joe Buck; **Cover Designer:** Keri Evans; **Cover Design Specialist:** Susan Rothermel Allen; **Photographs (interior):** Human Kinetics unless otherwise noted.; **Photo Asset Manager:** Laura Fitch; **Photo Production Manager:** Jason Allen; **Senior Art Manager:** Kelly Hendren; **Illustrations:** © Human Kinetics, unless otherwise noted; **Printer:** Walsworth

Printed in the United States of America

10 9 8 7 6 5 4 3

The paper in this book was manufactured using responsible forestry methods.

Human Kinetics
1607 N. Market Street
Champaign, IL 61820
USA

United States and International
Website: **US.HumanKinetics.com**
Email: info@hkusa.com
Phone: 1-800-747-4457

Canada
Website: **Canada.HumanKinetics.com**
Email: info@hkcanada.com

E7917

Tell us what you think!
Human Kinetics would love to hear what we
can do to improve the customer experience.
Use this QR code to take our brief survey.

CONTENTS

Part VI   Special Topics

FOREWORD

Reflections on Sport Science

September 2019

Michael H. Stone, PhD

Department of Sport, Exercise, Recreation, and
  Kinesiology
East Tennessee State University
Johnson City, TN

Past and Present

Although many may make this mistake, science is not a debate where the side putting on the best show wins. Science is in reality a search for truth and clarity. Atlas did shrug, and objectivity, a value in science that informs the practice of science and discovery of scientific truths, should be highly valued.

From early in my life my interest was focused on biology and especially centered on trying to understand everything about strength-power training and athletic performance that I could. As I made my way through school and into college I could not help but be impressed with the extraordinary contributions that science and engineering had made in a variety of areas that impact people's lives. As popular as sport has been over the years and as big a business as it has become, I have wondered and still do wonder why more importance has not been placed on "sport and science."

It is easily argued that sport is one of the most important aspects of our life. For example: Turn on the 6 p.m. "News, Weather, and Sports"; whole magazines are dedicated to a sport or sports, newspapers and news websites have a sport section; many thousands of people watch sport on TV or attend competitions every week. Indeed, considering the great strides in technology, medicine/health, and generally making life more comfortable enabled by objectivity (science), a designed integration of sport and science should be a rational and logical goal.

During the last few years, roughly 1970 to the present, while there have been some great strides in sport science and strength and conditioning, there are many aspects that have not really changed. S&C coaches are still undereducated, undervalued, and with a few exceptions underpaid. Although some schools and professional teams are hiring "sport scientists and high-performance directors," they are greatly undervalued, often ignored. Unfortunately, many of them are very poorly trained to actually be sport

September 2019

William J. Kraemer, PhD

Department of Human Sciences
The Ohio State University
Columbus, OH

First, I am honored and humbled to have been asked to give my reflections on the evolution of sport science. I know there are many others with longer evolutionary tales and experiences with this term and concept, from Al Vermeil, to Bob Ward, to Gene Coleman, to Terry and Jan Todd, to a host of other colleagues in my generation. My colleague, Dr. Michael Stone, is giving you another view of this field's evolution. We each share with the men and women of our generation the events that shaped us. For me, I have been blessed by so many people who have framed my career and shaped my views about this field. So upfront, I apologize for the many names I cannot share in this foreword, especially my many graduate students who in reality define my career.

To provide any comprehensive insights to enlighten you on the evolution of sport science is an impossible task. Hopefully, this book will start to give some of the insights into the many dimensions of this evolving field. To that end, I acknowledge the limitations of my perspective and experiences but will try to capture some of these ideas. In my view, there were so many evolutionary trails that started on their own paths and merged to enhance one another in the continuing challenge to better understand the demands of a sport and help prepare athletes to perform better.

"Sport science": The words themselves in combination have been a paradox for years. In many ways, this continues. Winning is now, and science is slow. Can it provide the so-called quick fix or silver bullet so many coaches are looking for in today's highly competitive and financially rewarding field of sports to produce winners? For me, it means to take care of athletes and give them the guidance and tools that allow them to safely compete and realize their potential. As a former strength and football coach at the junior high, high school, and collegiate levels, I could see the benefits of a properly developed and implemented training program for both young men and women before it was even popular in the 1970s.

Michael H. Stone, PhD *(continued)*

scientists. Hopefully, this book and the move by the NSCA and other like-minded organizations toward certification will help drive the integration of sport and science, and a true push to educate sport scientists.

For the Future

While many readers may think this section is too philosophical or even esoteric, please consider:

1. How does the universe work? or maybe
2. How could the universe work?

The second question is perhaps more difficult as it requires considerable thoughtfulness, creativity, and even imagination. It requires a hypothetical/theoretical approach, but if you can begin to answer this question, the first becomes much easier.

One may wonder in pondering the second question: where humans are (and sport science is) going. Imagine the creation of the Star Trek Transporter and the ability of this device to reassemble humans (and other animals) into more than they were. This idea is without a doubt the dawn of the "New Eugenics"—the acceleration of human evolution—and it's not just the transporter; it's genetic manipulation, human interface/integration with artificial intelligence (AI). Whether you realize it or not, the new eugenics is upon us, with all of its possible benefits and hazards. Accompanied by all of the ethical and moral dilemmas that made the *Twilight Zone* and *Outer Limits* really good science futurism at times.

Imagine for a moment, a world that some of you will likely begin to experience in the not-too-distant future. A world that could have three distinct groups of humans. One "chooses" to allow the natural evolutionary process to take place; they die younger and still experience disease, but believe they take the moral high ground. A second group takes advantage of genetic manipulation (CRISPR-Cas9, orthogonal ribosomes, and beyond); they live longer, have less disease, run faster, jump higher, lift more, and are more intelligent. In a third, human intellect/cognitive function can be transferred to AI, your intellect and cognitive function could live perhaps until the universe dies, you could be as strong and fast as an artificial body would allow, and intelligence could be boosted exponentially both by genetic and AI manipulation. What would this mean for sport and sport science?

A third question arises: "Where did we (you) come from?" And perhaps more importantly, "What did you come from?" (Think about the second question.) Think about who you are now and what you want to be. Think about facing the larger questions of the future.

William J. Kraemer, PhD *(continued)*

While beyond the scope of this short foreword note to you, the field of physical education of yesteryear, sadly not today in most curriculums, provided one basis for what we now call sport science. Such curriculums with the required sciences of anatomy, physiology, chemistry, biomechanics, motor learning, exercise physiology, sports psychology, sports history, and coaching have set the table for the study of sport by students. Many of these students went on to become sport coaches and strength and conditioning coaches. Sadly, the rigor of physical education programs for science is missing from most curriculums. For me, such a rigorous major in physical education and health education gave me the scientific understanding of sport and basics to build upon. It was in essence the basic building blocks of sport science at the undergraduate level. Without such sciences the ability to think through the functions of the human body and how exercise might impact it is missing. Learning to work with people and teams of research professionals in a laboratory day-to-day was an important element for me to work my way through college in addition to being an athlete. Laboratory work with now-outdated technologies, which included breaking down maximum oxygen consumption tests, analyzing bags of air with a Haldane gas analysis apparatus, and analyzing heart rates from EKG strips, taught me early in my career the importance of numbers and data. This is so vital in any sport science program today.

The Olympic Games in conjunction with the world politics of the Cold War also fueled the drive to further develop training theories and examine athletes who were successful and promoted the embryonic concept of a sport science team of experts. Seeing my friend and college football teammate, Dr. Steven Fleck, become one of the first sport physiologists at the U.S. Olympic Training Center (OTC) in 1979, I saw the early impact on how the Olympic Games stimulated the concept of sport science. I also had the good fortune to benefit from grant funding to study sport. This again showed how important funding was to drive sport science forward and help athletes with more sophisticated views of their sport. Having had the opportunity to work with the OTC's Coaches College, I saw again firsthand how science education was such an important part of the equation and vital in any sport science program. Working with Dr. Vladimir Zatsiorsky at Penn State University for many years teaching a class in theory of strength training and writing a book together, we kidded about making "East meet West." I realized from the many stories how sophisticated yet simplistic the programs and principles were to achieve optimal training for sport

Michael H. Stone, PhD *(continued)*

While we normally address these types of thoughts and questions on a macrocosmic and futuristic scale, begin to think about them on a microcosmic and futuristic scale. All of you are interested and involved in sport science and coaching to a greater or lesser degree—how would these thoughts and questions affect your microcosmic world? Producing a better human being? Eugenics? Are you not trying to do some of this already?—training, dietary practices, for example? (Epigenetic alterations?) So where do you draw the line—or should you? Will the new eugenics produce super athletes? Is this the new ergogenic aid?—it's not that far off. Some of you will deal with these ideas more than as just thought questions. Indeed it is possible that sport will become passé as almost everyone could become an elite athlete (and more)—unless Stephen Hawking was right?

Another aspect is that hopefully these thoughts bring home the inevitability of a "brave new world" and perhaps a truly better one: A good student of history will note that most, perhaps all, alterations in our timeline and cultural evolution have often been pushed and even driven by a handful of people. These pushers often shared psychological characteristics. Most had great intellects, most had high standards and expected others to adhere to those (and were often surprised and frustrated when people could not live up to them), almost none were politically correct, and all had great passion and emotion, including frustration and anger, that drove their intellect. They also had flaws and quirks. For example: Isaac was able to stand on the shoulders of giants and look down on those he thought could not. He had extreme bouts of depression and outbursts of a violent temper; these same "flaws" likely drove him to *Principia* (look it up). Temujin (look him up) literally left pieces of himself over most of Asia while building an empire; Ludwig transitioned the classical to romantic and was described as irascible, often had fits of depression, was deaf for a good part of his life, but wrote *Eroica*.

I think a very important aspect is to remember, the Vulcan approach to important scientific, cultural, and historical alterations, and evolution of ideas does not always work for humans. Often great intellect, artistic gifts, and the ability to drive change are in turn driven by emotion and passion. That brings us to a final thought (this time). Do you have the passion and the intensity of intellect to drive sport science forward? Indeed, what can you be?

(End)

William J. Kraemer, PhD *(continued)*

performance. It opened my eyes as to how former Soviet and Eastern Bloc countries viewed sport and how teams of scientists used Western literature, advanced physics, and mathematics to develop technologies (e.g., electrical stimulation, EMG, and biomechanical analytics) to design periodization theories. Thus, support and funding for such efforts were in part driven by the Olympic Games. Sport science was a beneficiary and continues to evolve.

Medicine was the word more closely aligned with the word *sport*, but from sports medicine other fields had scientific interests not directly concerned with the medical aspects. Thus, the American College of Sports Medicine's new journal in 1969 was called *Medicine and Science in Sports*. Sports medicine had spread out into the associated fields of athletic training and physical therapy with specializations for team physicians and orthopedic surgeons all interested in the prevention and care of athletes. The prevention aspect of athletic training merged, as history would prove, nicely with the goals of the strength and conditioning professional. As a professor and director of research in the Center for Sports Medicine at Penn State, under the direction of Dr. Howard Knuttgen, I saw what an evolution might look like in sport science when we created what would really be the first sport science program at Penn State starting in the late 1980s. We found that some coaches and teams wanted to know more than just the injury and rehabilitation aspects of their sport. Working with many outstanding physicians and athletic trainers in this area I saw what a genesis of a program might look like in sport science that would be realized some 20 years later at Penn State. However, for me the realization of a fully integrated program in sport science came at the University of Connecticut, where for over a decade we had "Camelot." Coach Jerry Martin was the head coordinator of strength and conditioning, Dr. Carl Maresh was the chair of Kinesiology, Bob Howard was the head athletic trainer, and Dr. Jeff Anderson was the team physician. This allowed for the full integration of athletic and academic programs. However, I was reminded of another lesson in evolution—if a careful eye is not kept on the environment, in this case, leadership, the evolved organism can crash and burn and become extinct. Bringing lessons from that experience here at The Ohio State University I have seen a burgeoning program develop in sport science over the past 5 years, and Coach Mickey Marotti, our assistant athletic director, supporting this effort for further such integration and use of science in sports.

In my view it was the field of strength and conditioning with its long history of physical development and performance arising from the resistance training sports

William J. Kraemer, PhD *(continued)*

of weightlifting, powerlifting, and bodybuilding, as well as track and field, that pushed the need for greater understanding of athlete development and the different sports forward using the sciences to do so. For me, this field provided the evolutionary "big bang" for sport science bringing together all of the different elements needed. The paths merged and planet "sport science" was created. The development was seen in the founding of the National Strength and Conditioning Association (NSCA) in 1978 by Boyd Epley. This fueled the interest of strength and conditioning professionals who wanted to know more about the science of sports and physical development. My many interactions with Boyd and his longtime assistant, Mike Arthur, allowed me to see from the start how a program and organization could impact athletes and professionals. This was the genesis of sport science. The NSCA was thus energized to emphasize education with Ken Kontor appreciating its importance, certification with Dr. Tom Baechle, and research with its two major journals being *Strength and Conditioning Journal* (formerly the *NSCA Journal*) in 1978 and then in 1987 a research journal dedicated to the concept of the applied aspects of conditioning, *Journal of Strength and Conditioning Research* (*JSCR*). I had the opportunity to work with both journals, especially the *JSCR*, where I served as editor-in-chief for 30 years. This allowed me to see how the growth and need of applied research related to sport science worldwide.

Concomitant to all of this was the fact that funding would be the engine for progress. Funding was critical to all of the advances for all sciences, including sport science. Government grants are typically tied to understanding and improving health treatments, health outcomes, and fighting and curing diseases. Thus, research in sport and athlete training and performance was left to other sources of funding or merged into a health care line. Funding to study sport, while existing in some countries, was not a typical funding line in most countries around the world. I saw this when collaborating with my friend and colleague, Dr. Keijo Häkkinen, at the University of Jyväskylä in Finland. For many years in Finland, sports research was funded by various government entities but slowly shifted to health-related issues. Our passion for resistance training drove both of us to be very creative in our grants that included resistance training in health-related problems but also had relevance to sports. In combination with my former postdoc, Dr. Robert Newton, from Australia, I learned the importance of worldwide collaborations in this process for developing research globally. For many investigators it was just a passion, or as some have said, a hobby due to the fact that they were athletes in their youth. Examples of this abound. Thus, the sport science projects

they undertook were related to their scientific training and area of research. They then needed to find internal funding to get studies done. Again, Olympic Committees and various corporations played considerable roles in funding sport science as it related to nutrition, materials, apparel, or equipment.

Ultimately, it was the exponential development of technologies from computers that required buildings to house this technology, which now can be accomplished using a cell phone or laptop. Corporations in the U.S. and around the world continued to make advances in communications, computers, microcircuits, software, biology, and bioengineering, all of which fueled various aspects of sport science. The United States' space program, celebrating its 50th anniversary of putting a man on the moon, funded and accelerated technological advances that spilled over to all sciences including sport science from materials to computers to software to biology. From my experiences as the associate director at Penn State's Center for Cell Research, which was funded by the National Aeronautics and Space Administration (NASA) for the commercial development of space, I was able to see the history of NASA. Having been involved with three shuttle missions that carried experiments, I saw up close the meaning of "work the problem." Admiring the human accomplishment of putting a man on the moon by the end of the 1960s, one realizes it took tens of thousands of professionals and corporations each working on different detailed and minute aspects of the larger goal to achieve. Just putting together the Saturn V rocket was an achievement of enormous technological complexity. This represents a model of my view of the challenges we face in the development of the field of sport science. It takes a team to get the job done and use evidence-based practices in sport science.

The military research programs took an interest in soldiers' health when a U.S. Air Force physician, Dr. Ken Cooper, reported his aerobics findings back in the 1960s on cardiovascular risk markers. Then in the 1980s the realization that soldiers were a type of athlete arose from the world of strength and conditioning. "Soldier fitness" (and performance) became a coined term. Having been a captain in the U.S. Army stationed at the U.S. Army's Institute of Environmental Medicine, under the visionary direction of Dr. James Vogel and Dr. John Patton, I saw how focused research for task-related mission demands mimicked what athletes need from sport science. I used such experiences in studying men and women warfighters over 4 years when I entered into an academic career. Subsequent research that I was involved in for the Department of Defense continued this line of work for me. This included women's health and preparation for combat-related jobs to demands of special operations warfighters in the different branches of service. Each acted as a model for me as to how vital evidence-based practices are and again how it takes a team of scientists and professionals to figure it all out. It was more than just metrics, despite the book and movie *Moneyball* bringing math and modeling into the public consciousness. However, for numbers to be meaningful they would need both context and scientific validity for the prediction models to work.

I got into this field unknowingly as a young boy. I wanted to be a better football player and found out that one of my heroes, Jimmy Taylor, of Vince Lombardi's Green Bay Packers, lifted weights. From there, my story started like so many others had. I asked my father to take me to Sears to buy a set of weights. From that point, I became fascinated and even obsessed with questions as to how the body works. Two other Packer heroes of mine, Jerry Kramer and Bart Starr, found out from Coach Lombardi that there is no end, just the continued chase for perfection with the hope of catching excellence in the process. So it goes with my view of the evolution of sport science.

RECOMMENDED READINGS

Amonette, WE, English, KL, and Kraemer, W.J. *Evidence-Based Practice in Exercise Science: The Six-Step Approach*. Champaign, IL: Human Kinetics, 2016.

Shurley, JP, Todd, J, and Todd, T. *Strength Coaching in America: A History of the Innovation That Transformed Sports*. Austin, TX: University of Texas Press, 2019.

PREFACE

The *NSCA's Essentials of Sport Science* has been created with a very specific objective: to provide the most contemporary and comprehensive overview of sport science and the role of the sport scientist. Within the domain of sport, the application of science is becoming more apparent. Indeed, not only are universities and academic institutions scientifically investigating sport, but in today's sporting landscape professional teams, sporting organizations, and private training companies alike are embracing approaches that use scientific principles and procedures and the empirical rigor that they provide. The contents of this book, which have been contributed by globally recognized experts and thought leaders from the field of sport science, address every aspect of the sport scientist role, from understanding training theory and performing needs analyses, to conducting athlete monitoring and assessment, managing data and analytics, and educating and disseminating information. This book supports sport science practitioners working with athletes in applied settings, individuals seeking to develop their knowledge and understanding of sport science, academics and researchers, and professionals aiming to explore how their technical expertise can offer potential benefits to athletes and sporting organizations. In doing so, this book presents the most comprehensive insight into the application of sport science and the role of the applied sport scientist.

FUNDAMENTALS OF SPORT SCIENCE

Science is the pursuit of logical approaches to discover how things work within the natural universe, in which the application of systematic methods of inquiry allow us to generate knowledge, testable explanations, and understanding. **Sport science**, therefore, is the application of scientific theory to sport, or the study of sport using scientific methods of inquiry in the fields of human performance, athletic endeavor, and sporting competition. Unlike **exercise science**, which largely uses sporting techniques and exercise as mechanisms (i.e., independent variables) to investigate and better understand specific adaptations relating to human physiology, psychology, or biomechanics (or more than one of these), sport science seeks to induce adaptations to human functional capacity for the specific purpose of maximizing performance in sporting competition. Sport science activities do this by converting data into valuable information that can then be used to support decision making and influence performance outcomes. While the nuances of exercise science and sport science can be considered similar, they are also different. Indeed, while it is important to understand how human physiology responds to different exercise stressors, stimuli, and interventions (i.e., the physiological stress experienced during exercise and the adaptations that occur consequently to this stress), the fundamental objective of sport science is instead to maximize the performance potential for athletes to increase their likelihood of success (2). Therefore, sport science represents the generation and gathering of information using scientific methods of inquiry in order to support better decision making for the purpose of winning in sporting competition.

The potential for science to be applied to sport training and competition, and for it to make a positive impact on performance, is vast. As an umbrella term, sport science is a multidisciplinary construct that is rooted in physiology, biochemistry, biomechanics, nutrition, and skill acquisition; however, it also involves the use of statistics and broader fields of data science, analytics, and technology management. By integrating each of these respective technical disciplines in an interdisciplinary fashion, it is possible to use collective approaches to address a host of performance-based problems within the paradigm of sport training and competition (e.g., workload management, underperformance, energetics and fueling, or postgame recovery). By formulating hypotheses for specific performance-related questions, sport scientists implement scientific processes of inquiry, either in the field or within controlled laboratory settings, in order to draw specific conclusions that can then be used to manipulate training methods or competition strategy. At its foundation, sport science seeks to examine how different psychophysiological systems interact to maximize human performance within sporting competition, and how the manipulation of different training paradigms can then be used to optimize such systemic interactions.

APPLICATION OF SCIENTIFIC METHODOLOGY

The word *science* is derived from the Latin *scientia*, meaning knowledge. Knowledge is gained through scientific inquiry rather than supposition, theory, accepted practice, or subjective opinion (3). **Pseudoscience** is sadly rife within the sport performance world, where science-like claims are frequently made but with little **evidence** provided in support of those claims—or if evidence is provided, it is typically misinterpreted or presented with biased intent. Everyone can perhaps recall a drill or instruction that a sport coach implemented, and that when questioned as to the reason for having done this, the coach offered little in the way of evidence to support the rationale for its use and application. Indeed, an overreliance on anecdotal evidence, a lack of skepticism and critical thinking, and a tendency to ignore data that does not support entrenched traditions and commonly held beliefs is widespread in sport, even at the most elite levels. It is therefore critical that scientific methods of investigation and learning be upheld throughout the world of sport, such that accurate understanding and knowledge can be gained and that this knowledge can then be used to complement impactful decision making, influence more effective training methods, and shape competition strategy for the betterment of athletes' health, well-being, and performance.

At the foundation of sport science methodology are the guiding principles of scientific inquiry, namely **empiricism**, **rationalism**, and **skepticism**:

- Empiricism is the philosophy of science that emphasizes the use of evidence, especially as discovered through experimentation, and suggests that all hypotheses and theories must be tested against observations of the natural world rather than resting solely on *a priori* reasoning (i.e., something that can be known without experience or data), intuition, or revelation.

- Complementary to empiricism, rationalism represents a methodology in which the criterion truth is not sensory but instead is intellectual and deductive. Rationalism is the theory that reason rather than experience is the foundation of certainty in knowledge.

- Finally, skepticism is the philosophical school of thought that questions the possibility of certainty in knowledge. Skeptical ideology can be generalized as the suspension of judgment due to the inadequacy of evidence.

Regardless of their technical background or designation within the performance support team (PST), one of the primary differentiators of sport scientists versus other coaches and PST members is their inherent expertise and desire to pursue scientific methods of inquiry and to obtain accurate knowledge and understanding through objectivity and data insights. This scientific approach towards understanding the complex demands of sports performance, studying the body of evidence-based research, answering questions, solving sport-related problems, or developing new and innovative ways to operate is represented by a simple methodological approach:

Make an observation ➤ Define the problem (ask a question) ➤ Hypothesize (create a theory) ➤ Experiment (test or challenge) ➤ Analyze ➤ Interpret (conclude) ➤ Implement (action)

Within the world of sport, sport scientists, perhaps more so than any others, are the individuals who are motivated to use the fundamentals of the scientific method to draw conclusions and theories as to what is objective versus subjective, what is accurate or inaccurate, and how impactful or redundant a performance intervention is. At the most basic level, sport scientists use analytical strategies (i.e., systematic methodologies) to distinguish the "signal from the noise"; that is, they filter what is valuable and efficacious from what is useless and ineffective. The generic processes of gathering and applying knowledge to sport performance are very broad, largely because of the numerous sports that sport scientists can be associated with, the strategies and skills they perform, the physical and psychological training approaches that are used, and their ability to affect all aspects of training and competition (3). However, sport scientists are the individuals who undertake critical thinking in order to study and investigate concepts relating to athletic performance, and to then relay the findings of these investigations to athletes and coaches, such that athletes and coaches can use the findings to make better-informed decisions (see figure 1).

EVOLUTION OF APPLIED SPORT SCIENCE

Sport science, as with many other disciplines, started out as an academic pursuit within universities and teaching institutions, in which researchers and faculty investigated specific aspects relating to exercise, sport, or other fields of human performance. In its infancy, the most common practice for sport scientists was to

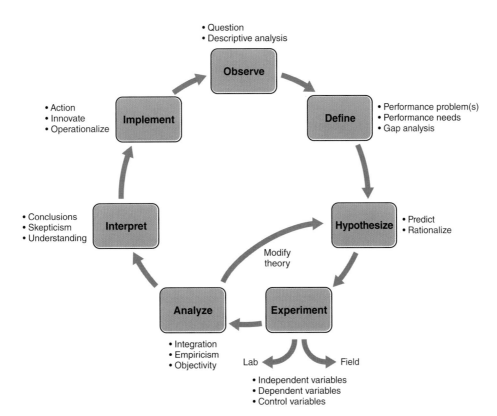

FIGURE 1 The scientific methodology loop for sport scientists.

perform "basic research," predominantly for the purpose of targeting publication of their findings in peer-reviewed journals or presenting their results to peers at academic congresses (or both of these) (2). This traditional approach provides outcomes, insights, and conclusions that can have some relevance to applied settings; however, on many occasions it can also have little applicability to sporting competition. With time, however, these professional scientists working in academic institutions offered their services to sport coaches in an attempt to understand sport and investigate ways to achieve a competitive advantage. Indeed, there are examples of early sport science projects that influenced sport science methods in today's competitive sporting arenas. For example, the work of academics at DePauw University shortly after World War II focused on documenting movement patterns during collegiate basketball and football games (5, 6). Upon reflection, this pioneering research can be considered the precursor to many of today's more sophisticated time–motion analyses that categorize and code the time athletes spend during a game walking, jogging, running, or sprinting at different velocities. Today, such analytics are used extensively to manage player workloads or as markers of heightened injury risk in professional sport teams around the world.

As the respective areas of technical knowledge and expertise have evolved, cross-pollination of theories and concepts has become more common, and even areas of business, human resources, management, medicine, and supply-chain logistics use "scientific approaches" to enhance their productivity. Sporting competition has been no different, and since approximately 2010, more and more sport organizations have realized that scientific expertise and data analytics can be of significant value. Indeed, more sporting organizations than ever before are recognizing the value of scientific approaches in the applied setting as a means to influence performance standards on both individual (i.e., athletes or staff) and organizational levels (i.e., team success and operational effectiveness). Consequently, sport science has evolved from a research-based pursuit of academics and university faculty into a method of investigation and inquiry that is performed throughout all sporting environments. Today, sport science approaches are used at the highest levels of professional and Olympic competition to directly affect performance and to aid practitioners in using the best available evidence at the right time, in the right environment, and for the right individual, in order to help athletes maximize their performance (1).

Evidence-Based Knowledge Versus Practice-Based Evidence

A central component of sport science is the development of systematic analysis frameworks to enhance performance through a process that includes data collection and analysis in order to drive insights and the communication of information (8). The undertaking of scientific thinking and methods of investigation (e.g., observation and description, controlled trials, literature reviews) serves as such a framework to generate knowledge and insight that can then shape decision making. A first approach, defined as **evidence-based knowledge** (EBK), in which information is generated through scientific study and investigation, allows practitioners to aggregate objectively informed rationales as to why certain methods and approaches are used. In practice, EBK indicates that strategic decisions have been informed by clear supporting information, reasoning, and objective data. Evidence-based knowledge is largely recognized as the gold standard approach to decision making.

However, in comparison, in the applied setting, sport scientists are often exposed to **practice-based evidence** (PBE); here, certain situations and contexts are not as controlled or structured as in traditional scenarios (i.e., laboratory and controlled studies). Instead, PBE often reflects the documentation and measurement, just as they occur, of patterns and characteristics. Practice-based evidence largely represents the process of describing or tracking certain performance dynamics and then reacting to situational responses while having less control over how they are delivered (7). If one considers the example of the professional sport team competing throughout a season, rarely would a sport scientist have the opportunity to implement a structured research study that reflects laboratory procedures with control groups, cross-over designs, or other recognized scientific approaches to isolate an independent variable's effect on the experiment. Instead, the method of collecting and analyzing PBE during the chaotic day-to-day activities of training and competition is often the most effective way to gain insights into performance regression or progression, understand adaptations consequent to changes in training strategy, or evaluate longitudinal changes in athlete health, well-being, and performance.

It is critical that sport scientists acknowledge the value of both EBK and PBE approaches and how each of them can provide valuable insights and information. In order to create EBK, sport scientists formulate hypotheses and then undertake structured investigations to test and contest these hypotheses. In PBE, this is challenging, and not always does the approach start with a clearly defined question that needs to be answered (i.e., hypothesis). Furthermore, sometimes sport scientists collect information from existing practices and afterward try to draw retroactive inferences from the information (e.g., injury audits, workload monitoring). The concepts of EBK and PBE perhaps represent the modern interface of applied sport science and the experiential nuances of sport coaching. Indeed, innovation and progression of coaching methods are often in advance of scientific rationale and understanding (i.e., coaches use drills and exercises to affect performance long before there is a body of evidence to support or refute their use). However, these coaching developments are fundamental to the evolution of any sport, with the trial and error of coaches adopting new techniques a key factor in advancing competition and training philosophy. Instead of rejecting this approach because it does not represent a traditional scientific methodology, sport scientists should embrace PBE, while at the same time recognizing that sport science must seek to implement the application of scientific principles to inform practice; therefore the pursuit of EBK principles, which adhere to the principles of scientific inquiry and critical thinking, should be embraced simultaneously (see figure 2; 4).

Interdisciplinary Approach

Central to successfully conducting sport science, or undertaking scientific endeavors within the domain of sport, is the acknowledgment that collaboration, team cohesion, and a sense of technical integration are fundamental. Scientific investigation must not get in the way of performance operations; investigation must instead enhance them. It must speed up decision making rather than slowing it down due to cumbersome procedures and methodologies. The sport scientist must also have a willingness to operate laterally across all the other PST services as well as upward to the technical coaching staff. Sport science collaborations must therefore be observed on three primary levels:

1. Services and support provided to the head coach and other technical coaching staff

2. Support given to the athletes

3. Integration and collaboration with other members of a multidisciplinary PST

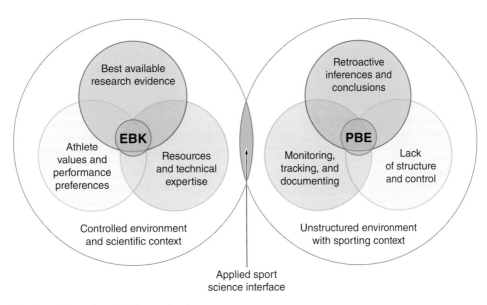

FIGURE 2 The interface of applied sport science.

Technical Coaches

From the outset, it is imperative that sport scientists accurately comprehend their role in supporting the technical coaching staff. It would be naïve to think that sport science expertise supersedes the decisions and perspectives of a head coach, even when those decisions may be perceived as largely subjective, anecdotal, or in conflict with known scientific findings. Instead, time should be taken to embed scientific methods and insight in a complementary and nonthreatening fashion, whereby technical coaching staff come to value the information that sport scientists provide. Head coaches and other coaching staff are often faced with complex decisions to make, which can range from regular process decisions (e.g., length of training sessions, game strategy, travel logistics) to more infrequent critical strategic decisions (e.g., team selection, equipment developments). Sport scientists possess the skills to support these complex decision-making processes, as they understand the methods of providing evidence, efficacy, or rationale upon which coaches can then formulate their own strategic approach. From the outset, any relationship with a coach needs to be built on trust as well as the ability to address very specific questions posed by coaching staff and the capacity to deliver comprehensible results and accurate information in a time-sensitive fashion.

Athletes

Sport scientists must establish an **athlete-centered approach** to their work, whereby scientific endeavors

and methods of inquiry are aligned with the specific needs of individual athletes. The professional relationships developed with athletes are often very different from those between the sport scientist and head coach or other technical coaching staff. However, trust and open lines of communication remain fundamental requirements if sport scientists are to optimize their impact and influence. Within the whole construct of sport, the athletes are the most important asset, and thus sport scientists must take the perspective that all their work is conducted for the purpose of supporting athletes to optimize their innate talents and maximize their genetic potential. Educating athletes such that they understand why scientific methodologies of investigation are being undertaken and become comfortable discussing and evaluating personal performance data, and also gaining their confidence that data will be handled with sensitivity and honesty, is essential to facilitating ongoing training and performance interventions.

Performance Support Team

Finally, sport scientists must embrace an **interdisciplinary approach** to working in collaboration with other members of a PST. By working horizontally across all performance services, sport scientists can apply their skills in monitoring and evaluation, data analysis, and data reporting and visualization, which can benefit multiple technical areas. Often it is the role of the sport scientist to work with other technical disciplines to identify and define their performance problems (i.e., research questions) and then formulate scientific approaches to create performance solutions (i.e., conclusions) using the principles of scientific investigation. As previously highlighted, it is necessary that the skills and attributes of a sport scientist be of great benefit and value to other technical disciplines that do not have the same expertise in using complex technologies, managing data, undertaking data analytics, and formulating conclusions around the efficacy of performance interventions.

COMPETENCIES OF THE SPORT SCIENTIST

If sport science is the study of sport through the application of scientific methods to the fields of human performance, athletic endeavor, and sporting competition, a sport scientist is a professional whose job is largely concerned with maximizing performance potential through the application of such scientific methods. Fundamentally, the sport scientist works to gather and interpret information that ultimately becomes knowledge for the purpose of supporting better decision making. The evolution of the sport scientist role reflects the increasing transition away from generalists on a sport team (e.g., technical coaches, physical trainers) to a team of experts, or specialists, who have discrete expertise and sophisticated knowledge of a sport or technical application (e.g., physiology, biomechanics, data science) that can serve to increase understanding. Therefore, it is largely the role of sport scientists to take complex data and applied research insights and translate this knowledge back to winning in competition by influencing strategy, tactics, equipment design, regeneration and rehabilitation activities, and operational logistics.

As the field of sport science continues to grow and becomes a more recognized discipline in sport performance (i.e., outside the academic environment), the role of applied sport scientists is becoming more common. However, there is still the need to understand what sport science encompasses as well as to understand what a sport scientist does. Examining current industry trends in the growth of professional sport scientist positions, it is apparent that sporting organizations are seeking two main profiles. The first focuses on individuals who possess expertise in one field or in particular fields of human performance, such as physiology, biomechanics, data processing or analytics, or in tracking systems and technology management. Often, the perceived notion of sporting organizations is to better understand concepts such as training load management, performance benchmarking, recovery and regeneration, or factors such as travel and sleep hygiene. All these areas can be considered critically influential in affecting athletes' availability or their potential to perform optimally (or both); thus sporting organizations are recruiting individuals to scientifically investigate and monitor them. The second type of profile is as a facilitator to integrate multiple disciplines; here the sport scientist has a holistic understanding of human performance. As people face the technology age and are exposed to the data tsunami that is now seen within sporting environments, sport scientists are also often called upon to manage large amounts of data (i.e., a data science emphasis). Indeed, in many sporting contexts there is an absence of staff in each technical discipline with the competency to handle technology (and manage data analytics) effectively, and therefore these tasks often fall upon sport scientists.

By embracing a multidisciplinary philosophy, it becomes possible to embed sport science into the infrastructure of any sporting organization, be it within the academic or applied setting, and to develop accepted methods of scientific inquiry that can directly influence sport performance. A key factor when engaging with or recruiting a sport scientist is the need for organizations and sport teams to employ individuals whose expertise and technical skills meet specific requirements and fill gaps in performance knowledge and understanding. Therefore sport scientists should be able to not only collect, analyze, interpret, and communicate data, but also employ a holistic approach to managing and combining information from all the technical disciplines.

CONCLUSION

In order to completely fulfill the meaning and value that the profession deserves, the sport scientist has to

1. practice hypothetical reasoning;
2. apply scientific principles of empiricism, rationalism, and skepticism;
3. foster competencies in statistics and data analysis, as well as reporting and data visualization on many occasions (but not as a general rule); and
4. possess sport-specific expertise.

Also essential to the role are behavioral characteristics and personal qualities, such as communication skills and a work ethic that promotes interdisciplinary approaches and working as a part of a team. There will be times when the sport scientist must act as an integrator of different disciplines and when the role implies interaction with different groups within the organization (e.g., management or front office, medical or health, coaching staff, analytics), and empathy with other technical coaches and PST members is vital. The purpose of this book is to offer a holistic overview of the technical expertise, skills, and knowledge required to operate effectively as a modern-day sport scientist.

ACKNOWLEDGMENTS

This textbook is the first iteration of the *NSCA's Essentials of Sport Science*, and it represents a seminal moment for the field of applied sport science. It serves to define the role of the contemporary sport scientist working across different genres and professional domains, and embodies the most comprehensive insight into the roles, responsibilities, and required expertise of those referred to as "sport scientists." The development of this book would not have been possible without the selfless contributions of a vast number of people. Most importantly, we wish to thank all of the contributing authors who have provided chapters in this book, sharing their respective expertise, as well as dedicating their precious time to formulate the most comprehensive body of sport science knowledge to date. We are truly grateful that you, the contributors, believed in our vision for this textbook and recognized the need to create a resource such as this for the global sport science community. We are also truly thankful that you have been willing to share your expertise and your wisdom so openly.

This book would not have been possible without the guidance and direction of Roger Earle from Human Kinetics. Roger, the energy and enthusiasm you have brought to this project has been the driving force behind us as editors from day one, and we are grateful for the support you have provided us throughout. Also, from Human Kinetics, we wish to thank developmental editor, Laura Pulliam, and managing editor, Miranda Baur, for your support throughout the copyediting and graphic design processes. To the NSCA, we appreciate that you allowed us to take editorial roles for this book, and for placing your faith in us to deliver your vision for the *Essentials of Sport Science* textbook. We hope that this text will become as fundamental a learning resource as each of the other books in the "Essentials" series. Thanks to Keith Cinea from the NSCA for his administrative support during the early part of this project, and to Eric McMahon for drumming up support and promoting this resource throughout the NSCA coaching community. We wish to acknowledge former NSCA president, Dr. Greg Haff whose bold idea was the initial catalyst to expand the NSCA's vision of sport science; without your commitment to the need for this type of resource, we wouldn't have arrived at this point. And thanks to the current NSCA president, Travis Triplett, and the NSCA board of directors who have followed through on the vision that Dr. Haff initially set in motion. Finally, we wish to thank all our sport science colleagues and friends around the world. The sport science and strength and conditioning communities are a truly special group of professionals, and we are privileged to serve you by providing what we hope is a valuable text to support all the amazing work you do for athletes, coaches, and teams across the globe.

DUNCAN N. FRENCH, PHD, CSCS,*D

I always say, "we don't work in a sports industry, we work in a people industry", and never more does that resonate with me than at the completion of this seminal textbook, for which I have had the pleasure of editing. Sporting competition and the pursuit of optimal athletic performance has become a hugely rewarding career for me. Either as a sport scientist, a coach, or now as a performance director, I feel truly humbled for the opportunities sport continues to present to me. Sporting competition is one of the most galvanizing activities in life, but it is the people I have met and the experiences that I have had along the way that made it so fulfilling.

I want to thank all the athletes and coaches that I have had the pleasure to serve over the years. I truly appreciate the trust and belief you placed in me, allowing me to play a small part in your success. Professionally, my greatest influence and the person who has shaped my beliefs and philosophies perhaps more-so than anyone else is a forefather of sport science and a founding member of the NSCA, Dr. William J. Kraemer. To this day I value your mentorship and your guidance greatly. To all my present and former colleagues working in sporting organizations around the world, I appreciate your camaraderie, your friendship, and the challenges you have offered me in striving to be the best I can be.

To my co-editor, my "partner in crime", and my very dear friend, Dr. Lorena Torres Ronda. While it has been a huge undertaking to deliver this text from its initial conception to the amazing resource that it is today for the global sport science community, I can't think of anyone I would have rather teamed up with on this project. You possess truly world-class expertise in sport science, which has been essential throughout this process, and your dedication and desire to create a special textbook have been unwavering. Most importantly you have always been there to support me with a kind heart and warmth as my co-editor and teammate. You have been right there with me throughout the challenging times and always offered support and a voice of reason. After working so closely together on this project for so long, I know I have a colleague and dear friend for life.

None of this would however be possible without the unwavering love and support of my family. Mum and dad, for so many years as a child you drove me all over the country to matches, tournaments, and sporting events. You were instrumental in providing me with every opportunity and sowed the seeds that grew into my passion and love for sport, athleticism, and human performance. To my brother, Stuart, who was always my sparring partner when we were boxing or kicking the soccer ball around in the back garden; you have always made life fun and lighthearted. My dear wife, Katie, you never doubt me and are a constant source of inspiration and motivation. You sacrifice so much in allowing me to pursue my passion and dedicate myself to my profession and my love for sport, sport science, and coaching. You keep me honest and bring love and laughter into my life when I consume myself with work and study. I appreciate all that you do for our family. To Alfie and Frankie, I'm sorry that daddy spent all those evenings tapping away on his computer and not playing games and having fun with you. Now that this book is finished, I promise I'll be there to run, jump, chase, lift, wrestle, roll, kick, and throw with you.

LORENA TORRES RONDA, PHD

The title of "sport scientist", as any other, does not make you one. It is the application of your values, principles, and knowledge, along with your experiences that actually shape your role. Most importantly, it is the impact you have on other people that will put you in the best position to apply sports science in your environment. "You do not fit people into jobs; You find the best people and fit the jobs to them" (S. Jobs). Titles do not create results; people do.

I want to thank all the colleagues, coaches, and athletes that have believed in me and that I have had the pleasure of working with and for. I want to give a special mention to Paula Marti Zambrazo, Ona Carbonell, and all the coaches and players at Futbol Club Barcelona Basketball. We won everything we competed for, and we had fun doing so! I owe another special thank you to RC Buford and Sean Marks, as well as the San Antonio Spurs organization, players, and coaches, for giving me the opportunity of working in the NBA, a world-class organization. I would not have become director of performance for an NBA team if you had not believed in me in first place. Last, but not least, thank you to all my colleagues and friends around the globe for sharing the happy moments, and supporting me when things are rough; you know who you are.

I also want to mention the people and organizations that have been a challenge and currently are a challenge. They neither believed or supported me but what they are probably not aware of is that they make me stronger, and thus better. I would not have become the professional I am today without those challenging people, moments, and experiences.

Thank you, Dr. Duncan French. Words cannot describe how grateful I am to have this fellow traveler during this journey. Readers of this book should know that the quality of it is largely due to the dedication Duncan has put into it. It has also been a real pleasure to have you as a co-editor and partner. You started out as my partner in this project, and now I can definitely state you are a lifelong friend.

To my girlfriends back in Spain, thank you for being so close and for everything else. And thank you to my family, to whom I dedicate this work. Thank you, mum, for always being present. I left you when I was 15 years old to pursue a dream in sports, and you have always supported me, guided me with your wisdom and your unconditional love; and Angela, my sister, thank you for being my best friend and the voice that guides me when I'm lost.

CREDITS

Figure 2.1 Reprinted by permission from T.O. Bompa and C. A. Buzzichelli, *Periodization: Theory and Methodology of Training* (Champaign, IL, Human Kinetics, 2019), 13; Adapted by permission from A.C. Fry, "The Role of Training Intensity in Resistance Exercise Overtraining and Overreaching," in *Overtraining in Sport,* edited by R.B. Kreider, A.C. Fry, and M.L. O'Toole (Champaign, IL: Human Kinetics, 1998), 114.

Figure 2.2 Reprinted by permission from S.L. Halson and A. E. Jeukendrup, "Does Overtraining Exist? An Analysis of Overreaching and Overtraining Research," *Sports Medicine* 34, no. 14 (2004): 967-981.

Figure 2.3 Reprinted by permission from S. Skorski, I. Mujika, L. Bosquest, R. Meeusen, A. Coutts, and T. Meyer "The Temporal Relationship Between Exercise, Recovery Processes, and Changes in Performance," *International Journal of Sports Physiology and Performance* 14 (2019): 1015-1021.

Tri-axial accelerometer equation Reprinted by permission from L.J. Boyd, K. Ball, and R.J. Aughey, "The Reliability of MinimaxX Accelerometers for Measuring Physical Activity in Australian Football," *International Journal of Sports Physiology and Performance* 6 (2011): 311-321.

Figure 2.4 Reprinted from M. Buchheit, "Monitoring Training Status With HR Measures: Do All Roads Lead to Rome?" *Frontiers in Physiology* 5 (2014): 73. This article is under Creative Commons CC BY.

Figure 2.5 Reprinted by permission from J. Vanrenterghem et al., "Training Load Monitoring in Team Sports: A Novel Framework Separating Physiological and Biomechanical Load-Adaptation Pathways," *Sports Medicine* 47, no. 11 (2017): 2135-2142.

Figure 2.6 Reprinted by permission from M.J.S. Buchheit, "Want to See My Report, Coach? Sports Science Reporting in the Real World," *Aspetar Sports Medicine Journal* 6 (2017): 36-42.

Figure 3.1 Based on Cananan et al. (2018).

Figures 3.2a, b Adapted by permission from NSCA, "Periodization and Power Integration," G.G. Haff, in *Developing Power,* edited by M. McGuigan (Champaign, IL: Human Kinetics, 2017), 36, 37.

Figure 3.2c Based on McGuigan (2017).

Table 3.1 Adapted by permission from G.G. Haff, "Periodization and Power Integration," in *Developing Power,* edited by M. McGuigan (Champaign, IL: Human Kinetics, 2017), 39; Adapted from Bompa and Haff (2009); Haff (2016): Haff and Haff (2012); Issurin (2010); Stone et al. (2007).

Figure 3.3 Reprinted by permission from J. Olbrecht, "Basics of Training Planning," in *The Science of Winning: Planning, Periodizing, and Optimizing Swim Training* (Antwerp, Belgium: F&G Partners, 2007), 191.

Figures 3.4 and 3.5 Adapted by permission from NSCA, "Periodization," G.G. Haff, in *Essentials of Strength Training and Conditioning,* 4th ed., edited by G.G. Haff and N.T. Triplett (Champaign, IL United States: Human Kinetics, (2016), 592.

Table 3.3 Adapted by permission from G.G. Haff, "The Essentials of Periodization," in *Strength and Conditioning for Sports Performance,* edited by I. Jeffreys and J. Moody (Abingdon, Oxon: Routledge, 2016), 404-448.

Figure 4.1; Figures 4.2a, b, c, d, e Reprinted by permission from P.B. Laursen and M.J.S. Buchheit, *Science and Application of High-Intensity Interval Training (HIIT): Solutions to the Programming Puzzle* (Champaign, IL: Human Kinetics, 2018) 12, 69, 70.

Figures 4.5, 4.6, 4.7, 4.8, 4.9, 4.10, 4.11 Adapted by permission from P.B. Laursen and M.J.S. Buchheit, *Science and Application of High-Intensity Interval Training (HIIT): Solutions to the Programming Puzzle* (Champaign, IL: Human Kinetics, 2018) 550, 551, 560, 561 559, 563, 562.

Figures 4.3a, b; Figures 4.4a, b; Table 4.1, Table 4.2 Reprinted from M.J.S. Buchheit, "Managing High-Speed Running Load in Professional Soccer Players: The Benefit of High-Intensity Interval Training Supplementation," *sportperfsci.com* 53 (2019): 1-5. This article is under Creative Commons Attribution 4.0.

Figure 6.2 Reprinted by permission from NSCA, "Administration, Scoring, and Interpretation of Selected Tests, M. McGuigan, in *Essentials of Strength Training and Conditioning,* 4th ed., edited by G.G. Haff and N.T. Triplett (Champaign, IL: Human Kinetics, 2016), 292.

Figure 6.3 Reprinted by permission from M. McGuigan, "Evaluating Athletic Capacities, in *High-Performance Training for Sports,* edited by D. Joyce and D. Lewindon (Champaign, IL: Human Kinetics, 2014), 10.

Figure 6.5 Reprinted by permission from NSCA, "Program Design and Technique for Speed and Agility Training," B.H. DeWeese and S. Nimphius, in *Essentials of Strength Training and Conditioning,* 4th ed., edited by G.G. Haff and N.T. Triplett (Champaign, IL: Human Kinetics, 2016), 544.

Figure 8.1 Reprinted by permission from R. Lovell et al., "Numerically Blinded Rating of Perceived Exertion in Soccer: Assessing Concurrent and Construct Validity," *International Journal of Sports Physiology and Performance* (2020).

Figure 8.2 Reprinted by permission from M.C. Varley et al., "Methodological Considerations When Quantifying High-Intensity Efforts in Team Sport Using Global Positioning System Technology," *International Journal of Sports Physiology and Performance* 12: (2017): 1059-1068.

Figure 9.3 Based on Buchheit and Simpson (2017).

Figures 10.4a, b, c, d; Tables 10.1a, b Based on Dwyer and Gabbett (2012); Suárez-Arrones et al. (2012).

Figure 10.5 Based on Malone et al. (2017).

Table 12.4 Data from Cohen et al. (2020); Hart et al. (2019); Cohen et al. (2014).

Figure 15.3 Reprinted by permission from A.F. Jackson and D.J. Bolger, "The Neurophysiological Bases of EEG and EEG Measurement: A Review for the Rest of Us," *Psychophysiology* 51 (2014): 1061-1071.

Figures 15.4a and b Reprinted by permission from P. Malmivuo, J. Malmivuo, and R. Plonsey, "Electroencephalography," in *Bioelectromagnetism: Principles and Applications of Bioelectric and Biomagnetic Fields* (Oxford University Press: USA, 21, 1995), 368.

Figure 15.5 Reprinted by permission from S. Motamedi-Fakhr et al., "Signal Processing Techniques Applied to Human Sleep EEG Signals—A Review," *Biomedical Signal Processing and Control* 10 (2014): 21-33.

Figure 16.1 Adapted by permission from J.P. Higgins, "Nonlinear Systems in Medicine," *Yale Journal of Biological Medicine* 75 (2002): 247-260.

Figures 16.5a, b, c, d, e, f Reprinted by permission from X. Schelling, J. Calleja-Gonzalez, L. Torres-Ronda, and N. Terrados, "Using Testosterone and Cortisol as Biomarker for Training Individualization in Elite Basketball: A 4-Year Follow-up Study," *Journal of Strength Conditioning Research* 29 (2015): 368-378.

Figure 17.1 Adapted by permission from R.M. Impellizzeri, S.M. Marcora, and A.J. Coutts, "Internal and External Training Load: 15 Years on," *International Journal of Sports Physiology and Performance* 14, no. 2 (2019): 270-273.

Table 17.1 Adapted from Mokkink et al. (2016).

Table 17.4 Based on Kellmann, Main, and Gastin (2017); Saw, Main, and Gastin (2016).

Figure 17.6 Reprinted by permission from A.E. Saw et al., "Athlete Self-Report Measures in Research and Practice: Considerations for the Discerning Reader and Fastidious Practitioner," *International Journal of Sports Physiology and Performance* 12, no. s2 (2017): S2-127-S2-135.

Figure 17.7 Reprinted by permission from C. Prinsen et al., "Guideline for Selecting Outcome Measurement Instruments for Outcomes Included in a Core Outcome Set," 2016. https://cosmin.nl/wp-content/uploads/COSMIN-guideline-selecting-outcome-measurement-COS.pdf; Based on Prinsen et al. (2016). This article is license under Creative Commons 4.0.

Table 18.3 Data from Buchheit and Rabbani (2014).

Figure 19.2 Reprinted by permission from J. Windt and T.J. Gabbett, "How Do Training and Competition Workloads Relate to Injury? The Workload-Injury Aetiology Model," *British Journal of Sports Medicine* 51, no 5 (2016): 428-435.

Figures 1, 2, 3, and 4 inside Table 19.1 Reprinted by permission from J. Windt and T.J. Gabbett, "Is it All for Naught? What Does Mathematical Coupling Mean for Acute: Chronic Workload Ratios?" *British Journal of Sports Medicine* 53, no. 16 (2019): 988-990.

Figure 19.4 Adapted by permission from T.J. Gabbett et al., "The Athlete Monitoring Cycle: A Practical Guide to Interpreting and Applying Training Monitoring Data," *British Journal of Sports Medicine* 51, no. 20 (2017): 1451-1452.

PART I

Training Theory and Process

CHAPTER 1

Performance Dimensions

Nick Winkelman, PhD
Darcy Norman, PT

Albert Einstein famously said that "we cannot solve our problems with the same thinking we used when we created them." In other words, if a group of people face a problem that came about as a consequence of their thinking, then they will need to change their thinking in order to solve the problem or avoid it in the future. To do this, people must have a mechanism for updating their own thinking or the thinking of others; otherwise they are destined to face the same problem over and over again.

WHY SPORTS NEED SCIENTISTS

Independent of the mechanism selected, one thing is clear: It needs to be fueled by information. Here, **information** is defined as knowable facts that reduce uncertainty about something or someone. Thus, for something to be considered information, it must have the potential to shift thinking and decision making. While this sounds simple, accessing a continuous flow of high-quality information is not always easy.

For one thing, the information needed to improve one's thinking must be measurable at some level. Assuming it is measurable, whether through qualitative or quantitative means, there must be a way of measuring it. If such a way exists, then one must take that raw information and analyze, visualize, and interpret it in a manner that, again, can refine the thinking of those it is meant to influence.

Historically speaking, the ability to maintain a continuous and up-to-date flow of information is a modern idea. Before computers, high-speed Internet, smart devices, and sensor technology, people's ability to rapidly acquire and integrate new information (beyond their own observations) was severely limited.

However, as the world ventures deeper into the 21st century, there appear to be no limits to technological advancement and the information it can offer. This actuality has forced every industry to adapt—acquire the right technology, staff, and skills—or die.

While some industries, like business, medicine, and transportation, were quick to change with the times, sport did not join the party until later. For example, in the past, if a sport team wanted to improve their understanding of an athlete's physiology, it was necessary to recruit the help of a university and a physiologist. This involved players having to take a day away from training to go to a lab and complete a battery of tests designed to assess key physical qualities. While many teams have used these services and continue to do so, the core limitations are scale, speed, and cost. That is, a team looking for real-time feedback on how a training intervention is affecting an athlete's progress will have little use for such an infrequent and impractical means of information gathering.

Knowing this, many businesses have emerged to fill the information gap, creating technology that brings the lab to the athlete. The turn of the century saw the emergence of wearable or portable devices that measure speed, strength, power, posture, readiness, heart rate, hydration, and sleep. With each passing year, new technologies are created, existing technologies improve, and more data is generated (see chapter 7). While the prospect of accessing real-time information on critical features of athletic performance is appealing to sporting organizations, it does present the challenge of finding someone to assess the technology, learn how to use it, and collect, analyze, visualize, and interpret the data that it produces. Add multiple technologies into the mix and the requirement for specialized individuals with discrete technical skills multiplies.

Recognizing this, sporting organizations have looked to their **high-performance unit** (HPU), sometimes referred to as the **off-field team** (e.g., strength and conditioning professionals, physical therapists, and nutritionists), to pick up the technological slack. While it is perfectly logical to think that strength and conditioning professionals should be responsible for the technology that measures running speed, physical therapists for the technology that measures groin strength, and nutritionists for the technology that measures hydration, a closer examination reveals a number of issues:

- The first issue is a matter of **time**. Spend a day shadowing a strength and conditioning professional, for example, and you are not going to see much downtime. When these personnel are not on the floor coaching, they are in meetings, and when they are not in meetings, they are writing programs and preparing the schedule. Outside of planned time for professional development, they do not typically have enough time to go through the process of assessing and integrating technology, let alone manage it on the ground. The same argument can be made for most traditional roles within the HPU.

- The second issue is a matter of **competence**. Many of the technologies that have already become ubiquitous in sport (e.g., Global Positioning System [GPS]) are still fairly new. For example, the two major sport GPS providers were founded in 2006 and 2008. Thus, many of the current department heads within sport HPUs have college graduation dates that predate the availability of this type of sport technology. Granted, while most personnel are familiar with the science on which these new technologies are based, they are not necessarily equipped to assess the validity and reliability of the technology; clean, analyze, and visualize the data it produces; and interpret the data within the broader context of all data collected on an athlete. These latter skills are as deep and complex as those germane to the roles within the traditional HPU, and therefore require specific competencies that must be developed or recruited.

- The final issue is a matter of **interest**. Generally speaking, the more interested people are in something, the more attention and effort they will invest. Hence, ask strength and conditioning professionals why they got into the profession and you

will get responses like "I want to help people," "I love to coach and help others achieve their goals," or "I've always wanted to work within sport." You do not hear things like "I want to work with new sport technology," "I love mining data to see how it can improve human performance," or "I want to work at the intersection between sport and innovation." While people with these interests exist, they do not tend to be those who fill the roles within a traditional HPU.

Therefore, if a sport organization wants to use technology and the data it produces to improve thinking, decision making, and therefore athletic performance, it will be necessary to find a solution to overcome issues of time, competence, and interest. Fortunately, a solution has been identified, and it exists in the form of the **sport scientist**, the newest member of the modern HPU.

THE HIGH-PERFORMANCE UNIT

Before discussing the role of the sport scientist, it is important to consider the evolution of the HPU and the roles that have traditionally existed within it. By exploring the inner workings of the HPU, one can draw a conclusion as to the necessity of the sport scientist and the nature of the role.

Before there was an HPU—"the team behind the team"—there were just athletes. As many sports shifted from amateur to professional in the late 19th and early 20th centuries, teams identified the need to have full-time sport coaches. These coaches were responsible for setting the performance directive (technical and tactical vision) of the team and, ultimately, helping them to win.

However, for a team to win, they must have athletes healthy enough to play. For this reason, medical staff were introduced to ensure that the health of the team was maintained. While this would have started with a team doctor, some combination of physical therapists (physiotherapist), athletic trainers, and massage therapists would have inevitably completed the medical arm of a sport team. Although it is difficult to identify when full-time medical staff became the norm within sport, organizations like the American College of Sports Medicine (ACSM) and the National Athletic Trainers' Association (NATA) were founded in the early 1950s.

Sporting organizations soon realized that optimal athletic performance required far more than simply playing the sport. Take American football, for example. Physical qualities like flexibility, strength, and speed are all important; however, the act of playing American football is insufficient for maintaining, let alone developing, these qualities. This is in no way a critique of American football specifically, or sport generally; rather, it is a recognition that for athletes to thrive in competitive sport, they require more than what is offered by playing it. This performance gap was inevitably filled with the professionalization of strength and conditioning in the late 1970s, which coincided with the founding of the National Strength and Conditioning Association (NSCA) in 1978.

In time, the nutritionist and, to a lesser degree, the sport psychologist would become recognized roles within the HPU. Interestingly, however, even though the American Psychological Association (APA) was founded in 1892 and the Academy of Nutrition and Dietetics (formerly the American Dietetic Association) was founded in 1917, it is still common to find sport organizations that subcontract or outsource their nutrition and psychological services rather than employ these professionals in a full-time capacity. While teams fully recognize the importance of nutrition and psychology, behaviors and budgets suggest that sport is still in the process of figuring out how to best use these key members of the HPU.

Ultimately, the HPU has evolved to meet the growing demands of sport and those who play it, with each role providing a central source of expertise for a piece of the performance puzzle:

- The **sport coach** establishes the technical and tactical vision that forms the basis for how athletes will play a game. This directive is then used to guide how athletes are physically and mentally prepared for their sport.
- The **strength and conditioning professional** uses this directive to build a physical development plan that will adequately develop or maintain the physical qualities required to deliver the sport coach's technical and tactical vision.
- The **doctor**, **physical therapist**, and **athletic trainer** medical collective collaborate with the strength and conditioning professional to make sure that training methods shown to reduce the likelihood of musculoskeletal injuries are integrated into the program (preventive) and that protocols are in place to deal with short-term injury and illness and rehabilitate long-term injuries (reactive).
- The **sport nutritionist** or **dietitian** ensures that all athletes consume the right quantity and qual-

ity of calories required to support their physical development and daily activity needs. Nutritionists are especially skilled at adapting nutrition plans to the dietary needs, wants, and limitations of the athletes they are supporting and thus are skilled in behavior change.
- The **sport psychologist** (or mental performance coach) works directly with athletes and coaches to ensure that they are developing and deploying the mental skills needed to consistently perform under pressure. Notably, **clinical psychologists** may also work within the HPU, providing direct support for athletes and coaches in the area of mental health.

Taken as a collective, the professionals in an HPU form an **interdisciplinary team** (IDT), in which each person's discipline, while unique, is interdependent on those of the other team members. Principally, this interdependence reflects the fact that just as biological systems are seamlessly integrated, so too are the disciplines that represent them.

For example, a rugby player who is malnourished may struggle to develop key physical qualities in the gym. If the physical qualities on which the position depends are underdeveloped, then the player's sport skill execution may suffer. If sport skill execution suffers, the player may develop movement compensations that could lead to injury. If injured, the player may start to lose confidence and find it difficult to cope with the new circumstances.

This example, and the many that could take its place, clearly demonstrate that if the body is an interdependent system, then the approach to developing it should be interdisciplinary. This reflects Aristotle's statement that "the whole is greater than the sum of its parts." In the case of the IDT, the whole emerges out of the interactions among the parts as opposed to the independent actions of the parts.

Hence, for an IDT to function optimally there needs to be a clear delineation between **independent** and **dependent** responsibilities. The former responsibilities are siloed and do not overlap with other disciplines. For example, a physical therapist does not consult the nutritionist on how best to manipulate a hip. The latter responsibilities are shared and overlap with other disciplines. For example, when an athlete is returning from injury, the strength and conditioning professional should work with the medical staff to design a program that is appropriate for the injured region and the stage of rehabilitation, while the nutritionist should be involved to ensure that the caloric needs of the athlete are progressing in line with the rising demands of the program.

As simple as this sounds, many HPUs struggle to strike the right balance between siloed and shared thinking, defaulting to the former more often than they should. In the authors' experiences, HPUs that function optimally rarely do so by chance alone. Rather, the members of the IDT consciously design a working environment that is integrated, allowing the right people to get the right information at the right time, so they can make better decisions (see chapter 30). To do this, three features of the work environment should be considered.

1. The first feature of a successful IDT relates to their **people**. At an individual level, each person must be competent in the job, be clear in communication, and have a desire to learn. If people are not competent in their job, they will struggle to build trust; if people cannot communicate, they will struggle to be understood; and if people do not want to learn, they will struggle to develop. While these individual qualities are essential, they do not guarantee that people will work well together. For this, the organization needs to create a glue that connects those within the IDT. This glue is often referred to as a **shared mental model** (SMM), which is nothing more than an established set of values and behaviors that align to a common vision and are upheld by all who enter the work environment (7). For example, the word "integrity" reflects a common value that is included in many a vision statement, and the word is plastered on many a gym wall. However, if that value is not clearly defined and anchored to key behaviors, then it will be nothing more than just that—a word on a wall. Thus, to bring integrity to life, an IDT could define it as characterizing "a person who is dependable, honest, and does what they say they'll do." The IDT could go one step further and identify the behaviors that they feel embody a person with integrity: taking responsibility and doing what you say; living your values and challenging others to do the same; and communicating with empathy and honesty. Ultimately, the conditions within and between people will determine, to a large degree, whether an IDT will be successful.

2. The second feature of a successful IDT relates to their **process**. In this case, the process is the documented way in which information is gathered, shared, decided on, and acted upon. Principally,

each information source within an IDT should involve a documented process that covers the journey from collection to dissemination. For example, if a team collects strength data, there should be a documented process outlining the standard for the collection, cleaning, storage, analysis, visualization, interpretation, and dissemination of that data. That said, having a documented process for dealing with all information sources is only the first step. Effective IDTs must also have a process for integrating and making decisions based on that information. For most, this is achieved through the creation of a weekly schedule that manufactures the necessary opportunities for communication among members of an IDT. Some of these meetings will involve the whole IDT, while others consist of smaller functional groups (e.g., medical, strength and conditioning) or discipline-specific meetings. Although organic conversation is also important, the best IDTs do not leave this collaboration to chance.

3. The third feature of a successful IDT relates to their **place**. Here, place represents the physical environment that the IDT works in. Specifically, if the strength and conditioning team is in the gym on the bottom floor, the medical team is in the therapy area on the second floor, the sport coaches are in their office on the third floor, and the nutritionist and sport psychologist are in a different building altogether, then scheduling interactions becomes challenging and the likelihood of organic conversations is minimized. This is not to say that an effective IDT has to be in the same office, even though some organizations are moving this way; however, proximity will have a material impact on the frequency of communication, which further affects the quality of the working relationships that are built.

By recruiting and developing great people, establishing a process that maximizes the quality of information sharing and decision making, and creating a place that promotes collaboration and communication, sport organizations create the potential for a successful IDT (6) (see figure 1.1). However, for this potential to be realized, sport organizations must recognize and account for an inconvenient truth about human behavior—humans are biased and, unless alerted not to do so, they tend to overvalue their own knowledge and experience, leading them to nudge decision making toward their own line of thinking (4). This is not done with malice or selfish intent; it is simply a phenomenon

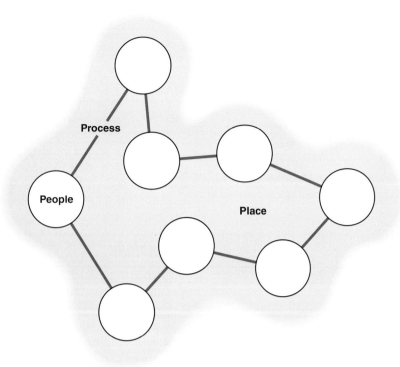

FIGURE 1.1   Considerations for building a successful interdisciplinary team.

of the human mind. People deal with the present by sampling their past and, as it turns out, they tend to trust their own experiences more than those of others.

This is not a problem when one is making a decision that is isolated to one's area of expertise (e.g., a strength and conditioning professional deciding how much load to program for a squat). But issues can arise when a complex decision must be made, requiring insights from multiple disciplines (e.g., deciding when an athlete is ready to return to competition after a soft tissue injury). If the decision is left to opinion and to domain expertise, parties are likely to default to their own perspectives. In these instances, the strongest personality in the room will likely sway the decision, or the designated lead will use that authority to make the call. This is not to say that logic and expertise are not important—they are. However, they are often insufficient when one is dealing with the complexities of the human body.

At this juncture it becomes clear that in addition to establishing the right people, process, and place, a successful IDT also needs a shared mechanism for effective decision making that can be injected into the process itself. As mentioned earlier, this mechanism is dependent on accessing a continuous flow of relevant athlete data and having a person capable of mining that data for objective insights. These objective insights can be used to debias, which is to say, integrate the decision-making process, connecting disciplines to a common source of informational truth.

This leads the discussion back to the need for a sport scientist—a person capable of working across disciplines, data sets, and decision makers. By helping the IDT develop data systems, ground interdisciplinary interactions in objectivity, and rigorously apply the scientific method to answer performance-related questions, the sport scientist is an essential addition to the IDT and the modern HPU.

THE EVOLUTION OF THE SPORT SCIENTIST ROLE

Although sport science informs every discipline within the HPU, the sport scientist has traditionally come from an academic context and specialized in a single scientific domain (e.g., biomechanics, physiology, or motor control). While this type of sport scientist exists to this day, playing a central role in increasing understanding of sport science, it is important to separate this individual's role from that of the sport scientists who are now being embedded into sport organizations, particularly at high levels of performance (1).

The career path of this latter sport scientist has evolved rapidly over the last decade. Early in the 21st century, all data collection and interpretation were handled by the discipline responsible for the application of learning in those areas. As technology evolved and data became part of the day-to-day conversation, sport organizations realized that there was far more benefit in the information than could be realized if left to a single discipline (e.g., strength and conditioning or medical) to manage. This left sport organizations with three options:

1. Distribute the responsibilities of a sport scientist across the IDT
2. Convert a member of the IDT into a sport scientist and rehire the position
3. Create a sport scientist position and go through an external hiring process

The order in which these options are listed provides a good approximation of how the sport scientist role has progressed since approximately 2010. Early on, sport organizations had to absorb the responsibilities and distribute them across the relevant IDT members. In time, a member of the IDT showed interest in sport science and demonstrated a capacity to drive sport science within the organization. As the dependency on the information this member was collecting grew, the organization allowed the IDT member to spend more time operating in a sport scientist capacity. Inevitably, this behavior matured into a role, and the member became the full-time sport scientist. While this is still how it is done in many sporting environments, academic programs are starting to catch up, producing professionals who have gone through a curriculum that is specifically designed to prepare students to step into the modern sport scientist role (1).

To be clear, the role of the sport scientist in sporting organizations is still evolving. Reflecting this is the authors' observation that no two sport scientist roles are the same. For some teams, the sport scientist still operates in a dual role: part sport science professional and part strength and conditioning professional. For other teams, the sport scientist is an isolated role, solely responsible for managing a team's sport technology, data, and insights. Despite these differences in role, the responsibilities of the sport scientist appear to be stabilizing across sport organizations.

Responsibilities

If the role of the sport scientist had a mission statement, it would go something like this: "To connect the IDT to the right information at the right time, so they can make better decisions." This is not to suggest that sport scientists cannot be a part of the decision-making process—they are. However, their primary responsibility is to be a constant source of objectivity in a world that heavily depends on the subjectivity of discipline experts. To generate this objectivity, three responsibilities appear to be consistent across sport scientist roles.

Technology

As alluded to earlier, the first responsibility is around sport technology. The sport scientist needs to have the theoretical background and the practical knowledge to evaluate both the scientific efficacy of sport technology and its practical utility in the context of a given sport (see chapter 7). In some cases, a sport organization will ask the sport scientist to test a new technology that has been brought to the attention of the IDT (e.g., a new sleep monitor). In other cases, the sport scientist will be asked to lead an innovation group responsible for identifying technology that can help solve or inform specific problems the sport organization is facing (e.g., how much sprinting should the athletes do each week?). In either case, the sport scientist needs to ensure that the technology is solving an actual problem the team is facing, rather than providing a solution for a problem that does not exist (2, 8).

Once a technology has been evaluated and purchased, it will be the sport scientist's job to work with the appropriate members of the IDT in designing a process document, outlining how the technology will be used and integrated into the IDT's day-to-day workflow (8). In some cases, the sport scientist will be directly responsible for managing the technology. For example, if a new force platform is purchased and used for jump analysis, it is reasonable to expect that the sport scientist would be the one running the jump testing and managing the data collected. Alternatively, the medical team might purchase a new camera system to screen movement quality. While the sport scientist would have provided support in the evaluation of the technology, the medical team is likely to be the discipline managing the application of the technology in the work environment.

While many sport technologies exist, the following is a short list of those that sport scientists should be familiar with:

1. The **athlete management system** (AMS) is the sport science hub for most sport organizations. Normally, this is a web-based application or software that is principally designed to store, organize, analyze, and visualize a diversity of data sets (e.g., strength data, speed data). Most AMS include apps that allow sport organizations to collect data via smartphones and tablets (e.g., subjective and objective monitoring data). Practically, the AMS is used to inform conversations pertaining to athlete readiness and training load management.

2. The **force platform** and other **force instrumented devices** are used to indirectly assess the readiness of the neuromuscular system and adaptation to training stimuli. The affordability of force platforms is such that sport organizations can now assess the kinetic features of jumping alongside jump height. What is more, novel devices designed to measure groin strength and hamstring strength, for example, have now been instrumented with force transducers and can be used to measure small changes in strength. It is rare to find a sport organization that does not have one or more of these devices that the sport scientist will be responsible for managing.

3. The **inertial measurement unit** (IMU) is a generic sensor that many sport technologies use to assess kinetic and kinematic features of movement. The IMU consists of an accelerometer, gyroscope, and magnetometer. Companies have created IMU-enabled sensors that can go on the body or a barbell, for example, and provide an indication of movement velocity. This data, typically reported in real time on an accompanying app, can be used to give athletes an indication of movement speed and to track training loads within the gym.

4. The **Global Positioning System** (GPS) uses a combination of IMU technology and satellites to triangulate the position of an athlete, typically 10 times a second or 10 Hz. With varying levels of accuracy, this allows the unit to measure metrics associated with running distance, velocity, acceleration, and deceleration. GPS is now ubiquitous in team sports because it provides an accurate representation of the training load being imposed on the athlete. Similar data is being produced for indoor sports or when sport is played indoors, using non–satellite-dependent technology (e.g., optical tracking and IMU algorithms).

While other technologies exist and are covered throughout this text (see chapters 7 and 9-15), those just discussed represent some of the key data-producing devices that a sport scientist can be expected to use and manage within the sport environment.

Data

While it is important to understand and manage the various sport technologies, this simply serves as a means to an end. That is, the value sporting organizations seek is in the data the technology produces. Once data is collected, sport scientists need a way of organizing, cleaning, analyzing, and visualizing the data produced (1, 2). While most single-purpose technologies come with software that allows a sport scientist to visualize the data collected (e.g., force platform), they are rarely designed to statistically analyze that data, and they most certainly do not integrate with other data sources. These latter needs can be fulfilled using some sort of data management system. Traditionally, this is done using Microsoft Excel or, often today, an AMS. While the former is flexible, it can quickly become overloaded with the amount of data being stored. The latter, on the other hand, has virtually no limits to the amount of data that can be stored, but there are serious limits on the flexibility a sport scientist has in analyzing the data.

Both of these problems have been solved by business intelligence software (e.g., Tableau or Power BI), which allow large data sets to be cleaned, integrated, analyzed, and visualized using superior statistical and design flexibility. What is more, these systems are scalable enterprise solutions, which means that the sport scientist can design and update data visuals (i.e., dashboards) while all other IDT members access and interact with the data from their own computers. Although business intelligence software provides superior storage, analytical, and visualization capabilities, it is not, by design, statistical software. Thus many sport scientists use statistical programs (e.g., private or open-source software) to statistically analyze or model data trends (e.g., how training load relates to injury risk). This is quickly requiring sport scientists to develop a suite of skills akin to those of a statistician or data scientist (8).

Interpretation

While technology management and data analytics are central responsibilities of the sport scientist, most would agree that interpretation is where the excitement is. While interpretation can quickly turn into a subjective free-for-all, the sport scientist can stay on the right side of objectivity using the mental model shown in figure 1.2.

It is helpful to categorize the knowledge a sport scientist would use to support interpretation as follows. Category 1 is what one knows or knowledge that is supported by objective evidence (3). This type of information, which includes quantitative data, should be used to inform decisions. Category 2 is what one thinks one knows or knowledge that is unsupported (i.e., intuitions) or supported by subjective evidence (i.e., experience) (3). This type of data, which includes direct observation, should be used to add nuance, context, and perspective to discussions. While this type of knowledge can be used, in part, to inform decisions, it is subject to bias and, until confirmed, should rarely be the only source of information that decisions are based on. Category 3 is what people know they do not know, or domains of knowledge that they know exist but have no evidence or experience to reference. Similarly, category 4 is the unknown, or domains of knowledge that people do not know exist. Collectively, categories 3 and 4 represent the knowledge one can access only by asking questions and identifying the best path to answering them.

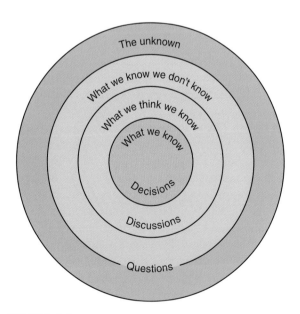

FIGURE 1.2 A mental model for improved decision making.

Where possible, the sport scientist should be the source of objective truth and seek to expand the overall objective knowledge of the IDT (category 1). When objective truth is not available, the sport scientist should leverage theory, logic, and direct experience to support decision making (category 2). Notably, the sport scientist's primary responsibility is to support the IDT's ability to ask and answer questions and therefore reduce that which is collectively unknown (categories 3 and 4). Ultimately, the more sport scientists turn relevant unknown information that exists within categories 3 and 4 into known information that can exist within categories 1 and 2, the greater their contribution will be. It is at this point that the sport scientist can turn back to technology and data to chip away at the unknown, one focused question at a time.

Skills

While the responsibilities outlined here represent the hard skills that a sport scientist needs to be successful, a number of soft skills are essential to bring those technical responsibilities to life. Notably, due to managing multiple technologies and data sets, the sport scientist needs to be very well organized, effective at time management, and able to prioritize (5). These skills amalgamate to ensure that the responsibilities noted earlier are executed at the speed of sport. Once they have been executed, the sport scientist must be able to communicate results and insights to a diversity of stakeholders with varying levels of sport science knowledge. As such, the sport scientist must know the material well enough to deliver clear, simple messages and answer any number of challenging questions. Further, the sport scientist needs a high level of **emotional intelligence**, as self-awareness is central to knowing how to calibrate the message to the IDT member it is intended for (4). This also allows sport scientists to adapt within a conversation when it is obvious that their message was not delivered at the right level or with enough clarity. Ultimately, sport scientists need to know the "how" to clearly translate the "what," because the knowledge they gather is of no use if not understood by the entire IDT.

CONCLUSION

It is clear that sport continues to evolve. Central to this evolution is the ability to use a continuous flow of high-quality information to guide the athletic development process. Since the turn of the century the sport scientist has emerged as the best person to manage the information that comes from each discipline within the IDT. By capturing, cleaning, organizing, analyzing, and visualizing this data, the sport scientist infuses objective truth, where available, into the decision-making process. In this way, sport scientists are a key role in what connects all of the IDT members. In a way, they are the hub, centrally collecting the critical data and insights that flow from each department, aggregating them into a collective view of the athlete journey. This allows them to shuttle that information back to each department, ensuring that the collective IDT receives the right information at the right time so they can make better decisions.

RECOMMENDED READINGS

Heath, C, and Heath, D. *Decisive: How to Make Better Choices in Life and Work.* New York: Crown Business, 2013.

Kahneman, D. *Thinking, Fast and Slow.* New York: Farrar, Straus and Giroux, 2011.

Senge, PM. *The Fifth Discipline: The Art and Practice of the Learning Organization.* New York: Doubleday/Currency, 1990.

Sinek, S. *Leaders Eat Last: Why Some Teams Pull Together and Others Don't.* New York: Portfolio Books, 2017.

Syed, M. *Black Box Thinking: Why Most People Never Learn From Their Mistakes–But Some Do.* New York: Portfolio/Penguin, 2015.

CHAPTER 2

Training Load Model

Stuart Cormack, PhD
Aaron J. Coutts, PhD

Athlete monitoring is often an essential role of the sport science practitioner. The primary reason for monitoring athletes is that the information obtained can be used to guide decisions about future training (i.e., controlling training). Following the process of athlete monitoring allows practitioners to better understand the complex relationships between training, injury, illness, and performance outcomes. This chapter presents the foundational concepts that underlie athlete monitoring and discusses the various tools that sport scientists can use. It also presents methods used for analyzing and interpreting the data provided by athlete monitoring systems.

MANAGING THE TRAINING PROCESS

While the range of physical qualities required in a given sport can vary considerably, the consistent aim of training is to progressively develop these qualities to enhance performance. In order to cause biological adaptation, the current capacity of the system must be disturbed (125). This disruption to homeostasis results in a transient performance reduction (i.e., fatigue) and is followed by a **supercompensation** effect whereby performance is enhanced (39) if the body is allowed to adapt. This physiological pattern of response to stress is described by Selye's **general adaptation syndrome** (see figure 2.1; 12), which provides a framework for the interaction between the imposed training stress, the acute fatigue response, adaptation, and ultimately a new level of homeostasis or performance (39).

A critical challenge for sport scientists and other practitioners is to balance the application of a train-

ing stress with appropriate recovery in order to allow continued adaptation (65). When these aspects are appropriately combined, performance capacity is enhanced; however, inappropriate combinations of training volume, intensity, and frequency can result in maladaptive states (65). As shown in figure 2.2 (65), this response is described on a continuum from the fatigue caused by a single training session, to overreaching (both functional and nonfunctional) occurring due to a period of intensified training, and finally to the development of overtraining syndrome, which is sometimes referred to as "unexplained underperformance syndrome" (22). Interestingly, functional overreaching, as the result of deliberately planned training (e.g., training camp or increase in training load before a taper), leads to a temporary performance decline in conjunction with high perceived fatigue (5) but is followed by a positive response leading to improved performance when recovery is appropriately managed (85). It should be noted that while overtraining syndrome is thought to develop as a function of continued high volumes or intensified training (or both) when an athlete is overreached, this progression may not always occur (65). It is also important to acknowledge that the overtraining syndrome is very rare in athletes.

As mentioned earlier, both a fatigue response and a positive adaptation response come from the appropriate application of a training stimulus. The interaction of these opposing effects is often referred to as the **fitness–fatigue model**, in which performance is a function of the positive fitness effect and negative fatigue effect, which both decay exponentially over time but at different rates (i.e., fatigue decays at approximately twice the rate of fitness) (8, 23, 99). Assessing fitness and fatigue, in addition to predicting performance, is

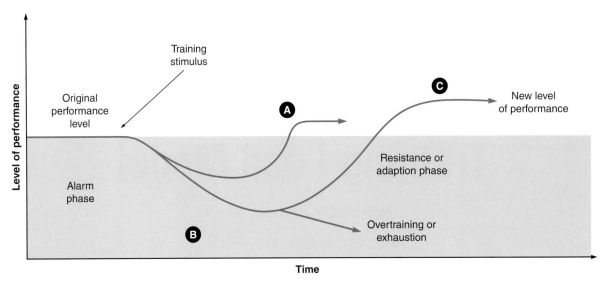

FIGURE 2.1   Selye's general adaptation syndrome.

A = typical training; B = overtraining; C = overreaching or supercompensation.

Reprinted by permission from T.O. Bompa and C. A. Buzzichelli (2019, pg. 13); Adapted by permission from A.C. Fry (1998, pg. 114).

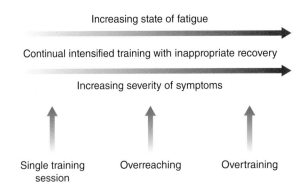

FIGURE 2.2   The overtraining continuum.

Reprinted by permission from Halson, S. L. and A. E. Jeukendrup (2004, pg. 961).

complex and is affected by numerous factors (13, 67). Some attempts have been made to model team-sport match intensity and performance using training load data (61, 62). However, it has been suggested that resultant estimates of fitness, fatigue, or performance obtained directly from the fitness–fatigue model may lack sufficient precision for direct application in high-performance athletes; in this situation, small changes in these outcomes can be very important (67). Despite these challenges, the fitness–fatigue model provides a suitable framework to guide approaches to monitoring athlete training and helps sport scientists ensure the proper application of a training dose at the correct time.

A key component of managing the training process is an understanding of the response or internal load that will occur due to a given training stimulus (also referred to as a training impulse or external load). This is known as the **dose–response** effect (8, 23). In general, a higher volume and intensity of training or competition (i.e., external load) will result in a larger acute fatigue response, although the type of stimulus (e.g., cardiovascular endurance, resistance training) will have a specific impact (i.e., internal load) on particular systems (e.g., cardiovascular, muscular) (126, 141). Critically, the impact of training on performance is not linear, and there is likely an inverted-U-shaped relationship between daily training load and resultant performance (23). It is important to note that the time course of the response to training and competition stress can vary from minutes or hours to several days poststimulus (126) (see figure 2.3). For example, the acute reduction in phosphocreatine stores with exercise may immediately limit performance, but phosphocreatine stores can be recovered between high-intensity efforts (126), whereas disruptions to the neuromuscular system may take 24 to 96 hours to fully recover (33, 126, 139). Furthermore, the response to a given exercise dose can be mediated by factors such as the training status of an individual athlete (76, 139). Specifically, the negative response to simulated and actual match play in team sports has been shown to be attenuated in athletes with higher levels of lower-body strength and aerobic fitness (76, 139). Given the potential for appropriate loading to maximize positive adaptations and reduce the risk of unintended outcomes, valid approaches to quantify this process are greatly needed (64).

DEVELOPING A TRAINING SYSTEM

Any training "system" includes all the factors important to performance, and can be considered to comprise those that directly influence the system (e.g., training and testing, load and fatigue monitoring) and those that support the system (e.g., training facilities and equipment) (12). While there are almost endless individual factors and combinations of factors, the development of an effective training system requires the integration of scientific evidence and a detailed understanding of the applied context in sport. As a result, high-performing training systems are developed with the input of both sport scientists and coaches. While the sport scientist can contribute evidence-informed approaches to planning, quantification of training and competition load, and physiological assessment, coaches can make subtle, but critical, day-to-day decisions and adjustments to the training process based on their experience and an in-depth understanding of the needs of an individual athlete at a specific point in time. This combined approach allows the development of appropriate underlying physiological qualities, as well as the technical and tactical requirements that are necessary for high-level performance.

The coach is generally responsible for setting the overall aims and philosophy that guide the development and implementation of a training system. Importantly, no single training system should be considered the template for all others, since each sport has its own requirements (nature of the activity, resources available, etc.), which guide the selection of the specific training and various load and response measures that are included in the system. In fact, the transfer of a training system from one environment to another without consideration for the context of the new environment will probably lead to unsuccessful outcomes. However, there are several key factors that underpin the most successful systems. These include, but are not limited to, clearly articulated system aims, detailed short- and long-term planning, regular assessment of progress relative to targeted aims followed by program adjustments as required, continual manipulation of program variables on micro (e.g.,

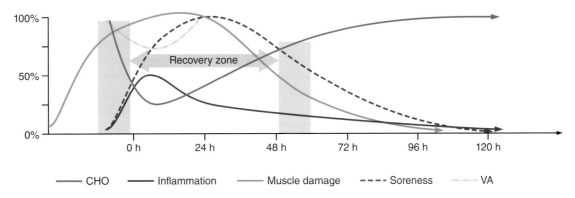

FIGURE 2.3 Physiological response to team-sport match play. Light blue bars represent the training stimulus, the lines the time course of carbohydrate resynthesis (CHO), inflammation, muscle damage, soreness, and voluntary activation (VA).

Reprinted by permission from S. Skorski, et al. (2019, pg. 1019).

session by session) and macro (e.g., training phase) levels based on the combination of valid and reliable measurement together with coach expertise, and the search for continuous improvement.

Furthermore, an important yet often overlooked factor common to successful training systems is the relentless pursuit of adherence to the fundamental aspects of training (e.g., evidence-based training program design, individualization of the training stimulus based on a needs analysis, progressive overload) on a session-by-session basis. The pursuit of these basic factors provides an important distinction between successful and unsuccessful systems, which are sometimes characterized by the pursuit of marginal gains without appropriate foundations in place.

QUANTIFYING TRAINING AND COMPETITION LOAD

A key component for both programming and monitoring an athlete's progression or regression is the quantification of **training load**. This process is critical for assessing whether an athlete is adapting positively to a training program (14). As mentioned earlier, external load refers to what the athlete has done (e.g., distance and speed of running, kilograms lifted), while internal load refers to how the athlete has responded to a given external load (72, 73). This internal response can be both physiological (e.g., heart rate, blood lactate) and perceptual (e.g., **rating of perceived exertion** [RPE]) (73). Ultimately it is the internal response to a given external load that drives the training outcome (72, 73). Importantly, measures of external and internal load should be used in combination to provide a complete picture of the training process and response (14). Furthermore, as mentioned earlier, a comprehensive understanding of the external load of a sport allows the development of specific training programs aimed at targeting the relevant underlying physiological qualities (e.g., aerobic capacity, speed, strength).

External load can be measured in a variety of ways depending on the sport or training modality (14). Technological advances such as camera systems and microtechnology (local systems and **Global Positioning Systems** [GPS]), often in conjunction with other sensors such as accelerometers and power meters, have made the quantification of various activity metrics in teams and in sports such as running and cycling relatively simple. While this process has become common, some critical elements should be considered with regard to the measurement of external load, and these are explored next.

The measurement of speed and distance metrics using GPS is now commonplace, and the validity and reliability of these devices have been extensively examined (21, 36, 75, 77). In general, higher-sample-rate (e.g., 10 Hz versus 5 Hz) GPS chips have demonstrated superior validity and reliability to lower sample rates, particularly for the measurement of high-intensity running efforts and accelerations (21, 75, 77). The sampling rate of these systems continues to increase, which may assist in further improving validity and reliability for the measurement of high-intensity events. Furthermore, the use of indoor stadiums has necessitated the development of indoor tracking systems such as **Local Positioning Systems** (LPS), which can provide information similar to that with GPS (131). Additional detail on these systems is provided in chapter 9. Furthermore, determining thresholds for classification of high-speed running, sprinting, and accelerations is challenging for practitioners regardless of the tracking technology employed, and doing this includes consideration of whether these thresholds should be based on team or individual values and whether they should have a physiological basis (134). Work in this area has used a movement sequencing technique rather than arbitrary thresholds to classify velocity and accelerations performed by elite netball athletes, and similar approaches in other sports may yield valuable insights (133). A primary driver for practitioners in deciding whether to use relative or absolute speed and acceleration thresholds is likely related to whether comparisons are being made between or within individual athletes. Furthermore, sport scientists and coaches should be aware that values transmitted live by the units and those calculated after downloading data can be different, and this may have significant implications for training or competition decision making (6). The impact of data processing (e.g., smoothing techniques) on measured variables should also be considered (137). Finally, a highlighted factor in the quantification of team-sport activity profiles is the consideration of average intensity versus peak intensity (41). Peak running intensity is substantially higher in relatively short time windows (e.g., 1 min) compared to the average intensity in a half- or full-duration rugby league match (41). This has important implications for the design of training programs targeted at developing the underlying physical qualities important for being able to perform at the required intensity; and in practice, both peak and average intensity should be considered. These and other considerations are discussed in more detail in chapters 9 and 10 of this book.

Given the chaotic nature of team sports, it has been suggested that speed and distance metrics may not completely quantify the full external load (15, 114). The reason is that many movements that are energetically costly and taxing on the neuromuscular system (e.g., accelerations, decelerations, change of direction, and contact) can occur at low speed and accumulate relatively little distance (15, 114). These activities can be measured with a variety of sensors such as high-sample-rate (e.g., 100 Hz or greater) triaxial accelerometers, gyroscopes, and magnetometers, and these accelerometers in particular have demonstrated high reliability and ecological validity (15, 30, 34, 97, 114). Manufacturers have tended to create their own metrics for values obtained from triaxial accelerometers, similar to the Catapult PlayerLoad™ calculation shown, but they all essentially represent a combination of individual vector values (15):

$$Player\ Load = \sqrt{\frac{\left(a_{y1} - a_{y-1}\right)^2 + \left(a_{x1} - a_{x-1}\right)^2 + \left(a_{z1} - a_{z-1}\right)^2}{100}}$$

where

a_y = Forward acceleration
a_x = Sideways acceleration
a_z = Vertical acceleration

Reprinted by permission from Boyd, Ball, and Aughey (2011, pg. 331-321).

Interestingly, changes to these metrics or the individual vector contributions to the overall value have shown promise in the ability to detect fatigue-induced changes in movement strategy (30, 97, 114). The use of this type of metric, in conjunction with traditional locomotor variables as measures of external load, may provide practitioners with additional insight.

Of particular interest is the fact that various manufacturers have developed algorithms to auto-detect specific sport events, such as fast bowling in cricket and tackles in contact sports, with reasonable accuracy (56, 71, 95). This may be useful in reducing the time and effort required for accurate measurement of external load, leading to more precise quantification and therefore assisting with both planning and monitoring of training and competition.

The frequent accelerations and decelerations performed in team sports can substantially increase the energy cost (42). In order to account for this, the concept of **metabolic power** was developed, which is based on the principle that the energy cost of acceleration is equivalent to running at a constant speed up an "equivalent slope" (42). As a result, numerous measures have been proposed; these include metabolic power (in categories from low [0-10 W/kg] to maximum [>55 W/kg]), total energy expenditure (kJ/kg), equivalent distance (representing the distance that would have been covered during steady-state running on a flat grass surface), and equivalent distance index (representing the ratio between equivalent distance and total distance) (108). While the use of metabolic power has undergone some investigation (37, 80) and has attractive practical aspects, its validity has been questioned for various reasons, including the innate error in measuring accelerations using positional systems (16, 19, 21).

In addition, work has focused on the detection of specific variables such as stride parameters and vertical stiffness from accelerometry (20, 49, 84, 101). This type of analysis may prove insightful for practitioners, although there is some conjecture regarding the impact of unit placement (i.e., scapular versus center of mass versus lower leg) on the ability to accurately measure specific variables (20, 46, 109).

Measurement of external load in endurance sports is also common (100). Sports such as running, cycling, and swimming lend themselves well to external load measurement via quantification of various combinations of speed, distance, and duration (100). In addition, the development of power meters has allowed easy measurement of power from pedal strokes in cycling (100). Readers are directed to part IV of this book for extensive coverage of this topic.

Because not all training occurs in the field, other training components also require quantification. For example, various indices of external load can be calculated from resistance training, including sets, repetitions, volume load, and device displacement velocity (124). An important reason for the quantification of resistance training load is the impact of volume and intensity of resistance training on muscular adaptation (110). These approaches can be used to both program and monitor resistance training load, although some methods arguably provide a more complete representation of external load than others (124). For example, the total number of repetitions performed (i.e., number of sets × number of repetitions) in a particular exercise provides a global representation of external load; however, it fails to account for the intensity (i.e., percent repetition maximum) (124). Accounting for the intensity in terms of load lifted by quantifying resistance training load as [number of sets × number of repetitions × weight lifted] somewhat overcomes the limitations mentioned earlier; however, it does not account for the intensity of the load relative to the maximum strength of the lifter (124). Therefore, quantification of resistance training load as [number of sets × number of repetitions × percent repetition maximum] may be most appropriate. Furthermore, the availability of measurement devices such as force plates, linear position transducers, and bar- and body-mounted accelerometers allows measurement of variables such as displacement, velocity, and power, which may also prove useful for both the programming and monitoring of resistance training (4, 9).

In addition to the measurement of external load, the quantification of internal load is a critical component of the training process. There are numerous approaches to this, including the use of both objective and subjective (often referred to as "perceptual") markers such as RPE, various heart rate indices, and biochemical markers. These measures are considered later in this chapter, and a detailed review of the assessment of internal load is provided in chapters 14, 16, and 17.

Fitness and Fatigue Response Measures

As mentioned earlier, notwithstanding the impact of numerous factors specific to the individual athlete (e.g., training history, genetics) and despite the relative simplicity of the general adaptation syndrome and fitness–fatigue models, performance is generally considered to be a function of the difference between fitness and fatigue (8, 23, 99). Due to this, there is extensive interest in assessing the response to training and competition in high-performance athletes (2, 64, 138).

One component of assessing the response to training is to assess the impact on specific fitness qualities. A detailed description of appropriate tests for each quality is beyond the scope of this chapter, and readers are directed to part IV of this book and other sources of information (25, 63, 135). While such tests are an important indicator of adaptation to the training stress, a potential limitation to their use on a regular basis is that they themselves may be fatiguing (e.g., tests of maximum aerobic capacity) and can therefore be difficult to fit in as part of crowded training and competition schedules. Accordingly, there is an increasing focus on monitoring fatigue status, sometimes referred to as **readiness** (121), in athletic populations (64, 138). Readiness has been defined as a "condition where an athlete has

no impairment of physical performance, no mental fatigue or excessive psychological distress" (121) and is challenging to achieve, particularly during crowded competition periods.

The first step in the monitoring process is to develop an understanding of what constitutes fatigue. Numerous definitions have been proposed; however, a common theme is a failure to produce or maintain the required force (or power) (136). This failure can result from both central (e.g., brain) and peripheral (distal to the neuromuscular junction) factors (136) and can last from minutes to days (47). The central and peripheral sites and processes that contribute to fatigue include (48):

- activation of the motor command (in the brain)
- propagation of the action potential through the descending motor pathway
- myofilament excitation-contraction coupling
- status of the intracellular milieu

There are, in fact, numerous models that aim to describe the underlying cause of fatigue attributed to physiological processes; these include the cardiovascular model, energy supply model, biomechanical model, neuromuscular fatigue model, muscle damage model, and psychological/motivation model (1). However, an important consideration in explaining fatigue is the role of the perception of effort in maintaining the required level of force output (89).

It has been suggested that exercise intensity and its modification due to fatigue are actually much more under central control than they are influenced by peripheral mechanisms (90, 105, 130), although this proposition has been criticized (148). An in-depth discussion of the psychobiological model of fatigue (89) and integrative governor theory (130) is beyond the scope of this chapter; however, readers are encouraged to explore these ideas further. In brief, the psychobiological model provides an elegant explanation for the modification of intensity whereby fatigue (exhaustion) occurs when the effort required exceeds the maximum effort the athlete is willing to exert, or when the athlete believes the effort has been maximal and feels it is impossible to continue (i.e., a conscious decision) (89). In contrast, the integrative governor theory suggests that both psychological and physiological factors limit performance with a particular focus on the subconscious avoidance of catastrophic failure due to severe disruptions to homeostasis (130). In addition, Enoka and Duchateau (48) have suggested that "as a symptom, fatigue can only be measured by self-report and quantified as either a trait characteristic or state variable" and that therefore "fatigue should not be preceded by an adjective (e.g., central)" (48). Nevertheless, practitioners are likely to be extremely interested in the site and mechanisms responsible for fatigue and its time course (116, 139). This has led to substantial efforts to develop valid and reliable protocols for the assessment of fatigue in athletes (138). An attractive proposition is the potential to assess fatigue via protocols that occur within the normal training and competition process, sometimes referred to as **invisible monitoring** (114).

An additional area of focus for both practitioners and researchers is that of mental fatigue, which has been defined as a "psychobiological state caused by prolonged periods of demanding cognitive activity shown to negatively influence physical performance" (91, 120, 128). It has been suggested that mental fatigue has greater potential to limit endurance performance as opposed to anaerobic performance, including the expression of maximal strength and power (140). Importantly, the reduction in endurance performance appears to be a function of an increased perception of effort (140). Reductions in running distance on the Yo-Yo intermittent recovery test and elevated RPE after a mentally fatiguing task have been observed in team-sport athletes (127). In addition, mental fatigue has been shown to impair technical performance in soccer players (7, 127). The implications of the impact of mental fatigue on performance include the development of recovery modalities to limit the negative impact of mental fatigue and the exposure of athletes to mental (i.e., cognitively demanding) tasks in order to prepare them for competition.

Performance Tasks

The utility of performance tasks to assess the response to training or competition (or both) has been extensively examined in sports such as Australian football, rugby league, cricket, and soccer (32, 33, 57, 70, 93, 106, 116). Much of this work has focused on the measurement of neuromuscular fatigue and has included assessments such as sprint tests (58) and the isometric mid-thigh pull (106). However, one of the most frequently studied is the countermovement jump (CMJ) (27, 30, 57, 60, 116).

A key component of understanding the usefulness of performance tasks for the assessment of fatigue is understanding both their validity and reliability. Readers are referred to the section later in this chapter and to chapters 7 and 8 for more detail on these statistical concepts. An often overlooked aspect of determining the suitability of variables is an analysis of how they respond to a given training or competition load (dose). In order for a variable to possess high ecological validity, it should respond relative to the dose of the prior stimulus (e.g., a reduction compared to a baseline value) and should also show a predictable or consistent pattern of return to baseline. Furthermore, and arguably most importantly, for a performance variable to be useful for the ongoing monitoring of fatigue status, an alteration in a particular measure (increase or decrease depending on the variable) following exposure to an appropriate load—one that persists up to a subsequent performance—should be reflected in a change in either exercise intensity or movement strategy in the subsequent performance.

There may be numerous reasons for the attractiveness of the CMJ for the assessment of neuromuscular fatigue, including its nonfatiguing nature, short duration, and common occurrence as a movement in many field and court sports, coupled with the increasing availability of technology (e.g., portable force plates, linear position transducers, inertial measurement units) to measure advanced CMJ parameters (see chapter 12). This is in contrast to the equipment and technical knowledge required for the gold standard measurement of central and peripheral neuromuscular fatigue, which requires electrical or magnetic stimulation (139). Furthermore, it has been suggested that movements involving the stretch-shortening cycle, such as the CMJ, may be particularly useful for studying neuromuscular fatigue (51, 104).

Countermovement Jump and Other Tests

Although variables obtained from a CMJ are routinely measured in an attempt to quantify neuromuscular fatigue, the research findings in relation to the sensitivity of these variables are not always consistent (33, 57, 58, 60, 88, 93, 116). There are numerous explanations for this, including, but not limited to, the actual fatigue effect of the performance (i.e., some performance tasks may not induce sufficient neuromuscular fatigue to allow measurement via CMJ), timing of the CMJ postexercise, comparison point (i.e., to a valid baseline), measurement equipment (e.g., force plate versus timing mat), variables chosen for assessment (i.e., outcome measures such as height versus variables such as flight time:contraction time ratio [33] representing movement strategy), and the statistical analysis approach. While a detailed review of the literature is beyond the scope of this chapter, a meta-analysis by Claudino and colleagues (27) examined the efficacy of the CMJ to monitor neuromuscular status and concluded that average CMJ height from multiple trials was more sensitive than peak values. Furthermore, it appears that variables from a CMJ representing a change in movement strategy may provide more insight than simple outcome measures such as jump height (33, 57, 58, 116). Therefore, it may be erroneous to conclude that fatigue is not present due to a lack of change in an outcome measure (e.g., jump height), since the maintenance of a specific outcome could be the function of a change in movement strategy that has been adopted by the athlete as the result of fatigue.

Interestingly, CMJ height decrement before a resistance training session has been correlated with the decrement in squat volume, suggesting that it may be useful as an indicator of fatigue and the athlete's readiness to undertake resistance training (143). These findings are supported by work demonstrating that 6 weeks of plyometric training regulated based on pre-session CMJ performance resulted in a lower training load without compromising performance adaptations (28). These findings suggest that sport scientists may wish to consider the CMJ before resistance training or plyometric sessions in order to optimize application of the training stimulus.

In addition to metrics obtained during a CMJ, sprinting, submaximal run tests, and maximal cycle sprints have all been proposed as useful for the assessment of fatigue status (54, 55, 58, 92, 147). For example, Garrett and colleagues (55) suggested the potential of a submaximal run test involving 3 × 50-meter (54.7 yd) runs completed in 8 seconds on a 30-second cycle in which variables from a triaxial accelerometer worn between the scapulae were obtained. The run protocol was completed 24 hours before and 48 and 96 hours after an Australian football match, and changes in various accelerometer metrics were observed 48 hours after the match. The authors concluded that these changes were representative of an altered movement strategy to achieve the required running speed in the presence of fatigue, and this approach warrants further investigation. Similarly, Wehbe and colleagues (147) examined the use of 2 × 6-second maximal cycle sprints for the assessment of peak power as a representation of neuromuscular fatigue following an Australian football match. The authors observed a reduction in peak power at 24 hours postmatch compared to prematch and suggested that a potential strength of this test is that it does not involve an eccentric component. However, the limited practicalities of this type of protocol may constrain its use in high-performance environments. It has also been suggested that 30-meter sprint time and maximum horizontal theoretical velocity (from the 30-meter sprint) may be more sensitive measures of neuromuscular fatigue than variables obtained from a CMJ following rugby sevens training (92); however, the findings may be related to the lack of sensitivity in CMJ variables chosen for analysis (i.e., height, power, force and velocity metrics) rather than limitations of the CMJ per se. It is also questionable whether a sprint test to assess fatigue is realistic in practice, because it may carry a risk of soft-tissue injury and requires substantial motivation to achieve a maximal performance.

Heart Rate as a Measure of Training and Competition Response

An increasingly common approach is to use resting, exercise, and recovery heart rate (HR) to monitor fitness and fatigue (11, 17, 81-83). Despite the relative ease of measuring HR, there is some complexity in the interpretation of observed results (11, 17), and the utility of these measures is likely dependent upon the sport and the frequency of measurement (17). It appears that improvements in heart rate variability (HRV) and heart rate recovery at rest and postexercise are indications of positive adaptations having occurred (11). A potentially confounding outcome is that postexercise HRV and heart rate recovery changes may also occur in overreaching, which emphasizes the need to consider the training context (i.e., recent changes in training load) and other measures of the response (e.g., perceptions of fatigue) to training to allow the correct interpretation (11, 17). Similarly, the inherent measurement error in these variables should be taken into account to determine the practical meaningfulness of any changes seen (17). Figure 2.4 provides some guidance as to which HR measures may be most useful in a given environment, and for more details, readers are directed to other chapters in this book (17).

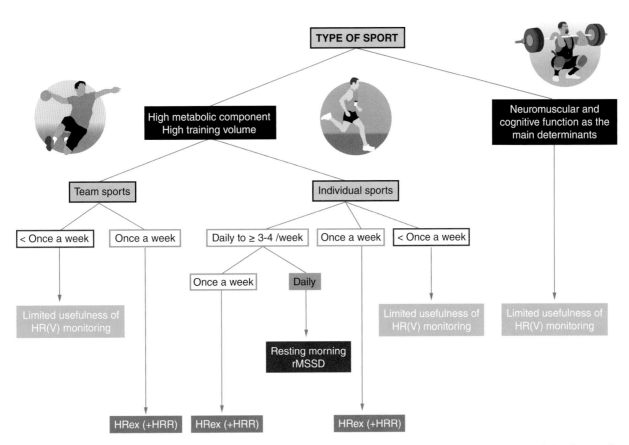

FIGURE 2.4 Decision chart for the selection of heart rate (HR) measures based on sport participation and implementation possibilities.

HR(V), heart rate variability; rMSSD, logarithm of the square root of the mean of the sum of the squares between adjacent normal R-R intervals measured after exercise; HRex, submaximal exercise heart rate; HRR, heart rate recovery.

Reprinted from M. Buchheit (2014, pg. 14).

Invisible Monitoring

While the use of standardized submaximal protocols is an attractive option for practitioners to assess the response to training and competition load, they still require that a specific activity be performed in addition to normal training, although they are minimally invasive and can be performed as part of a warm-up. An extension of this approach to assess the readiness of athletes to undertake further loading is the use of actual training drills, such as small-sided games; this is sometimes referred to as **invisible monitoring** (114). For example, Rowell and colleagues (114) found changes in select accelerometer metrics during a standardized small-sided game when soccer players were deemed fatigued (as determined by a reduction in the flight time:contraction time ratio measured from a CMJ). Critically, the altered movement patterns seen in the small-sided game were followed by an increased contribution of the mediolateral accelerometer vector to total PlayerLoad™ (a vector magnitude from the accelerometers in Catapult tracking systems), and the authors concluded that this likely represented a fatigue-driven modification to movement strategy (114). It seems that global speed and distance metrics can remain relatively unchanged in the presence of fatigue; however, the movement strategy adopted to achieve the same external load appears to change. From a practical perspective, this suggests that using variables that reflect a change in movement strategy, potentially in relation to global external load, may be informative.

Similarly, within-match changes of movement strategy inferred from changes to accelerometer-derived metrics in multiple sports suggest it may be possible to assess fatigue status during competition (10, 30, 96). As mentioned earlier, this could be in the form of custom metrics like PlayerLoad™, various stride parameters, or even variables such as vertical stiffness. Furthermore, as noted earlier, the continued development of automated event detection algorithms in microtechnology devices is likely to provide useful insight. The ability to access these measures in real time during competition or training may have implications for aspects such as substitution strategies and positional changes in various court and field sports for tactical purposes.

Psychometric Inventories

Monitoring the global psychological response to training and competition is an important component of a complete monitoring system (79, 122). Numerous psychometric questionnaires are used in sport, including the Profile of Mood States (POMS) (94), Daily Analyses of Life Demands for Athletes (DALDA) (119), Multi-Component Training Distress Scale (87), and Recovery and Stress Questionnaire (REST-Q Sport) (78). There are also specific questionnaires designed to assess isolated components such as sleep (44). Finally, the use of customized Athlete Reported Outcome Measures (AROMs) is commonplace in high-performance sport (122), and readers are directed to chapter 17, which discusses these scales and critical issues regarding their use in detail.

Integration of Internal and External Load

In addition to the potential usefulness of changes in specific external load variables for assessment of fatigue via changes in movement strategy, the integration of internal and external load (e.g., the total distance:individualized training impulse ratio) has also been proposed (3, 40, 53, 146). The general suggestion is that this type of metric provides an index of efficiency in that it represents the external load relative to the cost of performing this load (in the form of an internal load measure such as HR or RPE). Readers should refer to chapters 14 and 17 for more detailed information on measuring internal load. Further exploration of this concept appears warranted since it may provide practitioners with a more comprehensive understanding of the status of their athletes (3).

EXAMINING LOAD, INJURY, ILLNESS, AND PERFORMANCE INTERACTIONS

As discussed earlier in the section "Managing the Training Process," in simple terms, performance can be considered a function of the difference between fitness and fatigue (26), and attempts to model performance

due to the interaction of these two components have received considerable attention (8, 99).

The interaction between training load, injury, and illness has been extensively examined (43, 45, 59, 118, 149), including as the focus of a two-part International Olympic Committee consensus statement, which readers are directed to for more detail (123, 129). This interest is likely due to the demonstrated impact of injury on performance (68, 150). In general, it appears that load, injury, and illness have a relationship; however, both high and low loads have been shown to increase injury risk (29, 102, 107, 118), and it is likely that injury risk is mediated by a complex interaction of multiple factors such as training status, injury history, and load (including how it is measured). Despite its popularity, there are several critical conceptual and practical flaws in the acute:chronic workload ratio (ACWR) in relation to injury risk, including, but not limited to, the use of the acute workload within the chronic workload (known as *mathematical coupling*) and the use of rolling averages (86, 151). Indeed, research has shown that despite association, the ACWR has poor injury prediction ability (50). As a result, it is suggested that the ACWR not be used for this purpose (74). Nonetheless, it recommended that practitioners carefully plan and measure progressions and regressions in training load, and chapter 19 contains additional content relating to injury risk. This information, along with other athlete response measures and athlete and clinician feedback, can be used to guide decision making about managing training-related injury risks.

While minimizing injury risk is an important component of training program design, performance enhancement is the ultimate goal. Indeed, the most direct way to minimize injury is to stop training and competing altogether, but this is clearly not a logical solution. Given this, the application of a training dose required to elicit improved performance is a key focus for practitioners. Research in elite Australian football has demonstrated that distance and session RPE from training are associated with match running distance; however, the relationship between training load and match performance measured via match statistics was weak (61). Some work has demonstrated a direct relationship between fitness (Yo-Yo intermittent recovery test level 2 performance) and match performance (measured by ball disposals), as well as an indirect relationship between fitness and number of ball disposals through distance travelled at high intensity during a match (98). However, in general, while training load has some association with match running in Australian football (although not in a direct causal manner but probably due to enhanced fitness), the association with either coach rating of performance or match statistics is not as strong (121, 132). This suggests that assessing fitness capacity (with an appropriate test) in conjunction with training load is a valuable approach.

The relationships between training and performance outcomes in team sports are very complex, and it is unlikely that these can be easily identified. A review examining the association between training load and performance outcomes in team sports concluded there was little clear association between external training load and performance (52). However, high-intensity internal training load represented by activity at more than 90% of maximum HR was the best indicator of aerobic performance (52). It is recommended that training load constructs be purposefully selected based on sound conceptual frameworks and also that measures whose measurement properties (i.e., validity and reliability) have been established be used. Importantly, external load in terms of metrics such as distance run should not be confused with performance (i.e., match impact assessed by skill involvements or coach ratings of performance).

DEVELOPING LOAD MONITORING SYSTEMS AND STRATEGIES

Given the extensive range of methods and variables available to practitioners for both programming and monitoring training load and fatigue, the challenge is to select measures with demonstrated validity and reliability in the specific environment of interest (113). In the applied context, validity is important not only in comparison to a criterion or gold standard measure, but also from an ecological perspective (see following section for more specifics on statistical issues in monitoring training load). Although a foundation of any monitoring system is the ability to accurately quantify the training dose (121), microtechnology provides a potentially overwhelming number of external load variables that are not all uniquely useful (133, 144). Furthermore, the development of a system for athlete monitoring should involve the quantification of training load coupled with assessing the individual response, which is then used to guide decision making regarding future training volume and intensity (35, 121).

As described earlier, there are numerous options for assessing internal and external load, and sport scientists are advised to familiarize themselves with the specific advantages and disadvantages of the various measures given the context of their environment. Critically, there are very few, if any, approaches that should be universally applied (arguably perhaps apart from the routine measurement of session RPE).

External Load Measures

An important consideration in the selection of external load metrics is whether there is a conceptual justification and consistent association between any of these measures and performance or injury (see previous section and chapter 19) (121). In addition, it is important for sport scientists to ensure that external load metrics provide important and unique insight (133, 144). For example, research in field and court sports using advanced statistical approaches has allowed the identification of key parameters to quantify training and competition load (133, 144). This kind of analysis can reduce the burden on practitioners because it allows them to concentrate on only the most important metrics, which may reduce the likelihood of making a decision based on a variable that is ultimately not important (145). This should include consideration of locomotor load (i.e., speed and distance) and metrics that account for other movements (141). Finally, from a monitoring perspective, it is ultimately the response to a given external load that should be assessed.

Internal Load Measures

Although a group of athletes can undertake a similar external load, the internal response is likely highly individual (122). As addressed earlier in this chapter and covered in detail in chapters 14 and 17, there are numerous approaches to measuring internal load, including objective (e.g., HR) and subjective (e.g., RPE) methods. It is likely that a combination of these approaches, including the integration of internal and external load, will prove most useful; however, the context of the environment should be the driving factor behind the decision to use a particular approach.

General Monitoring System Components

In addition to the selection of individual variables that make up a monitoring system, some general system components should be considered—specifically, a combination of locomotive and mechanical external load and **session Rating of Perceived Exertion** (sRPE) (121), because it is unlikely that a single variable can capture the complexity of training and competition load (145). Figure 2.5 provides one example of a comprehensive monitoring approach (141). A fundamental requirement of a good monitoring system is that it be as noninvasive as possible to avoid adding to the challenges of the high-performance sport environment (66).

Athlete buy-in is fundamental to ensure that resources are appropriately used, and the purpose of the monitoring program and its impact on training and competition need to be fully understood by athletes, coaches, and other stakeholders (66). These aspects are important because both a lack of feedback and the suggestion that training modification decisions might be unfair are potential drivers of poor compliance (103). In order to limit these possibilities, the results of any monitoring program should be clearly communicated to athletes, coaches, and other staff with a specific emphasis on individual-level analysis and the use of reporting that is both visually appealing and

as easy as possible to comprehend (113). This may be partly achieved with a combination of color-coded formatting and the use of clear diagrams and figures.

An important consideration for sport scientists is that there is a tendency to overvalue the importance of variables obtained from new technology (e.g., GPS) or complex protocols (particularly for the assessment of internal load) when it can be argued that subjective metrics, in the form of self-report, are as good as if not better than most other measures. Ultimately, an approach that incorporates both biological and psychological components likely presents the best methodology (66).

Statistical Issues in Monitoring Training Load

A key foundation of any load and fatigue monitoring strategy is the use of appropriate methods of statistical analysis. Critically, traditional approaches such as null hypothesis testing for the determination of

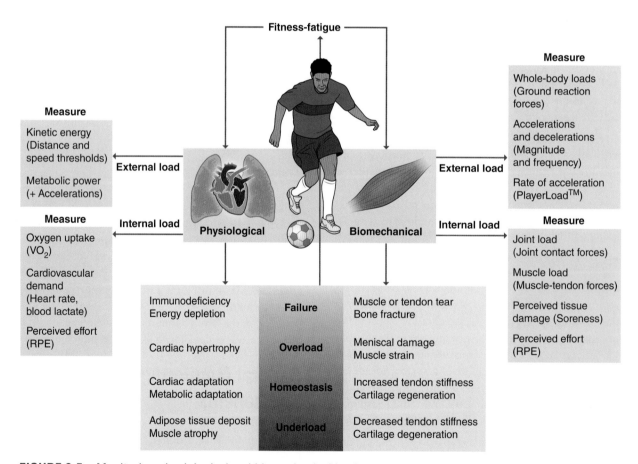

FIGURE 2.5 Monitoring physiological and biomechanical load.

Reprinted by permission from J. Vanrenterghem et al. (2017, pg. 2135-2142).

statistical significance are likely inappropriate in high-performance settings (18, 113, 152). Although analysis at the individual level is likely the most relevant in high-performance sport, there are instances in which group analysis (e.g., positional comparisons, rookies versus senior players) may be required. Similar limitations apply to the use of traditional approaches in group analyses as apply to individual assessment (112, 142). In any case, appropriate statistical analysis allows accurate determination of benchmarks, baselines, and boundaries from which comparisons can be made (113).

Whether analysis occurs on a group or individual level, an important consideration for practitioners is the fact that uncertainty exists in any measure, and this uncertainty, often represented in the form of confidence intervals, should be considered in any analysis (69). Readers should refer to chapter 18 for more detailed information on these topics; however, a brief review of key concepts as they relate to load and fatigue is included next.

Validity

As suggested in preceding sections of this chapter, variables used for the purpose of monitoring load and fatigue need to be both valid and reliable. While the validity of a measure should be assessed via comparison to a criterion or gold standard test (known as criterion validity), an evaluation of the impact of the variable on the training process is also critical (known as ecological validity) (18). Validity can be represented by various statistics, including a correlation, the typical error of the estimate (which is the difference between the field and criterion measure), and bias (which describes the degree to which the field measure tends to over- or underestimate compared to the criterion) (69).

Reliability

Similarly, reliability can be represented by a specialized correlation coefficient, the standard error of the measurement, as a **coefficient of variation** (CV%) (which is the variability of test–retest scores), and the change in the mean score between repeated trials (69). Quantifying reliability of variables used in load and fatigue monitoring is a key step in the ability to determine meaningful change.

Meaningful Change

While a detailed exploration of this concept is not possible here (see chapter 18), in essence, for a practitioner to be confident that the change or signal between time points on a particular variable is meaningful, the change must exceed the noise or error in the measure (e.g., as measured by the CV%) (18). A closely related concept is that of the **smallest worthwhile change** (SWC) or **minimal difference** (MD), which represent the smallest change in a metric for a given athlete that is likely to be of practical importance (18). Numerous methods are appropriate for calculation of the SWC or MD, depending on the metric and the context; however, it is generally a fraction of the between-subjects standard deviation from a repeated reliability trial (18). Although in many cases, measures of training load and fatigue lack the resolution to detect the SWC, they may still be useful because the regular variation in these measures such as the week-to-week change (also known as the signal) exceeds the CV% or noise (38). Assessing the magnitude of change relative to the CV% and SWC results in a range of potential qualitative descriptors, from "unclear" (where there is potential for the change to be simultaneously positive and negative) to "trivial" (where the change is too small to be practically important) and "positive or negative" (where the change clearly exceeds the CV% and SWC in one direction or the other). Figure 2.6 provides a graphical representation of how the CV% can be used to assess if meaningful change has occurred (18). This is a particularly important consideration for load and fatigue monitoring since it maximizes the likelihood that any change in status has been accurately determined, which has obvious effects on training program manipulation.

Numerous other approaches to the statistical representation of individual load and fatigue monitoring variables are possible, including the z-score, standard difference score (111), and standard ten (STEN) score (24). These approaches involve variations of standardizing the individual athlete's score relative to the spread of the group's scores, and thus allow scores to be presented relative to the group (or a predetermined standard if desired). All these statistics can be easily calculated in spreadsheet software and plotted in a figure to provide a visual representation that is meaningful to coaches and athletes.

Advanced Statistical Approaches

As suggested previously, it is beyond the scope of this chapter to examine this area in detail. However, sport scientists should be aware of the increased use of advanced analytical approaches to examine training and competition load, as well as fatigue. In particular, the use of these approaches to examine interactions with performance or injury (or both) and identifying

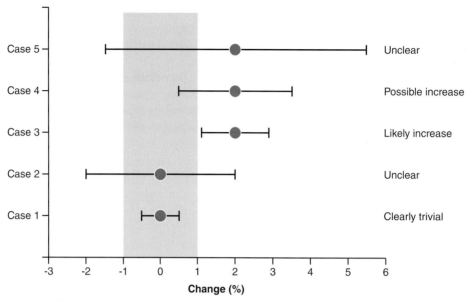

FIGURE 2.6 Interpreting change in individual performance data.

Reprinted by permission from M.J.S. Buchheit (2017, pg. 39).

unique external load variables are becoming more common (61, 115-117, 133).

CONCLUSION

A comprehensive understanding of both internal and external training and competition load is essential for the development of an effective training model. The ultimate aim of quantifying the internal and external load of training and competition is to optimize the stimulus applied to the athlete; as such, monitoring load and fatigue should not be viewed as the process of reducing the load. A variety of tools are available to sport scientists for the measurement of load; however, it is imperative to understand the appropriate use of a specific tool before applying it to a particular context. Importantly, the value of subjective perceptual assessment of the response to training and competition should not be underestimated. Similarly, the validity and reliability of measures of external load should always be considered. Finally, an effective system is likely to comprise the routine collection and analysis of a small number of key metrics that are then used for the ongoing manipulation of individual training loads in order to maximize the likelihood of achieving performance outcomes, including reducing the risk of injury. In the practical setting, this approach should be pursued in preference to overly complex modeling using large numbers of variables in a likely unsuccessful attempt to achieve such things as injury prediction. Similarly, the pursuit of overly simplistic explanations that look to describe complex interactions between training load, performance, and injury with reductionist approaches (e.g., one number to describe an athlete's fatigue and recovery or readiness status) should be avoided.

RECOMMENDED READINGS

Impellizzeri, FM, Marcora, SM, and Coutts, AJ. Internal and external training load: 15 years on. *Int J Sports Physiol Perform* 14:270-273, 2019.

Robertson, S, Bartlett, JD, and Gastin, PB. Red, amber, or green? Athlete monitoring in team sport: the need for decision-support systems. *Int J Sports Physiol Perform* 12:S273-S279, 2017.

Ruddy, JD, Cormack, SJ, Whiteley, R, Williams, MD, Timmins, RG, and Opar, DA. Modeling the risk of team sport injuries: a narrative review of different statistical approaches. *Front Physiol* 10:829, 2019.

CHAPTER 3

Periodization and Programming for Individual Sports

G. Gregory Haff, PhD

One of the key aspects of sport performance is guidance of the training process such that the individual-sport athlete is able to perform at the highest level at major predetermined time points. The ability to achieve these goals is largely affected by the long- and short-term programming strategies employed as part of the training process (57). The process of organizing these various programming strategies, and aligning them with the targeted performance goals and timelines, is the planning construct referred to as **periodization**. While the employment of periodization strategies is widely accepted by coaches and sport scientists (29) as a foundational practice for developing athletes, there are many misconceptions about periodization and its use in real-world individual-sporting scenarios (49, 50, 54). Central to the confusion is the false belief that periodization is a rigid programming construct that does not account for the individual athlete's ability to adapt to training stressors (50) and that periodization and programming are synonymous (48, 54). Fundamentally, periodization is a process used to organize the individual athlete's training (23). This is an evidence-based ongoing reflective process that is used to evaluate the current training status of the athlete and inform future program development. Central to this construct is the ability to systematically engage in an athlete monitoring process (see part III of this text) (23) and rapidly interpret the collected information to provide the coach with information (see chapter 22) that can be used to guide programming decisions (14). Due to their unique skills in collecting, analyzing, and interpreting monitoring data, as well as their understanding of the scientific process, sport scientists play a critical role in periodization and programming.

PERIODIZATION: AN INTEGRATED MULTIFACTORIAL CONSTRUCT

Many discussions on periodization center on implementation of the athletes' physical training program (1, 54) without consideration of other factors that can significantly affect their development and readiness for competition. Ultimately, periodization is an integrated process that combines all training components into a comprehensive structure that allows physical training factors to be matched with nutritional and recovery strategies in order to optimize performance (8, 57). Additionally, there has been increasing emphasis on including other factors, such as psychological (or mental performance) and motor skill development as part of the overall periodization plan (57). Similarly, Bompa and colleagues (8) suggest that truly optimizing the process of periodizing an athlete's training requires the integration of numerous interrelated factors. Due to the highly integrated nature of periodization, an interdisciplinary support team is often employed to optimize the training process of the individual-sport athlete (discussed further in chapter 30).

ROLE OF THE SPORT SCIENTIST IN AN INDIVIDUAL SPORT

The sport scientist plays an integral role as part of the individual athlete's multidisciplinary support team (40) by developing an evidence base for questions that the coaching staff has in order to inform the fine-tuning of the athlete's preparation (41). Conceptually, this multidisciplinary team of professionals work together to help manage the athlete's preparation and competitive performances. Central to this approach is that it is athlete focused, coach centered, and team supported (63) in order to leverage a variety of experts to optimize the athlete's preparations (12).

Norris and Smith (63) suggest that this multidisciplinary team approach is a central component of the modern philosophy of a well-structured periodized training plan that is appropriately designed to guide athletes through their preparation and competitive periods. This approach should help to dispel the false belief that periodization is a rigid or fixed form of training methodology (63). The key to this process is providing coaches with up-to-date interpretations of the ongoing monitoring process and to provide coaches with information that can inform their construction of the selected training interventions (14). Additionally, the sport scientist has the capacity to provide the coach with information on any facet of the training process based upon a foundation of research and knowledge.

In addition to overseeing the monitoring process and interpreting the data collected, the sport scientist continually examines the evolving body of scientific knowledge in order to determine what may add value to the training process. Based on a critical evaluation of emerging areas of research, the sport scientist can make informed recommendations about new training interventions, recovery, or nutritional methods that may be considered candidates for the athlete's overall training plan by the team supporting the coach (42).

PERIODIZATION AND DESIGNING A PLAN

Even though periodization is widely considered an important tool for guiding an athlete's training, there is currently no universally accepted definition of the concept within the scientific and coaching literature (23, 49). While some authors simply refer to periodization as planned training variation (25), others suggest that periodization serves as a directional template that operates as a systematic and methodological planning tool for guiding the athletes' training (63). As a directional training tool, periodization is sometimes referred to as a methodology for sequencing different training units (e.g., training cycles) to guide the athlete toward a desired state and a preplanned result (45). The reference to sequencing of training within the periodization literature has

resulted in the false suggestion that periodization is a rigid construct disconnected from the reality of how an athlete adapts to the training process (49). This false belief is most notable within the strength and conditioning profession, since several authors have repeatedly referred to periodization as overly rigid and an unbending concept (19, 49, 54). In reality, instead of being classed as a rigid concept, periodization is better explained as a scaffolding framework around which specific training programs are formulated to address specific needs and situations (57). Thus, the essence of a periodized training plan is the ability to make sound programming decisions that leverage combinations of training methods and consider the athlete's current performance profile in order to optimize the training process. It is in this way that sport scientists play a critical role in the process in that they provide the multidisciplinary team with quantifiable metrics from which training is guided within the context of the established periodization plan.

Periodization Versus Programming

The key issue that sport scientists and coaches must consider is the differentiation of periodization from the practice of programming (see figure 3.1). As noted earlier, periodization is the scaffolding framework from which programming interventions are designed and implemented. Central to this process is the ability of the sport scientist to leverage monitoring data about the athlete's current state and model the rate of improvement to help the coach become more agile in programming decisions (22, 23). As such, periodization is a macro-management strategy that serves as a training blueprint, from which the sport scientist and coach forecast and assign periods of time that target specific fitness-, skills-, or performance-related factors (22, 57). As seen in figure 3.1, the process of forecasting is simply establishing training objectives that are aligned with training cycles (e.g., micro-, meso-, and macro-cycles and annual and multiyear cycles) (63) and are based on the athlete's needs and objectives in order to inform programming decisions (22).

Programming therefore delineates the modes and methods that are used to structure the training stimulus the athlete is exposed to (22). This is best illustrated by training variables as shown in figure 3.1, such as volume or intensity or both, which are most commonly associated with physical training and the strategies that are employed to program physical

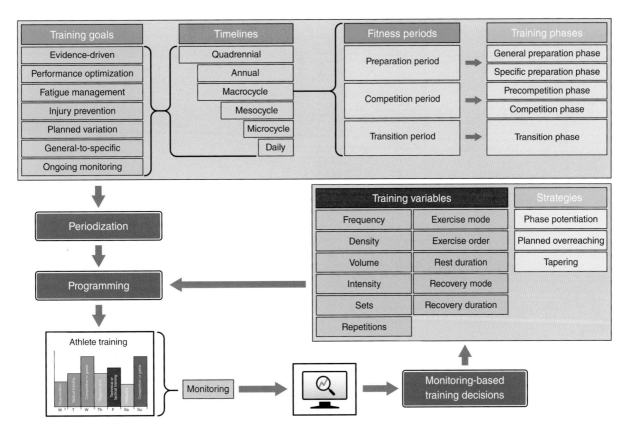

FIGURE 3.1   The symbiotic relationship of periodization, monitoring, and programming.

Based on Cunanan et al. (2018).

training interventions. As noted by Plisk and Stone (67) in their seminal article on periodization, it is clear that "**programming** is an operation of strategic thinking which is best accomplished when ongoing monitoring is integrated into the periodization process." While the programming of physical training is commonly discussed when one considers the periodization of training, it is also important to note that other factors, such as recovery, diet, mental skills, and technical and tactical training can all be integrated into the periodized plan (57). The establishment of training programs or strategies that target the optimization of these various factors are all part of a holistic periodized training plan.

Periodization and Planning the Training Process

In examining the periodization literature, it is clear that numerous models can be used to plan the training process, which can include the parallel, sequential, and emphasis models (see figure 3.2; 31).

Parallel Training Model

A **parallel training model**, as shown in figure 3.2*a*, involves training all factors simultaneously within one training session, training day, series of training days, or microcycles (31). This approach is sometimes referred to as the concurrent or complex parallel approach (9). Generally, this approach works well for youth, novice, or developmental athletes; it may not be beneficial for intermediate to elite athletes (31, 62). One of the main issues with the parallel approach is that as athletes progress, the training volume or load that they are exposed to must increase in order to continue to stimulate adaptation. This may be problematic, because athletes have limited levels of training tolerance, and these increases may exceed an athlete's ability to tolerate training (45) and eventually result in a state of overtraining (31, 62). Because intermediate to advanced athletes require greater stimuli to stimulate adaptation and increases in performance, it may be necessary to employ different planning strategies (31, 67).

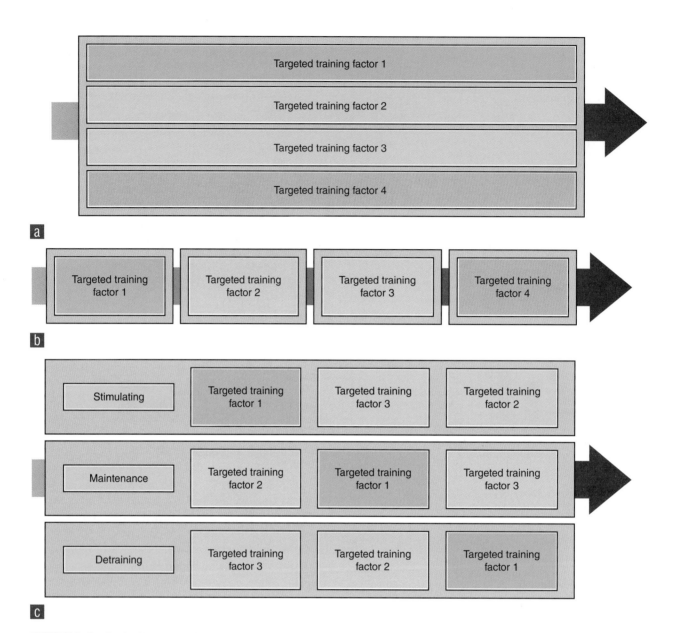

FIGURE 3.2 Periodization and models of planning: *(a)* parallel training approach, *(b)* sequential training approach, and *(c)* emphasis approach.

Figures *a* and *b*: Adapted by permission from Haff (2017, pg. 36, 37). Figure *c*: Based on McGuigan (2017).

While some issues can occur with parallel training models, a sport scientist may choose to employ this model during certain times of the training year with an individual-sport athlete. For example, during a transition period, when a multilateral approach is warranted, it may be beneficial to use a parallel training model in order to target all of the key training factors simultaneously within the training period. Additionally, if the athlete is required to undergo a particularly short preparatory period before a long competitive period, the use of a parallel training model may be justified (9). A sport scientist who makes this choice will most likely then shift toward an emphasis training model during the competitive period.

Sequential Training Model

An alternative planning method is the **sequential training model**, as shown in figure 3.2*b*, which is also referred to as block modeling (43). This model sequences individual factors or a limited number of training factors in a logical pattern to guide training toward a targeted outcome (31, 62). Sequential training models are commonly used in individual sports such as weightlifting (79), cross-country skiing (78), cycling (24, 72), track and field (65) and cardiovascular endurance sports (44). Conceptually, this approach enables the athlete to undertake higher training loads and intensities in sequential patterns that allow for the development of a specific training outcome (31). As the athlete moves through the sequence of training focus, some training factors are no longer emphasized, resulting in a reduction in the development of those factors (62) and in a progressive degree of detraining. The degree of detraining for a de-emphasized training factor is largely affected by the duration between exposures to training that focuses on its development (31). While some proponents of this strategy suggest periodic introductions of "mini-blocks" to allow training factors to be retained, it is possible for some athletes to benefit from a planning approach that modulates the factors being trained within a sequential model (31, 73).

Emphasis Training Models

The **emphasis**, or pendulum, **training model**, as shown in figure 3.2c, incorporates aspects of both the parallel and sequential models of periodization (31). Specifically, this model allows for several training factors to be trained simultaneously (i.e., parallel model) with a varying emphasis over time (i.e., sequential model) in order to stimulate or maintain adaptations or allow detraining to occur (81). Proponents of this model suggest that the emphasis on a given training factor should be rotated every 2 weeks in order to optimize performance capacity (81). This model of periodization

is ideally suited for intermediate to advanced athletes who have to compete in congested competition periods. While more typically employed in team sports (73), the emphasis model has also been suggested for individual sports such as track cycling (62) and sprinting (26). A classic example of the emphasis model is the vertical integration model for sprinting presented by Francis (26). In this example, six training factors are simultaneously (parallel model) trained and have varying degrees of emphasis (sequential model) that align with the targeted training goals.

Hierarchical Structure of Periodization

As a scaffolding structure, the levels of periodization contain a series of hierarchies that are used to organize the various time periods associated with the athlete's short-, medium-, and long-term training plan (29, 63). Conceptually these various structures are nothing more than interrelated levels of planning that help align the training interventions programmed for the athlete, with the targeted goals established for the athlete by the multidisciplinary team working with the athlete (29). Most commonly, the periodized training plan comprises a total of seven interrelated levels, which include the multiyear training plan, annual training plan, macrocycle, mesocycle, microcycle, **training day**, and **training session** (see table 3.1; 29, 33).

TABLE 3.1 Periodization Hierarchy

Level	Name	Duration	Description
1	Multiyear plan	2-4 years	A long-term plan outlines the progression of training goals over several annual plans. The most typical multiyear plan is the quadrennial plan (i.e., 4 years).
2	Annual plan	1 year	This outlines an entire year of training. It can contain 1-3 macrocycles.
3	Macrocycle	Several months to a year	This consists of the competitive seasons, which include the off-season, pre-season, and in-season. It is composed of multiple mesocycles.
4	Mesocycle	2-6 weeks	This is a medium-sized training cycle that is most commonly 4 weeks in duration. This cycle is sometime referred to as a block of training. It is composed of multiple microcycles.
5	Microcycle	Several days to 2 weeks	This smaller-sized training cycle is most often represented as a week (i.e., 7 days) of training. It aligns with the mesocycle goals.
6	Training day	1 day	This is a day in which training is undertaken and is aligned with the microcycle goals.
7	Training session	Minutes to hours	This is a period of time within a training day that contains specific training units. Multiple sessions within a day are defined as having >30 min rest between them.

Adapted by permission from Haff (2017, pg. 39); Adapted from Bompa and Haff (2009); Haff (2016): Haff and Haff (2012); Issurin (2010); Stone et al. (2007).

Multiyear Training Plan

The **multiyear training plan** is a central component of the long-term development of athletes (34) and is designed to project the intended pathway toward the long-term goals established for the individual athlete (see figure 3.3; 64). Central to the development of the multiyear training plan is the establishment of various performance markers, or benchmarks determined by the sport scientist and coaching staff that serve as targets to be achieved across the duration of the plan (7). Conceptually, the multiyear training plan is largely a long-term athlete development plan that serves to scaffold the athlete's development over time (34). While this plan sets the framework for the athlete's long-term development, it is important to note that it is not rigid and can be modified depending upon the individual athlete's rate of progress.

The most common multiyear training plan, or **quadrennial plan**, is composed of 4 years of training, which for the individual-sport athlete aligns with the Olympic Games cycle (29, 46, 74), high school sports (46), and collegiate sports (29). Regardless of the plan's length, the ultimate goal of the multiyear plan is to establish the long-term development pathway for athletes' targeted training goals so that they are able to develop specific physiological, psychological, and performance outcomes at predetermined time points (29, 46).

Annual Training Plan

The **annual training plan** establishes the sequential training framework for the entire year and defines the targeted developmental and performance goals for the individual athlete (11, 29, 74). The structure of this framework is based on the athlete's level of development (10, 11), the training objectives established for the multiyear training plan (21, 46, 64), and the athlete's competitive schedule (11, 29). Classically, the load progression across the annual training plan moves from higher volumes and lower intensities toward lower volumes and higher intensities and more technical or tactical training as the objective of the plan shifts from preparation toward a competitive focus (29, 36).

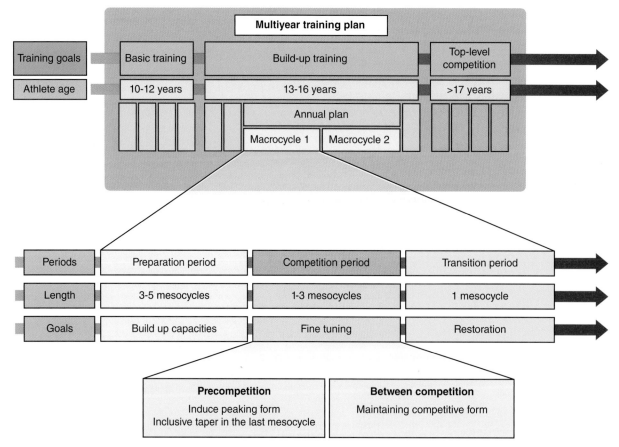

FIGURE 3.3   Example of multiyear training plan for swimming.

Macrocycle

When the annual training plan contains one competitive season it has traditionally been referred to as a **macrocycle** (11, 29). Due to the complexity of modern athletes' competitive schedules and the fact that many individual-sport athletes compete in multiple seasons (29, 38) suggests that macrocycles should represent seasons. For example, a collegiate distance runner might run cross country in the fall, indoor track in the winter, and outdoor track in the spring for a total of three competitive seasons. As such, this athlete's annual training plan would contain three seasons, which would divide the annual plan into three macrocycles.

Structurally, the macrocycle may be divided into distinct training periods and phases that help sequence the training goals within the annual training plan as well as help guide the development of the individualized training plan (see figure 3.4).

Specifically, there are three major periods in each macrocycle, including the preparation, competition, and transition periods. The primary focus of the **preparation period** is the development of the physiological, psychological, and technical base from which peak performance is developed during the **competitive period** (29). The **transition period** serves as a link that bridges between multiple macrocycle or annual training plans. During this period, the primary goal is to maintain fitness levels and technical skills while providing recovery and regeneration (35). It is important to note that if this period involves reduced training for too long (i.e., >2-4 weeks) the athlete will require a much longer preparation period in order to be ready for the subsequent competitive period (29).

These periods are further subdivided into more focused phases of training (i.e., **general preparation**, **specific preparation**, precompetition, main competition, and transition phases), which help the coach integrate, manipulate, and sequence the training goals that guide the programming process (see table 3.2; 35).

The general preparation phase is marked by higher volumes of training performed at lower intensities, with a wide variety of training methods used to develop general motor abilities and skills (29). After the completion of this phase, the athlete will typically begin a specific preparation phase that is designed to deliver more sport-specific training for the purpose of elevating the athlete's overall preparedness toward levels required for competition before entering into the precompetition phase (21). The precompetitive phase links the sport-specific and precompetition phases. This phase often contains simulated competitive events, or unofficial competitions, which are used to develop sport-specific fitness as well as gauge the athlete's performance levels. The structure of the main competition phase is largely dictated by the structure of the competitive schedule and is designed in a manner that maximizes competitive success at key competitive engagements. After completing this phase, the athlete will move into the transition phase, which will serve as a linking phase to the next macrocycle or annual training plan.

Mesocycle

A **mesocycle**, or block of training, is a medium-duration training plan, 2 to 6 weeks in length (29, 31, 33); 4 weeks is the most common length (29). It is important to note that mesocycles are sequenced and interlinked in order to guide the training process. There are numerous ways to plan a mesocycle, which are largely structured based on the training goals and the results of the various monitoring and performance

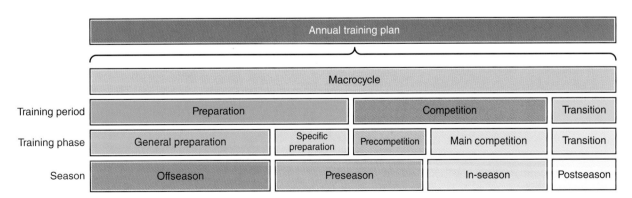

FIGURE 3.4 Relating seasons to classic periodization training structures.

Adapted by permission from Haff, G.G. Periodization. In *Essentials of Strength Training and Conditioning, 4th ed.*, Haff, G.G. and Triplett, N.T., eds. Champaign, IL: Human Kinetics, 592, 2016.

TABLE 3.2   Defining Periods and Phases Used in Periodized Training

Levels of planning	Comments
PERIOD	
Preparation	This is the period of training within a periodized training plan that targets the development of a physiological, psychological, and technical base from which peak performance is developed. It contains both general and specific preparation phases.
Competition	This period of training within a periodized training plan targets the maximization of competitive performance. It contains both precompetition and main competition phases.
Transition	This period of training within a periodized training plan serves as a link between multiple annual training plans.
PHASES	
General preparation	This occurs earlier in the preparation period and focuses on the development of a general physical training base. This phase is marked by higher volumes and lower intensities performed with a wide variety of exercises. Residual fatigue can be high as a result of the higher volumes of training.
Specific preparation	This phase occurs later in the preparation period and is marked by a shift in training focus toward more sport-specific training methods. There is a general shift toward more intensive training and lower training volumes during this phase.
Precompetition	This links the specific preparation and main competition period. During this phase simulated and exhibition events may be used to practice competitive strategies and gauge the athlete's progress.
Main competition	The main competition period is the phase of the annual plan with the competitive season. The main goal of the season is to maximize competition at the key competitive events.
Transition	A lower volume and intensity phase of training is used to induce recovery and prepare the athlete for the next preparation period.

testing that is incorporated into the periodized training plan.

The incorporation of performance assessments (e.g., isometric midthigh pull, vertical jump), continuous monitoring of the training process (e.g., session rating of perceived exertion, training load, sleep, body mass), and other laboratory tests (e.g., sport performance, kinetics or kinematics or both, hormonal or metabolic status or both) can be used to model the athlete's progress (18). These data can allow the sport scientist to give recommendations about what the athlete's training needs are in the next training block so that the training strategies can be adjusted at the microcycle level. For example, the athlete may display an unexpected reduction in performance, such as a reduction in the flight time to contraction time in the vertical jump (20), and changes in biochemical markers, such as reductions in testosterone (T), cortisol (C), or the T:C ratio (52), that are indicative of possible overreaching or overtraining. In this case the coach can decide to provide additional recovery in the next mesocycle (74). Conversely, if the athlete is demonstrating particularly good responses, such as reduced biomarkers associated with stress (e.g., decreased cortisol, increased glutamine) (52) or performance increases (56), the mesocycle addressing the targeted training load for the next mesocycle can be refined to provided additional training stimuli (74). Thus the sport scientist's ability to analyze and interpret the ongoing monitoring and testing program is essential to the programming decisions that are made at the microcycle level.

Microcycle

The **microcycle** is often considered one of the most important levels of planning in the training process since it contains very specific training objectives that are structured into individual training sessions (32). The most common microcycle length is 7 days; however, in the competitive phase, shorter microcycles lasting as little as 2 or 3 days can be used to accommodate a congested competition schedule (29, 35). Ultimately, a series of interconnected microcycles is designed to deliver specific training structures that are aligned with the goals set forth for the mesocycle.

Numerous microcycle structures can be used in the development of a training plan (74, 80), which can generally be classified as preparatory or competitive (see table 3.3; 64).

Fundamentally, these various microcycles are interchangeable planning structures that are used as part of

TABLE 3.3 Classifications of Microcycles

Period used in	Type	Phases used in	Description
Preparatory	Introductory	General, sport-specific	• Reestablish or establish general or sport-specific skills • Introduce new skills and training activities or introduce sport-specific skills • Elevate performance capacities
	Ordinary	General, sport-specific	• Contains lower loads performed with submaximal intensities • Loads gradually and uniformly increase across successive micro-cycles
	Shock	General, sport-specific	• Also known as *concentrated loading* • Targets general or sport-specific conditioning when used in the preparatory period • Contains a sudden increase in training volume and intensity • Best used with more developed athletes
	Recovery	General, sport-specific	• Contains a marked reduction in training loads • Designed to induce recovery and reduce accumulated fatigue
	Model	Sport-specific	• Used to model competitive environment • Structured to familiarize the athlete with competition by simulating competition
Competition	Model	Precompetition	• Reproduces the rest and efforts found in competition • Models the competition
	Precompetition	Precompetition	• May contain higher training volumes earlier in the microcycle that decrease across the microcycle • Special attention given to recovery • Focuses on sport-specific training
	Competition	Main competition	• Contains competitions • Designed to optimize performance • Includes training sessions structured to align with the competition schedule
	Recovery	Precompetition, main competition	• Contains a marked reduction in training loads • Designed to induce recovery and reduce accumulated fatigue

Adapted by permission from G.G. Haff (2016, pg. 404-448).

the programming process to target the training goals included in the mesocycle. For example, four inter-linked microcycles can be structured in order to create a mesocycle that is used within the preparation and is designed to increase the athlete's working capacity:

Introductory ➤ Ordinary ➤ Ordinary ➤ Recovery

Introductory ➤ Ordinary ➤ Shock ➤ Recovery

Shock ➤ Ordinary ➤ Ordinary ➤ Recovery

Shock ➤ Recovery ➤ Shock ➤ Recovery

If, however, the athlete is in the competitive period, a series of microcycles will be sequenced around the competition demands:

Model ➤ Precompetition ➤ Competition ➤ Recovery

Numerous microcycle sequences can be constructed when the athlete's training plan is being designed. However, a central consideration is that the microcycle sequence can be adjusted based on the monitoring data collected and interpreted by the sport scientist. For example, the coach may have planned the following microcycle sequence in which shock and recovery microcycles rotate:

Shock ➤ Recovery ➤ Shock ➤ Recovery

In this scenario, as part of the ongoing monitoring program, the sport scientist could determine that after the first recovery period the athlete has not achieved the requisite level of recovery needed to undertake the next shock microcycle. In this case the microcycle sequence can be altered to ensure that the athlete has the requisite level of recovery before engaging in the next shock microcycle, resulting in the following microcycle sequence for this mesocycle of training:

Shock ➝ Recovery ➝ Recovery ➝ Shock

Fundamentally, in order to alter the sequence, the actual training sessions (i.e., external training load) in each microcycle are modified or adjusted based on the athlete's internal training load.

Considerations for Indoor and Outdoor Individual Sports

While the periodization process is not different between outdoor and indoor sports, the sport scientist can play an important role in helping the coach optimize the individual athlete's preparedness for specific outdoor or indoor competitive environments.

When one examines outdoor sports, environmental factors are an important consideration and where possible should be addressed within the periodized training plan. If an athlete's competition period includes several engagements that are in very hot environments, the sport scientist can advise on acclimatization (16), pre-event cooling strategies (2), or hydration strategies (5) that can be integrated into the athlete's preparation plan. For example, the incorporation of short-term (5 days) heat acclimatization strategies into a periodized training plan can reduce heat strain, and periodic short reacclimatization (2 days) strategies between competitive engagements can further enhance performance and heat tolerance (16). Another strategy the sport scientist could employ to prepare the athlete for competitions in hot environments would be to incorporate other heat mitigation strategies. For example, precooling techniques can be integrated into the training plan to familiarize the athlete with the techniques and test the response in order to determine how the athlete tolerates the strategy (2). If well tolerated by the athlete, these strategies could then be integrated into the competition plan for actual competitive events.

When one is comparing outdoor and indoor sports, another consideration is the surface that athletes train or compete on and the type of shoes they wear (53). As part of the preplanning process the sport scientist can evaluate various competitive and training venues to determine the qualities of the various surfaces and determine which footwear is most appropriate for maximizing performance while minimizing injury risk. Research suggests that although both footwear

and competition or training surface exert an impact on vertical instantaneous loading rates, it is the footwear that exerts the greatest effect (53). Thus the sport scientist plays a significant role in determining which footwear the individual-sport athlete will use on different surfaces.

SCHEDULE MANAGEMENT: OFF-SEASON, PRESEASON, IN-SEASON, AND CONGESTED SCHEDULES

With regard to the various time periods, or seasons, within the athlete's annual training plan, a number of integrated strategies can be employed to ensure that the sport scientist and coach are able to best guide the athlete's training. While most sport scientists and coaches focus on the periodization of the athlete's physical training targets, it is important that nutritional, mental, and recovery strategies, as well as skills-based training, also be considered. It is important that the training processes within the various seasons be managed in a multifaceted fashion. In this manner, training decisions should be informed by an integrated monitoring program (see figures 3.1 and 3.5 on pages 29 and 40; 37). It is important to note that each season will have different training goals, performance outcomes, and demands that need to be understood when one is interpreting any monitoring data collected.

Off-Season

The **off-season** is a critical time period that lays the foundation for the athlete's competitive season (30, 38). If the athlete is not exposed to an appropriate level of training load, the ability to optimize performance and reduce overall risk of injury during the in-season will be compromised. This period of the annual training plan generally has higher volumes and lower intensities of training, which emphasizes general training modes for overall development (27) and aligns with the general preparation phase. As athletes move through the off-season, their workload (i.e., volume and intensity) is gradually increased as work capacity improves and they move toward achieving the required **sporting form**, or level of **preparedness**, necessary for competitive success. Several key factors including retrospective assessment of the athlete's past competitive performances, performance testing, forecasted performance needs for the upcoming season, and physical assessments or medical screenings (or both) can be used to inform the off-season training targets and guide the athlete's sporting form toward the desired level.

During the off-season the sport scientist plays a critical role in conducting or overseeing the physiological and performance testing as well as the athlete monitoring program. When interpreting the performance and physiological testing results, the sport scientist provides the coach with quantifiable metrics that are known to align with the performance required by the athlete during the competitive season. For example, the sport scientist can use performance and physiological testing to predict the performance progression and align it with the forecasted performance needed to achieve a specific placing at key running events (6). This information can then be used by the coach to establish the time course of improvement required to achieve the targeted performance outcome and align specific training interventions with targeted outcomes.

As the athlete progresses through the off-season training plan, the sport scientist will continually monitor the athlete's psychological and physiological response (i.e., **internal training load**) to the training program (i.e., **external training load**). During the off-season, when interpreting the data collected within the monitoring program, the sport scientist must consider the targeted outcomes and what training interventions are being targeted by the coach. For example, if the athlete is doing large volumes of resistance training in order to increase muscle mass (i.e., hypertrophy training) a reduction in the rate of force development (RFD) typically occurs (66). If the sport scientist notes a slight reduction in the RFD during this time period, alarms should not be raised and programming targets should not be altered, since this outcome is expected due to the targeted priority outlined by the periodized training plan. The goal of the off-season period of the annual training plan is to establish the physiological and psychological adaptations required for higher levels of performance in the preseason and in-season time periods.

Preseason

The **preseason** is a time period that includes the classic specific preparatory and precompetition phases of the annual training plan. This period of training serves as a link between the off-season and the in-season periods of the annual plan. During this period, emphasis increases on sport specificity and the incorporation of **specialized developmental** and **competitive exercises** in an attempt to elevate the athlete's sporting form in preparation for the in-season time period. A central theme of this period is the elevation of sporting form in a manner that aligns with the goals established by the coach and athlete for the in-season time period.

As athletes move closer to the in-season time period, in what has classically been termed the precompetition phase, they are often exposed to test events or exhibition-type competitions (11, 29). It is important to note that competitive success is not the main targeted outcome; these competitions or exhibitions are simply used as sport-specific training and to help the coach evaluate the athletes' progress toward the outcomes targeted for the main competitive part of the annual training plan (29).

During this time period, the sport scientist continues to evaluate monitoring data and provide usable data from which coaches can enact training decisions. The sport scientist will also examine the athlete's performance in simulated competitions and exhibition events, giving feedback to the coaches so that they can dial in the athlete's competitive performance development. This feedback can include updating the performance forecast for the athlete to allow coaches to determine whether the athlete is progressing at the intended rate.

An additional role of the sport scientist is to help the coach evaluate, or assess, how the athlete responds to different pre-event strategies (e.g., unloading, tapering, carbohydrate loading) that can be employed before simulated competitions or exhibitions. Along the same lines, the sport scientist can develop various multifactorial recovery strategies that can be employed after a competitive engagement in order to optimize the athlete's recovery strategies.

In-Season

With regard to the global periodization plan, or scaffolding, the **in-season** is the time period in which the primary goal is managing cumulative fatigue, continuing to elevate performance capacity, and maximizing the athlete's competitive performance (29). Although this time period includes global training goals within the athlete's training program, the actual methods and training are typically manipulated based on the athlete's ever-changing needs. During this time coaches often use intuition to guide their programming decisions rather than implementing a specific plan or strategic decision-making model to modulate the training process (47).

An alternative approach is to leverage the various monitoring strategies that can be used to track the athlete's physical and mental status in order to inform programming decisions, modulate recovery strategies, and optimize the athlete's training process (71). In addition to monitoring of the athlete's training progression, programming strategies can be informed by examining travel schedules, anticipated competition difficulty, and the overall density of competition (70, 71). The sport scientist can use what is termed "big data technologies," such as machine learning and modeling techniques (see chapters 18 and 20), to interpret monitoring and competition data in order to provide actionable feedback to the coach so that informed programming decisions can be made (69). While this strategy is more commonly used within team sports, the techniques can also be used with athletes who compete in individual sports. These strategies may be even more important as the individual-sport athlete's competition schedule becomes more congested.

Congested Schedules

When the competitive density is high, the overall risk of injury or illness can be significantly increased (76, 77), which reinforces the need to have a structured periodization plan that outlines when key competitive events will be contested. The importance of carefully structuring the periodized plan to avoid these potential negative effects of dense competitive periods may be of particular importance for the individual-sport athlete, since there are no substitutes or replacements as in team sports. Ideally, the coach should minimize the number of high-density competitive time periods in the annual training plan in order to better manage the athlete's performance progression and minimize overall injury risk. However, this may not be possible for athletes who are professionally required to participate in saturated competitive calendars (75, 77). By mapping out these competitive engagements, the coaching staff and sport scientist can identify the periods of time within the annual plan that allow for integration of preplanned strategies into the overall periodization plan so that the athlete's training is better managed. With careful planning and targeted preplanned recovery strategies (e.g., nutritional

interventions and training load manipulation), the coach will be able to better manage the athlete during saturated competitive time periods.

Additionally, during these periods it is critical that the sport scientist and coach carefully monitor the recovery and training status of the athlete (55) in order to refine the training process and optimize performance while minimizing accumulated fatigue. When excessive fatigue is noted during saturated competitive time periods, many coaches significantly reduce training loads in order to facilitate recovery. Although fatigue will be reduced, it has been reported that risk of injury can increase if training loads are consistently reduced and appropriate training loads are not undertaken (15). To better handle these time periods, the sport scientist can provide the coach with quantitative and qualitative information about the athlete's current fatigue and recovery status. This information can then help the coach establish the training load parameters that best match the athlete's current status, as well as matching the training requirements that will minimize injury risk while maximizing performance capacity.

Fundamentally, the ability to manage congested competitive schedules is facilitated by careful preplanning, comprehensive monitoring programs, and the ability to manipulate the training plan to optimize the athlete's training program in accordance with the training goals established by the periodized plan.

PERIODIZATION AND PROGRAMMING FOR INDIVIDUAL SPORTS VERSUS TEAM SPORTS

While the periodization process is similar for individual- and team-sport athletes, there are some important points of difference that the sport scientist should be aware of. When working with individual-sport athletes it is far easier to align the training sequence to maximize preparedness while minimizing fatigue at climactic competitions. As athletes move through the competitive schedule it is not as critical that they win every competition as they can build their competitive performance capacity so that the main competition of the annual plan is considered the climactic target. Having a true climactic target (e.g., Olympic Games, world championships) allows the sport scientist and coach to better leverage sequential training models as the framework from which to develop a truly individual training plan for their athletes.

Conversely, team-sport athletes must win as many competitive engagements as possible across the entire competitive season in order to reach the sport's climactic event (e.g., championship, grand finale). From a periodization perspective, this requires the overall training process for the team-sport athlete to focus on the team requirements, which ultimately makes it much more difficult to truly individualize the training process in view of the nature of the competitive schedule. Therefore, the team-sport athlete's training program must balance the global needs of the team with the individual performance demands of athletes. Thus team-sport athletes may not get the optimal training stimulus to elevate their performance capacity to their own optimal level, especially when teams are larger (e.g., collegiate football). While this is a critical consideration, the fact that a group of athletes can contribute to the success of the team makes it possible to implement a rotation system—which will allow athletes who require additional recovery or restoration to cycle off the main competitive squad in order to ensure their availability later in the competitive season.

TAPERING

A key aspect of the training process is the ability to elevate the athlete's performance level at predetermined competitive engagements that are outlined within the periodized training plan (30). The process of elevating the athlete's performance is referred to as **peaking** and is accomplished via the preplanned reduction of overall training loads (13, 30, 68). This process is referred to as a **taper**, (30) which should be defined as "a progressive, non-linear reduction of the training load during a variable period of time, in an attempt to reduce the physiological and psychological stress of daily training and optimizing performance" (58). Central to the tapering process is the ability to optimize the athlete's fitness level while simultaneously dissipating fatigue and elevating preparedness (30).

The ability to stimulate even small increases in performance in high-level sports can have a significant impact on competitive success (30). For example, it has been shown that in the year leading into the Olympic Games, swimmers need to improve their performance by 1% in order to stay in contention for a medal (61). Fundamentally, there is a very small difference between winning and not achieving a medal in Olympic competition. In swimming, for example, as little as 1.62% can differentiate between first and fourth place (60). Elite track athletes can significantly alter their placing by using a tapering strategy to stimulate a 0.3% to 0.5% increase in performance, while a 0.9% to 1.5% increase in performance can improve a field (i.e., throwing) athlete's placing (39).

The employment of well-crafted tapering strategies can reasonably be expected to improve competitive performance by 0.5% to 7.0% in individual sports such as swimming, weightlifting, running, throwing, and cycling (30). While tapering strategies are important tools for maximizing the performance capacity of athletes, it is always critical that sport scientists and coaches remember that the foundation of a taper is established during the off-season and preseason training the athlete undertakes before the in-season time period (30). If the athlete does not train hard enough or is unable to establish a robust foundation, the ability of a taper to maximally peak performance will be limited.

If an appropriate training base has been established, the tapering period will be designed to reduce the overall training loads the athlete is undertaking in order to induce recovery and elevate performance (30). It is generally recommended that an individualized fast exponential taper be implemented to reduce the workload leading into a competition (3, 59). A workload reduction of between 41% and 60% is often recommended depending upon the pre-taper training volumes (30). If the pre-taper training workload is larger, fatigue will be greater, which would require a greater reduction in workload. A key tapering strategy is to use moderate to high training intensities while simultaneously reducing training volume. However, it is important to note that when training volume is reduced, the frequency of training should be maintained at ≥80% of pretraining taper training frequency (30). Finally, depending upon the pre-taper training workload, tapers can last from 1 to 4 weeks; the most common duration is 8 to 14 days.

DATA SHARING AND CONTEXT ADAPTATION

With regard to the multidisciplinary team approach to developing the periodized training plan for the individual-sport athlete, a central theme is the ability to share data with the coach so that an optimized and individualized training process can be developed. The periodized training strategy is developed based on historical training, performance data, nutritional analysis, and an individualized needs analysis. These data can then be used by the sport scientist as part of a deterministic modeling process coupled with performance forecasting (i.e., predictive performance modeling) that is used to give the coach actionable information, which can be translated into a training plan (see figure 3.5).

As part of this process the sport scientist will examine the periodization strategies used in previous annual training plans and the athlete's performance testing results in order to create a **deterministic model**. This model can then be used to identify the key biomechanical and physiological factors that relate to the athlete's performance, and if these key factors are trained, will result in their development and ultimately translate to an improvement in the athlete's performance (17). Once the deterministic model is developed and key deficiencies are noted, the multidisciplinary team will work to create the periodized training plan in order to align with the forecasted performance progression. Central to this process is the establishment of key benchmarks that the athlete will need to achieve at predetermined time points across the multiyear training plan and within each annual training plan.

Interest has been increasing in guiding the programming process by leveraging the sport scientist's ability to use machine learning (ML) (4) and artificial intelligence (AI) (18) to develop predictive models based on historical training data. The aim is to model the athlete's internal and external training load, performance progression, and overall injury risk in relation to a proposed training progression (4, 18, 28). An example is the use of artificial neural networks to model the effects of a preplanned 15-week resistance training program on changes in jumping performance (51). Based on these data, an optimized training progression can be provided to the coach. Conceptually, the development of an optimized training progression effectively gives coaches actionable loading progressions that can guide their programming decisions in order to make the training programs more accurate.

As the athlete progresses through the training plan it is also important to note that the sport scientist plays a critical role in the monitoring process. The ability of the sport scientist to monitor the forward

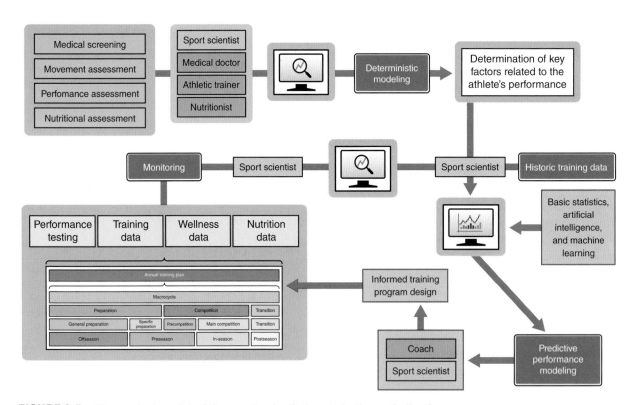

FIGURE 3.5 Theoretical model of the sport scientist's role in the periodization process.

Adapted by permission from Haff, G.G. Periodization. In *Essentials of Strength Training and Conditioning, 4th ed.*, Haff, G.G. and Triplett, N.T., eds. Champaign, IL: Human Kinetics, 592, 2016.

progression of the athlete's training, and then use AI and ML to interpret data collected as part of the monitoring process, allows for the training program to be continually fine-tuned. As part of this process, sport scientists engage in a constantly evolving predictive modeling process. Specifically, they examine the impact of the external training loads on the athlete's internal training load using actual training and monitoring data to constantly update the progressive model that is being used to inform the athlete's future training program (28). Based on the interpretation of the individualized monitoring process, sport scientists feed valuable information back to coaches so that appropriate modifications can be made to the athlete's training plan, in order to more accurately program the training interventions and optimize performance outcomes (4).

CONCLUSION

The ability to effectively periodize, plan, and program an individual-sport athlete's training process is largely dependent on a collaborative multidisciplinary support team that works with the coach to guide the athlete's training process. The sport scientist plays a central role in helping to develop the periodized training plan, which serves as the scaffolding from which planning and programming decisions are made. By using scientific methods, the sport scientist informs this process by providing the coach with actionable information that helps fine-tune the training process. The process is continually evolving, leveraging the sport scientist's ability to interpret performance testing, monitor data, and perform detailed analyses of the athlete's progression toward the targeted sport outcome.

RECOMMENDED READINGS

Haff, GG. The essentials of periodization. In *Strength and Conditioning for Sports Performance*. Jeffreys, I and Moody, J, eds. Abingdon, Oxon: Routledge, 404-448, 2016.

Ingham, S. Seven spinning plates. In *How to Support a Champion*. UK: Simply Said LTD, 86-119, 2016.

Verkhoshansky, Y, and Siff, MC. *Supertraining: Expanded Version*. Rome, Italy: Verkhoshansky, 2009.

CHAPTER 4

Periodization and Programming for Team Sports

Martin Buchheit, PhD
Paul Laursen, PhD

The accurate programming of training in team sports, including diverse neuromuscular and energy-systems training, is a key consideration to avoid overload or to maintain an appropriate stimulus (or both) across the different training cycles (14). Indeed, an accumulation of neuromuscular load often arises in athletes from different training components, including **high-intensity interval training** (HIIT), strength-speed sessions, and tactical/technical sequences. Periodization and programming therefore need to be an integrated part of the training process, to either complement (6) or supplement (4) the other training contents. Importantly, the metabolic adaptations arising from various training programs tend to be similar irrespective of the actual format experienced over a couple of months of training (5). However, in the short term (i.e., microcycle level), the likely acute neuromuscular impact of different training formats may play a critical role with respect to both the neuromuscular adaptations and interferences that develop from supplementary training and match content. This occurrence may also influence injury risk. An approach to managing the different training formats, including HIIT methods, is discussed in this chapter.

A multitude of factors must be considered by the coach and practitioner to prepare any team for battle, including team sport–specific skills, team tactics, and player interactions. Additionally, for the conditioning coach, depending on the sport, different emphases on physical development will be needed, including speed, strength, and aerobic conditioning. One of the key factors that can be manipulated by a practitioner, forming a useful tool for optimal preparation, is HIIT. High-intensity interval training specifically consists of repeated bouts of exercise performed in one's "red zone," or at an intensity above the maximal lactate steady state, anaerobic threshold, or critical power-speed, separated by relief bouts of easy exercise or complete rest. This form of exercise training is believed to be one of the strongest and most time-efficient training modalities that can be used to improve overall fitness (8). Following short HIIT supplementation periods across various sports, substantial improvements in various fitness-related variables have been shown, including maximal oxygen uptake, maximal aerobic endurance performance, and maximal intermittent performance, as well as the ability to sustain high-intensity efforts over prolonged periods of time (8-10, 15, 22, 23).

While HIIT is generally programmed intentionally to improve these specific physical characteristics, the important neuromuscular load that may be associated with performing some HIIT sequences should not be overlooked. In fact, depending on the actual HIIT format, the neuromuscular load and musculoskeletal strain can be diverse, from low to very large, despite a similar metabolic stimulus.

This chapter begins by introducing the importance of defining biological targets in relation to the metabolism involved (aerobic or anaerobic or both, lactic metabolism) and the level of neuromuscular load experienced in various team sports and invasion games (e.g., basketball, soccer, handball, rugby). Subsequently it presents practical examples of how training integration can be used effectively within the weekly training cycle for team sports.

PHYSIOLOGICAL CHARACTERISTICS OF HIIT

To begin, this section introduces the overarching training philosophy for team sports, including appreciating "physiology first" through the HIIT types and how one can select multiple formats to achieve various outcomes as the context specifically requires. Working from left to right in figure 4.1 (26), once context is fully appreciated (this example highlights the context specific to soccer or football), it is necessary to consider training sessions that include different degrees of aerobic (green; metabolic O_2 system), anaerobic (red), and neuromuscular (black) stress or load. Different quantities of these physiological responses inherent to training content form HIIT types 1 through 6. Traditionally, many coaches and practitioners have fallen into the trap of assuming that a particular training format (e.g., short interval, long interval) will necessarily elicit a physiological response. As shown in figure 4.1, the same format, if programmed appropriately, can be used to target multiple HIIT types (different physiological responses). Thus, once you know what HIIT type you are trying to pursue in the session, simply select the "weapon" (i.e., HIIT format) of your choice to hit your target (the HIIT weapons are covered in detail in the next section). Understanding the HIIT types in figure 4.1 creates a window of opportunity for the sport scientist working with a team sport in terms of understanding how to best solve nearly any programming situation.

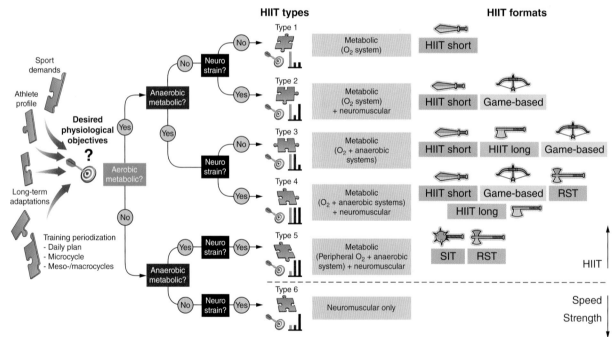

FIGURE 4.1 Decision tree for selecting the physiological targets of high-intensity interval training (HIIT), which should precede selection of the associated HIIT format. The six physiological targets include type 1: aerobic metabolic, with large demands placed on the oxygen (O_2) transport and use systems (cardiopulmonary system and oxidative muscle fibers); type 2: metabolic as with type 1 but with a greater degree of neuromuscular strain; type 3: metabolic as with type 1 with a large anaerobic glycolytic energy contribution but limited neuromuscular strain; type 4: metabolic as with type 3 but with both a large anaerobic glycolytic energy contribution and a high neuromuscular strain; type 5: a session with limited aerobic demands but with an anaerobic glycolytic energy contribution and high neuromuscular strain; and type 6: not considered HIIT, with a high neuromuscular strain only, which refers to typical speed and resistance training, for example.

THE HIIT WEAPONS

Now that a roadmap solution to develop physiological targets has been outlined, it is important to define the key weapons at one's disposal. As shown in figure 4.1, five key HIIT formats are used within the context of most team sports. These include long intervals, short intervals, repeated sprint training, sprint interval training, and game-based training or small-sided games, with general examples offered in figure 4.2 (26). For detailed information, the reader is referred to Laursen and Buchheit (26).

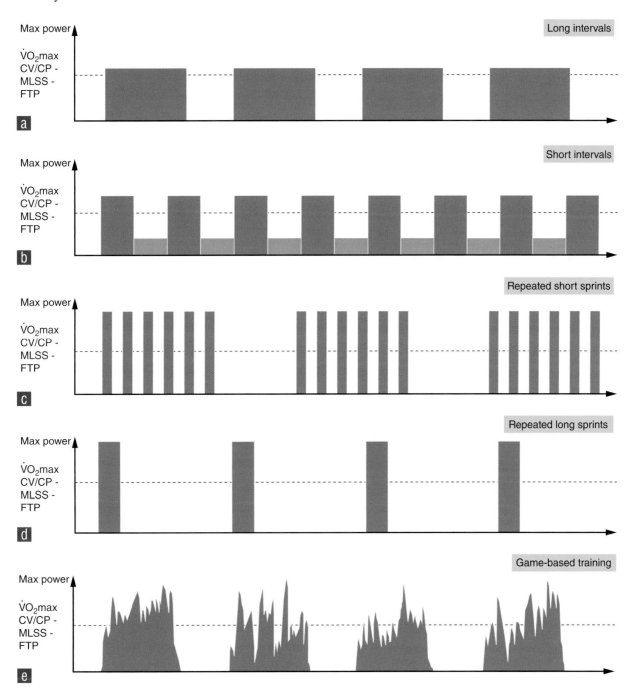

FIGURE 4.2   An overview of the five key weapons that can be used to form a physiological response with HIIT, including (a) long intervals, (b) short intervals, (c) repeated short sprints, (d) repeated long sprints, and (e) game-based HIIT.

$\dot{V}O_2$max, maximal oxygen uptake; CV/CP, critical velocity/critical power; MLSS, maximal lactate steady state; FTP, functional threshold power. Blue bars = effort intervals, green = relief intervals

Reprinted by permission from P.B. Laursen and M.J.S. Buchheit (2018, pg. 69-71).

Long Intervals

In general, long intervals use repeated bouts at the longer end of the intensity–time continuum, around the velocity/power (v/p) associated with $\dot{V}O_2max$ (95%-105%), 80% to 90% of the final velocity reached at the end of the 30-15 Intermittent Fitness Test (V_{IFT}, see later). The durations need to be longer than a minute to induce the acute metabolic and neuromuscular responses. For long intervals to be effective, they should be separated by short durations (1-3 min) of passive recovery, or longer durations of active recovery up to 45% of V_{IFT} or 60% of the velocity/power reached at the end of an incremental test, $V/P_{IncTest}$ (2-4 min). Long intervals can be used to hit type 3 and 4 targets (see figures 4.1 and 4.2).

Short Intervals

Short intervals use bouts of less than a 60-second duration, repeated in a similarly short time duration. Short intervals should be performed at between 90% and 105% of V_{IFT} (100%-120% $V/P_{IncTest}$), separated by less than a minute of recovery (passive to 45% V_{IFT}/60% $V/P_{IncTest}$), dependent largely on the lactate response you are after in the session (use longer passive pauses to lower the lactate response, type 1 to 4; see figures 4.1 and 4.2).

Repeated Sprint Training

Repeated sprint training (RST), or short sprints, is a weapon format that can be used to target more high-end capacities and comes with substantial neuromuscular strain. These formats involve 3- to 10-second efforts of an all-out maximal intensity, with a variable recovery duration ranging from short and passive to 45% V_{IFT}/60% $V/P_{IncTest}$. Repeated sprint training can be used to hit type 4 targets, and also the nonoxidative type 5 target (see figures 4.1 and 4.2).

Sprint Interval Training

Like RST, sprint interval training (SIT) involves all-out maximal sprinting efforts, but the durations of these are long, in the 20- to 45-second range. Such efforts are exceptionally taxing, and recovery is passive and long (typically 1-4 min). The SIT weapon exclusively hits the type 5 target, and therefore would not be a recommended weapon to use in the context of soccer (see figures 4.1 and 4.2).

Game-Based or Small-Sided Games

Game-based HIIT, or small-sided games (SSG), are ultimately game-based forms of HIIT using long-interval principles for time:recovery ratios. They tend to run for 2 to 4 minutes at a variable sport-specific intensity of effort. Recovery durations are typically passive and range from 90 seconds to 4 minutes. Game-based HIIT or SSG are highly versatile and can be used to target type 2, 3, and 4 responses. Ultimately, the sport scientist can be highly valuable in helping to monitor and program such game-based HIIT formats in order to hit physiological targets appropriately.

PROGRAMMING HIIT

Despite debate surrounding the feasibility (2), calculation (27), and overall value of the acute/chronic workload ratio (ACWR) for predicting injury incidence (19), it's well appreciated that we should maintain a stable and constant training stimulus to keep players fit and healthy. Conversely of course, large spikes in load, and especially high-speed running (HSR or HS) load, which may share an association with hamstring injuries (16), should be avoided. Additionally, results from a recent systematic review and expert-led Delphi survey of key football performance practitioners operating in teams from the Big 5 international leagues (i.e., Bundesliga, English Premier League, La Liga, Ligue 1, Serie A) have shown HSR management to be the most valued strategy for preventing lower-limb injuries (18). Here, we place special emphasis on the importance of HIIT supplementation in relation to HSR demands (more the neuromuscular load effect of these, and not only their metabolic stimulus per se). Guidelines for HIIT programming in terms of physiological targets, format, volume, and intensity are also provided.

Practical Example

Figure 4.3*a* shows the in-season HSR distribution measured in a soccer midfielder during both training and matches over a 5-week congested match period. While he repeatedly performed 600-800 m of HSR during the 5 first consecutive matches of that period, the coach decided to rest him for the 6th match (26th of September, bench). He then played 30 min as a sub on the 29th, was not selected in the squad on the 2nd of October (cup match for which he wasn't qualified), played again as a substitute on the 5th of October, and remained benched on the 8th (away game), before finally playing another full match on the 12th. If we were to only consider the loading pattern of HSR consecutive to his exclusive participation to training and matches, a spike would have been inevitable from the load associated with the full match on the 12th of October (i.e., ACWR >2).

Intervention Strategy

Figure 4.3*b* offers a viable strategy as to how HIIT supplementation (i.e., so-called compensatory training) permits the maintenance of HSR loading throughout the period where the player did not play much. While no HIIT was programmed on the 26th to enable recovery, compensatory HIIT sessions were

implemented subsequently in various contexts during the period of reduced match participation. The detail of the HIIT sequences, in terms of both the HIIT type and format are provided in tables 4.1 and 4.2.

The simple addition of four short HIIT sequences allowed the maintenance of a stable HSR load, which logically prevented the occurrence of a spike in load on the 12th of October, when the player completed a full match after a period of reduced match participation. This simple but likely efficient compensation strategy was either implemented on the fly, immediately after the match when the time and location allowed for it, or the following day at the training ground when the substitute player trained.

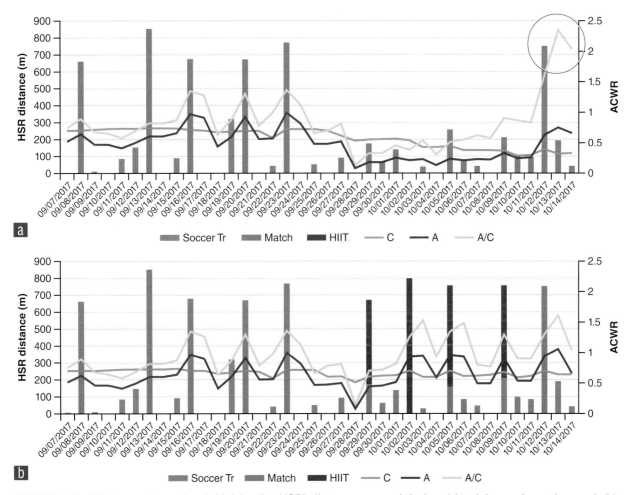

FIGURE 4.3   High-speed running (>19.8 km/hr, HSR) distance covered during *(a)* training and matches and *(b)* training, matches and supplementary high-intensity interval training (HIIT) in a midfielder (22 y-old, playing in a 1st division club) during a 5-week in-season period.

The acute (A) and chronic (C) load are calculated over 5 and 20-d periods, respectively. ACWR: A/C workload ratio. A spike (A/C >2) in HSR is shown with the red circle. GPS (training) and semi-automatic (matches) locomotor data were integrated with calibration equations (7). Note that while the match sequence is real, the actual dates have been changed to ensure anonymity.

Reprinted from M.J.S. Buchheit (2019, pg. 1).

HSR Volume to be "Compensated"

The appropriate target of HSR volume needs to be defined for each player at the individual level, based on typical match demands. This is illustrated in figure 4.4. Following its identification, the volume can be subsequently adjusted based on the day's context, i.e., whether the player had already performed some HSR as a substitute or not at all if he remained on the bench (see table 4.2).

In practice, the actual HSR volume of a given HIIT sequence can be easily manipulated and is related to the HIIT types and formats chosen (see figure 4.2). We recall for the reader that HIIT types refer to the physiological targets of the HIIT sequences, representing the degree of aerobic, anaerobic (lactic), and neuromuscular responses (26), while the formats refer simply to the work actually performed in terms of the distance, time, and number of repetitions (26). While type 2 (high aerobic and neuromuscular demands, low anaerobic contribution) or type 4 (high

aerobic, neuromuscular and anaerobic contribution) are required to incorporate HSR, they can be run-based only (see figure 4.5 and table 4.1, especially when performed soon after a match or game), or with ball integration if appropriate (see figure 4.6, likely individual and substitute training). These types 2 and 4 sequences are often supplemented with technical/tactical drills, or even type 1 HIIT sequences (high aerobic but low neuromuscular and anaerobic contribution) when necessary to increase the degree of metabolic conditioning without the neuromuscular load.

HSR INTENSITY: WORTH CONSIDERING?

An important point that has received very little attention within sport science literature is that for most of the HIIT options presented here, the actual HSR intensity (33-100 m/min over 6 min in the soccer example, see

TABLE 4.1 Examples of Two Position-Specific Run-Based Type 2 HIIT Sequences and Consecutively, the Associated Overall Daily Session

Position	Pattern (see figure 4.5)	# Repetitions	Distance/run (m)	HSR/run (m)	HSR volume (m)	HSR intensity (m/min)
MD Match volume: ~800m Peak 1-min Intensity: 45 m/min	A	4	65	50	200	100
	B	2	60	0	0	0
	C	6	55	35	210	70
	HIIT block	6 min	710		410	68
	Full compensatory session	6 min + 4 min (2 × B & 6 × C) (r = 2 min)	1160		**650**	**52 (over 12 min)**
FB Match volume: ~1300 m Peak 1-min Intensity: 60 m/min	A	8	65	50	400	100
	B	0	60	0	0	0
	C	4	55	35	140	70
	HIIT block	6 min	740		540	88
	Full compensatory session	6 min + 4 min (6 × A & 4 × C) + 2 min (4 × A) (r = 2 min)	1500		**1110**	**69 (over 16 min)**

HSR: high-speed running. Letters refer to the running patterns shown in figure 4.5. All runs are performed at 110% of player's V_{IFT} (speed reached at the end of the 30-15 Intermittent Fitness Test [1])—with running distance reduced as a function of the nature and number of changes of direction (2). r = 2 min: 2 min of recovery between sets.

Reprinted from M.J.S. Buchheit (2019, pg. 1-5).

TABLE 4.2   HIIT Programming During the Period of Reduced Match Participation

Date	Training HSR (m)	Match status	Match HSR (m)	HIIT HSR (m)	HIIT type and format
September 26	0	Bench	0	0	
September 27	91				
September 28	0				
September 29	0	Sub (30 min)	175	500	Directly on the pitch after the home game, run-based without the ball • Type 1: 8 × (20 s run 45°- slalom @ 90% V_{IFT}/ 10 s passive recovery) = no HSR • Type #4: 10 × (15 s @ 95% V_{IFT} / 15 s active-jog recovery) = 500 m HSR
September 30	65				
October 1	138				
October 2	1	Not selected	0	800	Individual session at the training ground • Type 2: position-specific HIIT with the ball (5 s run / 10 s passive rest). Depends on set-up, likely 2 × 10 reps = 300 m HSR • Type #4: run-based without the ball, 10 × (15 s @ 95% V_{IFT} / 15 s active-jog recovery) = 500 m HSR
October 3	34				
October 4	0				
October 5	0	Sub (30 min)	153	650	Directly on the pitch after the home game, run-based without the ball • Type 2: as per table 1 for MD = 650 m HSR
October 6	86				
October 7	46				
October 8	0	Bench	0		Away match and since the next game was in 4 days, no HIIT was performed that day
October 9	209			550	After technical session of the subs at the training ground • Type 2: position-specific HIIT with the ball (10 s @ 110% V_{IFT} / 20 s passive rest). Depends on set-up, likely 2 × 12 reps = 550 m HSR
October 10	106				
October 11	90				
October 12	0	Starter (full match)	756		
October 13	192				
October 14	44				

HIIT: high-intensity interval training. HSR: high-speed running. V_{IFT}: speed reached at the end of the 30-15 Intermittent Fitness Test (1). HIIT types refer to the physiological targets of the sequences, indicating the degree of aerobic, anaerobic (lactic) and neuromuscular responses (26). Formats refer to the work actually performed, in terms of the distance, time, and repetition number (26). Green indicates HSR requirements were attained; yellow indicates HSR was only met in part (i.e., substitute); and red shows an absence of load (i.e., benched) and thus HIIT gets supplements to counter the missed HSR load.

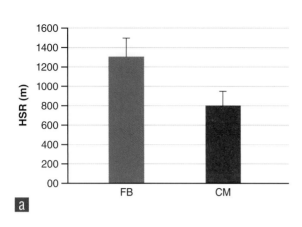
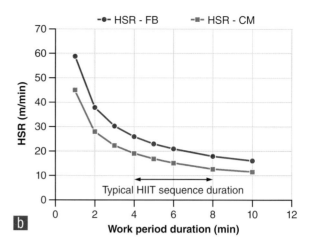

FIGURE 4.4 HSR volume *(a)* and peak intensity *(b)* as a function of different durations during matches for two positions (full back, FB; center midfielder, CM). Not surprisingly, the shorter the time period, the greater the peak HSR intensity. Also apparent is that in addition to a greater volume of HSR, FB show also a greater peak intensity of HSR compared with CM, irrespective of the period of interest (11).

Reprinted from M.J.S. Buchheit (2019, pg. 1-5).

figures 4.5 and 4.6) tends to be far superior over that of peak match demands during similar durations (20-25 and 15-20 m/min over 4 and 6 min, respectively, figure 4.4). In other words, when compensating HSR volume with HIIT (see figure 4.3), what is generally covered in a 90-min match is achieved in less than 15 min with HIIT. This means that match-specific HSR intensity is easily overloaded using HIIT—the question now being "how much does this really matter in terms of fitness development, match preparation, and injury management?" While evidence is still lacking, it may be logical to assume that extreme overload of HSR intensity (e.g., 100 vs. 15 m/min) may not be needed (or should even be avoided). Breaking such HIIT sequences into smaller effort sequences (e.g., 1-2 min of HIIT, then a rest period, then another short HIIT bout again) may lower HSR intensity near that of actual game intensity. However, the cardio-respiratory response may, in contrast, not be sufficient to enable desired adaptations (26). Practitioners may therefore need to decide on what needs prioritizing in the individual (i.e., metabolic conditioning [longer HIIT sets >4-6 min] versus match-specific HSR intensity [multiple shorter HIIT sets <3-4 min]). Alternatively, mixing different running patterns within the same HIIT block represents a viable option, such as alternating runs with large amounts of HSR (pattern A, see figure 4.5 and table 4.1) and runs where HSR is limited or even absent (pattern B, see figure 4.5 and table 4.1). For example, if straight-line and zigzag runs with various levels of changes of directions are

alternated over 6 min, the volume and intensity of HSR can be dropped from approx. 600 m and 100 m/min (straight-line only) to 300 m and 50 m/min, respectively. Similarly, if position-specific runs are alternated with different patterns/types of efforts (with or without the ball, including various turns, dribbles, passing) that prevent the attainment of high speeds, HSR running intensity can be dramatically reduced and made near equal to match intensity demands. In addition to be closer to match HSR intensity, this approach can allow players to exercise for longer periods of time without accumulating excessively large HSR volumes, which in itself could create a spike in load. For example, if an MD was to repeat 2 sets of 6-min HIIT (2 min recovery) including only straight-line runs, which in effect is only a moderate HIIT dose (26), he would likely cover >1.2 times his usual match running distance in no more than 14 min!

With players coming from the bench, for example in basketball or Australian rules football, HIIT supplementation immediately after matches or the following day is a practical and likely efficient strategy for the maintenance of a stable HSR load over the weekly cycle. Both the volume and intensity of HSR should be tailored for the individual (position and style of play) using typical locomotor match profiles (see figure 4.4). In practice, HSR volume can be tailored via both the absolute number of run repetitions and the pattern of these efforts (either with or without changes in direction that directly modulate HSR, see

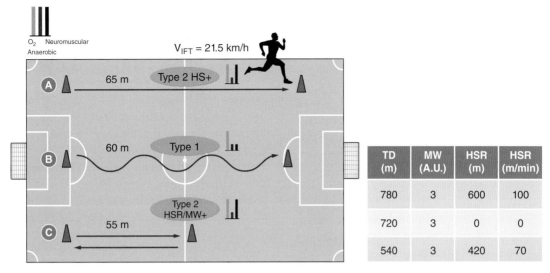

FIGURE 4.5   Example of three HIIT sequences with short intervals (10-s run/20-s passive recovery periods), performed either with or without turns at different angles to modulate both the amount and nature of the neuromuscular load (i.e., HSR and mechanical work, MW), which leads to variation between Type 1 and Type 2 (the latter being oriented either toward HSR or MW). The associated locomotor responses analyzed by GPS are provided for each 6-min sequence, as if the same running pattern was to be repeated 12 times (e.g., 12 × pattern A). TD: total distance; HSR: high-speed running >19.8 km/h; MW: >2 m/s^2 accelerations, decelerations, and changes of direction. V_{IFT}, Velocity achieved during the 30-15 Intermittent Fitness Test. Degree of contribution from oxidative (O_2), anaerobic (Ana), and neuromuscular (Neuro) systems are shown by the degree of green, red, and black bars, respectively (26).

Adapted by permission from P.B. Laursen and M.J.S. Buchheit (2018, pg. 550).

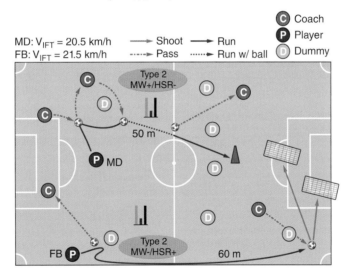

FIGURE 4.6   Example of two position (midfielder, MD and full back, FB)-specific HIIT with short intervals (10 s/20 s format, Type 2), based on V_{IFT}. The associated locomotor responses analyzed by GPS are provided for each 6-min sequence, as if the same running pattern was to be repeated 12 times. The FB can't progress because of an opponent (dummy), so he passes the ball to a coach/partner playing as a central defender, then runs along the sideline to receive from a second coach/partner another ball close to the box where he shoots into one of two mini goals (as if he was crossing). The MD comes close to the central defender to receive the ball, then to eliminate a defender passes and receives to/from a coach/partner situated on the sideline as an FB, before running forward with the ball where he passes to a second coach/partner and finishes his run toward the box, shooting into a mini goal. Note the large differences in terms of HSR and MW between the two position-specific efforts, which likely matches their match-specific loading targets (24) (greater HSR demands for FB, greater MW for MD). TD: total distance; HSR: high-speed running >19.8 km/h; MW: mechanical work >2 m/s^2 accelerations, decelerations, and changes of direction. V_{IFT}, Velocity achieved during the 30-15 intermittent fitness test. Degree of contribution from oxidative (O_2), anaerobic (Ana), and neuromuscular (Neuro) systems are shown by the degree of green, red, and black bars, respectively (26).

Adapted by permission from P.B. Laursen and M.J.S. Buchheit (2018, pg. 551).

figure 4.5 and table 4.1). While there is little evidence concerning the most appropriate HSR intensity for fitness maintenance, match preparation, and injury prevention, it makes intuitive sense to avoid a too high match intensity overload; this can be achieved while adapting running patterns within each HIIT block (see table 4.1). It is however worth noting that a volume of HSR accumulated across an entire game (1-2 hours) likely represents a different physiological and biological load than that accumulated in less than 15 min (HIIT)—whether both have the same effect on injury rate is unknown. We believe therefore it may be time for sport scientists to further consider the importance of the HSR intensity, and not simply its volume (20), when it comes to examining the relationship between load management and fitness level, as well as injury incidence. Finally, it could be argued that if the compensatory strategy presented herein is implemented successfully, computing the ACWR might not actually be required. Nevertheless, the ACWR might still be a useful guide for deciding on the most appropriate volume of HSR running needed for the compensatory prescription (e.g., 400 vs. 800 m).

SAMPLE TRAINING PROGRAMS

During the preseason (see figure 4.7; 26), there is a tendency to restrict locomotor load and high neuromuscular load during the first few days, using the most applicable SSG formats (6v6 and 8v8, possession [PO]) and type 1 HIIT with short intervals. On specific days, however, type 4 HIIT may be programmed, such as 4v4 game simulation (GS) during a strength-oriented session and HIIT with long intervals before 24 hours of rest.

In-season, 4v4 SSG (GS) are programmed during strength-oriented sessions, which may be the major HIIT format used with starters. For substitutes, however, these 4v4 GS are often complemented with run-based HIIT including various levels of neuromuscular constraints, depending on the timing of the following match, with greater emphasis on locomotor load with one (see figure 4.8, type 2 HS; 26) versus two (see figure 4.11, types 1 or 2; 26) games a week. Finally, note also that the overall training volume of work for the substitutes is adjusted based on their playing time the preceding day (i.e., they generally played for 5 to 40 minutes or did not play at all; see figure 4.3 on page 47).

INTEGRATION OF HIIT INTO THE WEEKLY TRAINING CYCLE

Beyond performing only HIIT (generally run around 18-22 km/h in soccer), sprinting maximally (17), or at least reaching velocities close to maximal velocity (28), is also required to cover the full HSR velocity range. In fact, while many fear that the implementation of maximal sprinting during team practice may lead to acute muscular strain, the reality is that sprinting itself is likely more the solution than the problem (17). In fact, typical strength work is unlikely to be intense enough to replicate sprint demands (29) (i.e., <75% of the electromyography activity reached during sprinting). This suggests that sprint-specific neuromuscular demands are unique and cannot be replaced by any other (isolated) muscular actions (17). While the management of HSR may essentially protect the integrity of the hamstrings, the importance of mechanical work (MW, accelerations, decelerations, and changes of direction), programming, and supplementation should not be overlooked with respect to other important muscle groups (i.e., quads, glutes, and adductors). Of course, all this is easier said than done, with the actual programming of such specific locomotor loads requiring particular attention in relation to typical team-sport training contents, match demands, and timing. The following are guidelines that coaches and sport scientists can use to appropriately program HSR and MW sequences in relation to technical training contents and match schedules (i.e., different weekly microcycles).

Within-Session Puzzle

The first aspect to consider when selecting HIIT types (i.e., physiological targets) and formats (i.e., actual sequences) (see figure 4.2 on page 45) is the neuromuscular demands of the tactical and technical sequences programmed within the same day or session (see figure 4.9). When a tactical session already involves large volumes of HSR, the best option to avoid overload of the posterior chain, and especially hamstrings, is probably to program either a run-based type 1 HIIT (with low overall neuromuscular load) or a SSG with high MW demand (in this case, a complementary load that loads the glutes, adductors, and quads). In contrast, when the goal is to overload the posterior

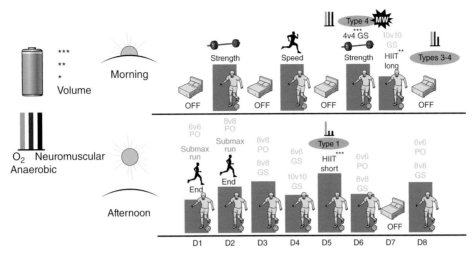

FIGURE 4.7   Example of preseason programming in an elite team (typically 1- to 2-week duration, but there is likely a friendly match during the second week that may replace the HIIT sequence with long intervals). The physical orientation of some of the sessions is given. Those with no indication have only technical and tactical objectives. Red: HIIT; orange: submaximal-intensity exercises. The blue bars refer to all technical and tactical training content in forms other than SSG. Run-based HIITs are always performed at the end of the session.

MW: mechanical work (>2m/s² accelerations, decelerations, and changes of direction); GS = game simulation; PO = possession.

Adapted by permission from P.B. Laursen and M.J.S. Buchheit (2018, pg. 560).

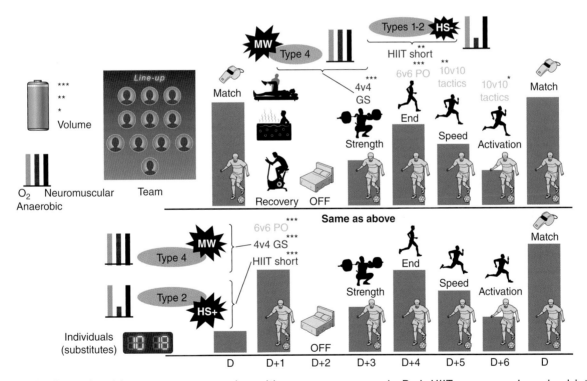

FIGURE 4.8   Example of in-season programming with one game per week. Red: HIIT; orange: submaximal intensity exercises. The blue bars refer to all technical and tactical training content in forms other than SSG. Run-based HIITs are always performed at the end of the session.

HS: high-speed running >19.8 km/h; MW: mechanical work (>2m/s² accelerations, decelerations, and changes of direction); GS = game simulation; PO = possession.

Adapted by permission from P.B. Laursen and M.J.S. Buchheit (2018, pg. 561).

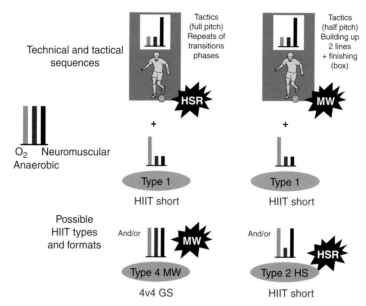

FIGURE 4.9 Typical framework for selecting the neuromuscular targets of a HIIT sequence in relation to the demands of the soccer-specific sequences of the same day or session. If the soccer-specific sequences already include HSR, HIIT may be more oriented toward (a) low or no additional neuromuscular load (type 1) or (b) MW (type 4) avoiding overload on the same muscle groups. In contrast, if the soccer-specific content already targets MW, HIIT could include (a) little or no MW (type 1) or HSR (type 2). HIIT types refer to the physiological objectives of the sequences, as shown in figure 4.2 (26).

Adapted by permission from P.B. Laursen and M.J.S. Buchheit (2018, pg. 559).

chain (as in preparing for the worst-case scenario of match locomotor demands [13]), a type 2 HIIT sequence targeting HSR could also be programmed (11). Finally, in the context of a technical/tactical session already involving a high MW load, using a supplementary HIIT sequence involving HSR is another good option to avoid overload, since it will likely overload different muscle groups than the technical and tactical sequence.

Between-Match Puzzle

This aspect, considering the training dynamics between consecutive matches during a season, requires a broader understanding of the entire program, and needs to take into consideration the previous match's locomotor load. Figure 4.10 shows the different training scenarios with various levels of HSR and MW loads, which all depend on both the amount of work performed during the preceding match (overall, related to minutes played, player profile and position [4]) and the number of days before the next match. Logically, the more minutes played in the preceding game, and the shorter the between-match microcycle, the less need for HSR and MW supplementation, and conversely. For starters who played a full game, there is likely no need for any supplementation when games are separated by less than 5 days. In

contrast, at the other end of the spectrum, substitute players having had more than five days to train before their next game should likely perform the full range of HIIT weapons (type 4, in the form of run-based HIIT and SSG targeting both HSR and MW), together with high speed efforts in the format of oppressive sprints to top up workloads to match equivalent volumes (see figure 4.11; 26).

CONCLUSION

In summary, the metabolic adaptations arising from diverse training content in high-performing team-sport players tend to be similar irrespective of the HIIT format or type experienced in most circumstances (10). Importantly, however, the neuromuscular response to various training contents, including match play, technical session, and strength work, as well as HIIT, has the most influential role with respect to the neuromuscular adaptation or interferences influencing injury risk. Thus, managing both HSR and MW, and their associated neuromuscular responses, is a key consideration needed to keep players fit and healthy throughout the season. The appropriate programming of these specific training sequences, targeting these two important locomotor loads, requires a thorough understanding

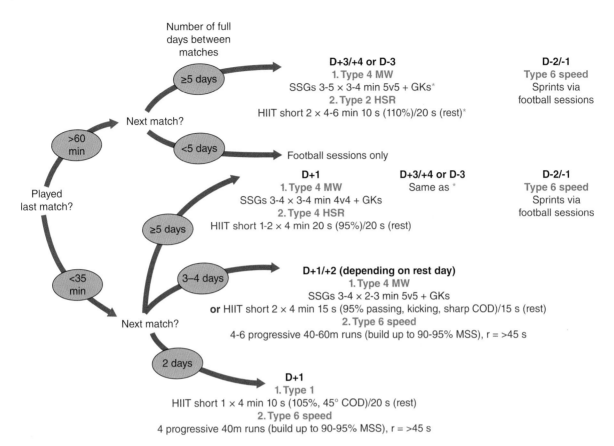

FIGURE 4.10 Decision process when it comes to programming locomotor loads, for example, high-intensity intermittent training (HIIT) including high-speed running (HSR) or mechanical work (MW) (or both) and sprint work, with respect to competition participation and match microcycle. Note that only those specific sequences are shown, with most sessions also including technical and tactical components and likely possession games. The different HIIT types are those presented in figure 4.2. Note that for all HIIT types involving a high neuromuscular strain, possible variations exist, that is, those more oriented toward HSR (likely associated with a greater strain on hamstring muscles) or MW (likely associated with a greater strain on quadriceps, adductors, and gluteus muscles). Type 1 can be achieved, for example, using 45° change of direction (COD), which is likely the best option to reduce overall neuromuscular load (decreased absolute running velocity without the need to apply large forces to change direction, resulting in a neuromuscular strain that is lower than straight-line or COD-runs with sharper CODs [21]). The percentage provided for short HIIT refers to the percentage of V_{IFT} used for programming (1) (V_{IFT} is the speed reached at the end of the 30-15 Intermittent Fitness Test). Note that individual adjustments should be made in terms of HIIT volume programming with regard to player profile and position (4, 26, 18).

MW: mechanical work (>2m/s² accelerations, decelerations, and changes of direction); HS: high-speed running (>19.8 km/h); SSG: small-sided games; GK: goalkeepers.

Adapted by permission from P.B. Laursen and M.J.S. Buchheit (2018, pg. 563).

Fanchini M, Pons E, Impellizzeri F, Dupont G, Buchheit M, McCall A. Exercise-based strategies to prevent muscle injuries. *Muscle injury guide: prevention of and return to play* from muscle injuries. 2019; Chapter 1:34-41.

of both match and technical sequence loading, and needs to be adjusted in light of the number of days between matches. While the monitoring of HSR and MW during matches and training sessions using appropriate technology (i.e., tracking systems [12]) is important, the anticipation and understanding of the HSR and MW demands of the various HIIT types and formats available (see figures 4.1 and 4.2) are vital for selecting the most appropriate puzzle piece placement.

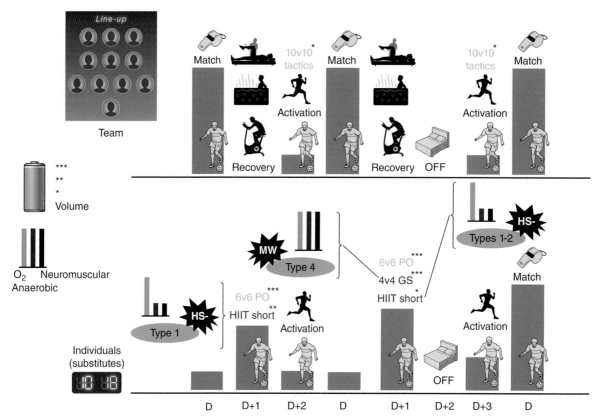

FIGURE 4.11   Example of in-season programming with two games per week. Red: HIIT; orange: submaximal intensity exercises. The blue bars refer to all technical and tactical training contents in forms other than SSG. Run-based HIITs are always performed at the end of the session. MW: mechanical work (>2m/s² accelerations, decelerations, and changes of direction).

Adapted by permission from P.B. Laursen and M.J.S. Buchheit (2018, pg. 562).

RECOMMENDED READINGS

Buchheit, M. Programming high-speed running and mechanical work in relation to technical contents and match schedule in professional soccer. *Sport Perform Sci Rep* 69:v1, 2019.

Buchheit, M, and Laursen, PB. High-intensity interval training, solutions to the programming puzzle: part I: cardiopulmonary emphasis. *Sports Med* 43:313-338. 2013.

Buchheit M, and Laursen PB. High-intensity interval training, solutions to the programming puzzle. Part II: anaerobic energy, neuromuscular load and practical applications. *Sports Med* 43:927-954, 2013.

Joyce, D, and Lewindon, D, eds. *High-Performance Training for Sports.* 2nd ed. Champaign, IL: Human Kinetics, 2022.

Laursen PB, and Buchheit, M. *Science and Application of High-Intensity Interval Training: Solutions to the Programming Puzzle.* Champaign, IL: Human Kinetics, 2018.

PART II

Needs Analysis

CHAPTER 5

Key Performance Indicators

Marco Cardinale, PhD

Sport has become an industry in which large investments and resources are deployed to win championships and earn medals at major sporting events or professional leagues and tournaments. Professional sporting organizations are therefore run and operated as businesses that require continuous review and assessment of processes and procedures put in place to reach success. Furthermore, each athlete is considered an asset that requires support, development, and care to ensure the best return on investment (ROI).

For these reasons, sport scientists should have a deep knowledge and understanding of the demands of the sport, the intricacies of rules and regulations, the specifics of the equipment, and the details of competition schedules in order to develop the best possible program. Moreover, once the overall demands are well defined, it becomes fundamental to be able to assess each athlete's characteristics and determine strengths and areas of improvement in order to develop individualized training plans, as well as ascertain their standing within the team or group context and among peers.

ANALYSIS OF THE SPORT

The concept of a **key performance indicator** (KPI) comes from the business world and is defined as a quantifiable measure used to evaluate the success of an organization or employee in meeting a performance objective (PO). In the sport setting, a PO may be winning a league, tournament, or other championship, achieving a specific time, distance, or mass lifted in centimeter-gram-second (CGS) sports, or beating the opposition in tactical events. Therefore, before determining KPIs it is fundamental to understand the expected PO of the team or athlete involved and whether it is realistic or not.

In CGS sports, it is possible to access historical databases of events and performances at various levels. International federations keep detailed databases of competitions and rankings that can be used to determine a PO or check yearly trends and find out what it may take to win a medal at a major competition. A number of authors have also analyzed the trends of results in specific events at the Olympic Games and have presented performance trends that may also be useful for determining POs (see table 5.1). World trends in various sports have been analyzed by Berthelot and colleagues (5, 6), who also provided some prediction and results trends in certain events. An attempt to analyze the evolution of swimming results has also been conducted (34), providing understanding of world-class performance standards. Finally, in some sports (e.g., triathlon, swimming, running events) there are now examples of performance analyses that may help with predicting POs at various levels (3, 37, 44, 50). In such sports, it is advisable to start the analysis from the result that is required before performing a detailed analysis of the demands and devising the appropriate training plan. In fact, it is fundamental to know exactly what level of performance the athlete needs to achieve before working out the **determinants of performance**. A clear definition of the PO is the first step in determining the realistic chances with respect to what the athlete can and should achieve and the potential rewards (e.g., medals at regional, national, and international competitions).

The information available in CGS sports can also be used to govern a performance pathway for athletes to track their progress and to benchmark what their performance might produce in terms of rewards (i.e., medal color, finishing position). Indeed, some federations have employed athletes' results tracking to determine their selection criteria and establish

TABLE 5.1 **Examples of Results Databases That Can Be Used to Develop and Track Performance Objectives for an Athlete**

Database	Web link	Notes
International Amateur Athletics Federation (IAAF)	www.iaaf.org/results	Results from official competitions from pre-1997
International Weightlifting Federation	www.iwf.net/new_bw/results_by_events	Official results database
Union Cycliste Internationale	www.uci.org/track/rankings	Official results database and rankings
World Rowing	www.worldrowing.com/events/statistics www.worldrowing.com/events/results	World Rowing statistics and results databases
World Athletics statistics and rankings	www.bluecattechnical.uk/iaaf	Free app to analyze official world athletics results
	www.worldathletics.org/stats-zone	Athletics statistical repository
Weightlifting database	iwrp.net/global-statistics	Weightlifting database data
Olympic sports and professional and collegiate sports databases	www.olympic.org/olympic-results	Official database of Olympic results
	www.sports-reference.com	Data about professional and collegiate sports
Swimming rankings and results	www.swimrankings.net/index.php?page=home www.fina.org/results	Swimming rankings and results databases

ratings and chances of medaling at major competitions (e.g., see British Triathlon selection criteria (10) and United Kingdom athletics performance funnels [48]). Work from the author's group (7, 8) and others (47) in athletics has started to show the typical development curves of results in various events and can be used to track the development of each individual athlete against international standards in an effort to determine that athlete's chances on the international stage, as well as to possibly predict senior performances. This chapter presents options for assessing, reporting, and visualizing POs.

The approach to be taken in non-CGS sports (e.g., team sports, acrobatic and artistic sports, combat sports) must still begin with gathering information on performance outcomes required to excel at a given level. In gymnastics, for example, the code of points determines how athletes are scored (16); therefore knowledge of difficulty values and elements is fundamental in order to determine what the athlete is capable of, what the focus of training should be, and how many points the athlete can realistically achieve. A similar system is in place for figure skating disciplines, in which points are scored according to program component scores and medals are awarded to the highest-scoring athlete or pair (depending on the event) (36).

In team sports, POs for individual players can be identified according to various aspects such as playing position or the athlete's role on the team (technical, tactical, social responsibilities). Thanks to extensive data now available, in many sports it is possible to identify specific performance outcomes for top performers. For example, in sports in which goals are scored and goalkeepers are part of a team, typical save rates are analyzed and reported (e.g., team handball, field hockey, water polo, soccer). In volleyball, passing accuracy and attack efficiency, as well as reception attempts and errors, are recorded. In basketball, many data are publicly available on shooting percentages, passing rates, distance covered, and movement characteristics (33). Major League Baseball provides detailed statistics on many aspects of the game (31), as does the National Hockey League (32). In the years to come, it is expected that all sports will have publicly accessible databases and statistics indicating what the athletes do and how well they do it; therefore it should be easier to define a performance profile at various levels of competition delineating what the athlete needs to be capable of in order to succeed. Team data are less relevant in this context, since the information gathered by the sport scientist should be used within the scope of developing an individualized training program aimed at improving athletes' abilities and maximizing their performance. However, for improving team performance, it is fundamental to have access to detailed data on how the team performs against different opponents and in special situations. Such information is fundamental for individual and team goal-setting purposes (not only in terms of the necessary physical abilities but also specific elements of technical and tactical aspects), and also for defining how the sport science support team can provide interventions to improve performance.

SPORT DEMANDS

Once POs are clear and can be defined, the next step is to gather information about the demands of the sport and how they affect performance. By understanding the demands of a sport, sport scientists can better devise the best training plans and identify specific performance strategies. Physiological, psychological, technical, and tactical demands of the sport should be well defined and clear to the coaching and support staff. This information is fundamental to establish the general direction of the training program and any sport science intervention aimed at improving performance (e.g., nutritional interventions, movement optimization, warm-up strategies, clothing, and technology strategies), as well as to highlight areas that may require further investigation or additional assessment (or both). A systematic approach should be taken to define the major determinants of performance and understand the specific training requirements needed to prepare the athlete (see table 5.2). This information may reside in the peer-reviewed scientific literature, especially for popular international sports. However, it may be challenging to find this information for lesser-known sports, new sports, or sports in which significant rule changes have occurred (e.g., the introduction of the libero in volleyball, the rule change of starting the game from the center in handball). Also, data presented in the scientific literature should be considered within the context of the experimental constraints and participant characteristics. In fact, the scientific literature is full of observations and experimental work conducted on lower-level athletes. Since elite athletes represent a small percentage of the population and usually present extreme physiological phenotypes and display exceptional skills and abilities, one should take care when extending research findings to these athletes. The best approach should always be to directly quantify how the individual athlete copes with training and competitions in order to determine the best course of action.

Coaching manuals are also a good resource; however, the practitioner should always consider accessing primary sources in peer-reviewed journals when possible to find the most valid, reliable, and up-to-date information on each sport.

When information is lacking, incomplete, or simply irrelevant, it is important to use expertise to measure the performance demands and understand the physical requirements necessary to excel in a sporting event. Without this information, it is largely impossible to create a suitable training plan, because the objectives pursued may not be the actual objectives and could therefore actually reduce the chances of the athlete's success. This is a good approach to adopt even when scientific information is available, since the end goal of each sport science intervention should be evidence-based, appropriate for what the athletes are trying to achieve, and based on factual information. The sporting world is full of anecdotal information and "evidence" that is perpetuated in coaching and athletic communities without proof, sometimes leading to inappropriate training paradigms that stifle performance development. Furthermore, since each sport has its own subculture and fixed mindsets, it becomes extremely challenging to innovate and move forward. Evidence gathering and relevant data collection and analysis might help in changing fixed mindsets and approaches when a modus operandi is well established and strong preconceived notions exist. Usually such data can produce paradigm shifts in a sport and contribute to a change in attitudes and the procedures used to prepare athletes for competition.

DETERMINANTS OF SUCCESSFUL SPORT PERFORMANCE

Sport performance is complex, and for this reason it is important to develop a holistic approach to determine what can positively affect a performance outcome in a given sport. One of the initial attempts to define the **determinants of performance** was made by Hay and Reid (20), with a simple scheme in which a sporting result was underpinned by factors affecting the result. Following their work, several sporting events and activities have been analyzed and deterministic models developed to help guide coaches and sport science practitioners in defining appropriate training interventions (2, 13, 46). The outcomes from deterministic models are precisely established through known relationships among variables, without any room for random variation. In such models (mostly

TABLE 5.2 Summary of Relevant Information Required to Analyze a Sport

Information sought	Importance	Source
Physiological demands (e.g., heart rate, oxygen uptake during competition, metabolic pathways involved, distance covered, accelerations, decelerations)	This information is required in order to devise appropriate training strategies aimed at improving key physiological variables determining sporting success. This information also informs nutritional strategies in training and competition.	• Scientific literature • Coaching manuals • Coaches' knowledge and experience
Technical requirements (specific movements performed, frequency, successful technical executions, etc.)	The information is helpful to assess technical abilities specific to the sport as well as develop resistance training plans able to enhance the speed and quality of execution of technical skills.	• Scientific literature • Coaching manuals • Coaches' knowledge and experience
Tactical requirements (e.g., pacing strategies, collaboration with teammates, how to cause errors in opponents)	This information provides details on what the athlete needs to be able to produce in competition to succeed, what cues the athlete needs to develop, and what extremes of movement skills might be required to be able to perform technical movements within tactical requirements.	• Coaching manuals • Coaches' knowledge and experience
Psychological skills (e.g., anticipation, visual skills, anxiety or arousal, reaction time)	This information might inform specific assessments required to ascertain the athlete's level as well as devise interventions aimed at maximizing performance.	• Scientific literature • Coaching manuals • Coaches' knowledge and experience
Equipment characteristics (e.g., sleds, shoes, wearables, implements)	A detailed knowledge of the equipment used for training and competition is fundamental to advising the athlete on what is appropriate and advantageous. Also, knowledge of equipment might help develop individual solutions or adapt and identify the most appropriate equipment for the athlete (or both).	• Coaching manuals • Coaches' knowledge and experience • Rulebook
Health aspects (e.g., injury risks, environmental challenges)	Knowledge of injury risks in a sport is required to design preventive strategies and target training plans to prepare the athlete to perform while reducing injury risk. Also, environmental, equipment, and rules challenges potentially affecting health should be well known by each sport scientist to develop appropriate strategies.	• Epidemiological studies • Coaches' knowledge and experience • Athlete's own medical history • Medical practitioners
Rules and regulations	The knowledge of rules and regulations, qualifying standards for major events, selection criteria, and reasons for disqualification should be well known by each practitioner involved in the sport, because this information can often determine winning and losing as well as the appropriateness, relevance, and possibilities for specific interventions in competition.	• Official rulebooks (making sure to read the most up-to-date version)

derived from biomechanical studies), the relationship between a movement outcome and its biomechanical determinants is analyzed and defined. Such an approach has merit as a pedagogical and structured way to describe and define what determines performance in a specific activity. However, researchers have criticized deterministic models for being too rigid in sporting environments (18) and have instead suggested dynamical systems theory as a viable framework for modeling athletic performance.

While complex approaches are developed to define and determine performance, sport scientists should work with the coaching staff to define the performance model of the given sport using a simple and consistent framework that directs specific interventions, develops KPIs, and tracks progress and activities using a common language. For that to happen, deterministic models can be considered a useful frame of reference. To be effective, this framework should be defined with input from the coaching staff in order to reflect the way they work, and then used as a guide for defining all training and competition interventions and drive routine assessment of KPIs to make sure everyone is on track to develop the aspects affecting the POs.

Engaging the coaching staff in the modeling process helps clarify terminology, discuss evidence, capture coaching philosophies, and reach a common understanding of what performance consists of for the group of athletes involved. Without coaching staff engagement, there is a risk that such an approach will become a framework that is not ultimately used to influence performance. Also, once the determinants of performance are defined and are clear to the coaching staff, they should be communicated to the athletes, so that everyone can be aligned with clear POs underpinned by a visible performance plan.

As discussed previously, this process can start only when a clear, realistically achievable PO has been defined. The PO is the driver of the plan and the ultimate goal. After that, using a reference table (see table 5.2), it is possible to start detailing the knowledge about the sport and discuss how each aspect is coached and how it is assessed. This information is key to developing clear, measurable, and achievable KPIs.

In the example provided in figure 5.2, the 800-meter run has been used as the target sport, with a hierarchical model used to define parameters. The hierarchical model is used to identify respective performance determinants and specify the details of each determinant. In this example, two areas have been highlighted: the physiological determinants and the health aspects. What is known from the literature is that elite performers in middle-distance running should possess very good aerobic capacity due to the

energy contribution of the aerobic pathways (9, 25). Work on elite performers has also highlighted the importance of speed, anaerobic capacity, and anaerobic speed reserve as other performance determinants (40, 41, 42). Health aspects affecting middle-distance runners include well-known injury risks linked to training load or biomechanical aspects of running gait or both (4, 14, 29), as well as upper respiratory tract health (12, 21, 35). An extensive literature search and fact finding regarding these aspects should be performed and summarized schematically to discuss with the coaching and support staff. The aim is to determine how best to address these aspects, and most of all to agree on how frequently to conduct assessments and check progress.

Once all aspects are defined and described, it is possible to start documenting the training interventions necessary to improve each of the determinants and to start building a coaching library that addresses the tools used to improve performance for a particular athlete. The KPIs can now be described (see the workflow in figure 5.1 and an example of detailed KPIs in figure 5.2), and assessment protocols can be put in place to benchmark the athlete, identify strengths and weaknesses, and assess the athlete's progress over the course of the sporting season.

It is important to state that this process is dynamic; with new knowledge, evolution of coaching plans, or changes in athletes' performance, things will change and new determinants might be added, intervention priorities changed, or innovative approaches generated. The primary scope of this process should be to define performance and identify its determinants, and to make this visible and accessible to the whole

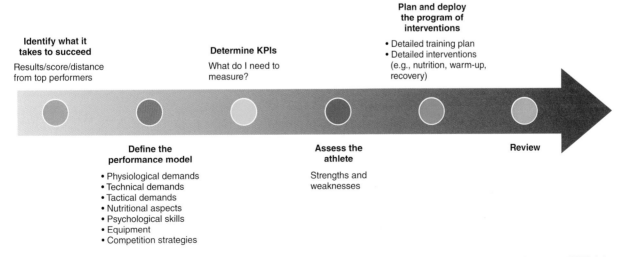

FIGURE 5.1   Schematic diagram describing the process to define and use key performance indicators (KPIs) in a sporting setting.

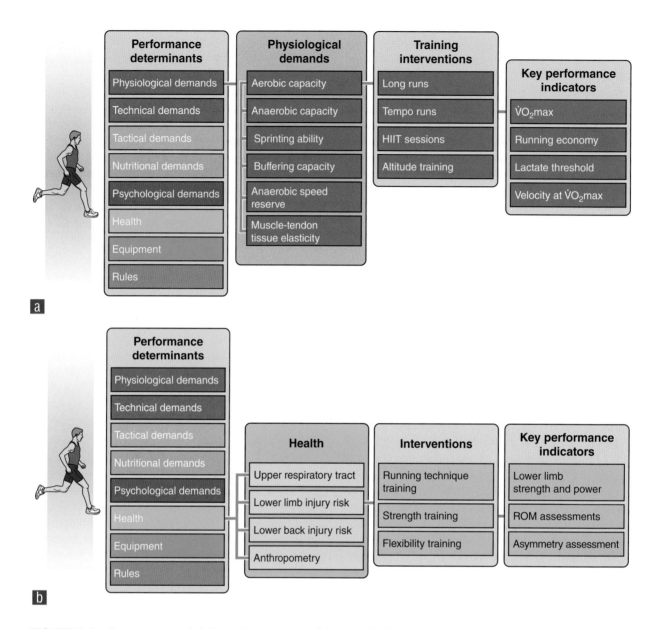

FIGURE 5.2 Sample deterministic performance model for an 800-meter runner leading to the definition of key performance indicators to assess progress. The sample determinants used are *(a)* physiological demands and *(b)* health. This is a simple example of how to establish a working framework, not an exhaustive or detailed presentation of determinants.

staff working with the athletes, as well as the athlete themselves. This will ensure that all support plans for athletes are aligned to a PO and are part of an agreed-upon action plan.

ORGANIZATIONAL AND GOVERNANCE ASPECTS

As previously discussed, sport scientists should be familiar with the technical terminology used by the coaching staff and athletes, the rules and regulations, equipment details and characteristics, and the typical routines in training and competition. This knowledge is fundamental in order to operate at any level, and it is something that cannot be learned simply by taking a university course but is the result of experiential exposure. Every sport has its own subculture, jargon, and terminology, and understanding the intricacies and standards of operation help in formulating the best course of action. Terminology, the lexicon, and jargon are of particular importance, since many sport-specific terms are used to define particular movements or activities. Also, in many coaching courses, scientific terminology is sometimes inappropriately used or modified, and this may cause dissonance with the true scientific meaning. It is therefore of utmost importance to become familiar with the working context of many areas—from rules and regulations, typical routines, and ways of operating, to the terminology used.

Clubs and sporting organizations tend to operate with routine processes and procedures, as well as defined beliefs and philosophies. Therefore, it is crucial to understand the heritage of an organization, its expectations, and its evolution, as well as its vision and mission—what it is seeking to achieve and how. It is important to recognize that every group of athletes and each organization has a way of operating and a belief system and philosophy that have evolved over the years, and that this is the result of its own subculture within the sport. Knowledge and understanding of this belief system provide the sport scientist with relevant cues to work within the group culture and help everyone contribute to its evolution.

Effective support requires consideration of several aspects. The level of the athletes, their expectations and commitment, their history in the sport, and their current environment are all important elements to be taken into consideration. Only a full understanding of such aspects can guide the practitioner to devise a set of interventions and assess progress against accepted and realistic KPIs and POs. The human element should not be discarded, and sole reliance on testing and data-gathering activities might yield insufficient information for the sport scientist to operate effectively. A deep understanding of each athlete's history, values, previous achievements, experiences, and ambitions, as well as beliefs, sociocultural norms, and behaviors, can provide better details to effectively implement interventions and develop a culture of responsibility. This would include using KPIs as a way to track progress and identify areas for further improvement. It is advisable to work directly with athletes and build a trusting relationship, as well as with the coaching staff and support staff, since these personnel may have particular insights regarding specific aspects.

National identity and sociocultural norms are an important aspect of operating in the sporting environment today. Working abroad or with multicultural teams is not uncommon, and understanding the national context and the sociocultural norms helps in developing effective working practices, as well as in identifying interventions that may be difficult to accept or implement due to local social norms.

Finally, while developing KPIs for the athletes and coaching staff, sport scientists should be aware of how such information is communicated to the stakeholders in the organization, how it is protected and made secure, and how it may be communicated externally. When policies are not in place, they should be developed to make clear how the information generated by the assessment of various KPIs affects day-to-day activities, and also how it is protected and shared to avoid litigation or inappropriate use of performance data or both. This context is evolving, and it is likely that specific guidelines will be established in the future. In United States health care settings and in biomedical research, biometric data are governed by regulations on informed consent, the Health Insurance Portability and Accountability Act (HIPAA), and other data privacy assurances. Elsewhere in the world, specific regulations exist for medical records and informed consent. However, biometric data collected in professional sport and consumer sectors remain largely unregulated and unexamined. Furthermore, the sport scientist should be aware that the collection and storage of biometric data by employers and third parties raises risks of exploitation, as well as employee discrimination when these data are used in the contract renewal context or termination decision making. With the evolution of professional sport, these issues have become more important, and the sport scientist should be familiar with the local regulations and organization policies (26, 43).

KEY PERFORMANCE INDICATORS IN SPORT

Key performance indicators should always be measurable, objective, and actionable. They should be useful for influencing performance planning relating to sport performance.

In summary, a suitable KPI should

- provide objective evidence as a valid and reliable measure,
- inform better decision making,
- offer a gauge to assess performance changes over time,
- provide information to benchmark one person's performance versus that of others, and
- inform attainability of POs.

Since all sports are different, KPIs should be specific to the sport, to the group of athletes, or the level of resources available to determine them. There is a tendency to use KPIs mostly to define physical fitness levels of athletes, possibly because technology makes it easier to assess fitness qualities such as strength, power, and speed in sport-specific movements. However, the sport scientist should work with the coaching and support staff to develop and determine KPIs specific to the group of athletes involved and to make sure that relevant measures are used for any decision-making process.

Skill-Based KPIs

Skill-based KPIs are relatively easy to determine in acrobatic and aesthetic sports (e.g., gymnastics, figure skating, synchronized swimming) in that a clear points system exists according to how specific skills are executed. In these sports, the sport scientist should be familiar with the details of how high scores are obtained and help develop the assessment framework to appraise these skills routinely in training and provide the athlete and the coach with a measure of progress. This type of analysis relies mostly on a combination of qualitative and quantitative measurements. The qualitative assessments should be carried out by technical experts (e.g., coaches and judges) and, ideally, in combination with video analysis. Quantitative assessments should rely more on wearable technology, motion capture systems, video analysis (with appropriate procedures typical of biomechanical assessments), and specialized equipment (e.g., force platforms, electromyography).

The key for each type of skill assessment is to provide useful information that can affect subsequent coaching interventions. For this to happen, the main criteria are data collection procedures that minimize disruption to training and competition, ease of access to information, rapid reporting, and, most of all, valid and reliable assessments that can be used to determine the degree of progression.

Acrobatic sports require very precise assessment of the skills required to succeed and are therefore better suited to the use of advanced **biomechanical techniques** with specific instrumentation in order to increase accuracy and possibly develop modeling approaches that predict the outcome of technique changes. In particular, since elite performers seem to demonstrate less variability of technique in key aspects (22), it is important to have measurement systems that are sensitive to small changes; therefore the use of 2D or 3D video analysis and a combination of wearable sensors are often the preferred route.

Key performance indicators for skill-based analysis should be clearly defined according to a reference framework, and then assessed against it. The terms of reference should be the optimal execution of the skill according to the point system of the sport, as well as past performances of top performers for benchmarking. For this activity, a model template should be drawn that identifies the high-scoring form for each phase of movement; the next step is to perform a comparative analysis on the athlete using video analysis or a combination of wearable technology. In such assessments, joint angles in key positions, relationships between different joint angles, segmental velocities, and other biomechanical parameters tend to be the KPIs of interest; therefore, particular care should be taken to collect data correctly using appropriate techniques and procedures to make sure the data can actually be used to assess the athlete. Indeed, even in today's sporting landscape, video is often poorly collected, with no reference frame and incorrect camera angles, and resolutions that lead to errors in measurement and incorrect interpretations or assumptions made.

In sports in which skills are not the outcome but are part of the athlete's toolbox, things become more complicated. Therefore the analysis of complex sport skills is usually conducted to improve technical and tactical outcomes (e.g., assessing the takeoff and running of a long jumper, the kicking technique of a Taekwondo athlete, or throwing techniques in a quarterback), to reduce injury risk (e.g., landing strategies, analysis of side-stepping techniques), or to assess the effectiveness of equipment (e.g., shoes, skis). Such approaches involve assessing a movement sequence relevant to the specific sporting context, and therefore care should be taken in developing the correct assessment procedure, the definition of what constitutes a KPI that can be tracked effectively, and, most of all, how the KPI can be used to produce effective interventions. While technology is helping to move the measurement gold standard from the laboratory to the field, inherent variability occurs when sporting movements are assessed within the live sporting context. Consequently, while some level of validity and reliability can be obtained in some sports (e.g., athletics events, weightlifting) and appropriate KPIs can be developed and tracked (e.g., running speed, takeoff angle, speed of the barbell), more challenges arise when open skills need to be assessed in chaotic sports. For example, a large body of evidence has been produced to understand cutting and change-of-direction maneuvers, which are common skills in team sports and invasion games. Most of the work has been conducted via simulating game conditions in the laboratory (19, 45, 52), and clear guidelines and reference data are available. However, only rarely has the use of opponents been introduced in this type of assessment (30). Unsurprisingly, these data show increased lower limb movements and forces, demonstrating clearly that simulations in a laboratory setting may not reflect what happens in the context of the actual sporting event. The most important aspects to consider when defining KPIs are always related to the validity and reliability of the measurement. Without a valid and reliable measure, such efforts should be discarded. All sports require the application of cognitive, perceptual, and motor skills to varying degrees, and the current consensus seems to be that aside from aesthetic sports or sports with closed skills, challenges lie in defining usable skill-based KPIs in team sports (1).

Finally, consideration should be given to the use of technical models that are particularly popular in many sports, including track and field athletics. While the best techniques have been analyzed and reported for years (and, apart from the technique change in the high jump introduced by Dick Fosbury, have not changed much), these should be used only as a general guideline to drive the training process and qualitatively assess the athlete. Researchers have discussed the possibility of identifying optimal techniques as a reference for athletes (17), further strengthening the view that individual assessments should be implemented that recognize the large role that movement variability, stress of competition, environmental conditions, and other factors play when athletes perform skills and techniques in competition.

The purpose of assessing KPIs in technical and skill-based sports is to identify areas that improve performance, reduce errors, minimize the risks of injury, and optimize the technical execution of a skill. This is represented in figure 5.3.

Skill assessment should be conducted using a **holistic approach** in which both the perceptual-cognitive aspects and technical motor skills are routinely evaluated, given the reciprocal nature of the relationship between perception and action and the need to intervene to improve both aspects in the practical sporting setting. Most of the scientific literature has so far focused on assessing the skills progression by measuring the outcome of the skill performed rather than the contributing factors. This is possibly due to the limited technology and methods available to conduct such assessments outside of biomechanics laboratories. Some attempts have been made in assessing generic motor skills, with mixed success. However, work describing the Canadian Agility and Movement Skill Assessment has suggested that this approach is valid and reliable (28) if appropriately trained individuals conduct the assessments following the protocol details.

Researchers (15) also suggest the need to assess skills within a periodization framework similar to the assessment of other training and performance-specific KPIs. However, while theoretically sound, the real applicability of this approach is currently limited and the time requirements to conduct a thorough skill assessment are among the main reasons coaches do not spend much time conducting regular quantitative skill assessments. Some examples of well-defined sport skills are published in the literature, with relatively simple data-gathering procedures (e.g., tennis serve [27], table tennis [24], fencing [51]). The equipment of choice still remains the use of video analysis, and thanks to the lower costs of high-speed cameras and

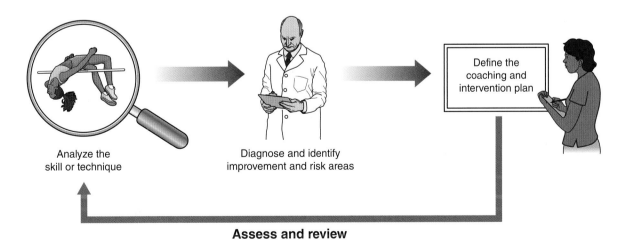

Analyze the
skill or technique

Diagnose and identify
improvement and risk areas

Define the
coaching and
intervention plan

Assess and review

FIGURE 5.3   Schematic diagram of the workflow to assess and review technical key performance indicators (KPIs).

access to some advanced applications, it is now possible to conduct detailed analysis of sport skills even with relatively low-cost solutions. Miniature wearable sensors are now permeating the market and in the near future may improve the ability to routinely assess sport skills using body sensor networks with immediate feedback—which may ultimately increase chances to infer meaningful approaches to improve performance. However, while some sports have plenty of examples of well-conducted studies (albeit mostly performed in noncompetitive situations in laboratories) to use as a reference, many sports, including "new" sports, have limited information. Therefore, it is the goal of each practitioner involved to develop an assessment framework that can provide the coaching staff with meaningful information to then correct and enhance skill execution during competitions.

Tactical-Based KPIs

Success in many sports is determined not only by an individual's tactical abilities, but also by the collective contribution to team tactics and strategy. In fact, in team sports and invasion games, winning is determined by the interaction of individual players, and how they respond to the activities of the opposition as well as how their tactics produce successful outcomes (e.g., scoring more goals, points). Historically, KPIs for tactical elements have been characterized by notational analysis and simple scouting techniques to assess effectiveness of specific sporting actions. Some sports have a long history of KPI collection and analysis, thanks to the ease of data collection and analyses during games. In basketball, for example, simple metrics like shots taken and scored, passes completed, blocks, and fouls have been used extensively. However, such metrics relate only to individual outcomes and do not take into account the collective tactical aspects. Thanks to advancements in things like video analysis and computing abilities, it is now possible to analyze collective tactical behavior in real time and mine successful outcomes to determine how each individual contributes to a collective outcome.

Since the introduction of multiple camera systems in stadiums (49), there has been a proliferation of studies and accessible data about the movement patterns and details of different roles within a team, as well as comparisons among teams, for a variety of sports. Notational analysis has moved to a more comprehensive approach to performance analysis whereby the notation of typical activities is accompanied by the determination of game outcomes and relationships between players to establish outcomes. In team sports and invasion games this is now an important aspect to be considered, since it may be used to identify strengths and weaknesses, as well as how changing players, positions, or tactical disposition may determine outcomes. Also, analysis may be used to identify weaknesses of the opposition and to determine better tactical approaches for beating them.

When one is determining KPIs for team sports, various frameworks can be put in place, specific to the sport being analyzed. Therefore it is virtually impossible to discuss all potential options in this chapter. However, as a general guide, it is possible to suggest the following areas of analysis to determine specific KPIs: tactical and strategy (e.g., patterns of play, formations, distance between players, formation efficiency), skills and technical (e.g., passing efficiency, shooting and scoring efficiency, interceptions), and technical-defensive or technical attacking to reflect particular phases of the game or sport. Good examples exist in the literature in some sports, such as the work on football by Hughes and colleagues (23), and can be used as a starting point. It is worth mentioning that in order to effectively assess and use the data for KPIs, it is absolutely fundamental to have well-organized and easily accessible databases in order to conduct appropriate analysis and build large enough datasets to be able to use advanced analytical techniques or artificial intelligence and data mining approaches to identify factors that really influence performance. After the publication of the popular book *Moneyball* by Michael Lewis and the subsequent movie, there was increased interest in "big data" in sport, with a race to develop performance analysis departments in top sporting franchises. Also, in Olympic sports, many organizations employ sport intelligence expertise to analyze the opposition and help identify weaknesses of opponents to exploit in international competitions. The working principles of the determination of meaningful KPIs can follow the same process previously discussed for individual sports (e.g., figures 5.1 and 5.2), with the first and most important activity being the breaking down of the sport of concern into clearly identifiable components and assessing how the individual players contribute to the overall team outcomes. While the importance of universal KPIs has been explored, more will be accessible in the near future. It is fundamental for practitioners involved in team sports to be familiar with data gathering, analytical techniques, and ways in which this information can help teams prepare better for competitions.

The analysis of KPIs requires a combination of video and human analysis. Furthermore, access and approval from international sporting bodies to allow players to use wearable devices in official competitions and allow public access to some of these data will mean that sport scientists will soon be able to improve their understanding of why and how some teams beat others. Work from Sampaio's lab in different sports (38, 39) suggests novel analytical approaches. Also, specific services provided by analytics companies are offering more opportunities for sport practitioners to improve their chances to positively affect performance in their team-sport athletes.

Individuals in team sports should be compared to their peers when one is analyzing KPIs and should be benchmarked against opponents in order to gauge not only their individual development, but also a realistic level of performance expected. Various techniques can be used to normalize, for example, fitness-related KPIs in teams (e.g., the use of z-scores, percentiles, and the like). However, for this to happen, databases have to be developed and routinely maintained, making sure that reliable and valid assessments have been performed using repeatable, clearly defined standard operating procedures (see chapter 8).

Determining and tracking individual POs or KPIs has been suggested to be an effective avenue to identify and possibly predict talent development in some sports. Analysis of competition databases indicates that in most events in sports like track and field, it is possible to succeed at a senior level without early specialization. For example, analysis of competition results databases has shown that most athletes reaching the elite performance level as seniors were not elite performers as juniors. Furthermore, many athletes winning medals at junior events do not repeat that level of performance when they compete as adults. All in all, it seems feasible to suggest that performance tracking and assessment of progression are necessary to determine if the progress young athletes make can lead them to high-level performance as adults. Some nations have made use of performance funnels to describe and assess an athlete's progression. Also, the use of results databases might identify performance trends in different events and predict the likelihood and necessary minimum requirements of reaching medal potential in major events.

However, while performance data might help in determining how athletes develop from youth to senior competitors, more needs to be done to identify appropriate training methodologies and factors that may increase the chances of transforming potential

at a young age into success in adulthood. A few examples have been published (7, 8, 11) and suggest that practitioners develop performance tracking approaches using competition databases and qualifying and medal winning standards, and that they keep these up-to-date. Such approaches using a mixture of POs and KPIs can be very powerful for tracking and assessing progress, and potentially to predict the likelihood of success in specific events or disciplines (see figure 5.4).

Physiologically-Based KPIs

Physiological KPIs represent the physiological determinants needed in order to excel in a particular sport. As previously discussed, they should be identified when the sport is assessed through use of a detailed needs analysis and the performance model is clearly defined. The KPIs can be defined thanks to specific sport science literature searches, examples in coaching manuals, and data collected on the athletes themselves. While some sports have many resources and a great deal of available data on the physiological demands and relative ways to measure and determine the KPIs, most newly developed sports do not have these. It is critical for the practitioner to define the physiological demands of the sport or activity in question and, following a comprehensive assessment, determine the best protocols to assess the KPIs. It is important for the practitioner to identify two types of physiological KPIs:

1. Physiological KPIs periodically assessed to determine the progress of the athlete (e.g., aerobic capacity, lactate threshold)
2. Physiological KPIs used to monitor training and that are able to influence the training program on a daily or short-term basis (e.g., heart rate variability, blood lactate responses to specific workloads, heart rate responses to specific workloads, salivary biomarkers)

The example presented at the beginning of the chapter (see figures 5.1 and 5.2) represents a framework to determine the important KPIs that need periodic assessment and are used to determine if the training interventions used are producing positive effects in key areas that determine performance outcomes. While this is a necessary process to verify the effectiveness of the training process, it is important to put in place more frequent KPIs that can be used to make sure the athlete is on track, but also that the contents of

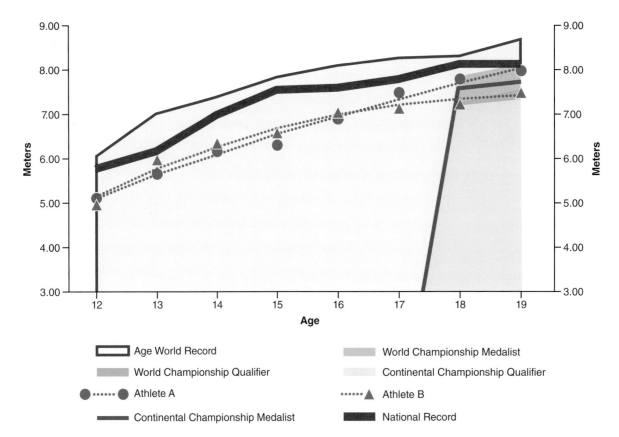

FIGURE 5.4 Example of a performance tracking graph of two athletes' progressions (long jump) from a young age according to typical progression curves, national records, world records, and qualifying standards.

the training activities are hitting the right targets and the athlete is coping well with the sequences.

For the purposes of monitoring training, the sport scientist can use KPIs to assess **internal load** (defined as the relative biological [both physiological and psychological] stressors imposed on the athlete during training or competition) and **external load** (objective measures of the work performed by athletes, their physiological responses during training or competition, or both) (see figure 5.5).

Internal and external load data can be collected to describe individual training sessions and help the coaching staff verify that physiological targets were attained (see figure 5.6). Alternatively, the data can be used to assess the accumulation of training load, as well as how the athlete responds to similar training sessions. This approach can be useful to develop a database of drills used by coaching staff and to characterize how athletes respond in order to improve individualized training programs or individual nutritional interventions.

With appropriate KPIs it is possible to develop some sessions that are repeated on a regular basis and then used as a way to assess the longitudinal development of an athlete within a season or multiple seasons. The role of the sport scientist is to work with the coaching staff to establish which KPIs are relevant, as well as which parameters can inform the coaching staff regarding how athletes are coping with training sessions or how the accumulation of workload is affecting their development. Consistent data collection with this approach can provide the staff with more evidence to develop better training activities. It also delivers more information for continuous debriefs useful to improve performance and to identify particular questions that can be answered with specific projects. A framework is provided in figure 5.7 with an example of how the process can look and how a training library may be presented following the analysis of specific KPIs in an athlete.

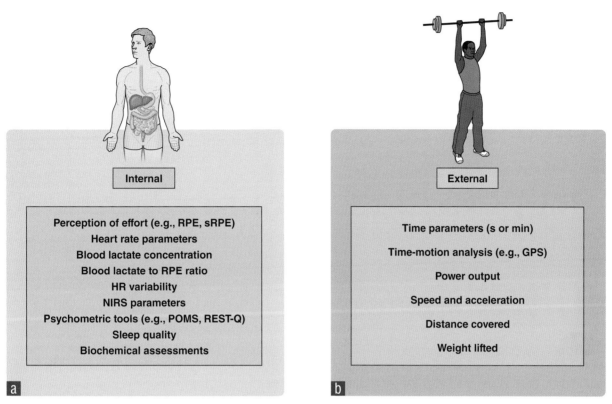

FIGURE 5.5 List of typical physiological key performance indicators (KPIs) used to assess *(a)* internal and *(b)* external training load.

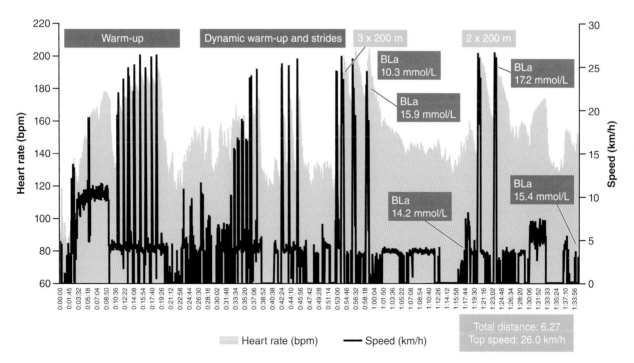

FIGURE 5.6 Example of a training session performed by a track and field athlete integrating physiological measurements of internal load (e.g., heart rate and blood lactate) with external load (speed and total distance with wearable technology).

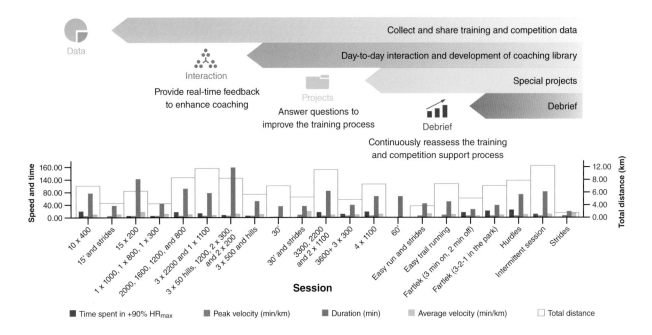

FIGURE 5.7 Key performance indicator (KPI) framework for the use of data in a sport setting with the particular aim to improve performance. This example is of an athlete's training library with specific KPIs collected over time to determine the physiological implications of different sessions.

Psychologically-Based KPIs

Psychological or mental performance KPIs can be generic (e.g., relevant to the overall well-being status of the athlete) or specific to the sporting discipline of interest (e.g., Profile of Mood States versus visual attention control in archery athletes). The collection and analysis of such information do require specific expertise, and it is important for the practitioners involved in this aspect not only to use the information to enhance performance (e.g., self-confidence, self-control, concentration), but also to identify potential pitfalls (e.g., overtraining, depression, lack of confidence), which may require more comprehensive psychological interventions to be carried out by licensed practitioners. Most KPIs can be quantified using well-known validated and reliable psychometric tools.

It is important to state that the version and format of any psychometric tools used should be validated in the scientific literature and that alterations of the questions, sequence, or anchors effectively invalidate their use. Also, the practitioner should not translate a psychometric tool in other languages but use validated translations to make sure that the data collected are of high enough quality to allow valid inferences.

RULES, CHARACTERISTICS, AND OTHER SPORTING CONSTRAINTS

A deep knowledge of the rules and characteristics of a sport is of paramount importance for effective interventions. Deep knowledge of the sport is a prerequisite in order to communicate effectively with the coaching staff, learn the sport-specific terminology, and also understand fully how athletes and coaches prepare for competition. The best source is still the rulebook of the sport in its international federation or national governing body. Also required is a deep understanding of how competitions work, the constraints, the level of access to the athlete, and the times and places and how the practitioner can operate. The restrictions around the Olympic Games and other events operating under accreditation systems may not allow some activities to be carried out (e.g., use of specific technology to assess competitions). It is the responsibility of the sport scientist to be fully familiar with such restrictions and constraints before preparing specific plans so that services are provided effectively in situ in competitions.

Finally, since sporting rules may be changed and may evolve, it is important to be aware of how the changes might affect sporting performance. Examples of rule changes in team sports (e.g., the introduction of the libero in volleyball, the introduction of fast center after a goal in handball, the rule changes in water polo) have clearly modified how such sports are played and consequently modified the physiological demands needed to succeed. Knowledge, understanding, and assessment of the implications of rule changes in sports is necessary to be able to plan more effective training interventions.

CONCLUSION

Sport has largely moved from an amateur pastime to a professional industry in which coaches and support staff are employed to improve the performance of athletes and reach successful outcomes in terms of medals, competitions, and championships won. Gone is the era of opinions and subjective approaches to training and performance interventions. As in business, it is important to define KPIs for athletes and teams, and also important for the strength and conditioning coaches, physiologists, sports medicine specialists, athletic trainers, nutritionists, and performance analysts to define the most important KPIs to track the performance of individuals or teams. Such an approach is also often required on the business side of sporting organizations to determine if an ROI is likely. Key performance indicators should be determined and assessed routinely to make sure the longitudinal development of athletes and teams is on track, to identify areas requiring intervention, and to assess the effectiveness of activities implemented to improve performance. Only an evidence-based approach and collective discussions based on a mixture of data and expertise can be considered as a useful strategy to advance performance in sporting organizations. For this to happen, assuming that expertise resides in key staff (e.g., coaching and support staff), data should be collected, stored, and analyzed in a systematic manner and then used to provide the necessary information for performance reviews and debriefs.

RECOMMENDED READINGS

Levitt, SD, and Dubner, SJ. *Freakonomics: A Rogue Economist Explores the Hidden Side of Everything.* New York: William Morrow Paperbacks, 2005.

Lewis, M. *Moneyball: The Art of Winning an Unfair Game.* New York: W. W. Norton & Company, 2004.

Mauboussin, MJ. The true measures of success. *Harvard Business Review* 90, 46-56, 2012.

Page, SE. *The Model Thinker: What You Need to Know to Make Data Work for You.* New York: Basic Books, 2018.

Schrage, M, and Kiron, D. Leading with next-generation key performance indicators. *MIT Sloan Management Review* June 26, 2018. http://sloanreview.mit.edu/kpi2018.

Silver, N. *The Signal and the Noise: While Most Predictions Fail—but Some Don't.* New York: Penguin Group, 2012.

CHAPTER 6

Profiling and Benchmarking

Mike McGuigan, PhD

Profiling and **benchmarking** are key starting points for the analysis of athletes. This chapter discusses how performance norms and benchmarking can be used by sport scientists. The profiling and benchmarking of athletes is a critical part of the process for informing training and programming. It also allows a complete picture of the athlete to be developed, including physical, psychological, technical, and tactical aspects. This has implications for athlete performance and injury prevention. Therefore, using data to inform short- and long-term decisions to support athlete development is also discussed.

ANALYSIS OF THE ATHLETE

Developing a profile of an individual athlete, team, event, or sport is a vital step in the training process that can be delivered by sport scientists to coaches and athletes. Many different factors need to be assessed within this process. The starting point of any profile is to assess the general demands of the sport, as well as the specific demands through different category analyses, such as playing positions, age groups, and level of competition, which can be performed using needs analysis (35). After this first level of the sport analysis, an individual profile can be developed and compared to the needs analysis. Using a "gap analysis," the athlete's current level can be compared to benchmarks. This enables the development of more systematic and objective training plans for athletes. The process can also aid athlete physical, psychological, and skill development, from early stages in the athlete's career. Therefore, growth and maturation need to be considered when one is implementing these processes in youth athletes. The ultimate value of these approaches is in allowing sport scientists to build up a

more complete picture of the athlete's current physical capacities that can then be benchmarked against known standards of performance. The approach can be applied across the physical, technical, tactical, and psychological domains. Individual- and team- or squad-based approaches can be used.

Benchmarking and profiling can be implemented for both short- and long-term programming; both aspects are considered in this chapter. Benchmarking and profiling can be applied within a single training session, within microcycles, or even within macrocycles. Also, long-term planning can be guided with these methods, both for the training year and over longer periods such as a quadrennial cycle.

MATURATION AND LONG-TERM DEVELOPMENT

For sport scientists working with youth athletes, it is critical to consider maturation and long-term development (26). According to the National Strength and Conditioning Association (NSCA) position stand on long-term athletic development, maturation refers to "progress toward a mature state and varies in timing, tempo, and magnitude between different bodily systems" (26). **Long-term athletic development** refers to "the habitual development of 'athleticism' over time to improve health and fitness, enhance physical performance, reduce the relative risk of injury, and develop confidence and competence in all youth" (26). Growth is particularly important during the early years of life and is defined as "an increase in the size attained by specific parts of the body, or the body as a whole" (26).

Effective profiling of youth athletes needs to take variations in maturation and growth into account.

Maturation and long-term development are also key considerations for talent identification. Several approaches can be used to measure maturation (29). Methods such as those proposed by Mirwald and colleagues (34) and the Khamis-Roche method (25) have been used to determine peak height velocity (PHV) and predicted adult height, respectively. **Biological maturation** rather than **chronological age** should be considered with profiling due to the large variation that can occur between individuals with regard to their development (28). Maturity status can be measured using age at PHV prediction equations from anthropometric measures (34). Calculating years from PHV has been widely used to measure maturation (34). Maturation offset can be calculated using age, sitting height, and arm and leg length (34). Previously it has been recommended that strength and conditioning professionals monitor body mass, height, and limb length quarterly in order to gain a comprehensive understanding of maturation rates (26).

Taking maturation into account allows more valid comparisons to be made between athletes (26). Developing age-appropriate assessments will also be important for sport scientists. Maturation and long-term development need to be considered when one is choosing appropriate assessments to be used for profiling and benchmarking. Monitoring of maturation provides sport scientists with critical information regarding development of youth athletes. Maturation can have a significant influence on different physical capacities (26). Training age can also be considered when the number of years spent training has been recorded. Having a good understanding of the differences can help sport scientists with both talent identification and programming.

Many challenges exist for talent identification that need to be considered by sport scientists. Chronological age is commonly used for benchmarking methods such as percentiles (see "Benchmarking and Data Interpretation" section). However, this approach has limitations because it does not necessarily take into account maturation of the athlete. Longitudinal research has tracked various aspects of athlete development (26). Most of the research has monitored physical aspects of performance. The multidimensional aspects of performance, including physical, technical, tactical, and psychological factors, should each be considered. Understanding how the factors interact during development can help drive more effective talent development processes.

PERFORMANCE NORMS

Establishing performance norms is vital for sport scientists when testing and monitoring athletes. **Performance norms** refer to the establishment of normative levels of performance. Clearly defining norms for performance provides a starting point for benchmarking and profiling. Normative data can be generated from the results of testing and assessments of physical, physiological, and other factors related to performance. Several aspects need to be considered when one is establishing performance norms, including sample size, sources of information, analysis methods, and data interpretation. Different options are available for establishing performance norms across different assessments. One of the challenges for sport scientists is the small sample sizes that are often encountered with testing, particularly when working with individual athletes. Therefore, establishing robust performance norms can be challenging. Specific statistical methods can be used to help overcome this problem (see chapter 18). A good starting point is to source data from the published literature. However, the context of the performance norms needs to be considered. The sport scientist may not be sure under what conditions the information was generated. Ideally, these data should be obtained from a similar population to ensure that the characteristics of the group being tested are similar. The equipment and analysis methods that were used to collect the data should be taken into account. Issues can arise when using performance norms from other sources for comparison, as most testing variables will be invalid if different equipment or analysis methods were used. For example, data obtained from a force plate, a linear transducer, or an accelerometer will not necessarily be comparable (36). As another example, using different methods of assessment to test speed (e.g., radar gun, timing lights, stopwatch) can give different results (18).

A series of steps can be followed to develop performance norms:

- Complete a needs analysis of the sport to identify the critical factors of performance.
- Perform a literature search to identify previous performance norms that may have been published for the sport.
- Ideally sport scientists should look to establish their own in-house performance norms to ensure validity of the data.

- Performance norms should consider maturation and long-term development when one is working with youth athletes.
- Adequate sample sizes are required for determining performance norms.
- Once testing is completed, the results can be compared to norms or benchmarks.

BENCHMARKING AND DATA INTERPRETATION

Benchmarking is another critical aspect for the interpretation of testing data. Having a clear understanding of the level of the competition and their physical profile is an essential part of the training process. Benchmarking refers to the comparison of an athlete's performance on a test against a standard. It is an objective process of defining performance and should be based on factors such as age, maturation, playing position, and training history. Benchmarking can also help to inform what adaptations to focus on in training to provide a competitive advantage over opponents.

As with determining performance norms, needs analysis of a sport is used to create profiles of different positions that can be implemented for benchmarking purposes. Needs analysis of specific events within the sport can also be used to create performance profiles. This differs from the athlete profile, which looks at the individual. The performance profile provides an overall picture of the sport or event. Benchmarking can be used for talent identification by identifying what aspects of sport performance determine success. Various aspects such as physiological, anthropometric, technical, tactical, and psychological data all contribute to performance. Therefore, the challenge is using methods that can measure the interaction between these domains. Methods such as principal component analysis (statistical method that reduces large amounts of data to smaller components) could help sport scientists to deal more effectively with issues such as multicollinearity (predictor variables are highly related). Future performance requirements of the event or sport should also be considered. While prediction is difficult in sport, sport scientists do need to attempt to understand where changes in future aspects of performance may occur when developing benchmarks (i.e., deterministic modeling).

The benchmark standard can be determined in different ways. One approach is to compare the score against elite or world-class performance in the given event or discipline. Development of gold standard models of performance based on competition data can be useful for informing programming (see "Using Data to Guide Short- and Long-Term Development"). The athletes' performance could be expressed as a percentage (or percentile) of the best performance. Best performance across different developmental levels is another method that can be used. For example, sport scientists could determine how performance on a test differs between high school, college, and professional athletes (1). Studies have been conducted that compare performance in physical capacities across a range of tests and athlete levels (1, 11, 43). Researchers have also investigated the physical characteristics of starters versus nonstarters in different sports (3, 51). By using benchmarking, sport scientists can build a picture of what different levels of performance look like for the sports they are working with. Appropriate benchmarking will follow a process of rigorously establishing targeted levels of performance for the variables being tested. Collecting large amounts of quality data increases the chances of developing more robust benchmarks.

Benchmarking and interpretation of data should include appropriate use of scaling (8). Allometric scaling has been proposed to control for differences in body size when comparing athletes (10). Simple ratio scaling using body mass is another common approach that is used (10). Some authors have suggested that constant scaling factors should be used, whereas others recommend basing the constants on the population being tested. Sports such as weightlifting (Sinclair formula [44]) and powerlifting (Wilks formula [49]) use validated scaling methods to compare athlete performance across different weight classes. By establishing coefficients, athletes of different body mass can be directly compared with the type of scaling determined by the test. Certain assumptions are made with scaling methods, and sport scientists need to check if these assumptions are being met to determine whether scaling is appropriate (46).

Data interpretation involves using appropriate methods to collect, sort, organize, and analyze the data (see chapters 20 and 21). When possible, the benchmarking should also occur on an individual basis. To assist with this, sport scientists often transform data to aid interpretation of the results. Methods that can be used include ranking data, z-scores, and percentiles (see relevant sections later in this chapter). Consideration of the individual results has the advantage of allowing for greater impact for each athlete.

A variety of ratios have been proposed for benchmarking and to aid data interpretation, some of which may potentially be used to guide programming (31). Examples include velocity-based training, dynamic strength index, reactive strength index, and eccentric utilization ratio, to name a few. While they can serve as a guide for programming, strength and conditioning professionals should not rely on a single ratio or benchmark as the sole basis of decision making with programming.

Another area in which appropriate benchmarking and data interpretation could be applied is rehabilitation and return to play following injury. Establishing accurate baseline data that allow for comparisons throughout rehabilitation will help to drive this process more effectively. Without this baseline information, it will be more difficult to develop appropriate benchmarks for return to performance. This is an area that highlights not relying on a single metric for decision making by sport scientists. For example, strength deficits and asymmetries, altered running patterns, or altered high-intensity metrics in team sports (e.g., sprint distance, distance at high speeds) have been shown to exist for long periods following injuries in athletes (7).

Velocity-based training is another approach that calls for sport scientists to use caution in applying blanket benchmarks. Factors such as the technology, methodology of assessment, and exercise performed can all affect metrics such as velocity (36). Individualized approaches for determining the benchmarks for both the athlete and exercise should be considered.

Test Quality

Testing and data collection are two of the most critical aspects of athlete assessment. Many different tests are available for athlete assessment and monitoring. Several factors need to be considered for choosing tests with applications for athlete profiling and benchmarking:

- Standardized testing
- Validity, reliability, and sensitivity to change
- Applicability and ease of use
- Test frequency
- Ability to conduct test with many athletes if needed
- Learning effect associated with the test
- Appreciating the error within the test

- Effectiveness of the testing information to improve athlete performance

Sport scientists should use high-quality tests that are reliable and valid and provide useful information. The sport scientist should be able to provide a strong rationale for why the test is being used in practice. A comprehensive needs analysis of the athlete and sport will provide the necessary background for designing the testing battery that is implemented. Tests need to be aligned to athlete monitoring and assess the determining factors known to influence success in the sport. Test quality will ultimately determine how effective the process is and the impact that the assessment can have. The quality of the test will have a significant impact on the validity and reliability of the test. Sophisticated methods of data analysis and interpretation cannot overcome poor test quality. Therefore, sport scientists need to be certain that they follow the necessary steps to ensure the quality of testing.

Tests should be used that are closely related to the underlying physical capacities of the sport or event in question. Performing a needs analysis of the sport, event, or specific position will help to determine specific tests. Sport scientists need to have confidence that the tests they are using with athletes are measuring the most pertinent aspects of performance (i.e., the determinants of performance or key performance indicators) (see chapter 5). However, it is also important to test general physical qualities such as cardiovascular or muscular endurance, strength, power, and overall athletic ability.

Validity is a critical factor for test quality. This refers to whether the test measures what it is designed to measure. Several different types of validity are of concern to the sport scientist. **Face validity** is the degree to which the test measures the variable it is intended to measure. **Criterion validity** is the degree to which the test is associated with another measure. Different types of criterion validity include predictive and concurrent validity. **Predictive validity** refers to the degree to which the test can predict future performance by the athlete. **Concurrent validity** refers to the degree to which the test results are related to other test results measuring the same physical capacity. Validity can be measured with statistics such as correlation. For example, measuring the relationship between the test and a gold standard measurement can be used to help determine criterion validity. See chapter 18 for more detailed information.

Another important question concerning validity is how well the test discriminates between different levels of performance. This will be critical for benchmarking purposes. For example, researchers have compared starters versus nonstarters (3, 51). Other research has investigated the validity of tests to discriminate levels of athletes (e.g., high school, college, and professional athletes) (1). Another essential question is how well the test relates to performance. Measuring the strength of the relationship between the test performance and match performance can provide insight into this aspect of validity. This has proven difficult in team sports.

Reliability is yet another crucial factor in relation to test quality. **Test reliability** is concerned with how consistent the test is. Various aspects of test reliability are as follows:

- Interrater reliability is the reliability between different testers. Testing needs to be consistent between testers.
- Intrarater reliability refers to the reliability or agreement for the individual tester.
- Intra-athlete variability is the degree of consistency between tests for individual athletes. Some natural variability will exist but needs to be minimized as much as possible.

Reliability of the test needs to be understood in the context of the population being tested. While the reliability of many tests is available in the published literature, sport scientists should determine the reliability in their own setting (i.e., with similar athletes in conditions under which they are usually assessed). To conduct an in-house reliability assessment of a test, these steps can be followed:

- Perform the test on a group of athletes (as many as possible, but at least 10) with multiple trials (three or four depending on the test).
- Repeat the testing under the same conditions several times. Depending on the test and how fatiguing it is, the time interval between retests may need to be 48 to 72 hours.
- Reliability statistics using the methods described in chapter 18 can be used to calculate within-session and between-sessions reliability.

Various statistics such as intraclass correlation coefficients, statistical error, and coefficients of variation can be used to determine reliability (discussed further in chapter 18). Sport scientists also need to be confident that the tests they are using provide consistent results and that the degree of noise associated with the test is low. Related to this is the sensitivity of the test. Sport scientists should be aware of the degree of change on the test that represents a meaningful change in performance. They should use tests that are best able to detect a real change in performance. Determining the coefficient of variation for the assessment and knowing the technical error of the test will help to inform this process.

The applicability of the test and how easy it is to perform in applied settings are also important considerations. While laboratory-based testing can provide highly controlled assessments, testing that can be conducted in the field is more ecologically valid.

Standardization of the conditions under which the test is performed will help to improve test quality. Several other aspects should be considered to address standardization:

- Adequate familiarization is provided regarding the test. This is critical for tests that involve higher technical demands and will help to control for learning effects.
- Consistent instructions are given before and during the testing.
- Adequate warm-up is completed before the testing.
- Time of day is consistent to avoid variations due to diurnal rhythms.
- Purpose of the test is explained to the athletes so they fully understand the reasons for the testing.
- Appropriate training is provided for the individuals conducting the testing.
- Testing instructions should be standardized, as these can influence test outcomes. Measuring rate of force development (27) and use of external or internal cues during jump testing (37) are examples of situations in which test results can be affected by instruction.
- Order of the testing should be established such that the potential impact of a test on subsequent assessments is minimized.
- The degree to which the test causes fatigue will help determine how frequently the testing can be performed.

Another important factor is when the testing will occur. Testing needs to be conducted regularly to provide maximum value. However, optimal frequency of the testing should be considered. It should be feasible to implement tests regularly, not just as a one-off event.

Ideally these assessments should be linked to programming and used to identify adaptations during key training phases. Using tests that have been widely used previously provides the advantage of having greater amounts of normative data available for comparison. However, sport scientists need to be careful not to let dogma dictate choice of test when better assessments become available. On the other hand, sport scientists should avoid changing tests too regularly. It may not be necessary to include all tests all the time; some need to be performed only occasionally. Therefore, the frequency of testing exists on a continuum, and the challenge is finding the balance between testing that serves a clear purpose and having no objective input via profiling and benchmarking.

Testing is rarely conducted as a single event but performed in conjunction with other assessments. When testing groups of athletes, the logistics of testing should be considered. Can the test be incorporated as part of training? Laboratory-based testing allows for athlete assessment under controlled conditions. However, accurate tests that can be conducted during competition and training under real-world conditions are critical for sport scientists. While the quality of the testing may be more difficult to control, valid and reliable field-based tests are available. Another advantage of field-based tests is that they are more specific. Tests that more closely assess the underlying capacities and aspects of sport performance will provide more useful information.

Sport scientists should consider whether additional tests are required and what extra information they provide. Performing several tests that are highly related may be unnecessary. The sport scientist should question whether a single test can provide the necessary information for a physical capacity or whether there is a need for additional tests. For example, when testing strength, is it necessary to perform a 1RM test in addition to the isometric mid-thigh pull test? While there may be a strong correlation between the two tests, a sport scientist may be justified in testing both, since one is informative for program design (1RM can be used to accurately determine percentages to train during various phases), while the isometric mid-thigh pull may be used as a more general, overall strength measure to accurately track adaptation.

The ultimate determinant of test quality will be whether it provides information the sport scientist can relay to the wider support team—information that can be used to improve the performance of the athlete. Therefore, testing needs to have a specific purpose.

Sport scientists should avoid collecting data just for the sake of collecting data.

Ranking

Use of **rankings** is a fundamental aspect of competitive sport. Since sports use ranking systems to measure performance, it makes sense that this approach should be incorporated into athlete testing. Various ranking systems can be used in athlete assessment. For example, ranking athletes on several aspects of a test can provide interesting insights into their strengths and weaknesses. This can be as simple as ranking the athletes within a squad from best to worst for a specific test. Athlete ranking systems could also place the individuals on a continuum for an event. Team sports present more of a challenge due to the multiple components that determine success in these sports. For example, athletes could be ranked in terms of physical, tactical, and technical components. Within the physical domain, rankings could be made for cardiovascular or muscular endurance, strength, power, speed, flexibility, and body composition, among others (see figure 6.1). Composite scores for the various domains can provide an overall summary, such as the Performance Index popularized at the University of Nebraska (42). Individual test results are critical, but overall scores may have application for talent identification and development.

Decisions need to be made about the tests for which rankings are used. Selection of metrics for reporting purposes also needs consideration. The type of scaling that should be applied before using the ranking is also something to factor in. Should relative-to-bodyweight or allometric scaling be used? Especially when the population or sample differs within the same team (e.g., basketball or American football can include very different body types on the same team; thus, aspects such as body weight, height, or limb measurements should be used as control factors). Sport scientists should also consider whom the rankings will be shared with. For example, it may not be appropriate to have rankings for physical capacity of developmental athletes on public display in the training facility without consent.

Within a squad of athletes, individuals may be ranked differently for specific physical capacities. Even with strength tests (isometric, dynamic, eccentric, and isokinetic), an individual may have different rankings. While studies have shown high correlations

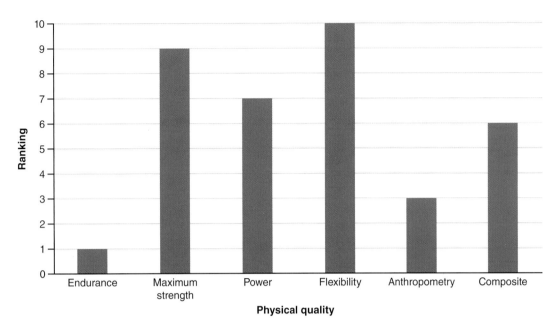

FIGURE 6.1 Rankings for an individual athlete for physical tests. Ranking is where the athlete ranked in the squad (N = 10).

between different strength measures across a range of populations (22), these are not perfect relationships and strength is task-specific (15). Athletes can be assessed using strength and power profiling and ranked for various aspects. For example, McMaster and colleagues (33) used a ranking system with a range of upper body strength and power assessments in rugby union athletes. The individual rankings can be used to identify strengths and weaknesses of players and implement plans to correct them. The study showed that ranking the athletes was able to provide insights into the upper body strength and power athlete profile (33).

Rankings can also be used for the comparison of athletes across different teams and positions. Many sports use ranking systems to rank athletes within different events and divisions (e.g., bodyweight) based on performance. Team sports also rank athletes based on different performance analysis measures to allow comparison between teams, individuals, and positions.

z-Scores

Several types of data transformation can be used by sport scientists. **Standardized scores** express the test result as a standard distance from the mean. For example, **z-scores** are commonly used by sport scientists so that test results can be expressed as the number of standard deviations away from the mean

(6). This standardization transforms the data so that zero represents the mean and one represents the standard deviation. These methods allow for comparison between and within athletes. Standardized scores present different tests and variables using the same scale and can provide more individualized approaches to data analysis. While summary statistics such as means can be used for establishing benchmarks, sport scientists need methods that can be applied on a more individualized basis, which allows for easier interpretation and comparison.

z-Scores can allow for comparison of the test scores when a group of athletes are tested. In this instance the athlete's score is compared to the squad or team. This is the formula:

z-Score = (Athlete Score − Team Average) / Team Standard Deviation

As mentioned previously, the z-score represents how many standard deviations and the direction of the score from the mean.

The athlete's score can also be compared to the person's baseline, which is a common approach used in athlete monitoring (47):

z-Score = (Athlete Score − Baseline Score) / Baseline Standard Deviation

Here the baseline standard deviation is calculated from a series of measures (e.g., three or four times during preseason). Calculating the measures over a set period, such as blocks of training or during a preseason, will help to account for variations that occur.

It is also possible to represent z-scores relative to predetermined norms or benchmarks (31). This approach can be used when testing squads of athletes, especially with small numbers. In these cases, having athletes unavailable for testing can have a large impact on the squad average. Therefore, presenting data relative to benchmarks can be more informative. The sport scientist could follow the process discussed earlier for establishing the benchmarks and use these, along with standard deviations determined from historical data, to calculate a benchmark z-score.

Interpretation of z-scores will be dependent on the context within which the sport scientist is working. This concept is discussed in more detail in the final section of this chapter. It is also useful to visualize z-scores with graphs. For example, histograms and radar plots can be used to represent z-scores (see figures 6.2 and 6.3; 11a and 24a). This enables coaches (and athletes) to view the data and visualize where the athlete has scored relative to the squad or baseline. The visual aspect makes it easy to see the strengths and weaknesses of the athlete and helps inform training program design.

T-scores are another type of standardized score that can be used. They are like z-scores except that they are calculated as follows:

$$\text{T-score} = (\text{z-score} \times 10) + 50$$

Therefore, the average T-score will be 50, with T-scores less than 50 being below the mean and those greater than 50 above the mean. The results will always be positive so they may be more easily understood by the end user.

Another variation of standardized scores is **standard ten (STEN) scores** (47). These convert z-scores to a score out of 10. which may be more intuitive. STEN scores can be converted from z-scores as follows:

$$\text{STEN score} = (2 \times \text{z-score}) + 5.5$$

In this case, the average z-score will be 5.5 with each STEN unit of 1.0 representing a standard deviation of 0.5.

Percentiles

Percentiles are another common method used by sport scientists. **Percentiles** are a statistical measure showing the value below which a percentage of results occurs within a group of results. Establishing percentiles based on large numbers of athletes' scores allows sport scientists to see where testing results sit relative to the population being tested. For example, tables and figures can be generated that will show which percentile band the athlete's result falls into (see figure 6.4). If an athlete is at a percentile rank of 70%,

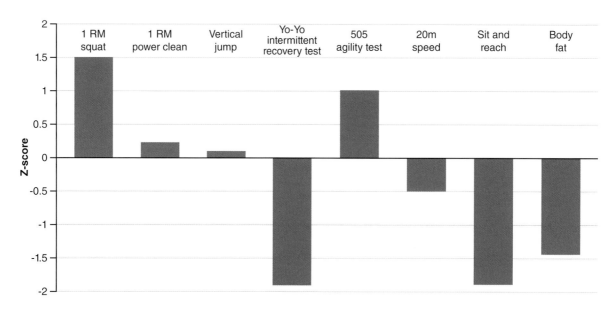

FIGURE 6.2 z-Score column chart representing standardized test scores across different fitness tests for an individual athlete. The zero represents the team average.

Reprinted by permission from McGuigan (2016, pg 259-316).

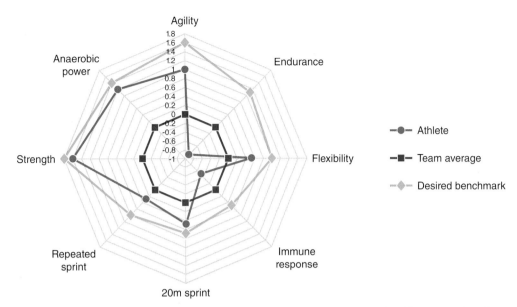

FIGURE 6.3 Individual athlete results compared with team average and desired benchmarks. Note that since this is an average of z-scores, the team average will always come out to zero using the traditional calculation.

Reprinted by permission from M. McGuigan (2014, pg. 10).

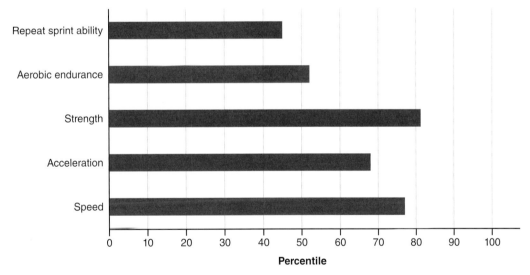

FIGURE 6.4 Percentiles for an athlete across a series of tests.

it means that 70% of the group had scores below the athlete's score. Tables have been developed and are available for different tests specific to various sports (30). The NSCA's *Essentials of Strength Training and Conditioning* provides examples of percentiles for different tests (30).

Percentiles are presented in a series of increments—for example, percentiles for 50th, 70th, 90th in a specific physical test. Percentiles can be deter-

mined across a range of levels and are commonly sex-specific, with age-based percentiles also available (30).

USING DATA TO GUIDE SHORT- AND LONG-TERM DEVELOPMENT

The most critical aspect of profiling and benchmarking is how the data can be used to guide short- and long-term decision making. Determining benchmarks so they can be used to guide short- and long-term decision making requires following a systematic process to aid development of performance. Collecting data is important for this process, but ultimately the information needs to be used effectively. Sport scientists should therefore avoid gathering data without a clear purpose. Through obtaining objective data from athlete assessments, targets can be set that will aid decision making. Having knowledge of how an athlete compares to peers who are the top performers can be an insightful way to identify gaps in performance and help to identify priorities for training. Benchmarking will then allow gap analysis of the athlete profile, which can enable more effective training program design. Regular and ongoing assessment may require adjustment of these targets. Ongoing evaluation is critical, and readjustment of training may be required. Effective profiling and benchmarking enable sport scientists to identify where the athlete currently is in terms of physical development. Then, the decision-making process will inform the development of the training program.

Benchmarking can provide objective information on when peak performance in terms of maturation is achieved. Researchers have analyzed when peak performance occurs across a range of sports, including weightlifting (45), powerlifting (45), and track and field (19). It is much more difficult to benchmark with team sports due to positional differences and varied demands with multiple physical capacities that need to be developed. Nevertheless, researchers have attempted to provide benchmarking for team sports such as Australian rules football (32).

Profiling can be used to identify strengths and weaknesses (31). Data collected during testing can provide information on these strengths and weaknesses relative to established benchmarks. The information can then assist decision making regarding the programming and what aspects need greater emphasis. For example, testing may identify a deficit for a general capacity such as change of direction (see figure 6.5; 11a). More in-depth profiling of a specific capacity such as power could show that an athlete is deficient in a specific area such as reactive strength. This type of information would assist the strength and conditioning professionals with decision making about what program to use in the next phase of training. For example, what is the effect of focusing on one specific aspect of performance? In other words, what is the correct dosage of training and which elements should be prioritized throughout the training cycle? Bench-

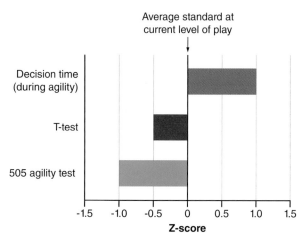

FIGURE 6.5 Strengths and weaknesses of an athlete through representation of standardized scores for perceptual-cognitive ability, maneuverability, and change-of-direction ability. Negative values indicate performance lower than average whereas positive values indicate performance better than average.

Reprinted by permission from McGuigan (2016, pg. 259-316).

marking and profiling are useful in this scenario as it allows the strength and conditioning professionals to optimally titrate the loadings on a regular basis. Rather than relying on one-off testing or testing before and after a longer training block, more regular assessments can provide ongoing feedback. The question arises as to whether to focus on strengths or weaknesses, or if it is possible to do both. Where this fits should be placed in the context of the periodization plan (chapters 3 and 4). While collecting data to guide short- and long-term development is important, the art of coaching should also be applied. Data should be used as a guide rather than applied rigidly all the time.

Force-velocity profiling is an example of a method that can generate profiling and subsequent training program design for improving those aspects of athlete performance (23, 24). The profiling allows the sport scientist to identify if an athlete is force or velocity deficient. Approaches such as force–velocity profiling also enable the use of training as testing. As mentioned previously, testing has traditionally been considered a stand-alone event with days within the program set aside for assessment. However, testing and monitoring can be incorporated into training sessions. Rather than adding burden on athletes, valuable information can be gathered during training and used to inform programming. Benchmarks would still need to be established in these scenarios to be able to achieve the most value from this approach. For example, with use of velocity-based training, identifying thresholds across a range of exercises will be required. The context and limitations of benchmarks and thresholds do need to be noted. These can be considered a guide to informing training program design rather than needing to be rigidly applied.

Benchmarking athletes longitudinally can be informative for sports. In team sports, this type of information can provide valuable detail on the makeup of squads by placing in context the individual development of players. Several published reports are available that include longitudinal testing data from several sports, including aerobic capacity (48), speed (17, 20), power (2, 20), and strength (2).

Various analysis methods are available for the short- and long-term analysis of data for sport scientists. The approach that will be used to analyze the testing data should be determined before using the test. Time series analysis can examine trends in performance and guide decisions, both short- and long-term.

When using data to guide programming, overreliance on single measures should be avoided. Athlete profiling and benchmarking requires painting a complete picture of the individual and team. Searching for a single metric that can be used to provide insight is appealing, but not practical. Only by considering a range of measures and where athletes sit relative to their strengths and weaknesses can this information be used to optimize the training program.

Case studies provide an excellent template for methods to guide short- and long-term programming. Published case studies are available that show examples of both short- (14) and long-term (4, 5, 40) approaches to athlete programming. Several reviews of how case studies can be used by sport scientists are available (13, 39). More published data on athletes would provide information regarding the use of performance profiling. Published benchmarks can be a starting point for determining levels of required performance at the elite level. Sport scientists should exercise caution when interpreting the findings since

the testing quality may vary across these published reports. In addition, different methods of data collection and analysis can make comparison between published datasets problematic. The goal for sport scientists should be to establish their own in-house set of benchmarks that can be used to inform programming.

Sport scientists can also use qualitative methods (16). Interviews, focus groups, and surveys are valid methods that can be used to inform and guide both short-term and long-term programming. Use of mixed methods and case studies can provide insights into the links between athlete assessment and programming. This process should include needs analysis, overviewing the athlete with the appropriate assessments, evaluating the effects of a training intervention, and evaluation for determining implications.

Long-term planning is also essential to consider with athletes. "Long-term" can refer to 1 year, a quadrennial cycle, or even an athlete's career. Periodization becomes even more vital with long-term development (see chapters 3 and 4). One scenario is to use the 4-year Olympic cycle when developing the training plan for Olympic sports. Another scenario could be with collegiate athletes in whom the development from freshman to senior is considered, from both a short-term and a long-term perspective. Transitioning athletes from youth and developmental levels to senior competitions can also be aided by the use of benchmarking and profiling. The frequency of assessments needs to be considered when it comes to long-term programming with the testing battery built into the periodization plan. Figure 6.6 shows the breakdown of potential uses of data for immediate, short-term, and long-term development.

Short-Term Examples of How to Use Data

As discussed previously, data is most valuable when it is used to inform programming on an ongoing and

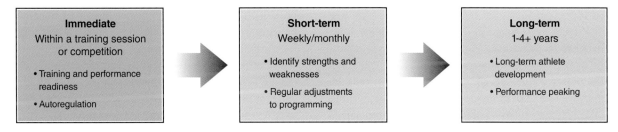

FIGURE 6.6 Uses of immediate, short-term, and long-term data to guide development.

regular basis. Strength and conditioning professionals can use data from regular testing to adjust the athlete training program. Incorporating testing within a session can enable immediate changes to training. For example, assessment of training readiness and measurement of current performance (velocity-based training) can occur during training sessions.

Various tools have been used for establishing training readiness. Measures such as wellness factors (fatigue, stress, sleep, muscle soreness), heart rate variability, neuromuscular performance (e.g., countermovement jump variables), and barbell velocity have been investigated (5, 9, 14). However, limited studies have demonstrated the efficacy of these approaches and their ability to influence superior training adaptations.

Athlete monitoring systems are discussed in more detail in part III of this book. Developing an effective monitoring system requires accurately establishing benchmarks for variables. Determining an adequate baseline is also vital. Benchmarking can be used for establishing levels if a traffic light system is adopted. Thresholds have been proposed by researchers whereby a z-score greater than 1.5 could indicate a cutoff (47). Some sport scientists use a traffic light system to help make decisions about whether intervention is required, using an orange flag and a red flag (38). For example, a z-score of −1.5 to 1.99 could be considered an orange flag and >−2.0 a red flag (47). However, it is important to note that these thresholds are arbitrary and are not validated by research. Until more research evidence is available, these thresholds should be considered a guideline, and the context of the setting worked in will help guide decision making regarding interventions.

Coaches and sport scientists also make in-game decisions using available data. Knowing the key performance indicators can help to drive this effectively. Performance analysis and the increased use of wearable technologies during games have provided the opportunity to use real-time data.

Within the course of a microcycle, data can be used to track progress and inform decisions about adjustments that can be made. Testing that occurs after just a few weeks can help to guide training emphasis for the subsequent training block. If an athlete is identified as being deficient in a specific physical capacity, then more of this specific type of training could be incorporated. One of the challenges of programming is the interaction of variables. Consideration needs to be given to potential effects of concurrent training

(chapter 4). The overall profile of that athlete should take into account how the physical capacities interact. Rather than just focusing on a single attribute, the interaction between aspects should be considered. For example, the relationship between fitness and body composition would be important for athletes.

Testing data can be used to inform programming on a short-term basis. For example, it has been recommended that benchmark levels of 0.60 to 0.80 be used for dynamic strength index (ratio of isometric peak force to dynamic peak force) (41). If the result is greater than 0.80, then it is suggested that the training focus should be on maximal force production (strength). If the result is less than 0.60, then more ballistic-type exercises should be programmed. However, there are limited training studies looking at this approach (9, 50). The findings of Comfort and colleagues (9) highlight the importance of not considering a ratio or threshold in isolation when making recommendations. The results need to be put in context and viewed alongside other testing results.

Using an applied example, a strength and conditioning professional could have athletes perform a 3RM back squat test and unloaded countermovement jump test. The athletes are subsequently ranked for 3RM strength and peak velocity on the countermovement jump test. Athlete A is ranked third (out of 15) for 3RM strength and 11th for peak velocity. Athlete B is ranked seventh for 3RM and fifth for peak velocity. The information could subsequently inform which areas to target in the training program. It is important to note that there may be limitations to relying only on one-off testing for decision making. The results need to be placed in context, and it may be appropriate to compare the results to historical data for the individual athlete.

Long-Term Examples of How to Use Data

Longitudinal tracking of performance is essential for determining the degree of adaptation, as well as providing insight into how well trained an athlete is. While one-off testing can be useful in terms of benchmarking, taking a long-term approach will allow for more in-depth understanding of the athlete. With youth athletes, the effects of maturation and growth can be better understood. Interestingly, elite athletes can continue to make long-term improvements, albeit smaller ones than less-trained athletes, in several physical capacities (2, 12).

Published reports in collegiate sports have demonstrated large changes in strength and power, but smaller changes in speed and acceleration qualities (21). Tracking these factors across the 4- to 5-year cycle can help with decision making regarding program focus for each year. Sport scientists also need to consider how training can transfer more effectively to improve match performance. A scenario could involve collegiate athletes, with a battery of physical tests used at the start of their freshman year to identify gaps and compare to established benchmarks. For example, the overall profile could identify that cardiovascular endurance is excellent, but strength and speed require work. This scenario would require short- and long-term planning. Regular checkpoints would be provided via testing. Throughout the athlete's college career, the physical profile can be updated and appropriate adjustments made to the training program.

CONCLUSION

Profiling and benchmarking are important components of athlete preparation. Sport scientists should be aware of the factors that determine test quality. They should consider physical, technical, psychological, and tactical factors when using profiling and benchmarking. Standardized scores such as z-scores are useful for presenting the results of different tests. The value of testing and monitoring data is its ability to inform short- and long-term athlete development.

RECOMMENDED READINGS

Buchheit, M. Want to see my report, coach? *Aspetar Sports Med J* 6:36-43, 2017.

Lloyd, RS, Cronin, JB, Faigenbaum, AD, Haff, GG, Howard, R, Kraemer, WJ, Micheli, LJ, Myer, GD, and Oliver, JL. National Strength and Conditioning Association position statement on long-term athletic development. *J Strength Cond Res* 30:1491-1509, 2016.

Newton, RU, and Dugan, E. Application of strength diagnosis. *Strength Cond J* 24:50-59, 2002.

Pettitt, RW. Evaluating strength and conditioning tests with z scores: avoiding common pitfalls. *Strength Cond J* 32:100-103, 2010.

Thornton, HR, Delaney, JA, Duthie, GM, and Dascombe, BJ. Developing athlete monitoring systems in team sports: data analysis and visualization. *Int J Sports Physiol Perform* 14:698-705, 2019.

PART III

Technology and
Data Preparation

CHAPTER 7

Technological Implementation

Lorena Torres Ronda, PhD

What is technology? **Technology** is the application of scientific knowledge for practical purposes, through use of the means, artifacts, devices, methods, and materials available to humans to fulfill a need, accomplish specific tasks, or solve problems.

Human evolution has been linked to the progress of technology since prehistoric times; however, the information technology revolution originated with Johannes Gutenberg's invention, the printing press (circa 1440), making information available to the masses and enabling an explosion of ideas (11). From then on, and with the invention of the microchip, the Internet of Things (IoT), WiFi, and mobile systems, information technology has evolved exponentially. The evolution of technology and the information it can provide have benefited all imaginable fields, including medicine, biomechanics, and physiology, disciplines directly linked to knowledge pertaining to sports. Measurement of core body temperature used to require an invasive technique (e.g., rectal temperature), but now it can be performed using a small pill. Today there are wearables, garments, patches, and watches capable of measuring cardiorespiratory function, movement patterns, sweat composition, hydration level, tissue oxygenation, glucose and lactate levels, and sleep patterns. Devices and applications allow practitioners to conduct biomechanical analyses that no longer require markers (e.g., motion digital analysis or marker-less systems), analyze the contractile properties of surface muscles, and measure real-time speed in weightlifting and its derivatives. There are tracking systems (e.g., semiautomatic video analysis; inertial measurement units [IMU]; radio frequency identification systems [RFID]; Global Positioning

Systems [GPS] that report the type, frequency, and intensity of movements in real time; and augmented and virtual reality systems [i.e., AR and VR])—and the list goes on (12). Technology is smaller, quicker, quieter, cheaper—in essence, smarter.

The essence of sporting competition consists of training, resting, competing, and repeating. Nevertheless, at the highest level of performance, technology is providing information that, just as has happened in other sectors, can be a "game changer." Technology in sport has been helping increase overall performance, including speed, mechanical efficiency or safety or both, or simply pure spectacle through sophisticated software, statistical algorithms, and data intelligence providing real-time AR, athlete identification, and statistics in a live broadcast. One can find examples in skiing equipment, swimming suits, helmets, bicycles that are more aerodynamic, motorbikes or canoes, training environments (e.g., VR and AR, Formula 1 simulators, wind tunnels), and plenty of other examples. Organizations and teams are continuously trying to achieve marginal gains and competitive advantage to win a championship or reach the number-one ranking. They are investing more and increasing budgets for research, development, and innovation. Furthermore, assessment and monitoring have dramatically changed with the evolution of technology and the knowledge it generates. Throughout this book, numerous chapters refer to technology and its current importance in the sporting context.

Under these scenarios, sport scientists and professionals involved in sport must know and understand how to select the most relevant and impactful technologies for their organization. This is not about technology itself; it is about how to use the right technology, at the right time, in the right way, and apply scientific knowledge gained from this technology for practical purposes.

The focus of this chapter, therefore, is to detail considerations about the implementation of technology, to provide a framework that guides organizations and professionals regarding technology implementation, and to discuss concerns pertaining to the use of technologies for certain purposes for which they might not be fully ready (yet).

THE INNOVATION PROCESS

Innovation is associated with technology, but technology is only a form of innovation. **Innovation** can be defined as the introduction of something new, an idea or behavior in the form of a technology, product, service, structure, system, or process (10). Technology, and the future of technology innovation, must yield scientific knowledge for practical purposes, and the artifacts, devices, equipment, or materials directed to this end should address performance gaps to accomplish specific tasks or to solve problems.

Innovation and the Combination of Knowledge

Innovative technological developments in sport require a combination of knowledge from different disciplines and a collaborative effort (also known as cross-disciplinary research) from specialists, sport scientists, engineering, and medical and materials sciences (3). As Arthur and Polak (1a) assert, the process of invention is almost entirely achieved by combining existing technologies, since "We find that the combination of technologies has indeed been the major driver of modern invention, reflected in an invariant introduction of new combinations of technologies engendered by patented invention." These phenomena reinforce the need for multidisciplinary support from and interaction between the different professionals involved in solving performance-based problems.

Innovation Process Stages

The innovation process follows a series of stages to either generate a new innovation, such as a new product or process to solve a problem, or adopt an existing innovation (carry out activities to further the use of the existing innovation). The stages are as follows (see figure 7.1; 10):

1. *Awareness.* Recognize a need and identify a gap in knowledge or performance. A potential mistake in this phase is determining the solution before identifying the performance problem.

2. *Interests (and evaluation).* Conduct research to develop knowledge bases and create or adopt solutions; identify suitable innovations (interest versus influence).

3. *Trial.* Investigate the product. The trial period is when one investigates the product in order to be able to answer several questions: Is there a potential competitive advantage to using this product for athlete development or organizational performance or both? Is it practical? Is the cost:benefit relationship a positive one? If the answers to this chain of questions are positive, one can move to the next stage.

4. *Adoption.* Propose some innovations for adoption; provide justifications for decisions.

The four stages of the innovation process are equally important. However, probably too often not enough attention is paid to the first steps; the implementation process is often introduced based on the last step (adoption). It is paramount to have a systematic process of asking questions, comparing answers, and making informed decisions about what to do next to improve conditions and performance. A good practice is to have a system in which the key stakeholders (i.e., multidisciplinary perspective) can assess the needs and wants (i.e., interest versus influence) of the organization. For both short- and long-term goals, it can be worthwhile to establish an organizational strategy to analyze sport trends, as well as trends in technology.

Four categories are included in an assessment of innovation needs (see figure 7.2; 10):

1. *Normative need.* This is defined by the experts in a particular field and refers to the standard or criterion against which quantity or quality of a situation or condition is measured. For example, if a whole league has a certain technology for the analysis of a game, having this technology is a normative need, since not having it could be a competitive disadvantage.

2. *Perceived need.* This is defined by those experiencing the need, who can be from different departments or can be professionals or specialists involved in the performance process. It refers to what they think or feel about the need. What

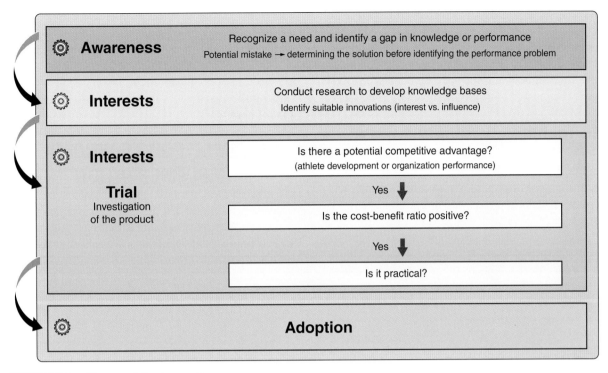

FIGURE 7.1   Stages of the innovation process.

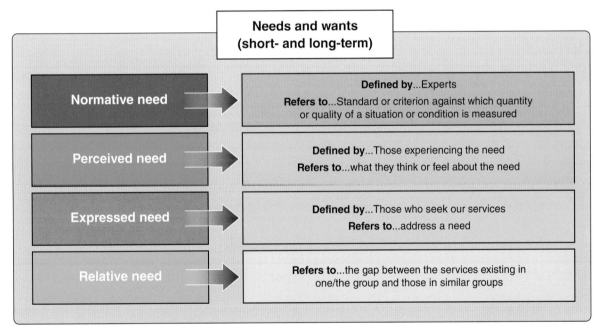

FIGURE 7.2   Needs assessment.

has to be clear at this point is whether a need is perceived after identifying a gap in knowledge or performance (or both) or whether it is perceived as a need because others are implementing that particular technology.

3. *Expressed need.* This is defined by those who offer the services and refers to addressing a need.

4. *Relative need.* This refers to the gap between the services existing in one group and those in similar groups.

The aspect to highlight when analyzing needs is to be clear about what these needs are (perceived need), regardless of what others may be doing to solve theirs (relative need). To do this, having deep knowledge of the environment and the specific context, as well as the problems that need to be solved, will be vital.

The Technology Adoption Curve

In some situations, the urgency for organizations to be at the cutting edge of new ideas and become early adopters of technology, as well as the momentum of technological advances that pushes them to chase the newest innovations, can place sport scientists in a difficult and challenging position (see figure 7.3). Often, sport scientists are attracted by the idea of introducing a new product, or even beta-testing the prototype of a product in a high-performance environment. This can be beneficial when working toward the validation of a product with technology companies or other third parties. However, skipping the process of vetting the product might place organizations in a compromising position. Instead, sport scientists should recognize when and with whom (athletes) it is worthwhile to experiment, such as

with youth or development teams. It is important to follow certain steps during the evaluation and trial stages of the process of technology implementation; otherwise, after a peak of inflated expectations there is a "trough of disillusionment," with people coming to recognize that the new technology will still require a lot of hard work.

ROADMAP FOR TECHNOLOGY IMPLEMENTATION

It has been proposed that the greatest invention in the past some 200 years was not a tool or a gadget, but the invention of the scientific process itself (4), which allowed humans to create things that could never have been discovered. The scientific method is a process of constant questions, change, challenge, and improvement that has the power to create myriad products and other advances, including technology. The role of the sport scientist in the scientific process is to ensure the implementation of technology using evidence-based support, through the fundamental components of scientific methodology and critical thinking (see preface and chapter 30).

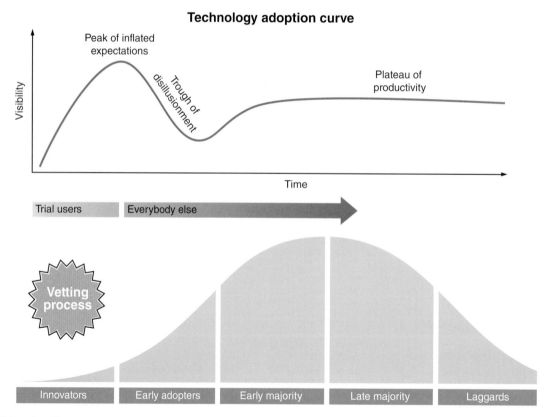

FIGURE 7.3 The technology adoption curve.

The Context

In his book, Christensen (2) proposed an organizational capabilities framework, in which he refers to three factors that affect what an organization can and cannot do when it comes to implementing ideas or new concepts: resources, processes, and values. The first, **resources**, includes people, equipment, technology, product design, information, relationships with brands, and the like. The second factor, **processes**, is the patterns of interaction, coordination, communications, and decision making that transform inputs of resources into products and services of greater value. The third and final factor, **values** of an organization, is the criterion by which decisions about priorities are made; they are the standards by which employees make prioritization decisions. Therefore, when one wants to implement new things, one has to analyze one's resources, processes, and values.

From the wide variety of technologies that will likely lead the future of technology development (each with very specific and different purposes), it has been suggested (2) that they can be clustered into services and processes, including, but not exclusive to, assessing, filtering, sharing, tracking, interacting, and screening (see figure 7.4). In the specific context of sport, one can also identify crucial areas in which technology is key to performance, with emphasis placed on describing, measuring, and defining performance and success (9):

- Key performance indicators (refining performance) (see chapter 5)
- Profiling or benchmarking (determining characteristics of elite performers) (see chapter 6)
- Identifying talent
- Monitoring training and competition performance outcomes (readiness and risk management; individual and team performance) (see chapters 9 and 19)
- Being aware of the context and the goals one wants to achieve with use of the technology (this is paramount)

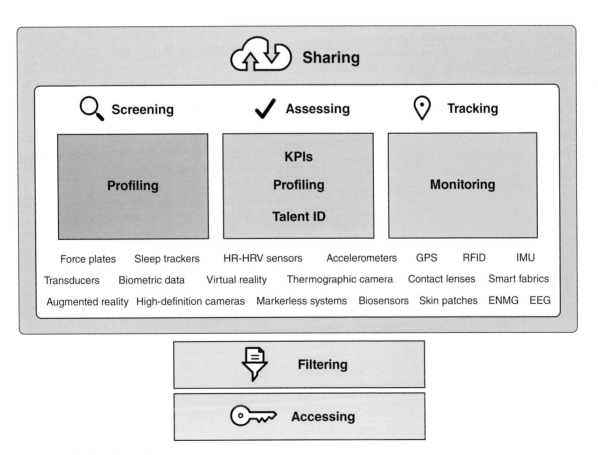

FIGURE 7.4 Technology clusters.

Data Collection

Before starting data collection, it is highly recommended that principles and values be in place that will serve as a framework for decision making. The greater accessibility to technology for monitoring and analysis of sport is sometimes accompanied by a fixation on metrics and pressure to measure performance. This does not happen only in sports and is common in different fields. What has been learned from other disciplines, and also sport, is that the problem is not measurement, but instead inappropriate measurement. What gets measured may have no relationship (e.g., causation, correlation, association, probability, prediction), or not the expected relationship, to what one really wants to know. The science of sport is relatively young; this, alongside the fact that technology and data analysis are not always well used, has meant that factors have been measured without a full understanding of the mechanism that one intended to study (e.g., physiological responses, mechanical analysis, statistics). As Muller writes in *The Tyranny of Metrics,* "[t]here are things that can be measured. There are things that are worth measuring. But what can be measured is not always what is worth measuring" (7). This does not mean that it is better not to measure than to measure, but it is important to study what is worthwhile measuring, or to measure what matters. The explosion of information seen today has shown that sometimes it takes time to translate information into useful knowledge: "We think we want information when we really want knowledge" (11). Consequently, the information provided by technology must be reliable, must be manageable, and, most importantly, must contribute to the decision-making process.

The Equipment

The performance of a product can be analyzed under the prism of competitiveness between products, which includes the following factors: functionality, reliability, convenience, and price (see figure 7.5; 2). When no product available can satisfy the market (i.e., the sport context), the criterion for choosing a product is functionality: One selects a product that could provide information and competitive advantage, and this causes one to adopt the technology. When there are two or more products that can meet functionality needs, people choose products and vendors on the basis of reliability. When two or more vendors satisfy the reliability criterion, the competition shifts to convenience and price.

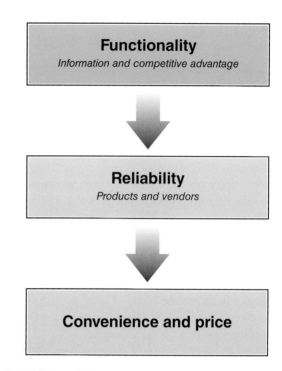

FIGURE 7.5 The performance of a product under the prism of competitiveness.

In the specific context of sport, there are other factors that require consideration. Notably, it is important to understand what the primary use of the technology will be (i.e., a needs analysis), what the technology claims to do, and whether it produces desirable outcomes. Also important are the aspects that might influence the performance of a device, which can be associated with accuracy (precision, resolution), calibration (time, cost efficiency), the setup (permanent, portable, both), the size, the location, and the like.

The athletes are the most important piece of the puzzle when it comes to sport performance. An organization can have the best facilities, the latest technology, or in-vogue wearables, but if the players do not want to use these resources and the technology is in a storage room or gathering dust, it will be of no help (5). Athlete buy-in is fundamental to ensure that technology is appropriately implemented. If one really believes in an athlete-centered or team-centered model, one must ensure that any technology, specifically a wearable, is athlete-friendly, minimally invasive, comfortable, ideally undetectable, and a part of the environment and more or less imperceptible, to the greatest extent possible. If one gives this matter even a moment's consideration and thinks about all the possible wearables and garments that an athlete could wear or use at the same time (since the technological companies tout all these potential advantages), the situation could become ridiculous. The sport scientist must therefore work to achieve unification of technologies with a single device able to offer multiple responses; "We keep adding sensors. We need to keep adding sense" (4).

As mentioned earlier, accessing and sharing are two of the main services that technology should (and will) help with. Therefore, it is important to consider certain processes such as means of importing and exporting data, data communication through application program interfaces (API), or other third-party integrations. Last, but not least, it is important to establish with vendors the duration of the service (contract), the necessity of maintenance, possible updates for both software and hardware, the people who will help when a product malfunctions, and education or continuing education programs.

Staff Involvement

High-performance environments comprise professionals from different areas related to health and performance (e.g., player development coaches, strength and conditioning professionals, physiotherapists, physicians, athletic trainers, sport scientists, psychologists, and nutritionists), and technology may affect more than one of these areas of expertise at the same time. A suitable combination of interdisciplinary and transdisciplinary teams will make the technology implementation process as efficient as possible.

This means that for successful implementation, it is necessary to involve all the professionals who will be using a technology with the athletes or players. They will need to have a good understanding of its use, methodological protocols, and the most relevant metrics they can use for (quick or deep) feedback. From the staff perspective, technology should eliminate progressively manual tasks and facilitate an integrated process between the different disciplines. When experts from different areas share the use of a single tool (a training process or, in this case, a piece of software or equipment), the feeling of belonging to a group is enhanced, the sense of being part of a greater collective is present, communication of the same message (unification) is enhanced, and there are great opportunities for sharing knowledge and competencies.

Data Quality

The lack of validity of some devices, as well as the lack of transparency of some companies reporting technology validity, requires that the end user consider the following questions (8):

- How thoroughly has the technology been evaluated?
- How strong is the evidence to determine that the device or technology is producing the desired outcomes?
- How much evidence exists to determine that something other than this device is responsible for producing the desired outcomes?

It is the responsibility of the sport scientist to recognize, analyze, and guarantee certain aspects relating to the validity of a technology, such as the strength of evidence, the validation, and the validation against the gold standard (or not). It is also the sport scientist's responsibility to understand the metrics and the rigor with which they are processed or calculated (or both); it is important to know the measurement error of the technology. Knowing this makes it possible to differentiate between the changes in performance resulting from training and from measurement error. Finally, importantly, the information provided by the technology must be manageable and reliable and must contribute to the decision-making process.

If the aspects mentioned here are not in place, technology should not be implemented, because implementation can waste time and money, potentially misguiding training decisions and putting at risk the credibility and reputation of the staff or organization.

Data Analysis

It is not the purpose of this chapter to present an examination of the different possibilities in the analysis of the information (see part V of this book), but from the perspective of technology implementation, there are certain aspects to keep in mind. As Michael Lewis states, "[w]e are getting better building our models, but we have to be aware of the limitations of our models" (6). Models (data analysis) are simplifications of the world. This is not a weakness; it is just something to be aware of. The analysis should not be limited to simplified reports that give a single value (or color code) to answer a question as complex as the state of the athlete, which will be determined not only by the individual's physical-biological status, but also by psychological and social state (1). Therefore, it is important to know what can and cannot actually be measured, the interdependence between different measurements, and the importance of the different variables in the decision-making process.

A characteristic trait of metric fixation is the aspiration to replace judgment based on experience with standardized measurement. There are situations in which decision making based on standardized measurement is superior to judgment based on personal experiences and expertise, and situations in which measurement combined with judgment could yield the most valuable outcome. Michael Lewis writes in *The Undoing Project*, "[w]e have to figure out what the model is good and bad at, and what humans are good and bad at" (6).

Due to the unceasing list of technological devices available on the market, there is a need for a common space for storing the data so that it can be analyzed in an integrative way. A number of companies offer products that allow data warehousing. From a practical point of view, these databases must allow the incorporation of data as new devices are implemented; they should provide for easy data loading (importing) and downloading (exporting), and they should note how the data is processed and analyzed before reports are generated.

Data Delivery

The essential "click," the last piece of the puzzle, is the means of delivering and communicating the information gathered from the technology. The data have to have a meaningful impact on the program. For this, it is necessary not only to guarantee the aspects described earlier, but also to contemplate who the different consumers of the information are, the timing for reporting, the communication channels, and the report format and its visualization, to mention some of the most relevant considerations. If the results are not communicated effectively, the device vetting process, the systematic technology implementation, the data storage, and the data analysis will have been pointless, since these efforts will not have contributed to the decision-making process nor demonstrated the usefulness of the collected data to the player. For a more in-depth review, see chapters 21 and 31.

DATA SECURITY AND TECHNOLOGY

With the possibility of collecting all types of information, including biometric and medical data, government institutions should seek to enforce strict information security policies and regulations aimed at protecting the confidentiality and integrity of athlete data gathered from wearables. As an example, in 2017 the National Basketball Players Association

(NBPA) and the National Basketball Association (NBA) created a joint advisory committee called the Collective Bargaining Agreement (CBA), with the following aims:

1. Reviewing requests by teams, the NBA, or the NBPA to approve a wearable for use, with the evaluation based on whether the wearable would be potentially harmful to anyone and whether the wearable's functionality has been validated

2. Setting cybersecurity standards for the storage of data collected from approved wearables

Related to the latter consideration, policies should include security standards for aspects such as administrative access and user accounts, remote access controls, encryption and treatment of biometric data, servers and endpoint infrastructure controls, and web and cloud interface security or physical security. This type of regulation will help to guarantee data security both in the use of technologies and in the security of the information.

Finally, to what extent does the use of certain technology contribute to competitive performance? Also, is the use of a sport technology advantage unethical? With technological evolution, technological revolutions occur; with biometric and genetic manipulation or the evolution of AI, technology becomes the new ergogenic aid to human performance. With it comes the need for ethical guidelines if the application of innovative sport technology is going to become the norm (3).

CONCLUSION

Unquestionably, the use of technology presents a great opportunity to obtain information (knowledge) using devices that are less invasive, lighter, more precise, smaller, safer, and cheaper than ever before. Based on both subjective and objective data collected with multiple tools (technology), the sport scientist can now potentially provide great feedback to coaches about athlete health, well-being, and ultimately performance. However, the implementation of technology is also a challenge. It is imperative to understand the usefulness, specificity, validity, and reliability of the tools implemented. It is obligatory to keep in mind that if a large part of the decision-making process is based on the information collected using these devices, the decision makers had better make sure they work (12). Although many companies claim to be the "Holy Grail" for athletes' superior performance or the cessation of injuries, the secret weapon is the athletes themselves. Anything extra will help and support reaching that extra 1%, but it is not the panacea to optimal performance. It is imperative to communicate with athletes that the information collected with technology belongs to them, as well as to build trust in the use of technology and information management. From the point of view of sport scientists, they build trust when they know how to convey that the coaches drive the program and that the technology supports making better-informed decisions. The challenge for technology companies is to provide multiple, integrative, and synchronized sources of information. Finally, even if technology has the potential to revolutionize decision making, training programming, and injury management, it will never directly affect the outcome by itself; the people who make use of the technology will ultimately have that responsibility.

RECOMMENDED READING

Christensen, CM. *The Innovator's Dilemma: When New Technologies Cause Great Firms to Fail.* 1st ed. Boston: Harvard Business Review Press, 1997.

Doerr, J. *Measure What Matters. How Google, Bono, and the Gates Foundation Rock the World with OKRs.* New York: Portfolio/Penguin, 2018.

Muller, JZ. *The Tyranny of Metrics.* Princeton, NJ: Princeton University Press, 2018.

CHAPTER 8

Data Hygiene

Matthew C. Varley, PhD
Ric Lovell, PhD
David Carey, PhD

The sport science profession serves to support athletes and coaches to maximize performance. Science requires the collection and organization of information in a systematic manner to create knowledge. Application of the scientific method involves identifying important questions or problems to solve, studying available resources, collating information, and determining the meaning or worth of the data or both (i.e., **evaluation**). The scientific method is underpinned by the rigor of the information or data collected.

This chapter serves as a guide for those who collect, analyze, interpret, and handle data in sport. It provides information on important aspects related to data hygiene, including the validity, reliability, and filtering of data. Further, it outlines best practices that can be adopted to maintain data integrity.

MANAGING DATA

Sport scientists commonly assess and monitor performance characteristics using objective information (e.g., distance, time, force, event frequencies), that is, empirical and verifiable data considered to reflect facts and unbiased by individual prejudice. Perhaps for the first time in the short history of sport science, technology proliferation means that the modern-day sport scientist is faced with the added challenge of prioritizing and filtering the overwhelming availability of objective data to inform decision making. This so-called data tsunami has evolved the requisite skill sets of budding sport scientists (11), who are now expected to demonstrate competence in data management, analytics, visualization, and communication (i.e., reporting). Indeed, the *Moneyball* phenomenon has led to the widespread recruitment of other professionals such as economists and data scientists into the sport science domain, providing expertise in objective data analysis for performance evaluation and solutions. In this highly desirable and saturated labor market, a unique selling point for sport scientists is their understanding of what needs to be measured and how data should be collected.

In this chapter **data hygiene** refers to the practices undertaken to ensure minimal error in the collection and storage of data. Given the large amount of data now available, data hygiene is of the utmost importance to sport scientists to ensure that decision making is based on high-quality data. The dynamic and evolving field of athlete performance presents several challenges that must be considered by sport scientists and all practitioners who deal with data used to support the athlete.

One challenge faced by sport practitioners is the management and integration of data collected from different sources. Interdisciplinary communication is essential in sport. Within the sporting environment, support staff can include coaches, sport scientists, strength and conditioning coaches, psychologists, nutritionists, physiotherapists, and physicians, all of whom will be collecting their own data. This data may come in various forms, including video, survey, medical, physiological, and technical, to name a few. Furthermore, all staff members may have their own way of recording and storing data, ranging from inputting data into a spreadsheet to writing notes on a sheet of paper.

Care must be taken to collate, clean, and maintain the integrity of the data. The ability to interpret data from each discipline in both an isolated and an integrated manner facilitates successful communication and provides holistic athlete support.

In the sporting domain, a challenge is presented by the rapid rate of development and uptake of technology. Increasingly sophisticated data is available to sport scientists; however, the value of this data must be understood and the limitations of its validity and reliability tested. Indeed, there is often a lag between the release of new technology and external validation studies (9). This is further complicated by the vast range of options for data filtering and processing, which is often not made clear to the user by technology manufacturers.

Another common risk pertaining to data hygiene is the fact that the individual who analyzes or interprets the data may not be the individual who collected the data. In many cases, data collection is performed by interns, university students, volunteers, or junior staff members. It is therefore critical that best practices for data hygiene be trained and implemented among all staff involved in data collection within the sporting environment.

Validity

Validity is the "degree to which a test or instrument measures what it purports to measure" (30). A sport scientist must be an expert in measurement validity as it pertains to athletic performance and monitoring. This is essential because the wealth of data now available needs to be understood so that the right data can be used to inform meaningful decisions.

The field of measurement validity is comprehensive; however, there are different types of validity, which becomes confusing as terms are used interchangeably in different occupational fields. A concise overview of measurement validity as it pertains to sport science is provided here, but readers are directed to several comprehensive resources for more in-depth information (30). Logical, face, and content validity each refer to rather obvious desirable characteristics of a measurement; that is, does the measure assess the performance trait or physiological response in question? Logical and face validity may be considered interchangeable terms, whereas content validity pertains exclusively to educational settings; for example, a midterm examination in sport biomechanics that tests knowledge and understanding of the curriculum delivered in the course (rather than a different topic,

e.g., human nutrition) would be an assessment tool that possesses inherent content validity. Two of the most relevant features of sport science measurement validity are criterion and construct.

Criterion validity is established when a measure shows a strong relationship to a gold standard (or criterion) assessment technique. Criterion validity is highly prevalent in sport sciences because practitioners are often interested in transforming rigorous laboratory-based measures into field environments in a pragmatic (feasible) way. Consider the criterion measure of aerobic capacity: maximal oxygen uptake ($\dot{V}O_2$max). Under known and standardized environmental conditions, volumes of expired air and the proportions of oxygen and carbon dioxide are measured as an athlete incrementally increases the exercise intensity, until volitional exhaustion. Careful evaluation of the data can identify velocities associated with transitions between different exercise intensity domains (i.e., mild, moderate, high, severe) and can be used to both benchmark the athlete and inform characteristics of the subsequent training process. The laboratory assessment is rigorous, but resource-intensive (equipment, expertise, time), and therefore not always feasible when one is dealing with a number of athletes. Accordingly, a wide variety of field-based, pragmatic estimates of aerobic capacity have been developed (e.g., Université de Montréal track test [20], multistage fitness [beep] test [21]). In providing evidence to support their criterion validity, researchers demonstrated strong associations between performance outcomes of these field tests (e.g., distance, speed, predicted $\dot{V}O_2$max) versus laboratory-determined $\dot{V}O_2$max (3, 20, 21). When evaluating the criterion validity of a new technology or measurement protocol, the modality of the criterion measure should be considered, and a thorough understanding of the relevant measurement principles is paramount.

When a strong relationship is observed for assessments of criterion validity, the sport scientist should then consider the magnitude of any differences between the surrogate and criterion measure. Using the aforementioned aerobic capacity example, the multistage fitness test estimates of $\dot{V}O_2$max were shown to be strongly associated with that derived from criterion laboratory assessments ($r = 0.81$), but the running velocity associated with this capacity was underestimated by approximately 3 km/h (3). The lower velocity is due to the repeated accelerations, decelerations, and changes of direction during shuttle running, but would arguably have substantial implications for programming subsequent training to maximize aerobic capacity.

Interpretation of the relevance of any differences presents a challenge to the potential user. Null hypothesis significance testing may determine if any difference is statistically significant, but this result relies heavily upon the size of the sample in the validity study and fails to consider what the end user or expert may determine as a practically worthwhile difference. Another approach used in sport science is to contrast the differences (or bias) with standardized thresholds of the between-athlete standard deviation of the outcome variable (normally taken from the criterion, or a baseline measure [2]). A novel and perhaps more attractive solution has been proposed (19) in testing the criterion validity of a Global Positioning System (GPS) for determining the peak velocity achieved during maximal sprint tests. The researchers first surveyed industry experts to inform their criteria for the acceptable degree of measurement error, contrasting this expert opinion with the measured difference in velocity between the surrogate (10-Hz GPS) versus the criterion measure (radar). This approach of defining satisfactory agreement in advance is strongly recommended since statistical analyses alone are unable to determine whether the magnitude can affect practitioner judgment or interpretation (4).

Irrespective of the analytical approach used to evaluate the magnitude and meaningfulness between-measurement differences in criterion validity studies, the relationship between bias and measurement range should be inspected. Plotting the individual measurement differences against their mean value is a useful and simple graphical method to visually investigate any relationship. Figure 8.1 depicts agreement data from a study evaluating a new measurement technique to collect ratings of perceived exertion (RPE), in which the numerical values were blinded from the athletes using a bespoke application (22a). In this example, the differences between the numerically blinded ratings versus the traditional verbal-report approach are uniform (systematic) across the RPE measurement range. In this situation, the sport scientist can adopt the new measurement tool by simply adjusting for the bias (here, 0.2 arbitrary unit mean difference). Where an association is present between the difference and the magnitude, further statistical investigation maybe warranted (e.g., Pearson product-moment correlation coefficient, or the nonparametric equivalent Spearman's rank correlation) (see chapter 18), and the sport scientist has the option to either consider data transformations (4) or elect not to use the new measurement tool.

Construct validity applies to any measurement domain in which a direct criterion measure is unavailable. One of the most widely studied areas in sport science is the construct validity of measures of athlete training load. In particular, RPE has emerged as an accurate and easily accessible estimate of an athlete's psychobiological response to an activity (exercise)

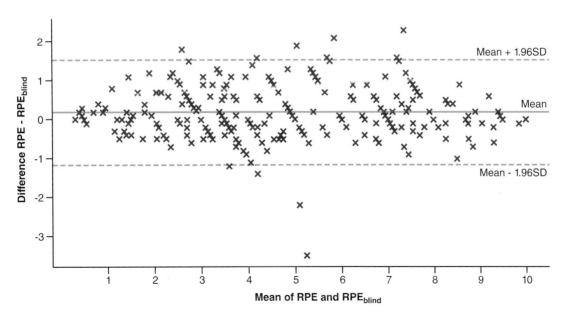

FIGURE 8.1 Visualization of between-method agreement.

Reprinted by permission from R. Lovell et al (2020).

stimulus. These ratings are subjective in nature, and they reflect holistic sensations integrated from signals originating in working muscles and joints and cardiorespiratory and central nervous systems (5). The numerical value presented by the athlete can be multiplied by the session duration to provide a training impulse (13). In examining the validity of this new and simple measure of training load, the researchers did not have a single criterion measure that represented the holistic biological and psychological sensations of the athletes, so criterion validity could not be examined. Instead, the researchers considered the theoretical framework in which the principle of the measurement belonged. If athlete RPE could be used as a measure of exercise intensity or training load or both, it could be expected to be related to other physiological responses (e.g., heart rate, oxygen cost, blood lactate accumulation) or measures of work (e.g., distance traveled, power output, velocity). Indeed, a number of studies have provided evidence of the construct validity of RPE as a measure of exercise intensity (6, 24) and training load (1, 17) in this fashion.

Concurrent validity of a measurement tool can be tested in a range of different ways, considering theoretically informed contexts in which the measured attribute would be expected to "behave." In sport science, these contexts might include, but are not limited to, the responses to fatigue, discriminating between athlete performance standards, identification of changes in fitness characteristics, and relationships to similar construct indices of performance. Therefore, establishing the construct validity of a new tool often requires a series of investigations to holistically evaluate whether the measurement behaves as expected in a holistic range of relevant contexts.

Technology advances and availability often precede independent validity studies. Moreover, in many performance environments (e.g., professional team sports), the sport scientist often coordinates a number of athlete tracking and assessment tools, synthesizing the information in a timely fashion for coach and athlete feedback and to inform characteristics of the next athletic development or preparation event (i.e., training, competition, recovery). In this environment, practical features of new technologies or software systems (i.e., athletic management systems) such as usability, workflow, and visualization may be valued more highly than the validity of the tool and its adherence to measurement principles. There are instances in sport science, particularly for self-report tools such as RPE and wellness, when athlete management systems have deviated from original measurement principles (15, 25), seemingly without the necessary validity checks and balances. For other tools, accuracy of the data may be influenced by the user's interpretation and degree of knowledge, training, and experience of the measurement (strength coach, athletic trainer, technical coach, sport science intern). These numerous challenges present a dilemma for the practicing sport scientist, whose role is to apply the scientific method to athletic performance, as constantly changing environmental factors and rapidly evolving hardware and software inhibit the application of systematic inquiry. Considering the rapid pace of technological development and proliferation in relation to the pace of the peer-review process, coupled with the heavily nuanced nature of performance environments, the modern-day sport scientist ought to take accountability for in-house validation of athletic assessment and monitoring procedures.

Reliability

While this chapter has addressed validity before reliability, reliability is the pillar of measurement precision; a test or instrument cannot be considered valid if it is not also reliable. **Reliability** refers to the consistency of a measure, often determined by the test–retest method, in which the assessment is performed two or more times within an appropriate time window. In research studies, the investigators use caution in standardizing the test conditions in an attempt to limit the impact of any extraneous factors acting upon the derived test result. These factors may originate from the measurement instrumentation, the environment or situation, the test administrator, or the participant being assessed.

Consider the example of tracking neuromuscular function to measure motor recovery following competition, often assessed using the countermovement jump (CMJ). In assessing the reliability of this test, the sport scientist invites athletes to perform the CMJ on two separate occasions separated, for example, by a week. The test–retest schedule may be designed to mimic the characteristics of the potential application, with 7 days ample to enable complete recovery from the test itself, but not so long as to invite potential performance changes due to training or detraining adaptation. Other athlete error sources between the two assessments (often known as biological error) might include such factors as the training schedule in the prior 72 hours, apparel, diurnal variation, warm-up characteristics, nutrition, sleep, hydration, experience of the test, and motivation. The sport scientist can take steps to limit the influence of these error terms by taking further measurements before the test, familiarizing the athlete, inquiring with the athlete, and developing repeatable pretest procedures. The CMJ can be performed indoors, which may address any weather-related environmental effects, but the immediate surroundings and particularly who else may be present (e.g., peers, coaches, etc.) could influence performance. The sport scientist ensures that the same jump mat or force plate is used between repeated assessments, undertakes the appropriate equipment calibrations, and ensures consistent assessment criteria (i.e., number of repetitions, inter-effort recovery, instructions and technique, motivational statements), but other sources of technical error (e.g., device limitations, signal or sensor drift) can be difficult to identify and quantify. Assuming that the same software and hardware are used throughout, human error in judging performance can be avoided for the CMJ, but it may be a cause for concern in other common sport science measurements such as event coding, anthropometry, or movement screening. The wealth of potential biological and technical sources of error may collectively create substantial noise in the measurement, making it difficult to detect true changes in test performance (signal). While research studies are rigorously designed and administered to reduce measurement noise and determine the true consistency of a measurement tool, their artificial nature may preclude translation of findings into routine industry practice.

Consideration of the unique characteristics of the performance environment and the rapid evolution in sport technology, reliability judgments cannot be formed exclusively from peer-reviewed research publications. Moreover, measurement consistency can often vary between individual athletes. Accordingly, application of the scientific method in-house can assist the practitioner in making informed and evidenced-based performance decisions. Sport science delivery rarely has the luxury of undertaking reliability assessments with high-performance athletes, especially when a number of different measurements are collected to holistically track athlete development or preparedness or both. Determining athletic performance capacities requires maximal effort from the athlete, a cost that ought to be carefully evaluated against the value-added of the information gleaned from the assessment. Therefore, capacity testing may be rarely scheduled at a sufficient frequency to enable the sport scientist to ascertain an accurate gauge of test consistency. In situations in which repeated maximal capacity tests can be administered, there are often threats to consistency of the assessment (e.g., environment, preparedness, scheduling, motivation). This uncertainty in determining true athletic capacities may have a profound impact upon subsequent exercise programming and necessitates consideration when one is evaluating results.

Perhaps owing to the challenges of determining reliability for physical capacity assessments in the high-performance environment, routine athlete monitoring in sport science has grown considerably. This trend has been facilitated by the proliferation and miniaturization of wearable technologies, but the approach facilitates more frequent touch-points with the athletes. This may create the potential to determine a true measurement signal, but the high-performance environment is rarely stable. Competition scheduling and travel requirements present challenges to consistency. For example, wellness ratings or tests of neuromuscular function and heart rate recovery are often used to evaluate recovery postcompetition, but their timing may differ considerably according to the event and training schedule, profoundly affecting the outcome measures and any subsequent assessment of test consistency. In contrast, while a high degree of consistency is desirable to identify true changes, frequently administered self-report measures (e.g., wellness, RPE) may lead to clustering, or a degree of stability that may render the measurement tool insensitive to the true dose–response to exercise stimuli (35). Objective monitoring tools such as tracking technologies (e.g., GPS, semiautomated tracking), heart rate variability, and inertial sensors (accelerometers) are less susceptible to athlete bias and potential clustering, but their metrics often suffer from a high degree of variability due to a range of situational factors (14), creating a degree of noise that makes it difficult to interpret meaningful changes.

In determining the test–retest reliability, repeated measurements taken from a group of athletes should be correlated with each other. If the previous example of CMJ assessment of neuromuscular function is reliable (consistent), the athlete with the highest jump height should perform well on any number of repeated observations, under the same assessment conditions. For reliability, the intraclass correlation coefficient is used to examine the consistency of the athlete's rank order, in which values greater than 0.90 are considered high, from 0.80 to 0.89 moderate, and below 0.80 questionable (32). However, for athletic populations with particularly homogenous results, or when the number of athletes tested is low, the correlation coefficient may be low, and should be interpreted with caution.

To quantify the random error that may be observed in repeated test observations, the most widely used statistic is known as the **typical error**, reflecting each athlete's variation (standard deviation) between test results while accounting for any systematic group differences. This value encompasses any of the sources of error identified earlier, and conceptually can be considered the typical noise in test results. The typical error can be quantified for a group of athletes but is particularly useful for monitoring meaningful changes in individual athletes over time. Again here, the outcome reliability statistics derived reflect the quality of the original data collected by the sport scientist. Data integrity and authenticity should be considered when one is evaluating reliability statistics; but in addition, the priority of the sport scientist is to facilitate (where pragmatic) test conditions that favor collection of the "true" value, thereby limiting potential sources of measurement error. (For further information regarding intraclass correlation coefficient and typical error, see the Hopkins article in "Recommended Readings" listed at the end of the chapter.)

As highlighted earlier in the discussion of measurement validity, expert opinion in conjunction with appropriate statistical tools is necessary to determine what might constitute a meaningful change. In the context of reliability, the **smallest worthwhile change** score can represent the signal that would affect the sport scientist's judgment or interpretation (see chapter 18), with typical error representing noise (16). If the noise in the test–retest CMJ result is less than the smallest meaningful signal, changes in jump performance can be detected with integrity. Unfortunately, this is not often the case in evaluation of human performance characteristics, and so any uncertainty is integral to both the process of evaluation and communication with athletes and coaches. When the magnitude of the signal and the noise are similar, the interpretation is more complex, and the user may require more repeated assessments or work to reduce sources of noise for the test to gain some practical utility (16). If the noise in the CMJ monitoring data is greater than the smallest worthwhile difference, the value added by the test is likely not worth the investment made by the athlete in performing the maximal test, the coach in adjusting the program schedule, and the sport scientist in setting up, testing, analyzing, evaluating, and communicating the results.

Where independent validity and reliability studies are published and available, skeptical sport scientists might ask themselves a number of questions before translating this new knowledge into their industry practice:

- Is the criterion measure or theoretical construct used to validate the technique appropriate and relevant for athletic purposes?
- Can the new knowledge created from the study's sample population be translated to my own sport science delivery context?
- Can I use the information gained from these field assessments to inform my practice? What subsequent impact will it have?
- Is this assessment logistically feasible for my performance environment?
- What factors might influence my interpretation of the results, and how can I operate proactively to limit bias or potential sources of error?

Filtering

In signal processing, a filter removes unnecessary information to reduce noise from a signal (23). **Filtering** can be applied to the many types of data that a sport scientist encounters; however, the most common is data derived from wearable sensors, motion capture systems, force plates, and other electronic sport technologies. These technologies detect a signal that is recorded and stored as data. Data that is unprocessed is typically referred to as **raw data**. Often the signal is subject to certain degrees of noise, which makes analysis and interpretation of the raw data difficult. The raw data can be processed or filtered to reduce any unwanted noise. This filtered data can then be analyzed to produce an output (an abstract representation of the signal). For example, a GPS can be used to detect satellite signals that are translated into raw velocity data. A filter such as a Kalman filter is then applied to smooth the velocity data. The smoothed velocity data can then be analyzed to produce an output or metric (e.g., distance covered at different running speeds or the number of sprint efforts performed). These metrics are then used by the sport scientist to inform athlete performance. Many different filter types can be applied to data, which may include exponential, Kalman, Butterworth, median, and Fourier. It is beyond the scope of this chapter to cover each filter in detail; however, many references are available to describe filtering techniques (33). This section briefly highlights the challenges associated with data filtering faced by sport scientists.

For several reasons, it is important that sport scientists be aware of the type of filtering that is being applied to the data they are collecting. Updates to hardware, firmware, or software may result in changes to the data filters being applied (8, 31). This can affect the metrics that are reported; for example, updates to GPS software were found to substantially decrease the number of acceleration (251 vs. 177) and deceleration (181 vs. 151) efforts being reported in football games (8). Some manufacturer software allows the user to choose the type of filtering that is applied or allows the user to select options that may automatically process their data in a specific manner. The implications of these options may not always be clear to the user, so it is important to understand how these decisions will change the data-filtering techniques. For example, figure 8.2 shows how data can change with use of different filtering techniques to derive acceleration from velocity (31). Finally, if sport scientists choose to filter the raw data themselves, it is important that they understand the types of filters available and the implications these will have on the metrics.

By understanding the effect that different filters have on their data, sport scientists can confidently compare their metrics to normative data, scientific literature, and their own longitudinal data. An understanding of the filtering that has been applied may assist with the interpretation of any large discrepancies or similarities between data sets.

An ever-growing number of metrics are available to sport scientists. A single type of technology may produce over 100 different metrics. This is further complicated by the fact that metrics vary between technologies, manufacturers, brands, and with software updates. Further, while these technologies provide their own metrics, many also allow sport scientists to produce their own custom metrics.

The challenge faced by sport scientists is that not all manufacturers disclose details around the data-filtering techniques that are being applied to their technology, often because this is considered intellectual property (22). Additionally, access to raw data may not be available, or the "raw" data that is available has already undergone prefiltering. This lack of

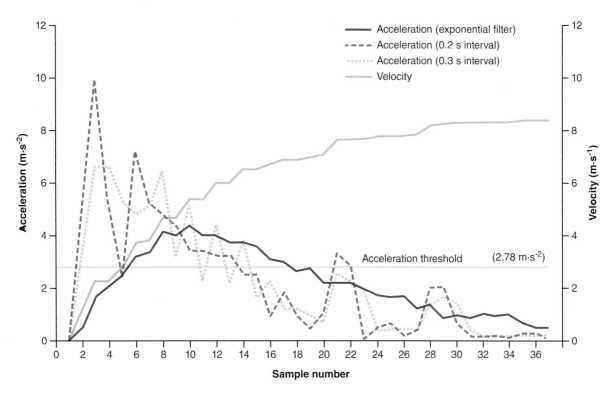

FIGURE 8.2 Global Positioning System velocity and acceleration data during a 40-meter sprint effort. The graph demonstrates how data can change with the use of different filtering techniques to derive acceleration from velocity. Techniques include deriving acceleration using a 0.2-second and 0.3-second interval and an exponential filter. The threshold used to identify an acceleration effort is indicated by the line running parallel to the x-axis at 2.78 m·s⁻².

transparency can have far-reaching implications for the interpretation, replication, and external validation of this data.

Sport scientists should understand and record information on the filtering techniques that are applied (by themselves or manufacturers) to their data. This information can be used to monitor changes in filtering techniques over time and to communicate filtering practices in their team and to the broader sport science community. Sport scientists should apply a consistent filtering method within a given season or period of time when comparing data to ensure that any observed changes are due to true change rather than changes in filtering technique. Sport scientists should perform due diligence with the metrics they decide to use, ensuring that they are meaningful and that the issues of validity and reliability discussed in the previous sections have been addressed.

MAINTAINING DATA INTEGRITY

Data integrity refers to the consistency, completeness, and accuracy of data, and it is an essential component at all stages of data collection, storage, processing, and analysis (18, 28). Common issues in sport science such as combining data from different sources, inconsistent labeling conventions, and uncertain filtering operations can compromise data integrity (27). The following sections provide recommendations and practices for maintaining data integrity when one is collecting, storing, and analyzing sport science data.

Central to maintaining data integrity is the concept of a reproducible data workflow. A **reproducible workflow** is one with enough detailed information that another person can exactly replicate it (i.e., could get the same output or results given the same input data) (26, 29). This property is important because it allows sport scientists to retrace their steps if they suspect an error has been introduced somewhere in the workflow. Figure 8.3 shows an example of a reproducible data workflow. Any operations applied to the data are clearly documented at each stage, and new versions of the data are saved to prevent overwriting the raw data (which would break reproducibility and prevent the sport scientist from correcting any error earlier in the chain).

Creating a data dictionary is a valuable step for any sport scientist collecting or analyzing data (7, 12). The **data dictionary** contains the definitions of all variables collected, as well as any naming or coding conventions. An example of a spreadsheet and data dictionary is shown in figure 8.4. A comprehensive data dictionary has many benefits (7, 12). It removes ambiguity if multiple people are collecting data that may have different naming conventions (e.g., a resistance training database in which a coach labels an exercise as "squat" and another as "back squat"), and it creates a permanent record of what is in the data, allowing for historical data to remain useful. The process of making a data dictionary before commencing data collection ensures a consistent approach to data collection from the start of a project and can help identify external or environmental variables that may be relevant to collect (e.g., weather conditions for outdoor field-testing data collection).

Data Storage

Saving and storing data or results is a necessary task at multiple stages in a reproducible data workflow (29) and can be accomplished in a variety of ways (see figure 8.3). Database management system (DBMS) software (such as MySQL, Microsoft Access, or MongoDB) may be required for large or complicated data sets, or if data needs to be shared among multiple users simultaneously (34). A DBMS forces the user to predefine the database structure (i.e., what variables will be collected and how they relate to each other) and has built-in controls that protect the integrity of the data (34). Sport-specific data management platforms (often referred to as athlete management systems) have emerged to address the increasing amount of data collection in sport. These platforms provide data integrity benefits similar to other DBMS but are also designed specifically for commonly collected sport data such as athlete wellness questionnaires or GPS movement data.

For small data sets, storing data in spreadsheets is a viable alternative (7, 12). Spreadsheet software such as Microsoft Excel does not enforce the same data integrity standards as a DBMS, so the sport scientist needs to be aware of the common pitfalls of storing data in Excel spreadsheets (7, 10, 12). Examples of poor and effective spreadsheet designs are shown in figure 8.5. Principles of good spreadsheet design include the following (7):

- Each sheet has a column containing a unique ID code referencing the participant. This allows integration of data collected from different sources (12). For example, merging a wellness and sleep monitoring database is straightforward if both contain a common player ID and date variable.

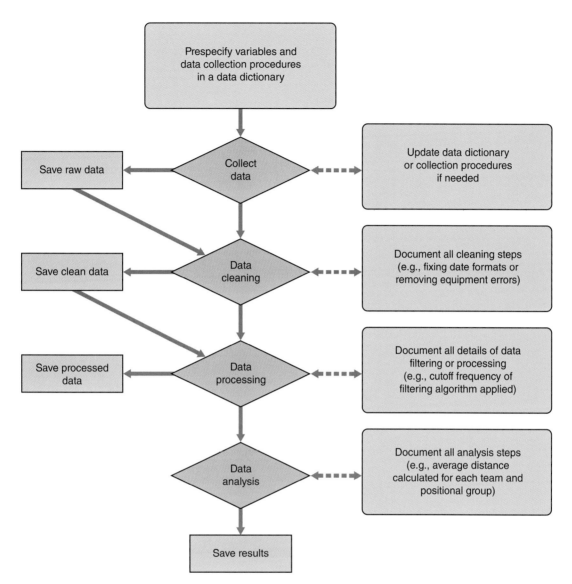

FIGURE 8.3 Documented and reproducible data workflow.

- Column names should not include spaces or special characters (e.g., *, #, $) and should not span multiple lines.
- Avoid any empty cells, columns, or rows. Missing values should be identified by a consistent convention such as N/A or NULL.
- Do not apply calculations, cell merging, or syntax highlighting to raw data files. This will prevent potentially overwriting the raw data and breaking the reproducible workflow. It will also make importing the data into analysis software such as R, Python, or SPSS more seamless.

Storing unstructured data such as images, video, or free text is a potential challenge for the sport scientist because these forms of data are not naturally storable in spreadsheet form. An effective alternative is to use a consistent filing format and create a spreadsheet containing the relevant metadata. For example, a video database of match footage could be stored and managed using a file system and accompanying meta-database as shown in figure 8.6.

It is also advisable to create backups of each different version of the data (raw, cleaned, and processed). This has become convenient and inexpensive with

	A	B	C	D	E	F
1						
2	ID	Date	Sport	Sex	Height	Weight
3	567943	04/03/2017	A	1	166	62
4	616852	22/05/2017	A	0	190	87
5						
6	186451	22/05/2017	A	0	184	79
7	168321	14/11/2017	B	1	172	76
8						

	A	B	C	D	E	F
1						
2		Variable	Definition			
3		ID	Unique identification code (6-digit)			
4		Date	Date that measurements were taken (Format: dd/mm/yyyy)			
5		Sport	Sport played by participant (A: hockey; B: basketball)			
6						
7		Sex	Sex of participant (0: male; 1: female)			
8		Height	Height of participant (cm) taken without shoes			
9		Weight	Weight of participant (kg) taken without shoes			
10						

FIGURE 8.4 Sample data set and accompanying data dictionary.

cloud-based services such as Dropbox, Google Drive, and Amazon Web Services.

Data Cleaning

Data cleaning is a necessary and important step before one analyzes or draws conclusions based on experimental data. Despite implementation of safeguards such as data dictionaries and consistent test procedures, it is still likely that any data collected will have some errors that need to be cleaned. Common things to look for in data cleaning include the following (27):

- *Consistent naming conventions.* Ideally all categorical data should have naming conventions prespecified in a data dictionary. However, it is common to see different terms used to refer to the same thing in data sets (e.g., "training" vs. "main training" vs. "Training" in a load monitoring data set). Similarly, it is important that all missing values be identified by the same flag.

- *Non-unique ID variables.* It is common to see participant names or initials used as an ID variable in sport science databases. This can cause issues if two people have the same name because the ID variable is no longer unique and cannot be used to properly merge data sets.

- *Date formats.* These are notorious sources of data cleaning issues. It is advisable to use the "DD/MM/YYYY" format (7). Storing dates in Microsoft Excel has compatibility issues between Windows and Mac computers that can be avoided if date columns are formatted as plain text (7).

- *Outliers.* These can be difficult to detect in some data; however, sport science data is typically collected from human participants, so some commonsense rules around physiologically plausible values can be applied (e.g., heights above 3 meters [3.3 yd] or running speeds above 20 m/s can be safely labelled as errors). Objective outlier detection rules (e.g., values more than 3 standard

	Player	Test 1 Date	Test 1 50 m sprint time (s)	Test 2 Date	Test 2 50 m sprint time (s)	Test 3 Date	Test 3 50 m sprint time (s)	Test 4 Date	Test 4 50 m sprint time (s)
		Test 1		**Test 2**		**Test 3**		**Test 4**	
6	J.Smith	17/02/2018	8.86	18/04/2018	7.29	18/08/2018	6.57	12/12/2018	6.86
7	S.Ford	14/03/2018	6.55	07/05/2018	injured	20/07/2018	6.44	06/03/2019	8.53
8	J.Brown	26/01/2018	6.79	16/04/2018	6.76	12/06/2018	7.76	23/03/2019	N/A
9	K.Adams	18/03/2018	7.60	12/05/2018	7.95	07/08/2018	missing	05/01/2019	6.38

	A Player	B ID_code	C Date	D Test_number	E Time_50m_sec	F Injured
2	J.Smith	P008	17/02/2018	1	8.86	0
3	S.Ford	P042	14/03/2018	1	6.55	0
4	J.Brown	P164	26/01/2018	1	6.79	0
5	K.Adams	P013	18/03/2018	1	7.60	0
6	J.Smith	P008	18/04/2018	2	7.29	0
7	S.Ford	P042	07/05/2018	2	NA	1
8	J.Brown	P164	16/04/2018	2	6.76	0
9	K.Adams	P013	12/05/2018	2	7.95	0
10	J.Smith	P008	18/08/2018	3	6.57	0
11	S.Ford	P042	20/07/2018	3	6.44	0
12	J.Brown	P164	12/06/2018	3	7.76	0
13	K.Adams	P013	07/08/2018	3	NA	0
14	J.Smith	P008	12/12/2018	4	6.86	0
15	S.Ford	P042	06/03/2019	4	8.53	0
16	J.Brown	P164	23/03/2019	4	NA	0
17	K.Adams	P013	05/01/2019	4	6.38	0

FIGURE 8.5 Example of *(a)* poor spreadsheet design for data collection and *(b)* effective spreadsheet design. Figure 8.5*a* contains merged cells (nonrectangular data), repeated column headings, non-unique row labels, unnecessary empty cells and formatting, column headings that start with numbers, and an inconsistent convention for identifying missing data. Figure 8.5*b* contains all of the same raw data but is in a format that can easily be imported into any data analysis software platform.

Name

- game-20180409.mp4
- game-20180421.mp4
- game-20180719.mp4
- game-20180811.mp4
- game-20181109.mp4
- game-20190127.mp4

File	Date_collected	Home_team	Away_team	Rain	Temperature	Time	Indoor
/home/Users/NSCA/Videos/game-20180409.mp4	09/04/2018	A	B	Y	20	19:00	N
/home/Users/NSCA/Videos/game-20180421.mp4	21/04/2018	C	A	N	15	15:00	Y
/home/Users/NSCA/Videos/game-20180719.mp4	19/07/2018	D	B	Y	31	15:00	N
/home/Users/NSCA/Videos/game-20180811.mp4	11/08/2018	B	C	Y	22	19:00	N
/home/Users/NSCA/Videos/game-20181109.mp4	09/11/2018	A	C	N	28	15:00	Y
/home/Users/NSCA/Videos/game-20190127.mp4	27/01/2019	C	D	N	19	19:00	N

FIGURE 8.6 Data storage and management system for unstructured video data.

deviations from the mean) can be helpful for flagging observations for further investigation but should not be used to immediately remove data or label it as erroneous. Data cleaning should be performed in a reproducible scripting language or clearly documented so that the steps can be followed and repeated exactly. For example, if some testing results have been removed from the data due to clear equipment malfunction, they should be explicitly documented so that another person can retrace the steps taken and arrive at the same cleaned data set. Importantly, cleaned data should not replace the raw data and should be saved in a separate location (29) (see figure 8.3).

CONCLUSION

The availability of data in sport continues to grow exponentially. The magnitude and complexity of this data requires sport scientists and all sport practitioners to have a greater level of data competency than ever before. Data can come from multiple sources; it changes rapidly as technology advances, and it must be communicated to many users. Considerations around data validity and reliability are of key concern to ensure that meaningful data is collected. Once data is collected, appropriate methods for filtering, cleaning, and storing must be determined and documented to maintain data integrity.

Sport scientists should ensure that they understand and can educate others as to the best practices of data hygiene. Decisions related to measurement selection, data collection, data filtering, and cleaning and storage should be made in a manner that is transparent and can be repeated by other sport scientists. Sport scientists should develop a strong culture of documenting and reporting among their colleagues in an effort to facilitate accurate comparisons across data sets over time and maintain a high level of data hygiene.

RECOMMENDED READINGS

Bland, JM, and Altman, DG. Measuring agreement in method comparison studies. *Stat Methods Med Res* 8:135-160, 1999.

Broman, KW, and Woo, KH. Data organization in spreadsheets. *Am Stat* 72:2-10, 2018.

Ellis, SE, and Leek, JT. How to share data for collaboration. *Am Stat* 72:53-57, 2018.

Hopkins, WG. How to interpret changes in an athletic performance test. *Sportscience* 8:1-7, 2004. www.sportsci.org/jour/04/wghtests.htm.

Malone, JJ, Lovell, R, Varley, MC, and Coutts, AJ. Unpacking the black box: applications and considerations for using GPS devices in sport. *Int J Sports Physiol Perform* 12:S218-S226, 2017.

Rahm, E, and Hai Do, H. Data cleaning: problems and current approaches. *IEEE Data Eng Bull* 23:3-13, 2000.

PART IV

External and Internal Load Data Collection

CHAPTER 9

Characteristics of Tracking Systems and Load Monitoring

Jo Clubb, MSc
Andrew M. Murray, PhD

Objectively capturing the time–motion activity profiles of athletes underpins a range of applications for the sport science practitioner. These require understanding the physical demands of practice and competition; stratifying these demands across playing positions, competition levels, age groups, and genders; and tracking athletes' loads over time.

Over time, the analysis of workload profiles within athletic populations has been a growth industry. The first objective motion analysis of soccer was published in 1976 by Professor Tom Reilly (45). That study involved a manual coded notation system of a single player's motion that was later validated with video analysis (45). Since then, improvements in technology have enabled the collection of such information for entire teams simultaneously, in a more time-efficient manner (see figure 9.1). Generally, options for tracking athletes fall into one of two categories, positional systems and wearable microsensors, both of which are covered in this chapter.

CHARACTERISTICS

Given the increase in tracking technologies available, it is pertinent that researchers and applied sport scientists understand the characteristics and interpretation of data from such systems to inform analysis and programming. The main characteristics and advantages and disadvantages of each are outlined in the following sections.

Optical Tracking

Optical tracking (OT) is characterized by the use of multiple cameras around the playing environment that record the positions of objects (which may include the athletes, referees, and the playing objects), infer the x- and y-coordinates of athletes, and create a two-dimensional reconstruction of movement patterns. These systems are constructed to ensure that at least two cameras cover every area of the playing surface for accuracy and resilience, with the separate outputs retrospectively combined into a single data set (19). The precise configuration of the number and location of cameras is dependent on the particular technology used and the venue in which it is employed.

Machine learning and computer vision techniques can then be applied to the raw data to calculate location information (37). Initially, these systems were only semiautomated, with quality control operators required to identify each player and verify trajectories (19). Such camera tracking systems, developed in the late 1990s, provided a leap forward since for the first time they enabled the simultaneous tracking of every player, the referee, and the ball throughout the whole game (13). Initially systems were deployed in soccer and rugby in open-air stadiums, but OT solutions are now found across an array of sports. Uptake has been increased by the emergence of indoor tracking solutions, necessary for sports such as basketball, ice hockey, handball, volleyball, and racket sports.

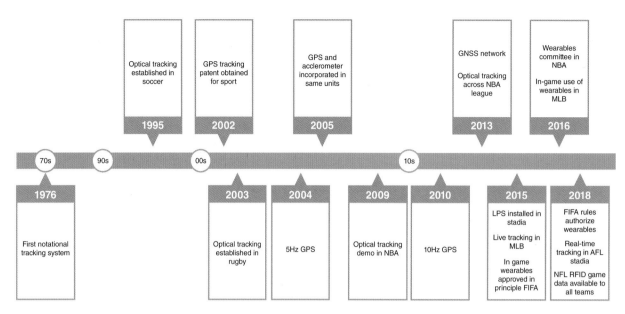

FIGURE 9.1 Timeline of highlighted developments in athlete tracking.

Due to regulations preventing the use of wearable technology in some sports or competitions, along with the desire to implement a noninvasive solution, optical solutions are appealing for athlete tracking. However, certain semiautomated multi-camera systems require 24 to 36 hours after the game to complete data processing. In contrast, some systems are now able to provide real-time solutions due to enhanced video processing and the development of mathematical algorithms first used in the military (13).

Nevertheless, disadvantages remain because OT systems can be costly and lack portability, with the installation of fixed cameras and a dedicated computer network required at the stadium, arena, or facility (19). Currently OT systems can generally be used only in competition since in order to function effectively the automation procedure requires an event such as a game or a match (i.e., composed of two halves or four quarters depending on the sport). This can necessitate the use of multiple systems per week to monitor performance. Moreover, the OT system may not connect to fixtures in away facilities. If the team plays at a location where the system is not installed, or if the opposing team (or the league as a whole) does not use the same OT provider, no data is collected for that game, or it is collected using other methods and cannot be directly compared with data from the home OT system. Therefore, teams may not acquire data when playing away from home. In addition, OT collects information in only two dimensions; thus, changes in vertical position (e.g., jumping demands)

are not quantified (52). Optical tracking systems are, however, capable of tracking the ball in team sports and can provide tactical information to coaches and athletes in addition to physical metrics.

Radio Frequency Identification

An alternative positional system is based on **radio frequency technology** (RFID). RFID was developed in a variety of civilian and military industries that require a precise means for tracking indoor position (2). This technology has since been applied to sport and evolved, from chips worn in shoelaces or straps around the ankle for mass running events, to tags typically worn on the upper body that are now mandated in some professional team-sport competitions (55). This system is characterized by antennae or anchor nodes positioned around the playing environment, which interact with the microchip transmitters worn by the athletes. The reception time between the transmitter and antennae is synchronized and used to determine location, with the data immediately processed by a central computer and made available for analysis (13).

Some have declared that such electronic transmitting devices are the future of sport performance analysis due to advances in accuracy and processing speed (14). One system, for example, enables positional measurements at over 100 Hz along with the integration of heart rate data and synchronization with video (13). An indoor positional tracking system, particularly with real-time data processing that enables immediate analysis, is an attractive technology to many sporting applications and organizations. Likewise, this technology may provide solutions for outdoor sports by overcoming issues such as changes in illumination quality with OT (13) and satellite signal connection in built-up stadiums with the Global Positioning System (36). Indeed, the performance of RFID has been demonstrated to be comparable in indoor and outdoor venues (47). However, RFID technology may be disadvantaged by susceptibility to potential electronic interference and signal instability, as well as the costs to install and to maintain a dedicated infrastructure (2). Furthermore, similar limitations to OT solutions exist with RFID, including a lack of portability due to static base stations and the restriction of data to two dimensions, though multiple anchor nodes at various heights can provide information in three dimensions (i.e., *x*-, *y*-, and *z*-coordinates). Unless the playing implement (e.g., ball, racket, bat) is also instrumented, it is difficult to provide tactical information via RFID systems unless it is supplemented with video technology to give contextual information.

Research has emerged on a particular type of RFID technology that may overcome some of the technical issues experienced. **Ultra-wideband** (UWB) technology is a type of radio frequency signal that has a bandwidth greater than 500 MHz, or greater than 20% of the center carrier frequency (2). By spreading information over a wide portion of the frequency spectrum, this technology can communicate large amounts of data while consuming little energy from the signal (2). Ultra-wideband may, therefore, provide a better solution than RFID due to low power consumption, as well as high precision, the ability of the signal to pass through obstacles, and greater resistance to interference (2).

Global Positioning System

The **Global Positioning System** (GPS) is a satellite navigation network that provides location and time information of tracking devices. The **Global Navigation Satellite System** (GNSS) is a collective term for all satellite navigation systems providing geospatial positioning with global coverage. Currently, this includes both the United States–based GPS (n = 24) and the Russian-based GLONASS (GLObal NAvigation Satellite System) systems (n = 24), which together comprise a network of 48 satellites. A GPS device, initially developed for military purposes, is a

receiver for a satellite network navigation system that determines location, velocity, and time. Within sports, GPS devices are typically worn on the upper back between the shoulder blades. Each satellite transmits low-powered radio signals with information on the exact time, from the onboard atomic clock, to the GPS device at the velocity of light (30). The signal transit time from the satellite to the GPS device is calculated by comparing the delay between arrival and transmission of the signal. The distance of the satellite from the GPS device is then calculated by multiplying the duration of signal transit by the speed of light (30). The physical location (latitude and longitude) of the GPS device can be trigonometrically determined when the distance to at least four satellites is available.

The sampling frequency is the rate at which the GPS device receives satellite signals. Initially, GPS devices used in sport operated at a sampling frequency of 1 Hz, or once per second (20). Technological advancements have included sampling frequency increases, and devices now commonly have a sample rate in excess of 10 Hz. The sport scientist should exercise caution, though, because some devices sample at lower frequencies and interpolate from an onboard triaxial accelerometer to increase sample frequency.

Inertial Measurement Units

GPS devices continually receive data and hence use power relatively quickly. A power-saving reduction in sample rate would lead to an associated reduction in accuracy; a solution to this problem is the application of accelerometers (41). Multiple transducer inertial measurement units (IMU) are housed within microelectromechanical systems (MEMS). One of those is an accelerometer (to detect movement). Commonly, there are also gyroscopes (to measure rotation) and magnetometers (to measure orientation). Such devices give a single sensor the ability to perceive movement in multiple dimensions that can be tracked on the Cartesian coordinate system (*x*-, *y*-, *z*-axes).

Accelerometry

Since the 1990s, the vertically mounted uniaxial accelerometer has been widely used to study energy expenditure outside the lab setting in free-living individuals. **Accelerometers** measure the deflection of a seismic mass between two electrodes caused by acceleration via capacitance (33). Triaxial accelerometers, which measure in three dimensions with sample rates in excess of 1,000 Hz, have become more commonly available. This has resulted in a number of studies comparing tri- and uniaxial accelerometers and various electronic pedometers to evaluate their efficacy as robust and valid measures of energy expenditure (28).

Accelerometers have proven to be a valuable tool in analyzing movement in the field in many situations (i.e., gait analysis or sport-specific technical assessments). Various approaches have been implemented to study human gait using accelerometry, with reference to the detection of gait events and spatiotemporal characteristics (21, 46). Traditionally these studies required multiple sensors to obtain data, but increasingly studies have focused on more practical approaches using fewer overall accelerometers or a single triaxial accelerometer, which is typically mounted on the torso. This single unit has been shown to be reliable for temporal stride characteristics and asymmetries (31, 32) and for distinguishing between different modes of locomotion (34). It was shown that variability in stride can be detected by commonly used

accelerometers and is associated with fatigue, soreness, and training load in a population of American football athletes (40).

While standard accelerometers refer to the integral of the vertical acceleration over a period of time, via counts, these cannot differentiate the intensity of an activity. This limits the effectiveness of commercial devices within elite settings, a limitation compounded by the lack of standardized reporting between systems. Triaxial accelerometers measure three-dimensional movements and have been used to quantify external load in team sports either separately or housed within MEMS (see figure 9.2; 5, 8, 35, 43).

Provided by the common manufacturers of GPS devices are various types of accelerometers that detect force in a single axis (which can vary based on their orientation) at different rates (±8-13 g; i.e., they can measure up to 8-13 times the normal gravitational acceleration), but they tend to have a lower collection frequency of 100 Hz (i.e., 100 samples per second) and

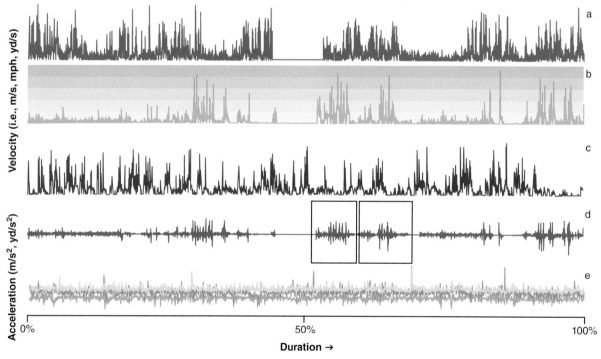

FIGURE 9.2 Across team sports the activity profile of athletes can be collected either by velocity *(a, b, c)* or via acceleration in a particular axis *(d, e)*. This represents the density of activity in the training session or competition and the subsequent analysis and feedback. Athlete sessions from basketball *(a)*, football *(b)*, and rugby *(c)* show the velocity, which can be measured in various units dependent on the practitioners and their preference; for football, a single axis of acceleration is shown *(d)*. For ice hockey, all three axes of acceleration are shown with a 10-point moving average *(e, forward = yellow, sideways = blue, up = orange)*. In all cases the duration has been normalized across each session, though typically these are reported relative to the elapsed duration of the session and can be reported in absolute or relative terms (e.g., per minute). Sessions are typically chunked by periods or drills to examine particular sections or rotations depending on the sport; see box within *(d)*. Thresholds or zones can be set for each athlete individually or the group as a whole using absolute or relative references *(b)*.

tend to be triaxial. While they produce variables that differ slightly across companies, most have attempted to measure workload exerted by the athlete by quantifying the sum of the individual triaxial accelerometer vectors and calling this "Player Load," "Body Load," or "Accumulation Load" (15). Typically, this measure of total effort is expressed in arbitrary units since it has been calculated as a scaled vector magnitude, which reflects the instantaneous rate of change of acceleration or mechanical stress ($accel_y$ represents anterior-posterior acceleration; $accel_x$ represents medial-lateral acceleration; and $accel_z$ represents vertical acceleration; t is time):

$$Player|Body|Acceleration\ Load = \sqrt{\frac{\left(accel_{y(t)} - accel_{y(t-1)}\right)^2 - \left(accel_{x(t)} - accel_{x(t-1)}\right)^2 - \left(accel_{z(t)} - accel_{z(t-1)}\right)^2}{100}}$$

Other accelerometers (e.g., actigraphs) have been used to detect movement patterns and infer sleep in the general population. Triaxial IMUs have been applied in elite sporting populations to further understand movement demands, particularly in indoor sport settings such as handball where GPS signals are unavailable (35). In running-based sports, inertial measurement units have been used to measure the force interaction between athletes and surfaces (51). In gymnastics, it has been shown that, due to the performance of multiple movements on a wide range of viscoelastic surfaces, the overall internal load on the gymnast can be estimated using an IMU (9). In baseball, a biomechanical system using a single IMU has been developed for the throwing motion that provides real-time metrics such as throw count, arm speed, maximal arm rotation, arm slot, and elbow varus torque. Across a number of pitches, shoulder flexibility, arm speed, and elbow varus torque (and likely injury risk) were shown to be interrelated (18). Similar approaches are now being taken by practitioners in American football to manage the throwing loads of the quarterback position.

Magnetometers and Gyroscopes

As previously mentioned, it is common to have gyroscopes (to measure rotation) and magnetometers (to measure orientation) within MEMS devices in addition to accelerometers. The **magnetometer** is essentially a compass that harnesses the magnetic field of the earth to determine orientation. By computing the angle of the earth's detected magnetic field and comparing that angle to gravity as measured by an accelerometer, it is possible to measure a device's heading with respect to magnetic north. The gyroscope measures changes in angular position or rotational velocity. Typically, it has three axes corresponding to pitch, roll, and yaw angles. Magnetometers and gyroscopes are complementary to each other. Typically, a magnetometer has poor accuracy for measuring orientation with fast movement, whereas gyroscopes alone can accumulate vast errors over time and require input on starting orientation since they measure only changes. Combining the inputs to these sensors allows for quick and accurate position and orientation determination with a low amount of drift over time.

Within the literature, gyroscopes have been used to identify collision events in team sports (22) by identifying periods in which the unit was in a nonvertical position and a spike in load was detected by the accelerometer. This allowed the development of a "tackle algorithm" that was subsequently used in various footballing codes to quantify the demands of the sport (23). While it has been shown that it is both possible and feasible to use accelerometer and gyroscope data to accurately classify sporting activities (57), the contribution of the gyroscope to classification is limited in relation to the accelerometer. The reason is likely that the location on the upper back is predominantly exposed to linear motions, as compared to rotational motions that gyroscopes measure. No study to date has assessed the validity and reliability of gyroscopes within wearable tracking devices, whereas several studies have been published on the accelerometer (4, 7, 27, 44).

KEY METRICS

Despite the differences in technology and computations, all the positional systems discussed ultimately attempt to track x- and y-coordinates of the athletes that are transformed into time–motion analysis. In team sports, the most common measures collected by practitioners have been acceleration (at various thresholds), total distance, high-speed distance, and metabolic power (1). These are typically "lower-level" metrics with a focus on distance- and velocity-based measures (see figure 9.3; 12).

Practitioners should be aware of the setup of their analysis software when tracking metrics longitudinally. The arbitrary thresholds used seem to reflect early time–motion analysis work without justification (42).

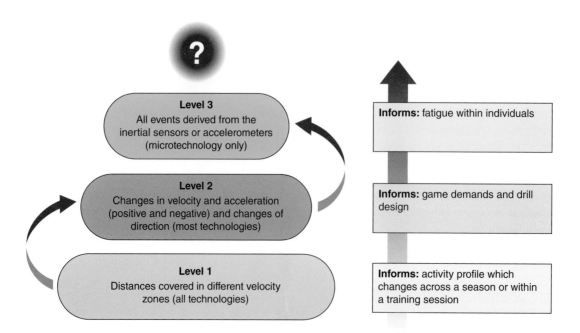

FIGURE 9.3 Classification system of athlete metric levels from tracking systems and how they can be used to inform different parts of the athlete monitoring process.

Based on Buchheit and Simpson (2017).

Work profile zones set by manufacturers for workload profiles can differ between sports, but in some cases are the same, without consideration given to the size of the playing field (see review articles that summarize zones in use for both speed and acceleration [16, 24, 52]). This may mean that in discussions of a particular zone or movement category (e.g., walk, jog, or high-speed), the meaning and interpretation of these data may not match between sport scientists or coaches. This is discussed more in chapter 10.

The two primary measures specifically from a GPS device that are used to monitor athletes are velocity and distance (see figure 9.2). These measures can be determined through two different methods: positional differentiation and the Doppler-shift method. Positional differentiation determines the change in device location to allow computation of the distance the GPS device has traveled over time. The velocity at which the GPS device is moving can then be measured by the change in distance over time.

Alternatively, the **Doppler-shift method** measures the rate of change in the satellite signal frequency (Doppler shift) caused by the movement of the receiver and uses a complex process to calculate velocity (49). Velocity calculated via the Doppler-shift method appears to have greater precision compared to positional differentiation (54). Distance can then

be calculated as the derivation of velocity (velocity multiplied by time). It is common for GPS devices used in team sports to determine distance through positional differentiation and velocity through the Doppler-shift method.

The interpretation of displacement-based variables assumes that the orientation of athletes and the loads exerted upon them are consistent (though this is not the case with differing conditions and with opponents present). Metabolic power-derived models may be more appropriate since they better reflect the large proportion of time typically spent walking or running within team sports and the differing metabolic costs when players are in possession of the ball or traveling backward, laterally, or accelerating (43). An immediate energy cost can be estimated for players at any point using their acceleration. The total cost can provide an estimation of overall energy expenditure throughout the activity or can be multiplied by velocity as an indication of metabolic power. There are reservations about the accuracy of metabolic power derived from GPS, because it has been shown to underestimate energy expenditure in team-sport activities that may compromise intense but static movements (10, 12). Alternatively, averaging the absolute accelerations (positive and negative) across an activity may be more appropriate to monitor session demands because it increases reliability without sacrificing sensitivity to change (17).

Incorporating the inertial sensor or accelerometry events is another level of analysis and interpretation (see figure 9.2). Player work profiles are heavily influenced by the context of training and competition (e.g., opponent, score line, rules, area). There are also playing position differences within team sports in terms of tactical and locomotor demands. Looking at accelerometry-based variables, which can give insight into stride kinematics and variability as well as imbalances and ground reaction forces (12, 40), may be more useful for longitudinal player monitoring.

With accelerometry, the combination of linear accelerations has traditionally been used to create an external training load variable from which one can infer mechanical stress due to the absorption of ground reaction forces (53). While the overall load is important, the ability of a torso-mounted accelerometer to identify asymmetries in stride characteristics has interesting applications in athlete monitoring. Both contact time and vertical stiffness measurements have been shown to identify differences between sides in stride characteristics to the same degree as an instrumented treadmill when ankle movement is constrained by taping (11). Also, more global measures of fatigue and stress inferred from accelerometry seem to detect changes in movement strategy (6).

One of the benefits of positional systems, as opposed to wearable microsensors, is the ability to also track the playing object (e.g., the ball or puck). Often, object tracking has been employed in a testing environment, for example to assess the efficacy of a training intervention on soccer ball shooting speed (56). However, such a stand-alone environment does not replicate the cognitive, emotional, technical, and tactical demands required to control and move the playing object in situ. The integration of such information can support tactical components and further develop understanding of the demands of the game.

Several studies have reported that both OT and RFID measures in situ have good reliability, displaying small absolute errors (<10%) (26, 50). However, such research also faces methodological challenges similar to those for assessing the accuracy of athlete tracking. Although every effort is made to "repeatedly simulate realistic situations," these studies often rely on machines to release the object at various speeds and trajectories. In one study, the peak velocity of one such machine was capped at 22.3 m/s, even though ball velocities up to 34 m/s were reached in the sport-

ing environment (50). Once again, however, it seems that the introduction of such systems preempts the reporting of relevant movement precision information. Object tracking via OT or RFID or both is already employed throughout many sports, including professional tennis, Major League Baseball, the National Football League, and European handball, and is to be introduced in the National Hockey League in the 2019 to 2020 season. Practitioners should maintain similar skepticism of technologies claiming to track playing objects with their positional systems and continue to critique research designs.

FUTURE DIRECTIONS

As technology has developed in line with Moore's law (speed and capability increase at an exponential rate every few years as the price falls), there has been an increase in availability and adoption. Currently, sport scientists in mainstream sports have the ability to easily collect and process data, but these abilities will continue to advance rapidly with new models and innovations. The dawn of the smartphone has seen the use of information about motion, position, and orientation, but currently these devices are still limited compared to wearable devices (25, 38). In the future the development of smart fabrics with embedded sensors may replace wearable devices or use on-phone processing to give real-time feedback (3).

CONCLUSION

The decision to select a tracking system for any sport scientist is complicated by the myriad of systems available. Some choices may be dictated by availability in stadiums or overall budget, but there are factors to be aware of when choosing a system to monitor player load. The level of information that can be obtained differs between the collection systems in its granularity and in how it can be used to support the athlete monitoring process. In some cases, different systems may be used in the training and competition environments. A consistent measure, either via the use of the same system or based on a good understanding of the interchangeability of system metrics, will undoubtedly help support practitioner decisions regardless of the sport.

The combination of systems can provide more in-depth outcomes and knowledge, as mentioned earlier. Combining different levels of technology can supplement and provide insight but is associated with increased costs in human capital and processing time to ensure valid and robust measurement. Any decision to combine systems should begin with a question and a clearly defined purpose. For example, a coach or practitioner may be interested in tracking fitness longitudinally or determining the level of short-term fatigue between games. Ultimately, the purpose and goals will likely influence the choice of systems or their combination. While in the future sensors may be fully embedded in garments, educating athletes on the purpose and importance of wearing their trackers will help encourage their engagement to ensure that the data is collected. The next task is analyzing the data in a way that is valid and reliable to help make informed decisions.

RECOMMENDED READINGS

Camomilla, V, Bergamini, E, Fantozzi, S, and Vannozzi, G. Trends supporting the in-field use of wearable inertial sensors for sport performance evaluation: a systematic review. *Sensors (Basel)* 18, 873, 2018.

Cardinale, M, and Varley, MC. Wearable training-monitoring technology: applications, challenges, and opportunities. *Int J Sports Physiol Perform* 12, 55-63, 2017.

Carling, C, Bloomfield J, Nelsen L, and Reilly T. The role of motion analysis in elite soccer. *Sports Med* 38, 839-862, 2008.

Malone, JJ, Lovell R, Varley, MC, and Coutts, AJ. Unpacking the black box: applications and considerations for using GPS devices in sport. *Int J Sports Physiol Perform* 12, 18-26, 2017.

McLean, BD, Strack, D, Russell, J, and Coutts, AJ. Quantifying physical demands in the National Basketball Association—challenges around developing best-practice models for athlete care and performance. *Int J Sports Physiol Perform* 14, 414-420, 2019.

CHAPTER 10

Analysis of Tracking Systems and Load Monitoring

Andrew M. Murray, PhD

Jo Clubb, MSc

The collection of tracking data will provide unfiltered information unless the context of the situation is accounted for, which can then enable a useful interpretation of the data. Management of this information requires an underpinning of reliable and valid analytical techniques to create knowledge that can affect the organization and its management of athletes. This chapter seeks to underline the analytical processes required to build upon the collection of training load and work profile information described in chapter 9.

VALIDITY AND RELIABILITY OF TRACKING SYSTEMS

For practitioners to have confidence in the data produced by tracking systems, they should have an understanding of the level of quality assurance in any outcome measures. The information provided should meet quality control specifications, including, but not limited to, validity and reliability (20). It is paramount that users be aware of the collection errors associated with each technology, along with having the ability to critique the methodologies and identify limitations of research relating to positional and tracking systems. With this understanding, practitioners will be well informed of the steps required to suitably analyze and interpret such data within the applied setting.

Despite the importance of measurement precision (i.e., reliability), the uptake of such technologies tends to preempt the publication of validation work. This "early-adopter" approach is perhaps not surprising

given the competitive nature of professional sports, along with the privacy of manufacturers' internal validation and "white papers" (not peer-reviewed) and consumer skepticism about such reports (48). This has led to researchers and sport scientists undertaking external validation studies on their own or with non-profit third parties (independent research) or both (46).

In addition, it has been acknowledged that validity and reliability are in fact not dichotomous classifications. **Validity** differs according to each variable, as well as the context-specific application of that variable (48). **Reliability** exists upon a continuum, requiring practitioners to understand how to calculate whether changes are meaningful in light of the reliability demonstrated (i.e., signal-to-noise ratio) (48). The discussions within this chapter emphasize the need for sport scientists to stay up-to-date with the literature validating such systems, conduct research, and, if possible, publish internal validation studies, as well as maintaining rigor within data collection (18). Practitioners should also be aware that firmware and software updates can affect data outputs, and examples of this are outlined later in this chapter. Therefore, validation is, and will remain, an ongoing process (14).

Positional Systems

As outlined in chapter 9, various solutions for positional tracking systems exist. Despite the differences in characteristics of such systems, many of them are employed across professional sporting settings, often with multiple types of systems used within the same setting. The application of Global Positioning System (GPS) devices was advanced by a wealth of independent research since its widespread uptake in the early 2000s, which provides a blueprint for validation research on emerging technologies. Technologies that later emerged may lack the same breadth as to their validity and reliability research base. Understanding the existing validity and reliability research, including the potential between-systems agreement (or disagreement), along with how to implement such analysis in-house, is necessary.

Optical Tracking

With the introduction of semiautomated multi-camera tracking systems in soccer in the late 1990s, much of the early validation was conducted in this sport (20). One of the first such studies aimed at validating an optical tracking (OT) system demonstrated excellent correlation coefficients during paced runs and sprints between the OT system and average velocity measured by timing gates (27). While understanding specific movement patterns relating to the game is important, clearly a predefined situation such as this does not truly represent all the demands involved. Furthermore, timing gates provide only average speed between specific points, rather than continuous sampling points. For further information on validation studies of OT solutions in soccer, see the review by Carling and colleagues (20).

Because the number of different OT solutions has increased, it is important to consider the measurement precision of the technology being employed. Such solutions may differ by the number and type of cameras used, the automatic tracking process, the manual quality control process, and the data treatment for determining displacement (47). The accuracy of OT systems that require a high level of manual intervention is dependent on the training and experience of the operators (9). Further limitations may include the quality of video, changes in illumination, frequency of instances of occlusion (i.e., where the direct line of sight between the camera and the tracking object is blocked, perhaps by the presence of multiple players in a small area), and restrictive conditions imposed by the stadium setup (steep stands in close proximity to the field of play is ideal; 5, 22, 23, 25).

Radio Frequency Identification

The later emergence of radio frequency identification (RFID) and ultra-wideband (UWB) systems has lim-

ited the availability of research in sports, and fundamental validity and reliability data has been described as scarce (48). However, it has been suggested that radio-based technologies may provide more valuable insight into instantaneous speed and acceleration data, owing to their enhanced accuracy compared to OT and GPS tracking (20, 66). Indeed, a 20-Hz RFID system demonstrated superior validity and reliability compared to both 10- and 18-Hz GPS using a team sport-specific circuit (37). However, more data was removed as outliers due to measurement errors, such as the devices running out of charge or poor signal strength, with RFID than with 18-Hz GPS; this will currently limit its use in applied practice (37), though the implementation environment should be considered because indoor sports cannot use GPS.

Studies on RFID technology have demonstrated that mean error of position estimates ranges between 11.9 and 23.4 ± 20.7 cm (55, 64). However, in a consistent finding, error increases with increasing speed (31, 55). This is graphically depicted in figure 10.1. Similarly, these systems have been found to be within 2% of the criterion measure, 3D-motion capture, for measuring mean acceleration and deceleration, but limited for the measurement of peak acceleration and deceleration (66). However, findings have been inconsistent in relation to the magnitude of error with increasing complexity of changes of direction (31, 55, 66). It has also been questioned whether positional systems can accurately measure instantaneous velocities (45, 55). Such outcomes are particularly concerning to practitioners given that the most physically demanding moments of the game, for example, high-speed (e.g., sprinting during a counterattack) or high-intensity movements (e.g., accelerating and decelerating to close down an opponent who is in possession of the ball), may be the most critical to performance (16, 20).

While positional systems are commonplace in some team-sport environments, research has also explored their application in individual events. Measurement precision must also be considered within these specific environments. Radio frequency identification has been investigated as a positional system solution for track running competitions, but has not yet demonstrated appropriate repeatability (84). Conversely, UWB technology has been deemed suitable for application in track cycling (49). Furthermore, research has established best practice positioning of the equipment by assessing performance and energy consumption with various tag and anchor positions (49). Elsewhere, the construction of an RFID system for open-water swimming competitions has been

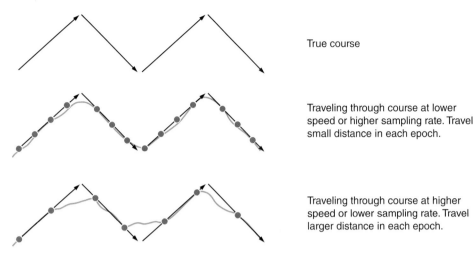

True course

Traveling through course at lower speed or higher sampling rate. Travel small distance in each epoch.

Traveling through course at higher speed or lower sampling rate. Travel larger distance in each epoch.

FIGURE 10.1   Schematic example of change in velocity or sampling rate (or both) and subsequent effects on positional tracking. Dots represent sample points. As sample rate falls at a given speed, athletes travel farther between sample points and so introduce more error or divergence from the analyzed compared to the true course. With a higher sample rate, the true and the measured course are closer. The same can be said for a given sample rate at higher speeds (traveling farther between sample points, more error).

presented, which enables a detection rate between 94.6% and 100% (83).

Global Positioning System

The latest models of most GPS devices appear to provide an adequate measure of distance and speed (10, 74). Therefore, sport scientists can have relative confidence in associated metrics (i.e., total distance covered and the breakdown of the distance within various speed thresholds). However, a familiar pattern in GPS validation research, as with positional systems, suggests that the precision of GPS to measure speed and distance decreases with an increased change in the rate of velocity, regardless of the sampling rate (1, 74). Validation research has associated a higher sampling frequency with an increased accuracy of GPS devices (74). While this may be true for 10-Hz versus 1- to 5-Hz devices, research comparing 10-Hz and 18-Hz devices has shown mixed results. One study showed no meaningful differences between the two sampling frequencies, whereas another demonstrated improved validity and reliability in the 18-Hz compared to the 10-Hz device (10, 37). It is worth noting that differences exist in the satellite systems that the respective technologies have access to, with the increased sampling frequency of 18 Hz used in devices that have access only to the United States GPS (10). This is opposed to the 10-Hz multi-GNSS device within that study, which is capable of tracking multiple satellite systems including both GPS and Global Navigation

Satellite System (GNSS) (10). While more research is necessary regarding the relative advantages of devices operating at higher sampling frequencies (>10 Hz), practitioners should have confidence in devices that operate at or above this threshold.

Rather than high absolute velocity, it is typically the actions that involve a high rate of change in velocity (i.e., acceleration, deceleration, and change of direction) that provide moments crucial to a game and its outcome. The measurement of these actions may, however, be associated with the greatest amount of error. Measuring instantaneous acceleration is a mathematical ideal limited by the sampling frequency of the device. Mathematically, as the denominator in the equation approaches zero, the limit of the rate is called a derivative. In this case acceleration (a) is a derivative of velocity (v):

$$a = \lim_{\Delta \to 0} \frac{\Delta v}{\Delta t} = \frac{dv}{dt}$$

Acceleration is the derivative of velocity with time (t), but velocity is itself the derivative of displacement (s) with time (38). Therefore, acceleration is the first derivative of velocity with time and the second derivative of displacement with time:

$$a = \frac{dv}{dt} = \frac{d}{dt} \times \frac{ds}{dt} = \frac{d^2s}{dt^2}$$

Calculating from the second derivative can compound calculated errors but is typically the way acceleration is calculated in GPS units that measure geographical position. Noise within the raw signal may be amplified (56, 81). For these reasons, positional data are often filtered to remove high-frequency noise (42, 56, 61).

Knowing the acceleration over time, one can work backward to calculate the integral of change in velocity via the first equation of motion (21, 38):

$$v = v_0 + at$$

Another consideration for sport scientists using GPS data in their monitoring practices is the signal quality. This can be affected by local weather, the location (e.g., within a densely populated area versus a remote location), and environmental obstructions such as trees close to training locations or particular stadium designs (e.g., partially covered) (46). Signal quality can be evaluated by quantifying the satellite number used to obtain the signal or the horizontal dilution of precision (HDoP) or both. The HDoP represents the precision of the GPS horizontal positional signal, determined by the satellites' geographical organization (46). Values range from 1 to 50, representing a ratio of the change in output location and the change in measured data, with 1 being ideal and under 2 excellent, whereas values over 20 are regarded as poor (82). Low values represent satellites far apart in the sky, with a wide angular separation giving the best positional information. While considering signal quality is a best practice in cleaning the GPS data, not all manufacturers make it available in their software. This can make it difficult to identify and potentially compensate for sections of poor signal quality within the collected data.

Drawing definitive conclusions on validity for tracking systems is problematic, given the variation in manufacturers, models, sampling frequencies, sport demands, variables assessed, thresholds used, and software and hardware versions (14). Specifically related to GPS technology, there are also many factors that can influence the validity, including the method used to calculate distance and velocity, the signal processing algorithms, the GNSS available, and the chipset technology used. Since these factors differ in GPS devices depending on the manufacturer, the GPS device model (within manufacturer), and the firmware version used (within-device model), the validation of these devices remains an ongoing process.

Sport scientists should consider if a suitable criterion measure was used to assess the GPS device when elucidating the results of validation research. When assessing speed, appropriate criterion measures

include a laser, radar, or 3D-motion capture system. Sport scientists should be attentive if timing gates are used to assess speed, since this will not provide a measure of instantaneous speed, but rather an average. When assessing distance, appropriate criterion measures include a theodolite, tape measure, trundle wheel, and 3D-motion capture systems. The movement scenario used in the methodology (i.e., predefined course versus complex and free movement) should also be considered.

The reliability of GPS devices is more complex to assess than validity. Within-device reliability would require nearly identical repetition of specific movement patterns. However, it is unlikely that human participants will produce with 100% accuracy the exact same movement patterns on multiple occasions throughout a sport-specific circuit (46). Therefore, most reliability research has investigated inter-unit (between units of the same model within manufacturer) and inter-device (between manufacturers) reliability. The 10-Hz GPS models from three different manufacturers have been compared for inter-unit and inter-device reliability when data was processed using manufacturer software (70). Inter-unit reliability was found to be poor for deceleration measures (coefficient of variation [CV]: 2.5%-72.8%), better with acceleration measures (CV: 1.4%-19.7%), and best for distance and speed measures (CV: 0.2%-5.5%). However, significant differences were observed between manufacturers for all measures (CV: −2.0% to 1.9%). While it appears that there may be some flexibility in device interchangeability using the same model, depending on the measures of interest to the sport scientist, the best practice of using the same device on a given player should still be applied where possible (39). It is apparent that data derived across manufacturers are not interchangeable, and caution is warranted when one is comparing such data.

In the applied setting of sport training and competition, it is commonplace for sport scientists to employ **real-time monitoring** of GPS data in order to provide the coaches or players (or both) with feedback relating to the volume and intensity of a session (46). Such feedback may be based on postevent data, downloaded directly from the device, whereas real-time data is derived via a specific receiver (6). Therefore, understanding the agreement between these data sets is essential. An early study in this regard published in 2010 (GPS frequency not specified, but thought to be 1 or 5 Hz) questioned the application of real-time data for decision making, given that only total distance displayed a signal greater than the noise (4). However, technology has developed since that study, and therefore two more investigations have reexamined the validity. This research has disagreed on the validity of real-time, accelerometry-derived data (6, 79). As with post-event velocity data, there is consensus that error increases with higher speed (see figure 10.1), but these data may still be used if the error is taken into account appropriately (6, 79). Given the paucity and inconsistencies of research regarding real-time monitoring, along with the variation in software and hardware available, conducting analysis within the applied environment that replicates the methodologies used in the literature represents best practice for practitioners using real-time data to assist with feedback and decision making.

Wearable Microsensors

As outlined in chapter 9, wearable microsensors have been employed since the early 1990s to capture movement outside of the laboratory setting for a variety of purposes. The primary purpose of wearable microsensors in sport is to further understand movement demands via integrated multiple inertial measurement units (IMU), which may include an accelerometer, gyroscope, and magnetometer. Although variation exists across manufacturers, typically workload is expressed as a summation of accelerometry load (see chapter 9) and a percentage contribution of the triaxial vectors. It is important to remember that changes in direction involve accelerations even if the velocity remains unchanged, so there is interest in the distinct accelerometry axes as well as overall load. Such metrics have demonstrated acceptable within-device and between-devices reliability in both laboratory conditions and field testing in Australian football (CV = 0.91%-1.9%) and during a standardized 90-minute soccer match play simulation (8, 11). Furthermore, the signal was shown to be greater than the noise, supporting the application of this metric to measure workload (11).

While accelerometers are worn on the upper body as part of microelectromechanical system (MEMS) units to enhance the signal communication with GPS satellites, the center of mass is considered the criterion location for measurement of overall body movement using accelerometers (33). Even though wearing GPS units between the scapulae is common in elite team sports (29), the cranial-caudal axis of the accelerometer will likely be only approximately equivalent to the global vertical axis (85) when the player is standing upright or performing movements in the vertical plane.

Any deviation from the anticipated vertical orientation of the device at contact will compromise the accelerometer's accuracy. For example, recreational athletes assume more crouched, forward-leaning postures during high-speed running trials (40). Indeed, in field hockey it is common to maintain a position of flexion when in possession of the ball. Investigations using IMUs have shown that 89% of the playing time is spent between 20° and 90° of flexion, with differences between positions (76). Despite this, the magnitudes of peak accelerations have been validated when an accelerometer is worn on the upper torso (85), which demonstrates that when it is placed according to the manufacturer recommendations, 10-Hz filtered data can assess peak accelerations with a CV of 8.9%. Similar units of a different brand have been shown to accurately identify temporal stride characteristics when compared to an instrumented treadmill (15). Contact time was found to be almost perfectly correlated between accelerometer and treadmill measures ($r = 0.96$), and large correlations were found for flight time ($r = 0.68$).

Between-Systems Agreement

Professional teams may be mandated to use a particular positional tracking system for competition, due to league limitations for permitted technologies tasked with in-game collection or league-wide deals with athlete tracking companies (48). Such systems may differ from those used internally to track practice sessions due to practitioner preferences, resources available, commercial agreements, or practicing and competing in different locations. Sport scientists may therefore be required to use multiple technologies throughout the season; thus, it is important to consider the agreement and potential interchangeability of data collected.

Research in soccer has demonstrated greater agreement between OT and augmented GPS, which has access to multiple satellites from the GNSS, compared to GPS alone (68). While this particular study suggested that tracking data from these augmented GPS devices and OT could be used interchangeably, best practice for practitioners remains conducting similar evaluations within their environment with their technology (68). Alternatively, another comparative study using a 90-minute soccer match found large between-systems differences across four commercially available tracking systems, specifically two OT and two GPS technologies (58). Such studies examine aggregated distances covered (e.g., total and high-speed) over the course of a match, halves, or

15- or 5-minute periods (or both), thus limiting the understanding of instantaneous speed and position accuracy. Furthermore, energetically demanding activities, such as accelerations and decelerations, often occur at low velocity; therefore assessing the agreement of high-speed distances alone omits this crucial information (67).

In an attempt to address limitations between different methods, Linke, Link, and Lames (44) assessed the validity of OT, RFID, and GPS against a 3D-motion capture system in three accuracy categories: position, instantaneous speed and acceleration, and key performance indicators [KPI; summated metrics (e.g., distance covered, mean or peak speed, peak accelerations)]. While RFID technology demonstrated the greatest position accuracy (with a distance root mean square error of 22-27 cm), there was a significant increase in error with fast changes of direction (44). In line with previous research, as speed increased, so did the magnitude of error in all technologies (44). The authors also showed a large margin of error in the KPI categories independent of the positional tracking system and thus recommended that sport scientists not make direct comparisons of summated metrics calculated from different systems (44).

Dismissing the ability to incorporate physical demands from practice with those from competition is unfortunate given the potential benefits of monitoring individual external loads over time, as well as planning training workloads based on competition demands. To overcome this, calibration equations for total and high-speed distances across four tracking technologies for different soccer situations (small area drills, medium area drills, and match play) have previously been presented (14). However, it should be noted that these equations were manufacturer- and model-specific, plus within-unit chipset changes and software updates can also influence the data collected (14). Consequently, best practice may involve practitioners repeating a similar protocol internally in order to establish calibration equations of their own.

ANALYSIS AND INTERPRETATION OF TRACKING SYSTEM DATA

Armed with an understanding of the validity and reliability of tracking systems available and employed within the applied environment, practitioners can turn their attention to analyzing such data and providing meaningful interpretations to coaches and athletes. Understanding the movement demands and planning

training accordingly remains the most fundamental application of tracking data. However, such information should always be considered within the context of the sport, the team, and the individual athlete. Finally, once the analysis has been completed and the interpretation established, it is the responsibility of sport science practitioners to communicate their message in an effective way through data visualization and interpersonal skills.

Time–Motion Analysis

An initial and fundamental step for analysis of tracking system data focuses on providing a descriptive summary of the time–motion activities within a particular sport and its playing positions. Reilly and Thomas (59) first described the average game distances of soccer players by position, and for the first time objectively demonstrated that midfielders covered the greatest distance and central defenders the least (goalkeepers were not included in the study). Similar work has since been conducted across a plethora of different team sports (3).

Such descriptive information can provide an overview of the physical outputs required in the sport, as well as quantifying the demands imposed across different playing levels (see figure 10.2). This understanding allows sport scientists to objectively prepare athletes for competition. In addition, such information can provide benchmarks that assist with planning of rehabilitation and return-to-train or return-to-play criteria. While people must not keep reinventing the wheel in relation to descriptive studies, tracking such information over time is required, given the evolution of such demands within the same competition (e.g., in soccer's English Premier League) (5, 13).

Beyond describing time–motion demands, research moved on to attempt to quantify the emergence of fatigue within the game in team sports. Initially, the distances covered between halves, 15-minute, or 5-minute segments in soccer were compared, with a view to understanding fatigue (20). However, research has demonstrated large variability in game-to-game demands, especially for the most demanding movements (i.e., high-speed activities) (32). Therefore, one cannot assume that fitness and fatigue are the sole determinants of game running performance. Factors such as tactical role, game interruptions, opponent, team philosophy, and technical purposes have been identified as influencers of individual game performance (12). For example,

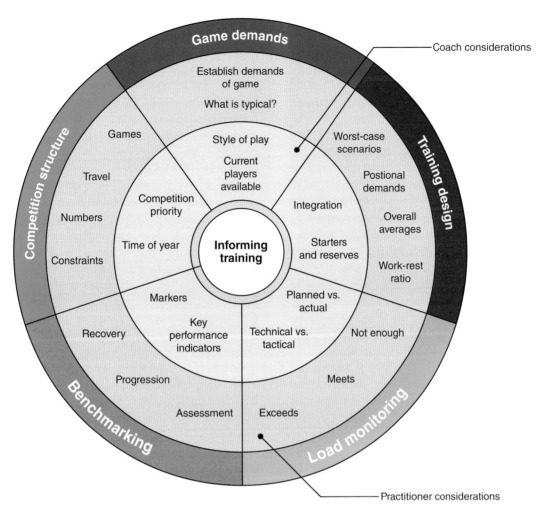

FIGURE 10.2   Feedback loop of the sport scientist and interdisciplinary team in monitoring training and game demands.

situational factors such as match outcome, points conceded, and weather conditions have been associated with increased physical performance in rugby sevens (36, 52). In addition, the effect of successive games on physical outputs during international tournament soccer influences individuals to different extents (73). Thus, time–motion analysis in isolation is not illuminating in terms of fatigue, and practitioners should consider contextual factors, along with monitoring individual athletes.

The traditionally reported physical metrics from positional systems in isolation have since been described as one-dimensional and "blind" distances (12). Thus, calls have been made to focus on an integrated approach that contextualizes such distances in relation to tactical activities (12). Such purposeful distances may make data more meaningful for coaches and players alike. Despite the drawbacks of the later emergence of tracking technology in certain

environments, sport scientists may be able to learn lessons from early-adopter sports and fast-track the integration of such data.

Workload Measurement

Quantifying competition time–motion demands has implications for physical preparation, and understanding them can assist practitioners with planning, implementation, and tracking of physical programs for training. For example, figure 10.3 demonstrates how a measure of load can be projected on a drill, daily, and weekly basis, constructed by using the average historic intensity of specific drills along with the expected times. Constraints, such as time and drill type, which may include number of players, the area of space afforded for the drill, work-to-rest ratios, and the absence or presence of coach encouragement, among other factors, can then be adjusted to achieve the load desired according to the periodized plan. Tracking data can then be analyzed, in real time or retrospectively or both, to compare the planned load to the actual load, along with assessing athletes on an individual basis. Such an approach has limitations in that the use of averages can obfuscate the data, especially in sports with large individual variation. This also considers only the physical demands of the drill or session or both, when other components of the preparation (i.e., technical, tactical, and psychological) also require consideration. Striving to integrate these different areas within planning and monitoring approaches should be the goal of the sport scientist working within an integrated support team in concert with the coaching staff.

Across sports, "workload" has been shown to relate to internal load measures (65) and is effective at distinguishing between the demands of competition and practice environments (50). In the absence of other time–motion analysis techniques, accelerometry-derived workload may provide a proxy measure of total distance, although using this derivate alone may lead to an oversight with regard to other energetically demanding movements (57). As such, accelerometry-derived workload may provide a suitable measure of load in sports with frequent collisions or directional changes (11). Alternate measures of load from the accelerometers that exclude the running components or look at individual axes in isolation have shown value in the literature in monitoring fatigue and response to training and competition (23, 62). For example, changes in the contributions of individual vectors to the overall player load have been shown in both simulated and professional match play (7, 8). In addition, associations between relative loading patterns and level of performance shown in netball suggest that players of different standard may have dissimilar movement characteristics (24). Analyzing the reliability of isolated movements rather than cumulative totals of workload shows much better results due to eliminating extraneous movements. Cumulative workload also fails to distinguish the impact and intensity of discrete actions and how these differ between individuals. One solution to this is to express intensity as a relative measure (workload per minute) that accounts for time on task and can apprise sport scientists when they look to inform subsequent interventions to modify practice (see figure 10.3).

It is rare that accelerometry or GPS variables are interpreted in isolation, particularly since MEMS units are commonly used to collect both concurrently. In particular training modalities it has been shown that a combination of relative load measures is required to interpret change and monitor progression (78, 79). Sport scientists do need to be cautious about the collinearity of variables (77) in any multivariate analysis; for example, overall load and total distance are highly correlated (3). Managing the data output to create valid decisions in a timely manner and influence the training process is key regardless of the monitoring system employed. Some more modern approaches look to combine metrics from both GPS and accelerometry systems to monitor load or neuromuscular efficiency by combining velocity and load as a ratio (17).

Tracking systems, however, measure only the physical output of athletes; such measures have been described as the **external load**. Integration of positional data as external load with **internal load** measures, which reflect the actual physiological cost to do the work, may provide avenues of interpretation relating to load monitoring, fitness, and fatigue measures (34). In addition, the physical demand from skill practice has traditionally been overlooked from workload aggregations. The application of wearable technology may therefore be used to understand the movement demands of such technical aspects and enable skill acquisition to be incorporated into the training program (30).

Speed and Velocity Change Tracking

Several studies have shown that GPS sampling at 10 Hz or greater can provide a relatively accurate measure of peak speed (10, 37, 60). In team sports this is beneficial to sport scientists who want to assess the peak speed of their athletes since they can take measures from within-game situations or, if testing formally, can do so without the use of additional equipment such as timing gates. Furthermore, because sport scientists may adopt relative speed thresholds to monitor their athletes, which may be based on peak speed, it would be best practice to identify peak speed using the same device that the relative threshold is going to be applied to. Consideration must be given to how often these peak speed values are revised and if a new value will retrospectively change the analysis of the season to this point, or moving forward. Research has shown that GPS can provide an acceptable signal-to-noise ratio to measure maximal acceleration also (41).

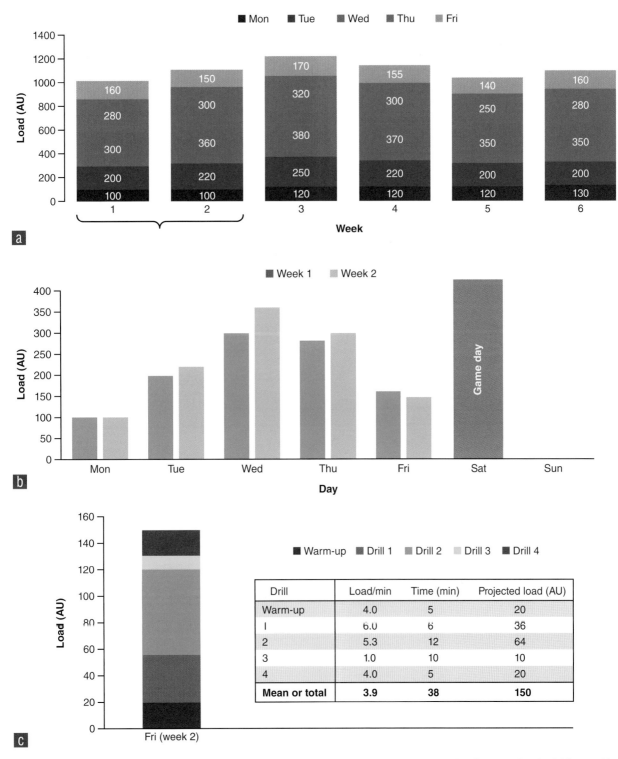

FIGURE 10.3   *(a)* Projected weekly team load in arbitrary units (AU), *(b)* projected daily team load within weekly microcycle showing the uncontrolled element of the game and the weekly loading cycle, as well as the difference within weeks, and *(c)* daily training plan showing individual drills and planned loading pattern for session.

In relation to high-speed activities, determining appropriate speed thresholds also warrants consideration for any sport scientist collecting tracking data. This also carries over when one is determining acceleration and deceleration thresholds. Manufacturers may define arbitrary thresholds within their proprietary software or provide consumers the ability to customize the number and ranges of velocity or acceleration thresholds or both, which has led to variability in those employed throughout research and practice

(see figure 10.4 and table 10.1; 3, 28a, 46, 66a, 67). This is seen across sports, with the greatest variation as the speed increases, but even then this transition point is not clear and is defined as jogging, striding, and high-velocity running (25). Practitioners should also be aware of the units in use ranging from m/s to kph, mph, and yd/s based on the continent or location. The goal is to highlight the effect of setting thresholds and how this affects the data considered rather than to provide advice on setting a particular threshold.

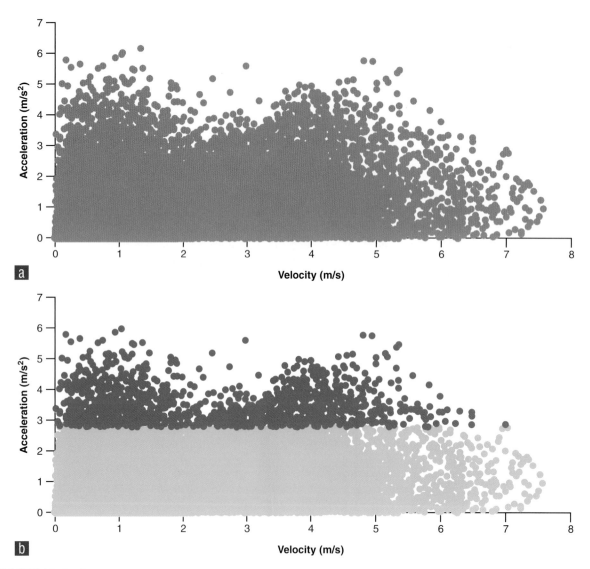

FIGURE 10.4 Examples of acceleration and velocity threshold for a single basketball athlete in a single session. Absolute accelerations are plotted against velocity for each sample point within the session. All data is shown *(a)* and then highlighted to indicate how it can be "cut" into high/low acceleration bands *(b), (continued)*

Based on Dwyer and Gabbett (2012); Suárez-Arrones et al. (2012).

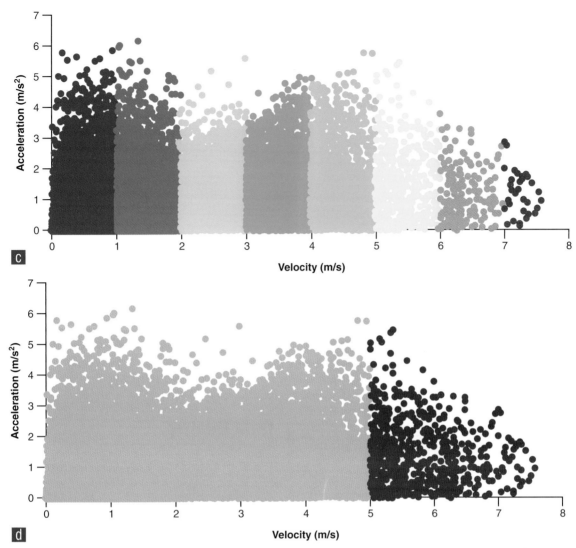

FIGURE 10.4 *(CONTINUED)*   specific continuous velocity bands *(c)* and high/low velocity bands *(d)*

Based on Dwyer and Gabbett (2012); Suárez-Arrones et al. (2012).

TABLE 10.1*a*   **Examples for Arbitrary Velocity Bands Across Sports**

		Stand	Walk	Jog	Run	Sprint
m/s	Soccer	<0.10	2.00	3.70	6.00	>6.10
	Rugby	<1.64	3.31	3.86	5.53	>5.56
	AFL	<0.10	2.40	3.50	5.60	>5.70
km/h	Soccer	<0.36	7.20	13.32	21.60	>21.96
	Rugby	<5.90	11.92	13.90	19.91	>20.02
	AFL	<0.36	8.64	12.60	20.16	>20.52
mph	Soccer	<0.22	4.47	8.28	13.42	>13.65
	Rugby	<3.67	7.40	8.63	12.37	>12.44
	AFL	<0.22	5.37	7.83	12.53	>12.75
Relative	Soccer	<10%	30	50	75	>90%
	Rugby	<15%	25	50	70	>88%
	AFL	<5%	10	40	65	>92%

TABLE 10.1*b* **Examples for Arbitrary Acceleration Bands Across Sports**

	Basketball	Football
A1	1	1
A2	2.5	3
A3	>4	>10
D1	–1	–1
D2	–2.5	–3
D3	<–4	<–10

Based on Dwyer and Gabbett (2012); Suárez-Arrones et al. (2012).

Malone and colleagues (46) present a thorough discussion regarding various approaches in which they urge practitioners to consider the justification for short- and long-term speed thresholds, and to use multiple physiological and performance variables based on routine testing to determine individualized speed zones. The merits of relative versus absolute zones are also worthy of consideration since these can alter the variable of interest (51), with some research showing a link between relative thresholds and an outcome of interest (54) and other research showing that it does not matter what sport scientists choose pending their method of analysis (69). Clearly, this inconsistency in threshold definition makes comparisons difficult.

There are further complexities in threshold definition to be considered (see figure 10.5; 46). The duration of a sprint is another important requirement when one is defining such metrics. However, there is confusion within the literature, with many studies not stating the minimum duration used (67). Using such a time threshold also leads to calculation problems such as not counting entries just under the threshold; in addition, a single sprint can potentially count twice if the velocity temporarily dips under the threshold. Also, the use of arbitrary bins may pose issues, given the occurrence of ambiguous descriptors using < and >, rather than ≤ and ≥, as well as the limitations of discretization of continuous variables (19, 67). Finally, when analyzing such data, regardless of the methodology employed to determine thresholds, it is also worth remembering that the precision of these systems is questionable at higher speeds and changes in velocities (44, 55).

Similar methodological considerations also apply when defining and tracking accelerations and decelerations. Using high-speed metrics alone may underestimate workload demands, given that energetically demanding accelerations and decelerations may occur at lower speeds (66, 72). Therefore, capturing the high-intensity activities is crucial, but, as with high-speed demands, there remains a lack of consensus regarding how to define such movements. Alternative data processing approaches to quantify the impact of acceleration and deceleration on workload have been explored to address this, such as providing an average acceleration-deceleration metric considering only absolute values (26) or determining the number of efforts undertaken (75).

Data Quality

While sport scientists can potentially extract the raw signal and conduct their own analysis using purpose-built software or computer coding options to automate a series of steps (28), they must also consider when to exclude data from analysis. While HDoP and the number of satellites connected to the GPS device can determine this, there may be irregularities in the velocity or acceleration traces caused by a loss in satellite signal, which can affect the signal but may not drop below a threshold for exclusion in terms of minimal satellite number. This can cause a delay in locomotion detection and a subsequent spike in speed. Whenever analysis is performed, sport scientists are encouraged to detail the specific criteria adopted and the amount of data that is discarded, as has been shown in Australian football (80).

INNOVATIONS IN DATA COLLECTION AND SHARING

Some sports have benefited from making player tracking data publicly available. For example, in the National Basketball Association (NBA), in-game OT information is shared with teams on a detailed level, as well as summarized data that is freely available to the public (48). This has enabled widespread analysis

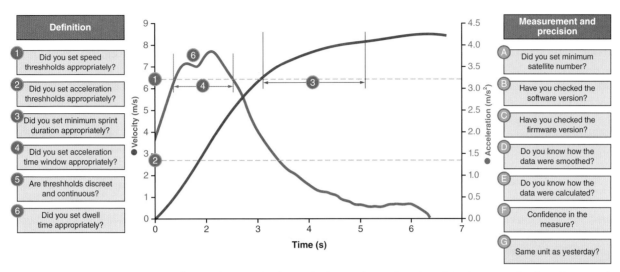

FIGURE 10.5   Workflow questions when analyzing velocity and acceleration data in a practical environment. Sport scientists should work through a number of these points when analyzing sprints or accelerations or both. They should have clear definitions of sprints or accelerations (or both) based on the thresholds (1, 2, 5), duration (3, 4) and, smoothing (6) of the data. In addition, a number of methodological considerations are given (A-G).

Based on Malone et al. (2017).

of in-game performance by groups outside of the organizations involved in the competition itself. The MIT Sloan School of Management coordinates a research paper and poster competition at its annual sport analytics conference, and finalists have previously explored open-access positional tracking data (53). In another example, publicly available NBA data was used to assess the differences in game performance between "all-star" and non-"all-star" players, as well as changes in performance based on game roles (63). In this instance, the positional data is already combined with notation data, thus enabling conclusions based on integrated physical and technical and tactical outcomes.

Teams may choose to publish research conducted in-house using detailed positional tracking information, with a view to advancing knowledge of the sport. Sport scientists may be wise to look to early-adopter sports, organizations, and individuals for forward-thinking ideas from emerging studies. Such research may have implications for understanding team tactics (2) and game preparation, and in-game management (22), for example. It is paramount that sport scientists looking to investigate similar concepts within their own environment maintain the practical application of such analytics. While such analysis may provide a competitive advantage within a specific environment, it may require investment in time and knowledge, along with incurring the potential for risks associated with conducting and implementing innovation.

In order to conduct such research, it may be beneficial, or even necessary, to explore partnerships between teams and external organizations. An example of this is embedded research, where sport scientists and PhD students split time across the team and academic environment. Collaboration between universities and sport teams has been encouraged to ensure academic rigor within data collection, as well as making certain that the research applies to the "real world" of professional sports (18). In addition, calls have been made for commercial agreements that permit pioneering research in order to better understand a given technology and its application within the sporting setting (48). As well as individual teams, governing bodies may engage in research themselves, such as the Fédération Internationale de Football Association's Quality Program for Electronic Performance and Tracking Systems and the establishment of the NBA Players Association Wearables Committee (48).

The validation of devices is an ongoing process, and new or updated models, brands, software, and firmware are released relatively frequently, reflecting the technological advances in the workload monitoring area. Consequently, when selecting or using tracking devices, practitioners are encouraged to monitor the literature for intelligence regarding their specific devices and obtain from the manufacturer as much detail as possible regarding the capabilities of the devices for their preferred metrics, as well as an indication of intended software and firmware updates. Being mindful of these updates and when they are applied within the context of the practitioners' season is important since an algorithm or firmware change that seems innocuous can change the inferences of a monitoring process, as mentioned in chapter 9. As systems develop, real-time event detection and classification will become commonplace and will combine technical and tactical information with simple load metrics. While there is already feedback based on the environment (71), there may also be real-time individual feedback on fatigue status or recovery using machine learning algorithms.

Practitioners must always keep the limitations and potential downsides to such technology in the forefront of their minds. While technical limitations around measurement precision are an ongoing consideration, the bigger picture surrounding technology and athletes also warrants attention. McLean and colleagues (48) outline concerns regarding data collection that have been discussed in relation to professional basketball but cross over to many environments. These include fears that the information is for the benefit of the team more than the individual. This highlights the need for practitioners to exhibit strong communication skills and build open relationships with athletes, which enables honest conversations in relation to positional tracking data. Furthermore, practitioners themselves have been warned of the pseudoscience used by some sport technology companies and urged to always consider whether collecting such information is unnecessary or a potential stressor for athletes (35). The motivation for using positional tracking data should never be solely to collect data, but to transform it into meaningful information that can assist in the preparation of athletes. Ultimately, the central goals of such data collection should always be to assist with improvements in availability, performance, and career longevity of each athlete.

CONCLUSION

The use of positional systems and wearable MEMS devices that enable the tracking of position within sporting activities continues to grow. Although the search for a competitive edge often tempts teams and organizations to become early adopters of technology, understanding the measurement precision of such data is essential. While the potentially increased precision provided by RFID solutions is attractive, the use of MEMS devices that incorporate GPS and accelerometers is here to stay in sport since it has taken the controlled lab environment to the applied setting of the field. While use of accelerometers as stand-alone items may increase, this will come only as software advancements make the signal processing and turnaround times easier and faster. Regardless of the system used, practitioners should be confident in the reliability of their measures and understand the impact of different updates or processing techniques on this. Only once the validity, reliability, and between-systems agreement have been established can data be applied for practical interventions such as stratifying demands based on groups, individual load monitoring, and rehabilitation or return-to-play markers.

RECOMMENDED READINGS

Gray, AJ, Shorter, K, Cummins, C, Murphy, A, and Waldron, M. Modelling movement energetics using Global Positioning System devices in contact team sports: limitations and solutions. *Sports Med* 48:1357-1368, 2018.

Leser, R, Schleindlhuber, A, Lyons, K, and Baca, A. Accuracy of an UWB-based position tracking system used for time-motion analyses in game sports. *Eur J Sport Sci* 14:635-642, 2014.

Linke, D, Link, D, and Lames, M. Validation of electronic performance and tracking systems EPTS under field conditions. *PLoS One* 13:e0199519, 2018.

O'Reilly, M, Caulfield, B, Ward, T, Johnston, W, and Doherty, C. Wearable inertial sensor systems for lower limb exercise detection and evaluation: a systematic review. *Sports Med* 48:1221-1246, 2018.

Scott, MTU, Scott, TJ, and Kelly, VG. The validity and reliability of Global Positioning Systems in team sport: a brief review. *J Strength Cond Res* 30:1470-2490, 2016.

Kinematics and Gait Analysis

Enda King, PhD

Chris Richter, PhD

How people move is fundamental to how they interact with their environment during everyday tasks and especially during athletic performance. Those involved in the coaching, athletic development, and rehabilitation of athletes are likely to carry out some form of informal subjective movement analysis during almost every interaction with an athlete. This may pertain to how the athlete executes a sport-specific task (e.g., golf swing or running mechanics), explosive exercise (e.g., jumping and landing), or strength exercise (e.g., front squat); the aim is to identify factors that may relate to injury or performance. However, this approach lacks the objectivity and consistency required to track changes within an athlete over a period to time, compare movement between athletes within a team or sport, or compare assessments between coaches or sport scientists examining the same athlete. The recording and analysis of the motion of objects is a subfield of biomechanics known as kinematics. **Kinematic analysis** provides coaches and practitioners the ability to objectively assess an athlete or group of athletes periodically. This enables the identification of barriers to, or improvements in, athletic performance, screening for injury-specific risk factors, and assessment of the effect of interventions or training programs on changing movement. This section describes commonly used kinematic variables and techniques required to capture and process kinematic data, as well as methods of analysis that are available today. It also outlines frequently used movement tests, with the key variables for each test or movement that have been identified relating to injury and performance. The chapter should enhance the sport scientist's understanding of the options available to objectively assess movement, the strengths and weaknesses of each method, and the key variables and tests to consider for assisting in the management of athletes.

KINEMATIC VARIABLES

Kinematics describes the motion of objects without assessing the forces that cause motion (known as **kinetics** and covered in chapter 12). The most commonly reported **kinematic variables** relate to the center of mass (CoM) (of an individual segment or the whole body), as well as linear and angular displacement, velocity, and acceleration.

Center of Mass

The **center of mass** is defined as the point that corresponds to the mean position for the concentration of the entire matter of a body (79, 106, 108). The CoM is an imaginary point that sits in the geometric center (the middle) of a regularly shaped and dense object (e.g., center of a ball). The CoM of an object with irregular shape and density is dependent on shape and mass distribution. When one is calculating the CoM of an athlete (object with interlinked irregular segments), the position of the center of each segment and their relative mass (anthropometric data) need to be considered (see figure 11.1). The CoM is useful because it reduces an athlete to a single point that can be described in a **global coordinate system** (two or three fixed axes that are defined in respect to the testing environment, such as vertical, forward-backward and sideward), allowing the application of basic physical principles (Newton's laws of motion). The CoM is commonly reported in millimeters or inches relative to a specific point (i.e., the origin of the global coordinate system).

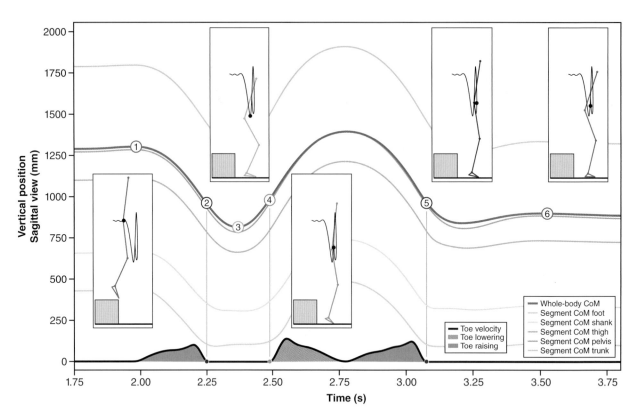

FIGURE 11.1 Whole-body and segment-specific center of mass (CoM) movement during a double-leg drop jump. The deep blue line represents the movement of the CoM during a double-leg drop jump. Shaded lines illustrate the vertical position of the center of the trunk, pelvis, thigh, shank, and foot segment. Using kinematic data, the vertical velocity of a toe marker (black line) can be used to identify toe-off (event 4) and impact (events 2 and 5), while the CoM can be used to identify the start of movement (event 1), end of eccentric movement (event 3), or the end of the drop jump (event 6).

Linear Displacement, Velocity, and Acceleration

Displacement, velocity, and acceleration are all inherently related to each other through Newton's laws of motion. **Linear displacement** relates to the movement of an object between two time points and is a vector quantity (i.e., has a magnitude [distance] and direction). If the task was to run in a straight line, the measurement would be along a single axis (e.g., 100-m sprint). However, sporting activities are rarely performed in a single straight line, and their description therefore requires two or three axes to describe the displacement of the athlete. In sport science, linear displacement commonly relates to how far an athlete has run, jumped, thrown, or kicked an object. Linear displacement can in turn be used to calculate the **velocity** of an athlete through differentiation (velocity = displacement / time). Athletic performance is commonly measured by examining average velocity over a specified distance or task (e.g., 100-m sprint) or at a specific point in time (e.g., the peak velocity in a sprint). Further differentiation of velocity calculates **acceleration**, which is the change in velocity over time (acceleration = change in velocity / change in time). This can be positive when an object is increasing velocity, or negative when the object is decreasing velocity (decelerating). In sport science, displacement (distance covered), velocity (in particular, maximum velocity), and acceleration (both positive and negative) are assessed as physical qualities. These kinematic variables are commonly used to monitor the training and playing loads of an athlete, as well as outcomes that can be targeted to train specific qualities within a session (e.g., high-speed running, in meters or miles). The relevance and interpretation of these variables with respect to individual sporting performance are different from sport to sport depending on the demands of the game. For example, the amount of high-speed running distance can be different between positions within a sport (e.g., goalkeeper versus midfielder) and between sports (Australian rules football versus American football). Similarly, in the 100-meter sprint, acceleration and maximum velocity are key metrics, whereas in soccer, acceleration and deceleration occur more frequently and maximum velocity may be less frequently achieved. The assessment of these kinematic variables can allow the sport scientist to monitor athlete load, identify deficits in performance specific to an athlete and the sport, and track changes in athletic development over time.

Angular Displacement, Velocity, and Acceleration

Angular displacement describes the movement of an object between two points around an axis of rotation creating an arc. In human movement analysis, this most commonly occurs during assessment of joint movement. Joint angles are calculated through the identification of individual segments of the body (e.g., trunk versus pelvis, femur versus tibia), the calculation of the joint center between those two segments, and the position of one segment relative to the other (joint angle reported in degrees). The direction of the angle reported relates to the position of the distal segment relative to the proximal segment (e.g., internal rotation of the femur on the tibia is reported as external rotation of the knee because it is external rotation of the tibia relative to the femur). It is usually described at a given time point (e.g., knee flexion angle at initial ground contact during a sprint) or by the magnitude of angular displacement (**range of motion [ROM]**) during a specific task or phase of a task (e.g., degrees of knee flexion during stance phase of sprint). Similar to linear motion, **angular velocity** is the rate of change of angular position of a rotating body (degrees per second), and **angular acceleration** is the rate of change of angular velocity (either positive or negative). Angular velocity and acceleration are commonly examined in relation to performance or injury risk during sport-specific tasks such as kicking a football (41, 52), club head speed during a golf swing (90), or humeral rotation during pitching a ball (38, 87).

ANALYSIS AND INTERPRETATION OF KINEMATIC DATA

A variety of devices can be used to record kinematic data, from simple to more complex solutions (com-

plexity rises with additional data points, dimensions, and segments). An example of a simple solution would be the use of timing gates to measure the completion time of a 100-meter sprint. This would allow only the measure of timed performance and the calculation of average velocity. The use of multiple timing gates across a distance could measure velocity and acceleration within specific phases (e.g., first 10 m, second 10 m). **Position tracking devices** (Global Positioning System [GPS] units) are more complex solutions since they record the position of an athlete multiple times within a time period in a two-dimensional coordinate system (e.g., a forward-backward, left-right axis). From this data, distance and direction, as well as velocity and acceleration, can be calculated. The most complex solutions are systems that collect data in three dimensions. A way to do this is to simultaneously film an athlete from different views (optical systems) or to combine a set of sensors that capture the velocity and rotation of the sensor unit attached to the body known as **inertial measurement units** (IMU) (see chapter 10). Optical systems can be separated into systems that track the position of a marker (**optical marker-based system**) and systems that identify the object to be tracked in the video and fit a predefined model into a silhouette (**optical marker-less system**). Table 11.1 examines the details of these three systems.

When using optical or IMU motion capture systems, a static trial is required at the start of testing. During the static trial the athlete is asked to assume a predefined position and the captured data is then fitted into a predefined anatomical model. Anatomical models can differ greatly in their complexity (e.g., some models have the foot as a single segment with no joints; others have it as a segment with multiple joints), and this is an important point for consideration depending on the movement and segment to be measured (79). While the principles behind optical and IMU motion capture systems differ, the position of a segment or object (e.g., the trunk) is commonly described with respect to a three-dimensional global coordinate system (x-y-z). The position and rotation of a segment can therefore be described and calculated by a 4-point × 3-axis matrix that consists of a point of origin as well as the end points of the lateral, anterior, and proximal axis of a segment for every recorded time point t (frame). This 4-point × 3-axis matrix can then be used to compute segments and joint angles via inverse kinematics or trigonometry (79, 106, 108):

$$segment(t) = \begin{bmatrix} origin_x(t) & origin_y(t) & origin_z(t) \\ lateralEnd_x(t) & lateralEnd_y(t) & lateralEnd_z(t) \\ anteriorEnd_x(t) & anteriorEnd_y(t) & anteriorEnd_z(t) \\ proximalEnd_x(t) & proximalEnd_y(t) & proximalEnd_z(t) \end{bmatrix}$$

TABLE 11.1 Motion Capture Systems

System	Method	Advantages	Limitations	Error potential
Optical marker based	Tracking of reflective markers	Most accurate	Restricted capture volume Marker placement required postprocessing	Gap filling Marker placement Camera movement Changes in sunlight
Optical marker-less	Image-based silhouette fitting	No marker or sensor placement time required	Restricted capture volume Transverse angle measurement	Camera movement Changes in sunlight
Inertial measurement units	Acceleration, rotation, and position of sensors	No capture volume restriction	Sensor placement required	Sensor placement Sensor drift

Optical Marker Systems

An optical marker-based system converts a collection of images of a set of reflective or light emitting diode (LED) markers from cameras with different views taken at a time point into positional data. As such, only motions (markers) that are in sight of the cameras (the capture volume) can be captured. The first step when recording data using an optical marker-based system is the static and dynamic calibration, which is performed to determine the position of the cameras and to set the global coordinate system. The purpose of the dynamic calibration is to estimate the relative position of the cameras to each other and is carried out by moving a known object (calibration frame) with three or more markers within the capture volume. The position of the cameras in relation to each other can be calculated from this step (using a process called triangulation) because the distance between the markers on the calibration frame is known and is the same across images even if it looks different in different views. When using the marker-based system, the number and the setup of cameras (their location and view) are vital, especially during more complex or dynamic movement assessments, because the position of a marker can be tracked only if a marker is captured by two or more cameras—and triangulation requires multiple views for calculation of the position

of a marker. If this is not the case, the position of a marker cannot be tracked, and this generates a gap in the positional data. The purpose of the static portion of the calibration process is to define the origin and axes of the global coordinate system. To do this, a calibration frame is placed within the capture volume, and the alignment of the markers on the frame is used to set the origin and axes of the global frame. Any movement or disturbance to the cameras after this calibration process leads to error in the calculation of the marker positional data.

Once data capture has taken place, marker-based systems require postprocessing (labeling, gap filling, and filtering) that is done either manually or automatically depending on quality of the data collected and software used. **Labeling** refers to the process of assigning and reassigning every tracked marker to the appropriate corresponding position on the athlete. **Gap filling** refers to the process of estimating the position of a marker during periods in which it was not tracked. Processes that can be used to fill gaps are commonly based on other markers or interpolation techniques. Filling a gap based on the information of markers on the same segment is the most accurate option, because the position of a marker can be calculated if three or more markers on the segment are present (segment fill) or estimated based on the movement of marker attached to the same segment (pattern fill). Less accurate options are interpolation techniques (e.g., spline fill) that use the existing data to estimate missing parts. An advantage of optical marker-based systems over others is their accuracy (less than 0.5-mm error) when set up correctly (58). Due to their high accuracy, they are often referred to as the gold standard in assessing position (95). Errors in kinematic data from optimal motion capture can originate from poor marker placement (resulting in poor fitting to an anatomical model), poor gap filling of marker trajectories (e.g., during the gap filling), changes in sunlight, and movement in camera position after calibration (see table 11.1).

Optical Marker-Less Systems

The basic principle of marker-less systems is the digital analysis of recorded images. This process detects and identifies the object to be tracked within the capture volume and generates the silhouette of the object by defining a border between the background image and the object (using a process called background subtraction). With multiple camera views these systems can detect the shape of the object in multiple dimensions to which an anatomical model can be fitted, with an increase in camera numbers improving the accuracy of the fitting. As with marker-based systems, marker-less systems require calibration. The advantage of marker-less systems over others is that there is no need to attach markers or sensors to the athlete; however, as with marker-based systems, they are limited to a capture volume. In comparison with marker-based systems during a squat task, a validation study reported differences (**bias**, which is a statistical term for the difference from an expected value) in peak joint angles of around 15° for sagittal plane angles of the trunk, pelvis, and hip joint between the marker-based and marker-less system, while knee flexion angles differed around 0.3° (75). Another study that compared these systems during gait reported biases in sagittal angles of 17.6°, 11.8°, and 12.9° for the hip, knee, and ankle, respectively. Furthermore, marker-less systems have difficulty accurately tracking rotational movements (e.g., humeral or tibial rotation) without any additional markers or sensors, leading to increased errors in these planes (e.g., errors in ankle rotation 7° [88%] or hip rotation 14.1° [129%], as well as knee rotation 22.5° [141%] or hip rotation 5.8° [207%]) (11, 75).

Inertial Measurement Unit Systems

The basic principle behind IMU systems (outlined in chapter 10) is to integrate the acceleration data from one or more accelerometers, gyroscopes, and magnetometers into velocity, which can be integrated into change in position or angle from the previous point. However, this process is susceptible to error because small errors (in measurement accuracy) are carried forward and accumulate over time. This phenomenon is known as **drift** and can be caused by environmental factors (e.g., heat, humidity). Kalman filters or gradient descent optimization algorithms are commonly used to remove the effect of sensor drift by fusing the sensor data (drift is independent across sensors).

With use of IMU systems, each unit stores its data onboard or sends it to a computer or both. With an onboard storage system, the user needs to upload the data after the test capture for postprocessing, while systems that send data directly to the computer can produce real-time views of the sensor positions, with or without avatar animations, and save data onboard in case of connection loss (data can be downloaded afterward). No labeling and gap filling are needed in IMU motion capture systems because of the attachment of the sensor to a defined body segment, so the sensor can never be "out of sight."

The advantage of an IMU motion capture system over alternatives is that there is no capture volume restriction, and these sensors are most appropriate when capturing colliding objects (e.g., rugby tackle), since no gaps or mix of two silhouettes occurs. However, like marker-based systems, they require sensor placement on the athlete, with inappropriate placement serving as a potential source of error during the anatomical model fitting. When comparing joint angles during walking and squatting captured simultaneously by IMU and marker-based systems, a validity study reported excellent similarity (coefficient of multiple correlation [CMC] and r^2 >0.75) between joint angle in the sagittal plane (hip bias = 15°, knee bias = 5°, and ankle bias = 10°), while frontal and transverse planes were judged acceptable (CMC and r^2 0.40-0.74) (2).

PROCESSING KINEMATIC DATA

Before the interpretation of the captured data, it needs to be processed and the variables analyzed need to be selected. Data hygiene is fundamental at this stage of processing in order to ensure that clean data can be used for analysis and interpretations (refer back to chapter 8).

Data Postprocessing

Before analysis and interpretation, kinematic data needs to be postprocessed because data capture contains noise and unwanted information (data before and after the task of interest). Noise relates to small random errors in the data (e.g., digitizing errors or skin movement) that can be removed using smoothing algorithms or filters (79). However, the filtering technique used should be considered carefully because it can affect the amplitudes of measures (53). Another crucial step is the identification of movement cycles and points of interest. For example, in gait analysis, identification of impact and toe-off is needed to compute general measures like contact time, stride length, or knee flexion ROM through stance. The identification of these points is based on the available data, and different approaches exist to detect ground contact and swing phase. After points or phases of interest have been detected, the extraction of key measures can take place.

Discrete Variables

A **discrete variable** is a metric that describes a key point or characteristic (e.g., knee peak flexion or peak vertical ground reaction force) of the captured movement. Kinematic variables can describe performance (e.g., jump height, jump length, ground contact or completion time or both) or movement characteristics. When describing movement, a discrete point is used to reduce the data (e.g., knee flexion angle) within a movement cycle to a singular measure to best describe that movement (i.e., maximal knee flexion angle or knee flexion angle at initial contact). The selection of a discrete point is usually based on prior knowledge (previous research or professional experience) or post hoc analysis. While discrete point analysis can be helpful in understanding movements, the selection of discrete points has the potential to discard important information (21, 23), to compare features that present unrelated neuromuscular capacities (80), and to

encourage fishing for significance (e.g., nontrivially biased nondirected hypothesis testing) (72). Due to potential information loss during discrete point analysis, other analysis methods that use all data within a movement cycle (**waveform analysis**) have been introduced.

Waveform Analysis

A number of methods of waveform analysis are commonly used in kinematic analysis, including statistical parametric mapping (72), functional principal component analysis (100), analysis of characterizing phases (20), point-by-point manner testing (20), and other techniques (12, 13, 82, 97). These techniques analyze the full movement cycle without discarding any data but require that the duration of all examined movement cycles be normalized to a fixed number of data frames. As such, waveform analysis requires an additional postprocessing step to ensure that the durations of all waveforms are normalized to a fixed number of data frames. For example, curves are often normalized from 80 or 111 frames to 101 frames (using interpolation), with each frame corresponding to a percentage within the movement cycle (0%-100%). Another factor for consideration is the neuromuscular quality used during a specific phase of the movement (i.e., contraction [eccentric and concentric] or acceleration [deceleration and acceleration]) that can be different at a particular time point between trials. For example, an athlete might have a short eccentric phase (0%-25%) and long concentric phase (26%-100%) during a specific trial but a longer eccentric phase (0%-50%) and shorter concentric phase (51%-100%) in the subsequent trial. Consequently, comparing phases around 30% to 40% of the movement may not be appropriate and could cause erroneous findings (80). This problem can be addressed using landmark registration techniques that align an event (e.g., start of concentric phase) so that it occurs for every trial at the same point in time (e.g., 37%) by altering time (changing time from a linear to nonlinear signal) using a time warp function (63, 83).

Coordination Analysis

A limitation of both discrete point analysis and waveform analysis is that they examine the magnitude of a measure or waveform as an individual entity rather than as one of several interconnected measures, which may cause the loss of important information regarding the interaction between joints and segments. However, understanding the interaction between joints and segments is valuable, as every movement is based on the interaction between segments that are not independent of each other. Examining coordination, the sequencing or timing of interactions between segments during a movement (47), seeks to overcome this limitation. Methods aimed at examining coordination include phase-plane plots (30), bivariate principal component analysis (34), and statistical parametric mapping (SPM) analysis (72). However, the analysis of coordination in sport science is in its infancy, and no evidence-based guidelines exist yet.

TESTS AND VARIABLES FOR KINEMATIC ANALYSIS

The purpose of this section is to outline the commonly used tests in kinematic analysis and the most commonly identified variables relating to injury (lower limb) and performance.

When one is assessing human movement, it is essential to

- select tests that will provide valid and reliable information relating to the athlete,
- understand which variables specifically relate to performance and injury risk within each task, and
- understand the potential sources of error specific to that test and method of analysis.

This is not an exhaustive list of tests or variables but should give sport scientists sufficient background and insight when they are considering what tests to include and the kinematic variables to measure in assessing their athletes.

Jump and Landing Tests

Jump and landing tests are probably the most frequently used tests in kinematic analysis relating to athletic performance and injury risk. Owing to the general ease with which jump and landing tests can be administered, as well as the highly meaningful nature of the data that can be acquired using such approaches, jump and landing tests present a valuable tool for kinematic analysis.

Athletic Performance

Jump testing is commonly used to assess how explosive or powerful an athlete is (62). Different jump

tests can be selected to target specific neuromuscular qualities. For example, countermovement jump height is commonly used as a measure of explosiveness since it is strongly related to peak power production (62). A squat jump is also a measure of explosiveness, but it minimizes the stretch-shortening component of the jump (98). In contrast, hop for distance places a greater focus on horizontal as opposed to vertical displacement, and may identify different impairments or deficits (7). Drop jumps from various heights are also used as a measure of explosiveness, as well as plyometric ability (efficiency in absorbing and transferring force) (91). Tests are generally carried out using a double-leg task (for maximal performance) or a single-leg task (for specificity or to identify asymmetries that may influence performance or injury risk). Jump height can be calculated if kinetic data is available via impulse-momentum or from kinematic data using flight time (video), displacement of the CoM, or velocity of CoM at toe-off. Errors can occur with each of these measures, though, since CoM displacement can be influenced by movement of the limbs (e.g., raising arms overhead) during task execution. Although flight time is a valid and reliable method of calculating jump height, it tends to overestimate jump performance compared to the other methods (4). Flight time can be modified by the execution of the test (e.g., if athletes land with more flexion of the kinetic chain than when they left the ground they will have a longer flight time, giving the appearance of greater jump height). It is important to be aware of sources of error and to have a consistent method of measurement across and within athletes over time for appropriate comparison (4).

Injury and Rehabilitation

Jump testing can be used not only to screen athletes for injury risk but also to assess athletes throughout rehabilitation especially relating to lower limb injuries.

Ankle Jump tests are commonly used in assessment after foot and ankle injury. Countermovement jump height has been reported to differentiate between those with more or less severe Achilles tendinopathy symptoms (89), and jump height deficits have been shown to persist for up to 6 years after Achilles tendon repair (76). Achilles stiffness has been demonstrated to influence drop jump performance, with greater tendon stiffness relating to shorter ground contact times and greater jump height (1). In addition, asymmetries in reactive strength and drop jump height are strongly related to asymmetries in ankle stiffness (54). Athletes presenting with chronic ankle instability have been demonstrated to have altered landing strategies with decreased knee flexion and increased hip flexion and external rotation to compensate for deficits at the ankle joint (9, 92, 93) (see figure 11.2).

Knee Kinematic studies relating to knee injury risk tend to focus on the landing or decelerative component of the jump. Kinematic variables at the hip and knee have been suggested to be a risk factors for **anterior cruciate ligament** (ACL) injury during a double-leg drop jump (35, 73). In addition, asymmetries in frontal and sagittal plane kinematics at the hip and knee have been demonstrated across a battery of jump tests after ACL reconstruction compared to the healthy limb and previously uninjured athletes (40, 45, 46). Athletes presenting with patellar tendinopathy have demonstrated lower peak flexion angles and angular displacement at the hip and knee during landing (81, 96). Differences in hip and trunk position during landing have also been demonstrated in female athletes with patellofemoral pain (77, 78).

Hip and Lumbar Spine Key kinematic variables relating to hip and groin injury tend to relate to the control of hip adduction. Increases in hip adduction

have been demonstrated during hopping in those presenting with athletic groin pain, and resolve to normative levels after rehabilitation in people who have a pain-free return to sport (31). In addition, it has been suggested to be a propagative factor in those presenting with lateral hip pain or gluteal tendinopathy (33). Athletes presenting with low back pain have been shown to have increased hip flexion and reduced knee flexion during countermovement jumps, potentially influencing loading through the lumbar spine (88).

Running Tests

Whether running is the main component of an athlete's sport (e.g., 400-m runner) or is a component of the sport (e.g., football), analysis of running mechanics can give insight into performance deficits and injury risk.

Athletic Performance

A wide variety of tests are used to carry out kinematic analysis of running. Most commonly these performance assessments are of linear velocity across

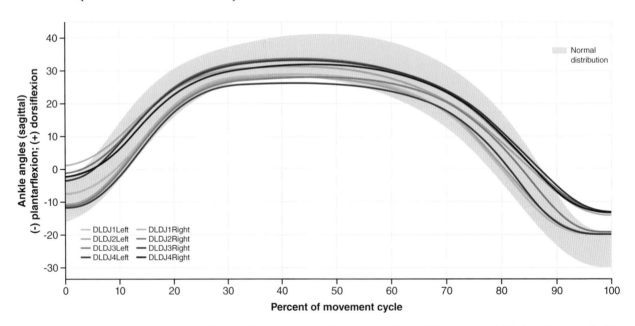

FIGURE 11.2 Ankle sagittal plane kinematics during double-leg drop jump. The orange (right) and green (left) lines represent drop jump trial with the gray-shaded area representative of the normal distribution of healthy athletes from a similar sporting background. In the chosen example, the data illustrates that the athlete presents with asymmetry dorsiflexion, with reduced plantar flexion on the right side during the impact and toe-off phases in comparison to the left side and normative data. This could be interpreted as a reduced capacity to absorb and transfer force on the right side during plyometric activity, reflecting insufficient physical recovery and potential increased reinjury risk.

various distances such as 5, 10, 20, and 100 meters. Average velocity, max velocity, and acceleration are key kinematic measures of running performance. These kinematics influence running performance and change as running velocity increases; step frequency (cadence) and step length increase, and ground contact time and vertical CoM displacement decrease with increased running velocity (10, 51, 55, 61, 65). The running speed when analysis is carried out and whether one is assessing continuous running (e.g., on a treadmill) or acceleration are important factors for consideration to ensure valid and reliable analysis. The ability to produce force, and the direction in which force is applied, also influence running performance. This is reflected in part by the relationship between toe-off distance (distance from CoM to toe at push-off) and faster acceleration times in both rugby players and sprinters (103). Although kinematic analysis should be performed throughout the running cycle, key measures are often assessed at defined time points, such as at initial ground contact (e.g., assessing overstride), midstance (defined by time or when ankle is directly under hip—assessing load absorption and running posture), and toe-off (e.g., pelvic tilt and control).

Injury and Rehabilitation

Analysis of running mechanics is key to identifying athletes who may be at risk of running-related injuries and for those athletes returning to play following rehabilitation.

Ankle   Kinematic variables during running have been associated with injury at the foot and ankle. Athletes presenting with chronic exertional compartment syndrome (commonly known as shin splints) demonstrated a number of kinematic changes after running reeducation relating to reducing overstride (tibial angle and hip flexion angle at initial contact as well as ankle dorsiflexion range and stride length) that led to a successful resolution of symptoms (8, 18). In relation to tibialis posterior tendinopathy, increased rearfoot eversion during running is consistently reported across the literature (64). Rearfoot eversion has also been suggested to have relevance in those presenting with Achilles tendinopathy, as well as knee flexion ROM, which was reduced from initial contact to midstance in athletes presenting with Achilles symptoms (5, 64). Changes in running kinematics with increased ankle inversion and plantar flexion angles, as well

as increased variability of movement in these factors, have been reported in people presenting with chronic ankle instability (14, 60).

Knee   The role of hip kinematics during running has been highlighted in various knee injuries. Greater hip adduction during stance has been demonstrated in runners with patellofemoral pain compared to those without (19). In addition, changes in hip adduction and contralateral pelvic drop have been demonstrated during the stance phase of running after a running reeducation program targeting patellofemoral pain, with these changes persisting at 1- and 3-month follow-up (68, 105). Increased cadence has also been demonstrated to reduce patellofemoral loads and may be an important factor for consideration in management of these athletes (104). Deficits in the control of ankle eversion and hip adduction have been reported during running in those with symptomatic patellar tendinopathy (32, 64). Changes in kinematics during running are commonly present after ACL reconstruction despite the fact that running is rarely a risk factor for ACL injury, with knee flexion ROM deficits during stance phase persisting up to 2 years after surgery (70).

Hip and Lumbar Spine   High-speed running or sprinting is the most commonly reported mechanism of hamstring injury, in particular during the late swing phase (69). Anterior pelvic tilt and trunk flexion during swing phase have been reported to be greater in soccer players who subsequentially suffered hamstring injury (84), with greater trunk side flexion reported in rugby players going on to suffer injury (42). In addition, kinematic differences relating to greater hip flexion, anterior pelvic tilt, and internal femoral rotation have been demonstrated between those with and those without a history of hamstring injury (15). Forward trunk lean has been suggested to increase the strain on the hamstrings during late swing phase and may also be a factor in injury (36). Changes in the kinematics of forward trunk lean and hip adduction have been suggested to influence running-related overload of the proximal hamstring tendons and gluteal tendons, respectively (6) (see figure 11.3). Overstride and anterior pelvic tilt have been demonstrated to influence the loading of the anterior hip symphysis pubis and should be considered during running analysis in athletes presenting with acute or chronic injury to the hip and groin (43). Reduced trunk and pelvis rotation coordination can also be detected between athletes with and those without low back pain (85).

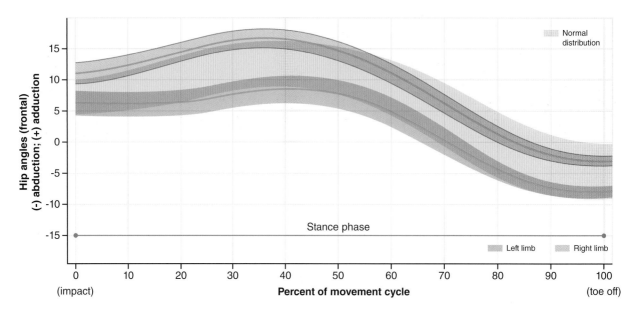

FIGURE 11.3 Frontal plane hip kinematics during running. The orange (right limb) and green (left limb) bold lines represent the mean of 100 running cycles with the shaded area on either side of the bold line representing the standard deviation of the cycles. The gray-shaded area represents the normal distribution of healthy athletes from similar sporting backgrounds. In the chosen example, the data illustrates that the right side collapses into more hip adduction from initial contact to midstance phase than the left side and in healthy athletes. This could be interpreted as a deficit in lateral hip strength and rate of force development, which may influence loading of the musculature on both the medial and lateral aspects of the hip as well as the tibiofemoral and patellofemoral joints.

Change-of-Direction Tests

The ability to efficiently change direction is one of the key components of athletic performance in field sports and also an important factor in influencing acute and chronic overload injuries, in particular to the lower limb. While these often encompass complex motor patterns, the assessment and diagnostic evaluation of change-of-direction attributes are valuable for defining fundamental characteristics that underpin performance.

Athletic Performance

A large number of tests examine change-of-direction (CoD) performance; such as the 505, 45°-, and 180°-cut, and pro agility tests (66). It is important to differentiate between the assessment of CoD during an anticipated movement, which is strongly related to physical capacity and movement competency (67, 74), and agility tests that are CoD in response to an external stimulus and have additional cognitive factors that influence performance (107). One of the challenges in assessing CoD performance is the variety of tests included with various distances and number of direction changes, making comparison difficult. In addition, there are increasing physical demands with more acute CoD angles (e.g., 45 vs. 180° [66]). A trade-off has been demonstrated between approach speed and the ability to execute more acute CoDs; its influence needs to be considered when one is setting up a test and comparing results within and between athletes (24). In addition, there is a strong relationship between performance in CoD tests and linear running speed, meaning that athletes who are quick in a straight line tend to do better in CoD tests (26). Furthermore, symmetry of CoD timed performance is poorly related to symmetry of biomechanical performance during testing, making performance time a poor outcome to use in judging movement efficiency during test execution (44, 46). As a result, both timed performance and kinematic analysis should be carried out when one is assessing CoD performance.

A number of kinematic variables have been reported to relate to CoD timed performance. Lower CoM facilitates easier transition in the horizontal plane (102), while greater lateral pelvic tilt, trunk rotation, and trunk side flexion have all been demonstrated to relate to faster CoD times (56, 102). In addition, maintaining the position of the CoM medial to the ankle and knee toward the direction of intended travel improved CoD times (102). Although the final stance phase is the most commonly assessed during CoD analysis, the penultimate step has also been shown to influence cutting performance and should be considered (25).

Injury and Rehabilitation

Change of direction is a common injury mechanism, especially in field-based sports, and its analysis is key in injury prevention and guiding athletes through rehabilitation.

Ankle   Change of direction is a common mechanism of injury for ankle sprains, with a combination of internal rotation and inversion at the time of injury (48, 71). Reduced ankle inversion angle has been demonstrated during CoD testing between athletes with and those without a history of chronic ankle instability, potentially as a protective mechanism or reflecting incomplete rehabilitation (28).

Knee   Kinematic analysis during CoD has focused on ACL injury and, in particular, on what variables increase knee valgus loading during CoD (see figure 11.4). Positioning the CoM toward the direction of intended travel, slower approach speed, and reduced cut width have all been demonstrated to reduce knee valgus load on the knee (22, 49, 99). In addition, a more upright trunk position with less trunk side flexion and rotation toward the stance leg reduced knee valgus loading (16, 17). Ongoing deficits between limbs after ACL reconstruction have been demonstrated, with increased knee external rotation and reduced knee flexion angles observed, despite no difference in CoD time (44).

Hip and Lumbar Spine   Change of direction has been cited as a common mechanism of acute groin injury and a contributor to chronic overload in those presenting with athletic groin pain (27, 86). Athletes who have been successfully rehabilitated from chronic athletic groin pain have demonstrated a number of

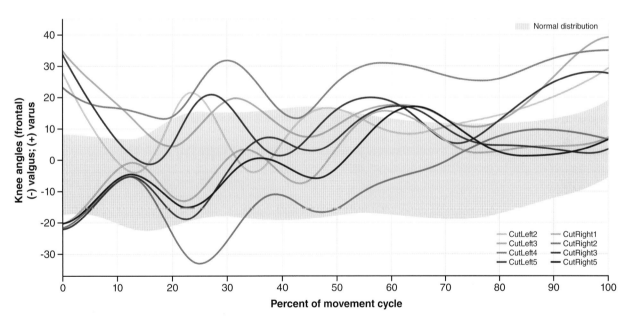

FIGURE 11.4   Knee valgus angles during planned 90° change of direction. The orange (right knee) and green (left knee) lines represent each trial of a 90° change of direction, with the gray-shaded area representative of the normal distribution of healthy athletes in similar sports. In the chosen example, the data illustrate that there is greater knee valgus on the right side at initial contact and through the eccentric phase of stance compared to the left limb and healthy athletes during the change of direction. However, it is noteworthy that although starting in greater knee varus at initial contact, the left knee makes a pronounced valgus movement through the initial loading phase of stance. This demonstrates the value of considering the entire shape and magnitude of a waveform rather than discrete points (e.g., initial contact). These observations could be interpreted as a deficit in frontal plane control of the left knee especially during the loading phase, which may influence the risk of anterior cruciate or medial collateral ligament injuries or loading of the patellofemoral joint.

kinematic changes during CoD after rehabilitation, including reduced trunk side flexion and pelvic rotation toward the stance leg, as well as reduced knee flexion and shorter ground contact times and greater movement of CoM toward the direction of intended travel, which may influence loading of the groin and anterior pelvis (43).

Considerations in Interpretation of Test Results

Once analysis is complete, one should consider a number of factors to improve understanding of the data when interpreting results.

Reliability and Sources of Error in Testing

The reliability of a test, and the data obtained from it, are key in any analysis, and the reliability of many of the tests outlined earlier has been reported (3, 37, 39, 59). However, a number of potential sources of error during testing are inherent to the setup of the test and its administration. Therefore, while a test may have been demonstrated to be reliable in a research setting, it is important that sport scientists review their own test results periodically to ensure that their execution of testing protocols is accurate, especially if multiple practitioners are involved in the testing process. The coefficient of variation (CV, the standard deviation divided by the mean) can be used to describe the variability of a measure within a testing session, and practitioners may find it useful to calculate CV while interpreting results to reconfirm the accuracy of the data collected.

Standard Deviation, Standard Error of Measurement, and Minimal Detectable Change

When interpreting data, especially kinematic variables, it is vital that sport scientists know and understand the variability, or standard deviation, of the variable measured. The **standard error of measurement** (SEM) is a measure of reliability and reports the magnitude of the spread of a variable around the true score (101). Changes in any variable less than the SEM can potentially be considered measurement error (29). The **minimal detectable change** (MDC $= \text{SEM} \times 1.96 \times \sqrt{2}$) is in turn calculated from the SEM and represents the smallest change in a variable required to reflect a true change in performance for an individual athlete. The values for SEM and MDC for a given variable will be different between tests and may be greater for more dynamic or complex movements (e.g., jump versus CoD). When interpreting results it is vital that the sport scientist be familiar with these values for each variable, specific to each test, because a difference must be greater than the MDC to be considered a real change and not measurement error (29).

Application of Kinematic Test Results

It is important when interpreting results not to extrapolate meaning that may be erroneous or represent misinformation. For example, the presence or absence of asymmetry of performance during jump (height) and CoD testing (timed) may not indicate asymmetry of kinematic variables throughout the kinetic chain, and therefore both movement and performance should be interpreted concurrently (44, 45, 46). Secondly, there can often be poor correlation in an individual variable between two tests (e.g., hip and knee angles during a single-leg squat and single-leg landing, or knee kinematics during landing and CoD) (50, 57). Therefore, a battery of tests is always preferable when one is creating a movement profile of an athlete (94). Finally, jumping, running, and CoD have strong ecological validity relating to field sports, but do not directly assess how an athlete moves in response to sport-specific demands or stimuli that require additional cognitive input. Therefore, caution is warranted when one is relating gym- or lab-based analyses directly back to the field.

INNOVATIONS IN KINEMATIC ANALYSIS

Future progress within the field of kinematic analysis will be related to further developments in technology and analysis methodology. With respect to technology, motion capture systems have evolved significantly and are likely to evolve further. The functionality of motion capture systems is expanding to facilitate the streamlining of large-scale data capture in every environment. This will help to bridge the gap between the laboratory, the gym, and the field and will enable more sport-specific analysis. This in turn will help expand understanding of underlying movement patterns that relate to injury and performance. For example, IMU sensors enable the capturing of movement during field-based tests or throughout a marathon race; marker-less and GPS systems allow the capture of kinematics in live game scenarios, while laboratories have started to use virtual reality to make their marker-based data capture more realistic while controlling the environment. While these technological advances enable practitioners to record more subjects and deal with a greater number of complex movements, and for a longer period of time, they also pose challenges. The biggest challenge will be the amount of data generated and the representation and interpretation of these data. Previous studies have commonly extracted just a few points of interest across a small to moderate number of subjects during a specific task; but when capturing data on the playing field or in other real-life situations with data capture over longer periods (e.g., capturing a marathon runner), higher-level data processing skills will be required.

In addition to developments in motion capture, there are also exciting developments in the methods of analysis of kinematic data, with a shift away from examining one variable at one joint at a point in time. Human movements are complex because the foot, shank, thigh, pelvis, and trunk are all interconnected and influence each other. Future work may give better insight into the coordination and variability of movements. Another trend is the differentiation of movement patterns, to identify the presence of more than one movement strategy within a cohort when exploring injury mechanisms (27). This may be done using machine learning techniques (linear and nonlinear) in sport science that can be trained to learn complex movement patterns that were previously hidden.

If these challenges are addressed correctly, practitioners might soon see the combination of advanced motion capture systems (e.g., combination of optical and IMU) and modern methodologies that will allow the provision of live feedback on motor performance and the risk of injury in game situations. The motion capture technologies and data analysis techniques introduced in this chapter have not reached their full potential, and kinematic data solutions will evolve rapidly in the coming years.

CONCLUSION

This chapter should provide the reader with a broader understanding of kinematic analysis, the variables it includes, and its relationship with injury and performance. To ensure appropriate use of kinematic analysis, valid and reliable data collection, as well as understanding the influence of various methods of analysis, is imperative. The opportunities for the expansion of kinematic analysis in the coming years are vast as the technology to streamline data becomes more readily available. While kinematic analysis can be extremely informative to the clinical or sport scientist, ultimately its best use is in combination with kinetic analysis, which is covered in the next chapter.

RECOMMENDED READING

Barton, CJ, Bonanno, DR, Carr, J, Neal, BS, Malliaras, P, Franklyn-Miller, A, and Menz, HB. Running retraining to treat lower limb injuries: a mixed-methods study of current evidence synthesised with expert opinion. *Br J Sports Med* 50:513-526, 2016.

King, E, Franklyn-Miller, A, Richter, C, O'Reilly, E, Doolan, M, Moran, K, Strike, S, and Falvey, E. Clinical and biomechanical outcomes of rehabilitation targeting intersegmental control in athletic groin pain: prospective cohort of 205 patients. *Br J Sports Med* 52:1054-1062, 2018.

Richards, J. *Biomechanics in Clinic and Research.* Philadelphia: Churchill Livingstone, 2008.

Stergiou, N, ed. *Innovative Analyses of Human Movement.* Champaign, IL: Human Kinetics, 2004.

Winter, DA. *Biomechanics and Motor Control of Human Movement.* Hoboken, NJ: John Wiley & Sons, 2009.

CHAPTER 12

Kinetics and Force Platforms

Daniel Cohen, PhD
Cory Kennedy, MSc

The kinetic analysis of mechanical function in humans has historically been conducted using force platforms embedded in the floor of research laboratories, in conjunction with kinematic measurement systems (i.e., motion capture, video analysis). However, the second decade of the century saw an exponential rise in force platform usage in applied settings by sport scientists, medical personnel, and performance staff, and this technology is now a common feature of many professional, Olympic, and collegiate sport weight rooms. The increased feasibility of force platforms as a tool to acquire detailed neuromuscular performance data during both dynamic and static activities is largely related to two key factors. Firstly, contemporary software and data processing tools now provide instantaneous feedback on performance standards, rather than requiring extensive data processing exercises. Secondly, the availability of portable force platforms is greater due to less prohibitive costs in today's marketplace (i.e., the cost of laboratory-grade technology is now cheap enough to be attractive to applied practitioners). Both these developments have meant that force platform assessments, which previously were largely limited to athlete profiling (such as pre- and postseason evaluations), now also feature as a means to monitor athlete neuromuscular status (69) and quantify acute and residual responses to training and competition load on a more frequent basis (71).

Force platforms provide information on **kinetics**, a term that refers to the forces applied to and by objects. These forces are measured using embedded load cells that include strain gauges, piezoelectric cells, or beam load cells. Force transducers themselves quantify force in Newtons (N) and sample the application of force at high frequencies (500-2,000 times per second) in order to produce force–time data. **Impulse** is the term used to describe the product of force and time (Newton-seconds [N·s]), or the area under the force–time curve, and it allows for better understanding of the changes in movement of the body in question. Acceleration, velocity, power, and displacement can also be derived from force platform raw data (see (51) for a description of such analysis), and this plethora of metrics provide intelligence on the output, underlying mechanics, and neuromuscular strategies adopted during human movements such as jumping, landing, and isometric muscle actions. While other tools like contact mats and optical devices can also be used to assess mechanical performance (e.g., jump height [JH]), these technologies primarily estimate performance outcomes using flight-time calculations as a proxy for JH measurement. In comparison, force platforms use the more accurate impulse–momentum relationship (45), which, unlike the flight-time method, is not affected by variations in methodological factors such as takeoff and landing position (45, 51).

In this chapter, **load–response monitoring** (LRM) refers to the tracking of an athlete's response to physiological load (e.g., training, competition, and other sources), the associated fatigue (characterized by performance deficits), positive adaptations in performance characteristics, and habitual neuromuscular status. The **fitness–fatigue model** (16), which is a central feature of many athlete monitoring programs, has led to a focus on the quantification of athletes using tools such as Global Positioning Systems (GPS) or rating of perceived exertion (RPE) (12). Force platform technology can provide a detailed characterization of individual athletes' response to load over time and can be used in conjunction with other load monitoring technologies or without these. For example, physiological measures such as heart rate variability (HRV) or subjective wellness questionnaires may complement measures obtained through force platform testing (53), and together these variables can provide comprehensive insight into the status of an athlete (i.e., physiological, mechanical, and perceptual).

The purpose of this chapter is to provide an overview of the primary applications for force platform testing in athletic populations. They include the following:

- **Profiling and benchmarking** characterize performance standards and the underlying mechanisms at a single time point for comparison within a group or longitudinally across time for an individual or group of athletes.

- **Load–response monitoring (LRM)** quantifies the acute, residual, and chronic neuromuscular responses to the stress of training, competition, and other sources.

- **Rehabilitation and return to sport (R-RTS)**, which may also be considered LRM, relates to the use of force platform data in assessing injured athletes and introduces metrics specific to rehabilitation. For this reason, it is treated separately.

PROFILING AND BENCHMARKING

The **profiling** of athlete populations provides an opportunity to establish key performance indicators (KPI) within a sport (see chapter 5), or a positional grouping, in order to track chronic changes over time that may be crucial for development. Force platforms can be used to profile and monitor athletes during both isometric (i.e., static) and dynamic muscle actions. These force platform–derived indicators may not be direct performance measures within the sport (see chapter 6), yet they can still provide critical insights that support athletic development and influence training strategy. For example, in many field-based sports, the vertical jump is often used to identify important physical adaptations (e.g., changes in lower-body power), even if the vertical jump itself is not a movement within the sport. The process of developing pertinent KPIs is an extremely valuable endeavor and should be implemented on a regular basis with respect to athlete profiling, because the transfer of training adaptations into sport performance is the primary goal.

While force platforms are among a number of tools used in athlete profiling, they provide valid, accurate, and detailed measures of neuromuscular performance. Table 12.1 shows examples of force platform use in athlete profiling. Tests include isometric mid-thigh pull (IMTP), countermovement jump (CMJ), squat jump (SJ), drop jump (DJ), and athletic shoulder test (ASH). Metrics include JH, reactive strength index (RSI), and rate of force development (RFD). The SJ, CMJ, and DJ provide global assessments of dynamic performance, and the IMTP and ASH test provide specific information on maximal and relative lower- and upper-body strength, respectively. All of these tests can also provide interlimb asymmetry measures (data not shown).

TABLE 12.1 Profiling Tests Using Force Platforms in Elite Sporting Groups

SPORT	GENDER	ISOMETRIC MID-THIGH PULL			COUNTER-MOVEMENT JUMP	SQUAT JUMP	DROP JUMP		ATHLETIC SHOULDER TEST
		Peak force (N)	Relative peak force (N/kg)	Rate of force development (0-200 ms) (N/s)	Jump height (m)	Jump height (m)	Jump height (m)	Relative strength index	Mean force (L/R)
Gymnastics	Women	1,590	32.1	2,280	0.27	0.25	0.26	1.6	100/100
Ice hockey	Women	2,800	36.3	4,400	0.32	0.28	0.30	2.0	120/120
Diving	Women	2,200	35.0	3,000	0.30	0.28	0.28	1.7	90/90
Diving	Men	3,500	50.0	6,000	0.48	0.45	0.45	2.3	140/140
Elite soccer	Women	2,600	40.0	4,000	0.35	0.33	0.36	2.1	90/90
Elite soccer	Men	3,200	46.0	7,500	0.44	0.42	0.44	2.4	140/140

Note: Data are approximate.

Isometric Tests

A variety of isometric tests can be performed using force platforms (see table 12.1 for some sample reference values). These are generally multijoint, fixed-position isometric tests (MJIT) for the lower limbs performed bilaterally on dual platforms, providing unilateral data collection. However, when dual force platforms are unavailable these tests can also be performed bilaterally or unilaterally using a single force platform. Also additional isometric tests are used in applied sport settings that measure single-joint muscle actions. The isometric tests most commonly used in current practice include the following:

- **Isometric mid-thigh pulls (IMTP)** are performed to replicate the "second pull" position of the weightlifting clean or snatch movements, with between 125° and 150° of knee flexion; participants pull against a fixed bar set anterior to the thighs (8).

- **Isometric squats (IsoSq)** are performed using a fixed bar in a squat cage at a knee angle of approximately 90° (10) or, when this is contraindicated by back issues, using a belt squat device that can reduce spinal loading (49).

- **Isometric leg press (IsoLP)** involves positioning portable force platforms onto the surface of a leg press machine, then fixing hip and knee joint angles at a predetermined position.

- **Isometric posterior chain (IPC)** is an assessment of isometric knee flexion and hip extension, typically performed supine with heels on a raised surface to create either 90° or 30° at the knee with differing contributions of the posterior chain musculature (60). It can also be performed in standing (54) or supine positions.

- **Athletic shoulder test** is designed to measure long-lever force transfer across the shoulder girdle at three different positions. These tests are of interest in the assessment of athletes who participate in sports with greater upper limb demands, or in R-RTS (4).

- **Isometric "calf test"** is performed under a fixed bar in a standing or seated position to preferentially involve the gastrocnemius or soleus muscles during plantar flexion; this test is used to simulate a key position in high-speed running.

Peak force (F_{peak}) is the most commonly assessed variable in isometric tests due in part to the high reliability of this metric, even with little familiarization (20). F_{peak} can be expressed as an absolute value (Newtons), relative to body mass (N/kg), or allometrically scaled ($N/kg^{0.83}$) where participant body mass is accounted for (67). The majority of isometric tests require low skill levels and can often be executed in a short amount of time, thus making them very practical in the regular assessment of maximum strength (i.e., F_{peak}) (24, 25). Indeed, F_{peak} in the IMTP and IsoSq have been shown to be strongly related to 1RM in the major compound weightlifting exercises for the lower body (26). Literature also indicates that isometric F_{peak} in MJITs may be correlated with sprint speed and acceleration qualities (13).

Rate of force development (i.e., the change in force production over a specific time period, or the slope of the rise in force) is another metric commonly assessed during isometric tests. Rather than determining peak output, like F_{peak}, the aim in measuring RFD is to capture force production during defined periods of an explosive isometric muscle action (1), and sampling can occur over any time period (e.g., 0-50 ms, 0-100 ms, 100-200 ms). Common practice is to sample over the first 100 or 200 ms following the onset of a muscle contraction. Early epochs, such as 0 to 75 ms, are most likely related to intrinsic and neural properties, while later RFDs are perhaps more influenced by contractile elements (1). While sampling windows shorter than 200 ms tend to have high amounts of variability, often making them difficult to infer performance changes from (13), with adequate familiarization and appropriate cueing their reliability can be improved and thus they can be useful in the assessment of performance qualities (36).

In MJITs, both F_{peak} and multiple RFD epochs have been correlated with sprint acceleration, sprint velocity, and change-of-direction performance (74). Consequently, sport scientists are encouraged to evaluate both these metrics as a means to profile and characterize training load response. Importantly, evidence indicates that IMTP RFD is more sensitive to acute and residual neuromuscular fatigue induced by competition (52) or training than F_{peak} (38). Furthermore, the later recovery of RFD characteristics following injuries when compared to F_{peak} suggests that practitioners should also consider interlimb asymmetries in RFD when quantifying deficits in neuromuscular function during R-RTS (2, 14, 68). IMTP or IsoSq F_{peak} may also be combined with CMJ or SJ F_{peak} to calculate the **dynamic strength index** (DSI = CMJ or SJ F_{peak} / IMTP or IsoSq F_{peak}) (12). This index reflects the proportion of maximum isometric strength an athlete produces under dynamic conditions and aims to determine an athlete's force–velocity qualities for the purpose of programming more efficient training interventions.

Dynamic Assessments

The CMJ, SJ, DJ, and single-leg jump (SL-CMJ) have all been widely used in athletic profiling for the assessment of dynamic performance (23), with the CMJ the most common force platform assessment used in applied settings. In the CMJ, SJ, and SL-CMJ, JH is the most frequently reported variable. In the DJ, which begins on a raised surface, contact time is also evaluated, further allowing the calculation of a **reactive strength index** (RSI = JH / contact time). It should be noted that RSI can be modulated by a change in either JH or contact time. Therefore, an athlete who maintains JH while spending less time on the ground will show a higher RSI, and the converse also applies.

Sport scientists should be aware of the protocols used to profile athletes' dynamic strength qualities. Major compound lifts such as squats, deadlifts, and weightlifting derivatives (3) can be performed on force platforms and provide bilateral outputs and asymmetries during these exercises. Elsewhere, loaded force–velocity jump profiling (41) or the Bosco protocol (11), or both, can also be performed; however, these assessments require only measurement of JHs or contact times. Since these output variables can be obtained using other technologies and therefore do not necessarily require force platforms, they are not covered in this chapter, and readers are directed to more detailed descriptions elsewhere (11, 42).

LOAD–RESPONSE MONITORING

Fatigue can be defined as a loss of strength or power or both, or an increased perception of effort to produce either (58), and is highly complex, with both central and peripheral origins. Therefore, while fatigue can be induced by metabolic and mechanical factors such as high-intensity eccentric contractions in high-speed running (47), lifestyle factors like sleep, stress, and poor nutrition can also contribute to performance deficits (65). While force platform tests may be used to quantify acute fatigue and fatigue resistance (e.g., assessing athletes before and immediately after competition or training), logistical and practical bar-

riers generally limit this application to individuals in R-RTS. However, force platform technology is commonly used to assess neuromuscular function in the days following intense training and competition to quantify the magnitude of residual fatigue, its duration, and the rate of recovery.

Various jump metrics exhibit residual fatigue effects 24, 48, and up to 72 hours after competition (23, 30). These changes likely reflect various types of fatigue, and determining whether alterations in specific metrics or parts of the force–time curve reflect specific types of fatigue is becoming better understood (75). Taking LRM measures at different intervals (e.g., 24 hours before, at 0 hours, and at 24 and 48 hours after competition) provides data to inform recovery strategies and training loads within the current or upcoming microcycle and can potentially influence player selection and deployment strategies. This data may indicate that an athlete requires a reduced training load, but could also highlight athletes coping well with the current physiological (competition + training) loads and indicate an opportunity to increase loading (18).

Based on their eccentric and stretch-shortening cycle (SSC) demands, the CMJ and DJ are considered the most appropriate jumps for LRM in high-intensity running or jumping sports (52). However, due to the greater musculoskeletal stress, or the perception thereof, athletes are often averse to frequently performing DJs as part of regular LRM strategies, especially during competition phases (i.e., in-season, tournaments). While there is less data on the use of the SJ in LRM (31), there may be some value in assessing this for athletes participating in activities that feature little SSC use. These might include rowers, swimmers, and athletes in various cycling events. The SJ could also potentially be used alongside the CMJ to contrast the response in the two tests and to distinguish SSC and eccentric fatigue from that of concentric muscle actions. Nonetheless, the widespread adoption of CMJs performed on a force platform since the core LRM test is currently justified based on practical considerations such as athlete familiarity, the volume of published evidence demonstrating its reliability (17, 31), and the sensitivity of CMJ performance metrics in the response to both acute and chronic loading (24, 29, 53).

Sport scientists are justifiably interested in tests that are highly specific to the actions in a sport, particularly when trying to profile athletes for future success. However, these activities typically have a significant technical element that introduces additional sources of variability in output beyond that related to the biological variability already present. Aligned with this, the most frequently applied protocol in LRM research (24, 30) involves minimizing upper-body involvement via performance of the CMJ with the hands on hips or while holding a wooden dowel across the shoulders. It is important that the sport scientists and members of the performance team understand the value of CMJ and other force platform test data in LRM, and that this value does not depend on its specificity to the athlete or sport in question (73). Instead, it relates to the capacity to detect relevant changes in neuromuscular status, which manifest as changes in CMJ metrics, and evidence that alterations in those metrics are associated with changes not only in jump performance, but also in other activities such as acceleration during sprinting (22, 39).

Isometric Tests in Load–Response Monitoring

In some sporting settings, for example, among heavier athletes or aging athletes with a history of knee pain or injury, there may be resistance to performing regular jump testing during the competitive season for LRM purposes. Because landing impact is often the principal concern for these athletes, isometric tests may represent an acceptable alternative. For example, in high-speed running sport athletes, IPC test use should be considered, as F_{peak} in this test is sensitive to acute and residual fatigue induced by soccer competition, with recovery shown 48 to 72 hours later (21), in line with CMJ recovery patterns. The IMTP also has potential LRM value in running sports (59) and in other athletic disciplines (66). In some team-sport environments, weekly LRM includes both CMJ and IPC testing to provide information on load response in different muscle groups.

Analysis and Interpretation of Load–Response Metrics

Performing a battery of force platform tests can provide a wealth of valuable metrics; therefore processes must be in place to convert all this into actionable data that can inform decisions made by the sport scientist and other members of the performance support team (see chapter 22). This section summarizes a selection of bilateral CMJ metrics that sport scientists should consider for LRM purposes (see figure 12.1). In

addition, variables featured in profiling and R-RTS literature (25, 35, 36, 68), but with limited published evidence to date in the context of LRM, are also included and referred to as prospective metrics.

Jump Height

Jump height is the most widely used and investigated CMJ metric in athlete profiling. This is partly due to the accessibility of methods to measure JH, and also the strong association between this metric and other aspects of athletic performance, such as sprint performance (39, 40). In addition, improvement in CMJ height may itself be a training objective relevant to sporting success (e.g., volleyball, basketball). There is also evidence supporting the value of JH in LRM research, showing that changes in JH can be used as an indicator of accumulated fatigue (40, 64) or readiness to train. Its use in informing modifications to a training plan to maximize adaptation has also been demonstrated (18, 19). While the following sections emphasize the importance of tracking other underlying metrics shown to have greater sensitivity than JH in LRM, JH remains a variable of interest in profiling and LRM.

Reactive Strength Index Modified and FT:CT Ratio

The flight time:contraction time ratio (FT:CT) (23) and reactive strength index modified (RSImod) are equivalent metrics, and as such only one of these metrics needs to be monitored (55). The FT:CT and RSImod are calculated by dividing the output (i.e., flight time or JH, respectively) by the time taken to produce that output (i.e., time to takeoff, also referred to as contraction time). If time to takeoff (TTT) is considered the input and JH the output, then FT:CT/RSImod could be considered an index of CMJ "efficiency" (see figure 12.1a). While these metrics are strongly correlated to JH, they represent a sufficiently distinct neuromuscular quality (5, 44), providing additional information about an athlete's physical characteristics. In some athletes, JH may itself be an important attribute; however, the ability to produce the output in a shorter time (TTT) also represents a positive adaptation, especially when related to speed performance (27). In addition, due to greater sensitivity to the acute and residual effects of competition and training stimuli (5, 29) than to JH,

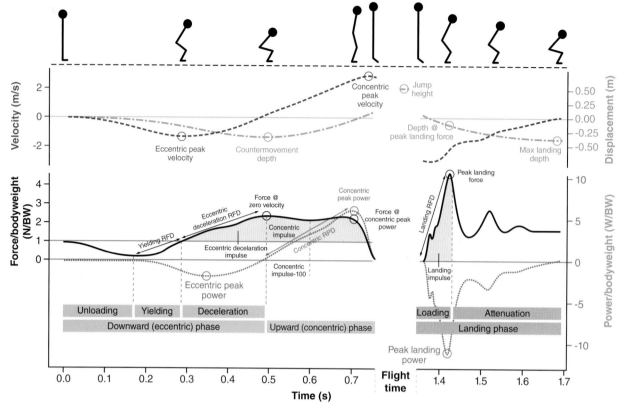

a Force (in N [Newtons]) and power (in W [watts]) are expressed as multiples of body weight (BW). RFD = rate of force development; RPD = rate of power development "Depth" refers to center of mass displacement. Concentric peak force is not shown; due to variations in the shape of the force–time curve, it occurs at different time points across the phase. Eccentric peak force typically aligns with force at zero velocity, occurring just prior to it. Italicized variables indicate that they are also examined across other epochs than those shown—concentric impulse also part 1 (first 50%) and part 2 (second 50%) time-wise; concentric RPD also 0-50 and 0-100 ms; landing impulse (landing to peak power) also landing to peak force and landing to landing +70 ms; landing RFD (landing to peak power) also 0-40 ms and 0-70 ms.

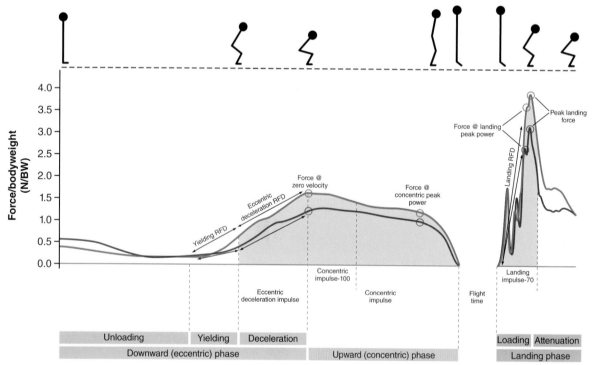

b Force (in N [Newtons]) is expressed as multiples of body weight (BW). RFD = rate of force development. Italicized variables indicate that they are also examined across other epochs (as per bilateral variables).

FIGURE 12.1 Countermovement jump metrics. *(a)* Vertical ground reaction force–time curve, velocity–time curve, power–time curve, and center of mass displacement–time curve, with selected bilateral variables highlighted. *(b)* Vertical ground reaction force–time curves for involved and uninvolved limbs 6 months after the athlete's anterior cruciate ligament surgery, showing asymmetries of interest.

 Special thanks to Richter C., Betancur E., and Taberner M. for their contribution to this figure.

FT:CT/RSImod should be the primary metric to track (beyond JH) in LRM.

The greater sensitivity of FT:CT over JH in LRM is explained by the observation that in some athletes neuromuscular fatigue manifests not in a reduction in JH, but in an alteration to jump strategy (34), expressed as a reduction in FT:CT/RSImod (see table 12.2). This change in strategy involves increasing net impulse, the principal determinant of JH, by extending TTT. This increase, which suggests that underlying neuromuscular fatigue is present, affects the athlete's ability to prestretch (47). Conversely, reduced values represent a positive adaptation indicative of a more efficient SSC, which can also occur independent of any change in JH.

Time to Takeoff

The maintenance of JH in association with a decrease in FT:CT is indicative of an increase in TTT or contraction time (CT), which in jump testing is defined as the time from the initiation of the countermovement to moment of takeoff (23). As TTT comprises the duration of the eccentric and concentric phases (see figure 12.1), an increased CT can be due to a change in the length of either one or both of these phases. In practice, eccentric duration is typically more sensitive to load (5, 25, 30) and therefore prioritized over concentric duration in LRM, but because the latter is also responsive in some athletes it should also be considered. While jump strategy metrics (FT:CT/RSImod) and their subcomponent durations predominantly feature

in the fatigue monitoring literature, improvement in these metrics represents a means of detecting positive responses to a training stimulus or to competition load that may not manifest in increased JH.

Force at Zero Velocity

In a CMJ, at the end of the countermovement, at the transition between the eccentric and the concentric phase, the velocity of the center of mass is zero (see figure 12.1a). In many athletes, force at zero velocity (FV0) is also the instant in which F_{peak} occurs. In some, F_{peak} may occur during the concentric phase, particularly in developing athletes and in sports that have a higher reliance on concentric force production characteristics. Decreased FV0 is observed after fatiguing exercise, which aligns with increased eccentric duration and CT, while beneficial increases in FV0 have been reported after training interventions (30).

Concentric Peak and Mean Power

Concentric peak power (P_{peak}), or the highest instantaneous product of force and velocity in the concentric phase, is commonly used as a metric in athlete profiling due to its associations with performance in various athletic tasks. The principal value of both peak and mean concentric P_{peak} is in profiling athletes and assessing chronic training adaptations, whereas neither of these variables shows consistent sensitivity to acute or residual fatigue and their use is therefore limited in LRM (30).

TABLE 12.2   Individual Responses to Training Load Before and After a Soccer Match in Various CMJ Variables

	CONVENTIONAL PROFILING				CMJ ALTERATION			CMJ PROSPECTIVE MEASURES		
	Jump height	Concentric impulse	Concentric peak power	Eccentric deceleration impulse	Reactive strength index modified	Eccentric duration	Concentric duration	Concentric impulse @ 100 ms	Concentric rate of power development	Eccentric deceleration rate of force development
Team mean change (%)	−1.7	−1.7	1.0	3.2	−4.2	1.5	−0.4	−1.9	−4.9	−11.5
Player A change (%)	−0.4	2.5	−2.9	1.8	−11.1	10.6	12.3	−9.3	−16.9	−25.3
Player B change (%)	0.2	−2.4	−0.5	−3.4	1.5	−1.2	−1.1	−3.0	2.1	−12.4
Player C change (%)	−5	−4.4	−4.6	−6.9	−21	27.3	4.1	−17.2	−9.6	−39.7

Note: Attention should be given to the individual variation compared to the team mean.

Prospective CMJ Metrics

Time-constrained variables such as time to P_{peak}, or the slope of the concentric power curve (i.e., rate of power development or RPD), show promise as performance metrics in LRM. Originally cited as metrics for athlete profiling and the assessment of chronic training adaptations (25), these prospective variables appear also to have greater sensitivity than P_{peak} in LRM (30) and in identifying post-RTS deficits (34). Concentric RPD and concentric impulse at 100 ms (i.e., from the onset of the concentric phase) aim to capture an explosive concentric quality in the early part of concentric phase of the CMJ. This might also be represented by the concentric rate of force development (i.e., RFD); however, its utility is questioned due to the shape of the force–time curve in the concentric phase of the CMJ, which undermines reliable calculation.

Other metrics that show promise include the following:

- **Eccentric deceleration impulse and RFD, eccentric power**, is the rate of force development during the deceleration (or braking phase).

- **Eccentric-to-concentric ratios of time or impulse (Ecc:Con)** provide sport scientists with a snapshot and the relative influence of training and injury on these CMJ phases.

It is crucial for sport scientists to understand that in addition to conventional output variables, time-constrained kinetic metrics are key to a deeper understanding of the response of healthy high-performance athletes to acute and chronic loads and in R-RTS.

REHABILITATION AND RETURN TO SPORT

While force platform testing has traditionally been the domain of the sport scientist or strength and conditioning coach, such assessments can also provide valuable information to medical staff and allied health professionals. Indeed, in combination with other performance data and clinical reasoning, bilateral, unilateral, or asymmetry data from dynamic and isometric tests can inform decision making on load and phase progression throughout R-RTS (68). It is well established that residual neuromuscular and biomechanical deficits identified in jump-land tests may persist for months and even years after RTS following anterior cruciate ligament (ACL) reconstruction, and that a reduction in these deficits is not strongly associated with the time elapsed since surgery (56). In addition, in elite sport, there is often pressure to expedite the return of athletes to competition, despite evidence that early return is associated with higher reinjury risk (33). Force platform data can therefore add critical objectivity by quantifying the individual's neuromuscular response to injury and rehabilitation, reducing dependence on time-based progression criteria and improving RTS decision making, and potentially outcomes.

As preinjury (i.e., baseline) unilateral performance data is often not available for athletes, interlimb asymmetry in measures of isokinetic or isometric strength, or performance in hop, jump, or agility tests calculated using the uninjured limb as a reference, is commonly used as an indicator of rehabilitation progress and RTS criteria (e.g., a limb symmetry index of <10%) (48). This approach, however, is potentially misleading, since performance in the healthy limb may also decline during rehabilitation, leading to an underestimation of injured limb deficit. Furthermore, after injury, significant interlimb kinetic asymmetries and biomechanical deficits are observed even in athletes who have achieved hop distance symmetry or normal JH performance (48). Benchmarking of neuromuscular performance should therefore be integrated in high-performance settings as a part of best practice and duty of care. Bilateral CMJs performed on dual force platforms allow the capture of performance and asymmetries in approximately 45 seconds (3-5 trials) per individual when using appropriate software, making systematic benchmarking feasible even when large numbers of athletes are present (i.e., team sports and military settings).

It is well documented that residual interlimb kinetic asymmetries in jump-land activities persist following lower limb muscle and ligament injury after RTS and competition (35, 43). In individuals evaluated with the CMJ 32 months after ACL reconstruction (ACL-R) (6, 7, 37), and in athletes following mixed lower limb injuries (36), the largest asymmetries were observed in the eccentric deceleration and landing phases. Hart and colleagues (35) also showed that in parallel with their greater sensitivity in LRM, alternative (FT:CT) and prospective jump variables (e.g., ConRPD, Ecc:Con ratio) may also show residual deficits post-RTS not detected by JH and concentric P_{peak}. This is evident in the case study of an elite soccer player, in which benchmark data and two time points during rehabilitation following a knee injury show a slower recovery of alternative and prospective than conventional performance metrics (see table 12.3). Therefore, these bilateral metrics should also be considered in evaluating rehabilitation progress and RTS, in addition to interlimb asymmetries.

Notably, in addition to increased JH and decreased concentric impulse asymmetry between rehab 1 and 2 (see table 12.3), this player also had a substantial increase in sprint speed. However, in contrast with the progress indicated by this data, increases in both peak landing force and eccentric RFD interlimb asymmetry are also observed, and represent important information to consider in decision making around progression to the increased eccentric loading and deceleration demands of high-speed change-of-direction activities (19a). This case study highlights that asymmetries in different phases may not correlate at a single time point (9), necessitating consideration of phase-specific asymmetries—and also that these phases may show different patterns of response to loading during rehabilitation.

Table 12.4 highlights mean asymmetries in selected CMJ variables in a sample of professional soccer players 6 months after ACL-R surgery (19a) showing substantial differences in the magnitude of asymmetry in eccentric, concentric, and landing phase metrics. Such differences in magnitude are also observed in healthy athletes (35). Based on these patterns and variations in asymmetry related to the demands of the sport, the use of universal asymmetry thresholds to identify excessive or abnormal asymmetry is not recommended. Instead, practitioners

TABLE 12.3 Selected CMJ Performance Variables in an Elite Soccer Player During Knee Rehabilitation

Variable	Healthy benchmark	Rehab 1	Rehab 2	Deficit % (relative to healthy benchmark)
Jump height (cm)	44.9	32.0	39.3	-30.4
RSI modified (m/s)	0.59	0.30	0.40	–32
Peak power (W/kg) / RPD (W · kg^{-1} · s^{-1})	58/264	48/154	56/206	–4/–22
Eccentric deceleration RFD (N · s^{-1} · kg^{-1})	82	25	48	–41
Eccentric/concentric peak velocity (m/s)	1.5/3.0	1.1/2.5	1.3/2.9	–14/–4

All values are mean of three CMJ trials taken at three time points. Healthy benchmark is a healthy preseason assessment. Rehab 1 = the first CMJ assessment performed during rehabilitation following a knee injury; rehab 2 = an assessment 6 weeks later in the rehabilitation pathway. RSImod = reactive strength index modified; RPD = rate of power development; RFD = rate of force development.

TABLE 12.4 Selected CMJ Kinetic Asymmetries (%) in Post-ACL-R and Healthy Elite Soccer Players

	Eccentric deceleration rate of force development		Concentric impulse		Peak landing force		Jump height (cm)	
Mean (± standard deviation) ACL-R/healthy	24.8 ± 15.4	20.0 ± 14.9 / 10.5 ± 8.2	18.6 ± 6.4	13.0 ± 6.5 / 4.1 ± 2.8	25.2 ± 14.7	16.5 ± 16.0 / 11.9 ± 8.7	35.3 ± 5.8	15.0 ± 2.0
Months post-ACL-R	6.0	8.0	6.0	8.0	6.0	8 .0	15.2	8.0
Player 1	28.0	6.0	20.0	11 .0	31.0	14.0	33.0	13.0
Player 2	8.0	27.0	23.0	17.0	6.0	1.0	22.8	11.0
Player 3	14.0	16.0	20.0	16.0	23.0	38.0	35.5	43.1

Mean values for healthy players and for players 6 and 8 months post-ACL-R. Values for selected players in the ACL-R sample show large interindividual variation in asymmetries and asymmetry trends. CMJ = countermovement jump, RFD = rate of force development; ACL-R = anterior cruciate ligament reconstruction.

Data from Cohen et al. (2020); Hart et al. (2019); Cohen et al. (2014).

should use sport-specific and phase-specific data if available, or determine values from within their athletes (without recent injury) as reference. Table 12.4 also shows the asymmetry profile in selected players within the post-ACL-R sample and demonstrates that the individual athlete may present with substantial differences in asymmetry values in each phase (19a, 19b, 35). Thus, testing can inform the sport scientist and medical staff on the phase-specific effectiveness of their exercise programming during rehabilitation. This information enables greater precision in the individualization of programming through R-RTS, and following return to competition, to address residual neuromuscular deficits.

Conditioning interventions aimed at reducing interlimb asymmetries in SL-CMJ performance in healthy athletes have been described previously (32). While asymmetries in these functional movements may represent strength deficits, the interlimb asymmetries observed during the performance of double-leg CMJ and other jump-land tests may in addition reflect compensatory strategies to avoid high rates of loading on a previously injured side (6). Furthermore, despite the greater loading demands of the SL-CMJ, it has a substantially lower eccentric velocity (and countermovement depth) that makes it less suitable than the CMJ for challenging deceleration capacity and therefore quantifying deficits and asymmetries thereof. These factors also partly explain the common observation that interlimb asymmetries determined in the CMJ and SL-CMJ often do not align (19a). Data from single- and double-leg tests may therefore provide complementary information that can inform rehabilitation programming. Importantly, Baumgart and colleagues reported that post-ACL-R, larger CMJ interlimb asymmetries in FV0, the eccentric deceleration phase (6), and peak landing force (7) were associated with poorer subjective function, while SL-CMJ JH asymmetries were not—suggesting that these are more sensitive markers of R-RTS residual deficits. Furthermore, while higher DJ relative peak landing force is a prospective risk factor for ACL injury or reinjury in female athletes (37), higher CMJ relative peak landing force may be a risk factor for overuse knee injuries in mixed indoor sport athletes (72). Single-leg jump peak landing force asymmetry and CMJ eccentric deceleration RFD have been identified as risk factors for lower-extremity injury in youth soccer (59a) and military cadets (52a), respectively.

The double-leg CMJ has the potential to be included relatively early in R-RTS, but as an athlete becomes more able to tolerate load, more demanding tests such as DJ, SL-CMJ, repeated jumps, and potentially SL-DJ may be added as a progression to the monitoring battery. Additionally, even before clearance for jumping, performing squats on dual force platforms can provide early information on the magnitude of asymmetries and compensatory strategies (15). Also, while unilateral or bilateral performance and asymmetries during these vertical jumps allow detailed quantification of limb capacity deficits and compensatory strategies during triple extension, kinematic analysis of these tasks may also be of value (63). Dynamic or isometric strength tests, including some of those described earlier, can further inform understanding of joint- or muscle-specific contributions to the overall deficits and progress through the rehabilitation progress.

TEST ADMINISTRATION AND PRACTICAL CONSIDERATIONS WITH FORCE PLATFORMS

When entering a new environment, sport scientists may be expected to persist with a pre-existing testing battery to allow comparison with historical team data. However, where possible, the sport scientist should attempt to integrate the best testing protocols available, considering sport specificity, athlete population, and current scientific literature and best practice. Many performance teams successfully undertake more extensive testing batteries two to four times per season, with short LRM protocols (i.e., CMJ or CMJ + an isometric test) used with high frequency—weekly, biweekly, or even daily. In LRM, using mean data based on adequate repetition ranges (3-5 for jumps, 2-3 for isometrics) is recommended over the result of the best trial when the objective is detecting change (18, 69), while maximal performances are also of interest from a profiling perspective. Robust baseline data combined with ongoing reliable and repeatable protocols is critical to creating a kinetic performance evaluation system capable of identifying meaningful change for both short-term and long-term monitoring needs.

Test familiarization, training history, and age are all factors that may influence performance variability across different sports and groups of athletes. Referring to the literature and sharing information between colleagues will aid in determining appropriate benchmarks for a given athlete cohort. While strict laboratory conditions may not be achievable in a high-performance sport setting, standardized testing conditions, clearly defined and consistent protocols, and coaching cues can improve reliability and increase confidence that changes observed can be interpreted as meaningful.

The following are testing conditions that can influence performance or confound interpretation of trends:

- *Test day relative to competition or intense training*: An example is comparing performance data obtained 48 hours after competition with data obtained 24 hours post.

- *Warm-up protocols*: Differences may exist in muscle temperature, preactivation, or acute fatigue elicited by varied length or content of warm-up protocols or both.

- *Time of day*: Due to circadian rhythms, performance is typically higher in the afternoon (70).

The inherent distractions of some testing environments, such as music, which can also positively or negatively affect effort and performance standards, are factors that are more difficult to control. Having an efficient workflow by installing force platforms in a convenient location (in or close to the gym) and minimizing wait times in group testing, positively affects the testing experience and enhances athlete buy-in. Providing timely, meaningful, and actionable insights to fellow staff and potentially athletes is as valuable as the testing itself (28) (see chapter 21). Communicating the significance of test results to current training sessions or competition schedule, and providing individual results in the context of group load responses, are examples of such practices (62). Some immediate contextualized feedback to athletes, referenced to previous performance or team leaderboards, can also be effective in promoting maximal efforts and improving reliability in these tests. While CMJ coaching may be as simple as saying "Jump as high as you can," an adequate velocity in the descent or countermovement is an important element to monitor. Therefore, familiarization should include efforts with an explosive descent. Regardless of specific coaching cues for the jump itself, two critical and non-negotiable aspects of any force platform protocol are quiet standing for accurate weigh-in and a 1- to 2-second stable period before each jump, thereby affecting the accuracy of the calculation of a number of key variables and as a means to precisely identify the start of the movement, respectively.

Allowing arm swing during jump assessments tends to produce a noisier (less stable) force–time curve, making it more difficult to accurately detect the start of movement and thereby reducing the reliability of some key strategy variables (36). However, as a practical exception to the CMJ no-arms recommendation, if the practitioner considers that use of the arms is critical in the particular environment, then implementing a protocol whereby the initiation of arm swing and knee flexion are synchronized time-wise can mitigate some of this noise.

INNOVATIONS IN KINETICS AND FORCE PLATFORM ANALYSIS

With increased force platform use in the daily training environment, an increase in applied research across different sports is anticipated, and with large data sets, analysis will continue to evolve in the coming years. Specific areas that will develop as the sport scientist increases the integration of this technology in applied environments include the following:

- *Analysis and visualization*: There will be wider use of raw force–time curve analysis using statistical techniques such as principal component analysis (PCA); overlaying of time-normalized and non-normalized raw force–time curves (75); comparison of force–velocity loops (25); and other methods of analysis aimed at identifying differences in kinetic patterns between sport positions within a sport, responses to specific loading (61), injury and rehabilitation (68), and characterization of different types of fatigue (75).

- *Isometric testing options*: Continuing creativity in positioning body segments and the force platform apparatus will expand the options for isometric force platform tests used in LRM and R-RTS. Assessments such as the IPC, ASH test, and isometric calf test are currently being integrated into LRM—other sport-specific test positions likely to be of interest for kinetic analysis.

- *Upper-body testing*: In addition to upper limb isometric tests, dynamic upper-body tests such as the plyometric push-up (46) and variations thereof will be increasingly integrated into profiling, monitoring, and R-RTS. Beyond conventional outputs of flight time and estimates of P_{peak}, the test may, in parallel with the CMJ, also provide measures of push-up efficiency (FT:CT), time-constrained impulse and force metrics (RFD), and left-right asymmetries, among others.

- *Assessment of fatigue resistance*: Quantifying the decline in dynamic or isometric force production or power outputs during strenuous activities may provide indices of strength or power endurance, an often overlooked neuromuscular performance characteristic. Furthermore, the ability to better quantify the "cost" of different training sessions could aid in planning and periodization in healthy athletes and inform progress in R-RTS.

- *Profiling sport skills*: Force platforms provide a means for exploratory analysis of the kinetic profile of sporting movements. Assisted by a biomechanist or performance analyst, insights can be gained on the force production necessary for successful completion of specific sporting actions. A good example of this is the work of Nagahara and colleagues (57), who used force platforms embedded into a running track to describe force production characteristics through an entire 60-meter sprint. Understanding performance of sprinting through first principles can allow practitioners to hypothesize as to the best methods of mimicking or modifying these force–time profiles with specific conditioning exercises. This type of analysis has also begun to be used in golf, baseball, softball, cricket, boxing, and karate (50).

CONCLUSION

The increased use of force platforms in the applied setting as tools to reliably measure the kinetic variables that reflect neuromuscular function and underlying movement provides practitioners with means to better understand physical performance, as well as the short- and longer-term responses to loading in both healthy and injured athletes. This information also supports the sport scientist's process of identifying sport-specific neuromuscular KPIs and in evaluating progression in an athlete or team. The rapid measurements and data processing, as well as the flexibility of this technology, also facilitate applied research and development of new tests and variables of interest in isometric, dynamic upper- or lower-body tests. Additionally, key elements of sporting actions can be interrogated mechanistically to provide information that complements kinematic analyses, further enhancing understanding of various sport actions.

A sport scientist with the ability to use force platform technology, interpret and communicate results across an organization, and also contribute to a culture where this data and the process of collection is valued by athletes, performance staff, and coaches alike can add immense value to a sporting organization. Along with the appropriate statistical analysis, short-term (e.g., daily, weekly) and more long-term (e.g., monthly, yearly) decisions around training and recovery can be informed by this data. Systematic benchmarking of neuromuscular profile with this technology and greater integration into R-RTS promise to enhance the precision of these processes, as well as musculoskeletal health outcomes of athletes.

RECOMMENDED READINGS

Beckham, G, Suchomel, T, and Mizuguchi, S. Force plate use in performance monitoring and sport science testing. *New Studies in Athletics* no. 3, 2014.

Buchheit, M. Want to see my report, coach? *Aspetar Sports Med J* 6:36-43, 2017.

Chavda, S, Bromley, T, Jarvis, P, Williams, S, Bishop, C, Turner, AN, and Mundy, PD. Force-time characteristics of the countermovement jump: analyzing the curve in Excel. *Strength Cond J* 40:67-77, 2018.

Coles, PA. An injury prevention pyramid for elite sport teams. *Br J Sports Med* 52:1008-1010, 2018.

Linthorne, NP. Analysis of standing vertical jumps using a force platform. *Am J Physics* 69:1198-1204, 2001.

Strength Tracking and Analysis

Jean-Benoît Morin, PhD
Pierre Samozino, PhD

When athletes want to change velocity (i.e., accelerate or decelerate) or movement direction (i.e., side-to-side or down and up), they have to project force into the ground. This stems from Newton's principles of dynamics. The same principles apply during acting on a ball, a racket, or an opponent, with force having to be applied to these various types of external mass. This force production should be as high as possible in many sporting activities (team sports, martial arts, or track and field) in which rapid movement changes are key performance indicators, or when athletes have to resist or overcome resistance, as in contact and collision sports. The athlete's maximal force output capability is thus one of the numerous components of sport performance and one of the most important traits in sports involving explosive and ballistic movements. Among the physical qualities of an athlete, this is what is commonly called **maximal strength**. In some languages, the same term is used for strength or force (e.g., "force" in French). However, the expression of maximal strength should not be confused with the force developed during a given movement performed with maximal effort. The latter does not reflect the maximal strength quality of athletes since it is specific to the mechanical constraints of the task (inertia, resistance). For example, the force, mechanical impulse, or power output developed during a maximal vertical jump is not a correct metric for maximal lower limb strength, since it also directly depends on the inertia and resistance offered by the athlete's body mass and weight (27). A given athlete may thus be able to produce more or less force depending on jump loading conditions, so these values may not characterize that athlete's maximal lower limb strength or maximal force production capabilities. The aim of this

chapter is to explore the important factors that relate to strength assessment and analysis, such that sport scientists can accurately evaluate strength qualities and consequently influence training strategy and sport performance.

SPECIFIC VERSUS NONSPECIFIC STRENGTH

If strength metrics should be independent of the mechanical conditions (i.e., load, resistance) in which they are assessed, they are inevitably associated with the body configuration, contraction modalities, and muscle groups involved in the movement used for testing and assessment. For example, measuring lower-body extensor strength (i.e., hip, knee, and ankle extensors) during a squat movement gives different values than if it were assessed in a seated position on a leg press ergometer, during cycling sprints, or when performing knee extensor isokinetic testing (34). The testing task should therefore be carefully chosen after consideration of what exactly needs to be assessed, especially with respect to kinematic and kinetic specificity. This goes from the strength of a specific muscle group (e.g., knee extensors) in very standardized conditions (e.g., using a leg extension machine to isolate the movement to a single joint), to the assessment of lower-body extensor strength during cycling (implying multiple joints) or the assessment of strength during rowing, which involves the whole body. The latter two provide more macroscopic strength indices that are closer to functional performance, while the former is more informative about the mechanical capabilities of the neuromuscular system of a given muscle group, nonspecific to any sport activity. When focusing on strength and conditioning and sport performance, strength assessment closely related to functional movement is of great interest. So, measuring what magnitude of force the lower or upper limbs are able to produce is common and yields direct practical insight to orient training and maximize performance. For this reason, this chapter focuses on such strength assessment, even if all the concepts and methods presented here can also be applied to other more specific strength diagnostics.

Among the various upper- and lower-body strength tests, it is worth distinguishing strength assessments that are specific to a given sporting activity from those that are nonspecific. The latter aim at evaluating the total force output that the neuromuscular system of the limbs is able to produce (i.e., **maximal capacity**). This reflects testing based on squatting, jumping, leg press, or bench press exercises, for instance. The interest is not to test lower limb strength in order to improve squat, jump, or bench press performances, but rather to assess the total force production capabilities during limb extension, independent of the specific skills of a given activity. Such nonspecific strength assessments contribute to performance in many sports. The associated **strength metrics**, which encompass almost the entire force output produced by the limbs, are easily transferred to different activities, and can refer to one of the athlete's general physical qualities. Some other types of strength evaluation are more specific to a given task (e.g., all-out cycling or running sprint tests). In these particular cases, for lower-body strength assessment, the entire force output developed by the limbs is not considered, only the force component that is oriented in the direction of the movement and thus effective for performance in the specific task. Examples include the normal force component applied to the pedal crank in cycling (8) or to the horizontal component of force developed onto the ground in sprint running (31). In these cases, strength measurements integrate both the total force developed by the lower body (referring to the nonspecific strength mentioned earlier) and the ability to orient it effectively (which rather corresponds to skills specific to the testing task). These strength metrics are very specific to the movement used for the test and thus less transferable to other movements compared to the nonspecific strength metrics. However, they are valuable when the targeted sport activity involves movements similar to the testing task, since they assess lower limb force production capabilities in the specific context of this task. This is the case when one

is assessing an athlete's strength during all-out sprint running tests for team sports or track and field disciplines involving linear accelerations (e.g., football, rugby, 100- or 200-m sprints, or American football). Both sport-specific and nonspecific strength testing are discussed in this chapter.

STRENGTH AS A VELOCITY-DEPENDENT CONCEPT

Beyond the task or muscle groups involved in testing, what does it mean to be a "strong athlete"? First and foremost, a central pillar of exercise physiology dictates that muscle force output depends on the movement velocity. In sprint cycling, for example, "being strong" while producing high levels of force when pushing on a pedal during the very first downstroke is not the same as "being strong" a few seconds later, when the highest possible levels of force onto the pedal are still needed, this time at a pedaling rate above 200 rotations per minute. However, in order to perform successfully, the objective of the cyclist should be to apply the highest amount of force in all possible velocity conditions throughout the sprint. The same line of thinking may be applied to many other sports or movements, like pushing a 200-kg bench press bar (very high force output, likely low velocity) versus a shot-put action (relatively lower force output, very high velocity output). Therefore, although strength is associated in the collective thinking with the maximal level of force output an athlete can produce (against very high resistance and in a very low-velocity context), it is critical to understand that maximal force, and therefore the strength capability, depends on the **movement velocity**. This pillar of human skeletal muscle physiology has been verified at the isolated muscle fiber level (15), during single-joint movements (3), and during multijoint sporting movements like vertical jumps and bench press, as well as cycling and running sprints (17). In complex tasks such as vertical jumping or sprinting, there is a linear decrease in the force output capability with increasing movement velocity (29).

The force–velocity capabilities of several hundred male and female athletes (from leisure to elite level) have been compared in 14 sports, and it was clearly shown that the maximal force capability at low velocities was, overall and within each sport, poorly correlated to the maximal force capability at high velocities (here termed velocity capability), especially in highly trained athletes (21). An illustration of this experimental result is shown in figure 13.1. Although exceptional athletes display very high levels of both force and velocity, the two ends of the force–velocity spectrum are not highly and systematically correlated, and being strong in a low-velocity context does not necessarily mean being strong in an intermediate- or high-velocity context. In addition, the higher the training and practice level, the lower the overall correlation between maximal force and velocity outputs, in both vertical jumping and sprinting modalities (21). For example, the authors of this chapter directly studied sub-10-second elite sprinters who were not able to produce a high level of force when performing a half squat (1RM below 120 kg), but could apply more force onto the ground than their peers when running faster than 10 m/s. They were definitely strong, but at the very high-velocity end of the force–velocity spectrum (maximal velocity phase of sprinting), not at the low-velocity end of the spectrum (i.e., half-squat 1RM test).

Consequently, coaches should avoid the unsubstantiated belief that a strong athlete (as quantified in classical maximal strength tests) will be de facto strong, that is, able to produce high amounts of force throughout the force–velocity spectrum. Instead, coaches should seek to assess and monitor the entire force–velocity spectrum of the athlete in order to get

the big picture of the athlete's strength within all the possible velocity conditions. In turn, since physical performance in specific tasks (e.g., sprint acceleration, upper-body push, vertical jumps) generally occurs within quantifiable velocity bandwidths, training could be based on the individual comparison between the sport task demands (in terms of velocity) and the athlete's force production capability (both outside and within this specific velocity zone).

Modern training, based on the physiological, neuromuscular, and biomechanical principles of force and velocity production, should include the assessment, analysis, and long-term monitoring of the force–velocity spectrum on an individual basis. Indeed, another clear research finding is that large interindividual differences in the force–velocity profile or spectrum orientation can be observed within heterogeneous groups of athletes from different sports, position, and level of practice (14, 21). This can help improve training practice, but also the prevention and rehabilitation process and the long-term physical development of young athletes. Finally, how this force–velocity profile changes in fatigue conditions (sport-specific or not) is key additional information for a more comprehensive description of the athlete's strength capabilities.

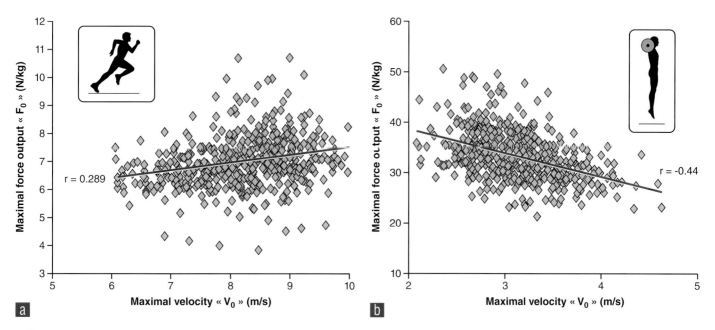

FIGURE 13.1 Correlations between maximal force and velocity capabilities: *(a)* correlation between sprinting maximal force and velocity outputs in the horizontal anteroposterior direction and *(b)* correlation between vertical jumping maximal force and velocity outputs. In both cases, the plot shows very large interindividual profiles, and rather low magnitudes of correlation.

Data was obtained from >500 athletes of varying levels (leisure to elite) in several sports (e.g., basketball, track and field, soccer, rugby, weightlifting, gymnastics).

FORCE–VELOCITY–POWER PROFILE

This section details the mechanical components and main variables of the force–velocity–power profile, and how they may be determined in vertical jumping and sprinting tasks. It then lists the key metrics and discusses how to analyze and interpret them for a more individualized assessment and training.

Force–Velocity–Power Profile Characteristics

Regardless of the task and muscle groups involved, the maximal amount of force that the neuromuscular system can produce during a movement depends on the movement velocity. As mentioned before, the alteration in force production when velocity increases is not the same for all athletes. When one focuses on concentric muscle actions (observed in most sports), this is described by the well-known inverse force–velocity (F-V) relationship. When explored using isolated muscles (and sometimes in monoarticular movements), the F-V relationship has been described by a hyperbolic equation (15, 46). However, during multi-joint functional tasks such as pedaling, squat, bench press, or sprint running movements, linear F-V relationships are consistently observed (17). This linear model is not a simplification of the more complex hyperbolic one. Instead, it is what has been experimentally observed each time maximal force production was assessed during a multijoint movement at different velocities. Researchers (37, 38) have shown that the F-V relationship is linear until at least 90% of the maximal theoretical force (38) and 80% of the maximal theoretical velocity (37), as shown in figure 13.2. This difference in models is likely explained, in part, by the different biological levels at which force production capacities have been assessed, from isolated fibers studied in vitro to sprint running on a track. The physiological, biomechanical, and neuromuscular mechanisms underlying the force measured at these different levels of exploration are different. When measured during multijoint movements, F-V relationships are a complex integration of the different mechanisms involved in the total external force produced during single-joint extension, which are not necessarily implied in the force produced by an isolated muscle. Such multijoint F-V relationships encompass individual mechanical properties of the various muscle-tendon units involved in the movement (e.g., intrinsic F-V and length–tension relationships, rate of force development, muscle-tendon stiffness), some morphological factors (e.g., cross-sectional area, fascicle length, pennation angle, joint lever arms), neural mechanisms (e.g., motor unit recruitment, firing frequency, motor unit synchronization, intermuscular coordination), and segmental dynamics (3). These properties describe not only the fascicle mechanics of a given muscle, but the overall dynamic force production capabilities of the entire limb, which can explain the differences observed with in vitro conditions for a single muscle.

The inverse F-V relationship should not be confused with the fundamental principles of dynamics stating that when the external force applied to a mass increases, the acceleration of this mass increases and so does its velocity. This positive association between the force applied to a system (e.g., athlete, ball, racket) and its resulting velocity is often the first intuitive idea about force and velocity. This is not in opposition to the inverse F-V relationship mentioned earlier, which refers to a decrease in the maximal force production capability of an athlete when movement velocity increases. Moreover, since **power output** is the product of force and velocity, the maximal power output an athlete can develop also changes with shifting velocity. For multijoint movements, this is described by a second-order polynomial function in the form of an inverted-U (see figure 13.2; 8, 36, 43). Both individual F-V and P-V relationships offer an overall view of the force and power output production capabilities during dynamic contractions. This is the athlete's **force–velocity–power** (F-V-P) profile (see figure 13.2). It represents a more complete view or spectrum than one, two, or three tests in specific conditions (for instance, 1RM squat, vertical or horizontal jump, 20-m sprints).

To determine individual F-V or P-V relationships, the athlete has to perform an assessment of a given task (lower limb extension, for instance) at different velocities, executed maximally regardless of the external resistance or velocity threshold. The only parameter that changes during the course of the assessment is the velocity, not the other movement modalities, and especially not the range of motion of the various joints involved in the test. In practice, different solutions exist to induce changes in movement velocity. Simpler methods consist of changing the resistance or inertia of the moving system (using additional load, elastic or pneumatic resistance or assistance), which by itself implies a change in the velocity (due to principles of

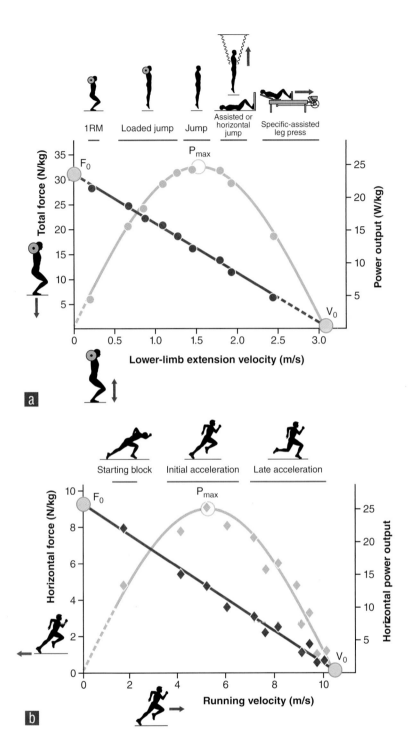

FIGURE 13.2 Typical force–velocity and power–velocity relationships obtained during *(a)* all-out ballistic lower limb extensions and *(b)* sprinting. The red (force) and pink (power) points correspond to averaged values obtained over the different all-out lower limb extensions or steps performed at different velocities corresponding to different conditions or phases of the sprint acceleration. Continuous lines represent the linear and second-order polynomial models associated with force– and power–velocity relationships, respectively, from which are estimated the main strength metrics: the maximal power output (P_{max}) and the theoretical maximal force (F_0) and velocity (V_0).

dynamics), as does the maximal force the neuromuscular system can develop (4, 43). It is also possible to set a target velocity using specific ergometers that adjust the resistance so that the velocity or the force produced are kept quasi-constant throughout the movement (47, 48). Force production and limb extension velocity have to be measured to obtain one value per limb and then establish F-V and P-V relationships. These values of force, velocity, and power that are considered to

determine the F-V-P profile during limb extension can be the instantaneous peak values observed during the movement or the values averaged over the entire movement (limb extension, for instance). Even if peak values are easier to detect, the averaged values make more sense when one is assessing the maximal force or power production capabilities over a single movement. In addition, peak values of force, velocity, and power do not occur at the same time during an all-out movement, and instantaneous values correspond to very specific anatomical and neuromuscular configurations and do not fully represent the entire dynamic capabilities of lower or upper limbs during a movement. Force–velocity–power profile testing is presented in greater depth in the next section.

Specific and Nonspecific Lower-Body Force–Velocity–Power Profiling

This section covers F-V-P profile testing for lower limb nonspecific (jumping) and sport-specific (sprinting) strength. All the considerations presented can be transferred to any other kind of movement (e.g., leg press, bench press, pulling, cycling, rowing). Note that, for practical reasons, F-V-P profiling in jumping and sprinting has been called vertical and horizontal profiling, respectively, due to the overall direction of the movement used for the test (21, 28). However, the associated strength metrics are not usable for force production alone in these respective directions. For instance, the nonspecific lower limb strength (i.e., vertical F-V-P profile) refers to the capability of lower limbs to produce force in the same overall orientation as the limb (e.g., during a vertical jump), but also during a start or horizontal push in swimming or propulsion phase in rowing. The sprint-specific strength (i.e., horizontal F-V-P profile) characterizes the force production capacity in an overall direction that differs from the limb axis, which is quasi-normal in relation to the lower limb when the sprinter is upright.

Measurement Methods for Nonspecific Strength

For assessing nonspecific strength, such as the strength of lower-body extensors, the F-V-P profile can be determined during acyclic movements, for instance, squat or jumps, by testing different trials with different loads or resistances. The greater the load, the lower the velocity, and the greater the force output developed by the limbs. Since the aim is to assess the athlete's maximal capacities, each trial must be an all-out effort. When possible, the movement should end with a ballistic takeoff for squats (or a throw for bench press). For squat (regardless of the type of squat performed or the type of barbell used), the different loading conditions can range from a vertical jump without additional load to a squat with the 1RM load (38). Between these two conditions, different loads

can be used during jump (or all-out push-off) tests. The range of motion during push-off should be standardized across the different loading conditions so that only the lower limb extension velocity changes. The starting position (or lowest position with use of countermovement) can be predetermined (at a given knee-joint angle, for example, to match sport-specific positions) or freely chosen by the athlete as the most comfortable position. The latter option is preferred by the authors of this chapter (16).

In order to determine the F-V-P profiles, at least four to six progressive loading (resistance) conditions are required that cover the largest range of velocities possible. The lowest load often corresponds to a jump without additional load, and the highest load is usually the highest load with which the athlete can jump (for quality of movement and risk reasons, loads for jumps lower than ~8-10 cm are not advised). To ensure acceptable reliability to determine the F-V-P profile, the range of velocities covered by the different conditions is more important than the number of conditions (11). When the athletes are familiar with this kind of testing, two different loading conditions (for instance, without additional load and with the load corresponding to an ~10-cm jump) may be sufficient (i.e., two-load method [11]). During vertical jumps, the condition without additional load corresponds to the middle of the entire F-V spectrum since body mass is actually a moderate load. To reach the velocity end of the F-V spectrum, modalities other than vertical jumping against body weight or additional mass have to be used. Pushing faster than during a squat jump can be achieved with the following methods: lower limb extensions performed with a horizontal direction (horizontal squat jumps [44]); assisted vertical jumps against resistance lower than body weight, which can be achieved with the use of elastic bands (10, 24, 45); or extensions of the lower limbs only (without trunk displacement to reduce inertia) during horizontal assisted push-offs (37) (see figure 13.2).

For each trial, force, velocity, and power variables can be measured using force platforms or kinematic (video, linear encoder, accelerometer) measurements, or both (12). In such a nonspecific strength test, almost the entire force developed by the lower limb is measured. For field testing, a simple method was proposed and validated to easily assess force, velocity, and power during loaded vertical jumps from only three parameters outside of the laboratory: body mass, jump height, and push-off distance (41). Its reliability and concurrent validity against force plate measurements have been tested several times during squat and countermovement jumps and has been reported to be very high (12, 16, 20, 35). A simple spreadsheet including the different computations is available online to allow athletes or coaches to determine individual F-V-P profiles and then obtain the different strength metrics (see next section) after entering the individual input data (push-off distance, mass, and jump height for each load condition). Finally, there are commercial smart device applications (2) that also make it possible to test some of the characteristics mentioned.

Measurement Methods for Sport-Specific Strength

For testing sport-specific strength, for instance, the strength of lower limb extensors during sprint running or cycling, the individual F-V-P profile can be assessed during cyclic movements from a single 6-second all-out effort (1, 6, 30). Each downstroke or step corresponds to distinct lower limb extensions performed at different velocities, and thus to different points in the F-V and P-V relationships. The gold standard methods used to compute F-V-P profiles involve tracks or treadmills (for running) and pedals (for cycling) that are equipped with force sensors (load cells or force platforms). To cover the largest range of velocities possible, the running sprint should be performed from a standing start to the peak velocity reached within the first 5 or 6 seconds, before fatigue induces a decrease in velocity. In the case of a single cycling sprint, the choice of the load is key to obtaining a large range of points that are well distributed over the entire F-V spectrum (9). During sprint running testing, the load usually corresponds to the body mass when performed over ground or to the resistance of the treadmill, which covers an acceptable range of the F-V spectrum (26, 36). The application of resistive load is possible (e.g., loaded sled [5, 7]), but not convenient for simultaneous mechanical measurements.

Movement velocity and the force produced by the lower limbs should be continuously measured to obtain a single average value per limb extension or step. In such sport-specific strength testing, the entire force produced by the lower limbs is not considered, but only the component in the direction of the movement, and thus the force component directly associated with the acceleration in the overall direction of the movement. In sprint running, this corresponds to the horizontal component of the force produced onto the ground (30). Thus, the F-V-P profile in sprint running informs the sport scientist of the lower limb capability to produce force, but also the ability to transmit and orient it effectively onto the ground (mechanical effectiveness of force application [26]). Sprint-specific strength includes these two capacities, which can be distinguished by specific indices during the sprint F-V-P profile testing (see the next section). To assess this lower limb strength specific to sprint propulsion, different methodologies have been proposed to measure horizontal force and velocity during all-out running acceleration (see [6] for review). Classical laboratory methods employ motorized or nonmotorized sprint instrumented treadmills (18, 30) or force plate systems (33, 36) for running and instrumented pedals for cycling (8). For field testing, a simple method, based on a macroscopic biomechanical model, has been developed (32, 42). This method is very convenient for field use since it requires only anthropometric (body mass and stature) and spatial-temporal (split times or instantaneous running velocity) input variables. It models step-averaged values of horizontal force, velocity, and power over an all-out sprint acceleration. The reliability and concurrent validity against force plate measurements have been shown to be very high in several studies (13, 25, 36). The split times and instantaneous velocity can be measured by various devices and lead to accurate measurements, provided that the initial accuracy of the device used is high for position–time or velocity–time data (32). Similar to what has been discussed previously for jumping, a spreadsheet is available online to easily compute the different variables characterizing F-V-P profile in sprinting from few inputs. There is a smartphone or tablet application that was designed and validated to compute the sprint mechanical variables using the present simple method from split times determined with the 240 frames per second slow-motion camera in Apple devices (39).

Key Metrics in Force–Velocity–Power Profiling

Force–velocity–power relationships characterize the dynamic maximal force production capabilities and can be described via different metrics that each represent a specific component of strength. These different indices are presented in detail in table 13.1 for jumping and sprinting F-V-P profiles. The most macroscopic index to characterize dynamic strength is the maximal power output (P_{max}). Yet incomplete, it gives the first big picture of the whole F-V-P profile. However, similar P_{max} can be achieved by two athletes presenting very different strength profiles characterized by different

TABLE 13.1 Definitions and Practical Interpretation of the Main Strength Indices Associated With Force–Velocity–Power Profiling in Nonspecific Strength (Jumping) and Sport-Specific Strength (Sprinting)

	What is it exactly?	What is it in practice?	How to compute it?	What are common values? From extremely low (leisure sport) to extremely high (elite level)
JUMPING				
F_0 (N/kg)	Theoretical maximal force output lower limbs could produce during an extension at null velocity (extreme force end of the F-V spectrum)	Lower limb force production capability at low velocities (strength at low velocities)	Force-axis intercept of the linear F-V relationship	From low to high: 20-50 N/kg; 1,100-5,000 N
V_0 (m/s)	Theoretical maximal extension velocity until lower limbs could produce force output (extreme velocity end of the F-V spectrum)	Lower limb force production capability at high velocities (strength at high velocities)	Velocity-axis intercept of the linear F-V relationship	From low to high: 1.5-6.5 m/s
P_{max} (W/kg)	Maximal mechanical power output lower limbs could produce during one extension (apex of the P-V relationship)	Lower limb power production capability (maximal power)	$P_{max} = F_0 \cdot V_0/4$ or apex of the P-V 2nd-order polynomial relationship	From low to high: 15-45 W/kg; 850-4,300 W
S_{FV} (N·s/m/kg)	Lower limb F-V mechanical profile	Orientation of lower limb force production capability toward force or velocity capabilities (balance between strength at low and high velocities)	$S_{FV} = -F_0/V_0$ or slope of the linear F-V relationship	From most force-oriented to most velocity-oriented: −29 to −3.5 (N·s/m/kg)
S_{FVopt} (N·s/m/kg)	Lower limb optimal F-V profile maximizing ballistic push-off performance	Individual optimal balance between force and velocity capabilities for maximizing jumping performance (best balance between strength at low and high velocities)	For detailed computations, see (46)	From most force-oriented to most velocity-oriented: −15-−10 (N·s/m/kg)
FV_{imb} (%)	Magnitude of the relative difference between S_{FV} and S_{FVopt}	Individual imbalance between force and velocity capabilities for maximizing jumping performance (imbalance between strength at low and high velocities)	$FV_{imb} = 1 - S_{FV}/S_{FVvopt} \cdot 100$	From balanced to completely imbalanced: 0-100%

	What is it exactly?	What is it in practice?	How to compute it?	What are common values? From extremely low (leisure sport) to extremely high (elite level)
F_0 (N or N/kg)	Theoretical maximal horizontal force output lower limbs could produce at null running velocity (extreme force end of the F-V spectrum)	Horizontal force production capability at low velocities (sprint-specific strength at low velocities)	Force-axis intercept of the linear F-V relationship	From low to top: 4-12 N/kg; 200-1,100 N
V_0 (m/s)	Theoretical maximal running velocity until lower limbs could produce horizontal force output (extreme velocity end of the F-V spectrum)	Horizontal force production capability at high velocities (sprint-specific strength at high velocities)	Velocity-axis intercept of the linear F-V relationship	From low to top: 6-12 m/s
P_{max} (W or W/kg)	Maximal mechanical power output lower limbs could produce during one step (apex of the P-V relationship)	Capability to produce power output in the horizontal direction (maximal sprinting power)	$P_{max} = F_0 \cdot V_0/4$ or apex of the P-V 2nd-order polynomial relationship	From low to top: 7-30 W/kg; 350-2,300 W
S_{FV} (N·s/m/kg)	Sprinting F-V mechanical profile	Orientation of horizontal force production capability toward force or velocity capabilities (balance between sprint-specific strength at low and high velocities)	$S_{FV} = -F_0/V_0$ or slope of the linear F-V relationship	From most force-oriented to most velocity-oriented: –1.8--0.4 (N·s/m/kg)
RF (%)	Ratio of force over a step	Proportion of the total force produced by the lower limb onto the ground that is directed horizontally (mechanical effectiveness of force application)	Ratio of the horizontal component to the resultant force produced onto the ground over a step	Different at each step; ranges from RF_{max}- 0
RF_{max} (%)	Maximal value of RF	Maximal mechanical effectiveness of force application (occurring at the first step) (mechanical effectiveness at low running velocities)	RF value of the first step (force plate measurement) or RF value modeled at time = 0.3 s (simple sprint method)	From low to top: 24-60%
D_{RF} (%·s/m)	Rate of decrease in RF when running velocity increases	Capability to maintain a high mechanical effectiveness despite increasing running velocity	Slope of the linear RF-V relationship (for time >0.3 s for the simple sprint method)	From low to top: –12 to –4 %·s/m

(left margin label: SPRINTING)

force production capabilities at low versus high velocities. The latter are quantified by the two theoretical extremums (force- and velocity-axis intercepts) of the F-V relationship (F_0 and V_0, respectively). The interest in considering these extremums, even if they are theoretical values, derives from the fact that they are independent from the loading or velocity conditions of measurement. This is not the case if strength at low and high velocity is assessed at two different velocities or in two different loading conditions (via two jumps at low and high load, for instance); the choice of the exact conditions largely influences the strength metrics. The orientation of the athlete's strength toward F_0 or V_0 is given by the F-V mechanical profile (S_{FV}) representing the individual ratio between force and velocity qualities (i.e., the slope of the F-V relationship). The F-V profile is independent from P_{max}, so it is necessary, in addition to P_{max}, to have a comprehensive view of the athlete's dynamic strength. Ballistic performances aimed at accelerating one's own body mass (e.g., jumping or all-out push-offs) have been shown to depend on both P_{max} and S_{FV}, with the existence of an optimal F-V profile (S_{FVopt} [20, 40, 43]). This optimal profile can be accurately determined for each athlete and is used to determine the F-V imbalance (FV_{imb}) toward F_0 or V_0, as well as the magnitude of the associated force or velocity deficits. These indices are interesting tools to individualize an athlete's training program aiming to improve ballistic performance. Similar indices to optimize sprint F-V-P profile have also been suggested, although they have not yet been published.

For sprint-specific strength tracking, P_{max}, F_0, V_0, and S_{FV} describe exactly the same mechanical features, except that they refer to the sprint-specific force production capability in the horizontal, anteroposterior direction. This set of variables integrates the athlete's nonspecific strength qualities and those more specific to running propulsion (mechanical effectiveness of force application). Additional metrics are thus necessary to characterize this ability to transmit and effectively orient the force onto the ground. The latter can be computed at each step by the ratio of horizontal component to resultant force (RF) (26). Mechanical effectiveness then can be well described by the maximal value of RF observed at the first step (RF_{max}) and its rate of decrease when velocity increases (D_{RF}). Individually quantifying the mechanical effectiveness can help distinguish the physical and technical origins of inter- or intraindividual differences in both F-V-P profiles and sprint performance, which can be useful to orient the training process more appropriately toward the specific mechanical qualities to develop.

Finally, due to its macroscopic level, the lower limb F-V-P profile fails to inform about all the strength indices underlying the main F-V-P metrics. For instance, the rate of force development, usually measured during an isometric exercise modality (23), is a key strength metric for explosive contractions. It is one of the mechanical underpinnings of F_0 and mostly V_0, and in turn of P_{max}. Even though the rate of force development is not discussed here, the authors of this chapter think that it should be measured in addition to the F-V-P profile to characterize a particular component of nonspecific strength (especially if explosiveness is targeted).

Analysis and Interpretation of Force–Velocity–Power Characteristics

It is important to build, analyze, and interpret the individual F-V-P spectrum beyond the basic performance analysis (e.g., jump height or sprint time). Understanding how to interpret the individual results is an important skill for the sport scientist, which, if done in the specific context of the athlete (e.g., level of practice, objectives, physical and training, or rehabilitation status, etc.), will allow more in-depth and evidence-based training programming. Of course, sometimes athletes show very similar profiles and mechanical outputs for the same level of jump or sprint performance, but most of the time individual athletes have profiles with different subcomponents, which is what makes the testing and tracking of physical capabilities and the quest for margins of improvements so interesting. At this point, the group or team average and normative collective data will be considered as a broad reference, since sport scientists first and foremost seek to improve or maintain individual players' capabilities, rather than group averages.

Mechanical Profile of Lower Limb Extension and Jump Performance

The first step in the analysis of the individual lower limb F-V-P spectrum with the method described in this chapter is to simply map the main mechanical variables described earlier. This will give a detailed picture of the individual's capabilities in the context of the test, which has not only immediate interest (describing performance and its mechanical underpinnings), but also a long-term impact (a time point within a development, training, rehabilitation process).

In the case of vertical jumping tests (typically squat or countermovement jumps) that allow analysis of the overall lower limb capabilities, studies have shown that jump performance (i.e., maximal jump height) was sometimes not a good indicator of lower limb maximal power (27). Several factors may confound the relationship between maximal power output and squat or countermovement jump height and should thus be considered for a thorough analysis: body mass, the push-off distance, and the F-V profile itself. For the latter, research has shown that for a given level of P_{max}, among the many possible profiles (i.e., slope of the F-V relationship), jump performance was maximized for an optimal value. In turn, any FV_{imb} will be associated with a submaximal jump performance, and thus a potential margin for improvement. Research in highly trained athletes showed that the best athletes were those who showed both a high P_{max} capability and a low FV_{imb} (i.e., an actual F-V profile slope close to their individual optimal slope [40]). The following example (see figure 13.3) shows two athletes with the very same jump performance (squat jump height of

27 cm), but very different F-V profiles and anthropometrical features. The analysis of these athletes is an example of how to interpret the F-V profile in the context of training for jump performance improvement. It is then possible to extrapolate this approach to other contexts, such as rehabilitation and return-to-play scenarios.

The interpretation here is that an improvement in these athletes' respective jump performance will likely result from different training programs, or at least different modulations of the training content. A similar one-size-fits-all training approach will likely result in suboptimal adaptations since these players show different mechanical components for a similar jump performance. In this particular case, as will be discussed later, Player A should follow a program that will decrease FV_{imb} (especially by improving the left side of the profile, i.e., more force-oriented profile) in addition to improving P_{max}. In contrast, Player B should follow a training program that will aim to shift the entire F-V curve toward higher levels of P_{max} while maintaining a similar, close-to-optimal profile.

Player A	
Squat jump height	27.0 cm
Body mass	90 kg
Pushoff distance	0.25 m
P_{max}	24.5 W/kg
FV_{imb}	40%

Player B	
Squat jump height	27.0 cm
Body mass	80 kg
Pushoff distance	0.35 m
P_{max}	20.0 W/kg
FV_{imb}	1%

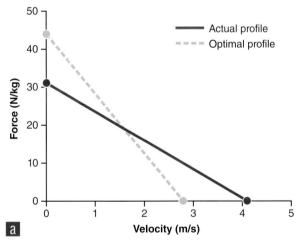
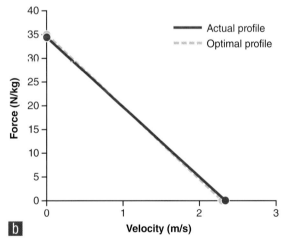

FIGURE 13.3   Two athletes with the same squat jump performance (maximal jump height of 27 cm) can show very different lower limb P_{max}, and vice versa. In this example, *(a)* Player A shows a 20% greater P_{max} but a large FV_{imb}, greater body mass, and a shorter push-off distance, explaining why Player A's jump performance is not greater than that of Player B; *(b)* despite the lower P_{max}, Player B shows an almost perfect optimal profile (FV_{imb} close to 0).

Mechanical Profile of Sprint Acceleration Performance

The very same analysis can be applied to sprint acceleration performance: Similar sprint time does not necessarily mean similar underpinning mechanical profile. Linear sprint acceleration performance (e.g., 30-m or 40-yd dash) can be interpreted as resulting from the following mechanical variables (see description earlier): P_{max} (determined by F_0 and V_0 values), RF_{max}, and D_{RF}. The following example (see figure 13.4) shows two rugby players with the same 30-meter performance, but very different underpinning mechanical profiles.

Player A shows a greater P_{max} and sprint F_0, partly explained by a greater maximal RF at the beginning of the sprint (49%). However, Player B shows a lower RF_{max}, but a better ability to limit the decrease in RF with increasing velocity (D_{RF} of −7.64% s/m versus −11.2% s/m for Player A). Player B is therefore able to produce more net anteroposterior force onto the ground for longer during the acceleration, and eventually reach a greater maximal speed in the last phase of the sprint. Should the testing distance be shorter or longer than the 30 meters chosen here, the interpretation of these two individuals' sprint capabilities, and the associated training recommendation, would likely differ. Sprint testing interpretation should not depend on the testing distance chosen. This is why the authors strongly recommend that sport scientists build and analyze the entire F-V profile, which is pos-

sible from data for a single sprint. In this example, the individual training should be at least in part tailored to the specific profiles, and thus needs, of Players A and B. Specifically, Player A should improve his ability to orient the force more horizontally with increasing running velocity (D_{RF}) and his horizontal force production capabilities at high velocity (V_0). In contrast, Player B should improve his maximal horizontal force output via a better ability to orient the force horizontally at very low running velocity (RF_{max}). In addition, if the lower limb F_0 of Player B in the jump profile is lower (force-oriented deficit or low F_0 value or both), his training content should target both his lower limb nonspecific maximal force output and his ability to transfer it in the specific sprint acceleration context. This supports the fact that even in sprint specialists, lower limb profiling using the jumping profile method helps to build a comprehensive picture of the athlete's capabilities and allows for better deciphering of the associated training needs and priorities.

Profile-Based Modulation of Training Content

When considering an entire team or group, this individual interpretation will surely make the overall analysis and interpretation challenging, but the large differences in interindividual profiles and performance make the potential for more effective training evident. An individually (or group, if several athletes show similar mechanical features) tailored program,

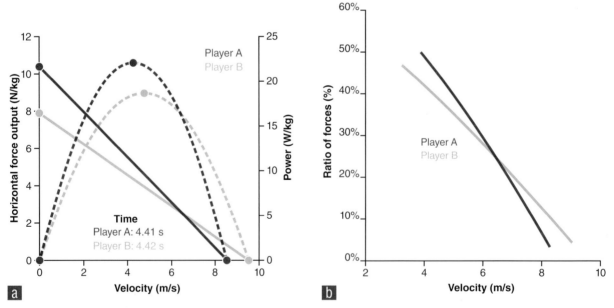

FIGURE 13.4 Two rugby players with almost identical 30-meter sprint performance but very different (a) force–velocity–power profiles and (b) ratio of forces as a function of running velocity. The force lines are solid and the power curve lines are dashed.

at least in part, can be built to both target and fix weak links and reinforce or maintain strong links in the mechanics performance chain (28). In contrast, it is likely that a one-size-fits-all approach (i.e., with no individual modulation of the training content) will induce suboptimal adaptations at the individual level, even if the average results are positive. The sport scientist must focus on individual effects of training, not only group average effects that could easily mask nonresponders or even negative responders. The first study to show the superiority of an individually designed program as a function of FV_{imb} to improve jumping performance was published by Jiménez-Reyes and colleagues in 2017 (19). The specific 9-week training program used induced (a) a clear and almost systematic decrease in FV_{imb} in the experimental group, and (b) substantial increases in squat jump performance by a larger magnitude and with much less interindividual variability in adaptations than for the control group (who had no individualization based on FV_{imb}).

Athletes have different individual F-V-P (and fatigue) profiles, thus different training needs. In addition, they will likely adapt differently to the specific training proposed (in terms of both magnitude and timing of responses). A modern, evidence-based approach to jump and sprint performance should therefore include these analyses (which is made easy thanks to field methods) in the strength tracking and monitoring process.

INNOVATIONS IN FORCE–VELOCITY–POWER PROFILING

The next frontiers that applied practice and research professionals are trying to cross are those pertaining to the most efficient training content and periodization (i.e., what type of resistance, exercises, training program, for what type of athlete and context?). A 2017 pilot study (19) on jumping included a fixed-duration program, and no information on the individual kinetics of adaptation within the 9 weeks or during detraining after program cessation. In 2019, Jiménez-Reyes and colleagues replicated the first study (22) and obtained the same results, but this time were able to take each athlete studied to that athlete's optimal profile zone after a variable number of weeks. They also showed that the magnitude of the initial FV_{imb} (in force or velocity) was correlated to the number of training weeks necessary; that is, the larger the imbalance, the longer it takes to reach an optimal profile zone.

In sprinting, the same questions must be answered (i.e., training content to effectively stimulate each part of the profile, best periodization approach, effects of fatigue), and especially that of the existence of an optimal sprint F-V profile similar to ballistic jumping movements. These studies are currently ongoing. In terms of periodization, the challenge will be to integrate a FV_{imb} reduction or maintenance program designed to eventually improve jump or sprint acceleration performance within the overall strength and conditioning, tactical, technical, and physical development of the athlete or team or both. Of course, this concerns only players (and teams) for whom improving ballistic performance or sprint acceleration (or both) is an objective. However, these approaches and methods can also be used to monitor the effects of other types of training (e.g., maximal force output training period) on the athlete's profile, and other types of physical events, such as postinjury rehabilitation, tapering periods, and postseason detraining.

Finally, in both cases, the future will also involve being able to collect in-game or in-race data, to make the F-V-P testing even more realistic and sport-specific. Some scientific studies, for example, show that it is possible to estimate muscle force output during running with portable, light, and convenient technology (25). Although the current tests are already simple and are applied to sport-specific movements (jumping and sprinting), it is just a matter of time before the methods discussed in this chapter are embedded into wearable sensors and deliver accurate, real-life data in the actual context of practice.

CONCLUSION

Performance in several sports that include ballistic actions (i.e., actions during which the aim is to propel an object, a limb, or the overall body as fast as possible under specific sport constraints) is highly determined by impulse and mechanical power output. Athletes' power output depends on their force and velocity capabilities and on the level of force they are able to produce in the specific velocity context of the sport action. Thus, a comprehensive assessment of an athlete's strength should explore the entire F-V-P spectrum. Although not yet available for all types of sport actions, this analysis and monitoring is now possible for vertical jump, bench press, and sprint acceleration exercises, thanks to simple methods validated against gold standard laboratory measurements. These methods require only inputs that are usually measured during field testing (jump height, sprint times or velocity) and affordable devices. By bridging the gap and removing barriers between laboratory (science) and field (practice), research has also suggested that an individual approach to F-V profiles could allow a much more in-depth analysis and interpretation of each athlete's strength, performance, and their underpinnings. This information may in turn be used to guide and improve training, monitoring, and rehabilitation interventions.

RECOMMENDED READINGS

Blog articles: https://jbmorin.net/category/blog/

Jiménez-Reyes, P, Samozino, P, and Morin, JB. Optimized training for jumping performance using the force-velocity imbalance: individual adaptation kinetics. *PLoS One* 14:e0216681, 2019.

Morin, JB, Jiménez-Reyes, P, Brughelli, M, and Samozino, P. When jump height is not a good indicator of lower limb maximal power output: theoretical demonstration, experimental evidence and practical solutions. *Sports Med* 49:999-1006, 2019.

Morin, JB, and Samozino, P. Interpreting power-force-velocity profiles for individualized and specific training. *Int J Sports Physiol Perform* 11:267-272, 2016.

Morin, JB, Samozino, P, eds. *Biomechanics of Training and Testing: Innovative Concepts and Simple Field Methods*. Cham, Switzerland: Springer International Publishing, 2018.

CHAPTER 14

Heart Rate and Heart Rate Variability

Joel Jamieson

Though the first recorded measurement of heart rate is generally attributed to Herophilus of Alexandria, Egypt (circa 335-280 BC) (32), its use in sport did not begin until more than 2,000 years later with the advent and launch of the first wireless electrocardiography chest strap by Polar Electro in 1983 (26). In the subsequent decades, the analysis of heart rate and related metrics such as **heart rate variability** (HRV), a measure of the variation of beat-to-beat intervals over a specific time, has become increasingly commonplace throughout the field of human performance (6, 13). The rise of a multitude of mobile applications, along with the widespread availability of accurate, low-cost monitoring devices, has only served to fuel the broader use of heart rate–derived metrics as potential indicators of internal load, as well as changes in both fitness and fatigue (25, 85).

Despite this increase and the relative ease of measurement across various training environments, there remains a lack of agreement in the literature and among coaches as to best practices and the ability of these metrics to help drive decisions related to managing both acute and chronic loading over time (64, 66, 67). For example, though a variety of methods and formulas have been proposed as simple and practical means of calculating training load from heart rate data, such as training impulse (TRIMP; see "Modeling Training Load Using Heart Rate and Heart Rate Variability" section), first proposed by Bannister in 1991 (5), none have been adopted as a gold standard or gained widespread adoption.

One potential cause for inconsistency in the literature relating to practical use of heart rate monitoring may be the highly dynamic nature of heart rate and related metrics, along with the multitude of influences, both internal and external, that drive them (13). The simplicity of heart rate and HRV as single numbers belies the complexity and sensitive interplay between the external environment and the many dynamic biological systems that influence them.

THE REGULATION OF HEART RATE

The delivery of oxygen to tissues and cells throughout the body is a fundamental requirement of metabolism and is thus necessary to sustain life. Because of this, heart rate is tightly controlled by a vast array of overlapping feedback loops across multiple biological systems that ultimately lead to regulation and maintenance of energy homeostasis (1). Without these processes and regulatory mechanisms, heart rate would be confined to its intrinsic value of 100 to 110 beats per minute (bpm) (43), set by the spontaneous firing rate of cells in the sinoatrial (SA) node, and would be poorly suited to meeting the varying energy demands across different environments. Underpinning the regulation of heart rate is the **autonomic nervous system** (ANS) and its drive to maintain the internal state within the limits necessary for metabolism at all times, while simultaneously striving to meet the immediate needs of the external environment (56). The ANS regulates heart rate through the autonomic nerves and its two branches: the sympathetic and parasympathetic nervous systems (69).

Within this regulatory context, activation of the sympathetic branch of the ANS stimulates the release of a cascade of hormones such as norepinephrine, along with other signaling mechanisms that cause an increase in heart rate, and thus oxygen delivery and aerobic energy production. This increase occurs in response to either real or perceived stressors within the external environment, including these:

- Physical stressors, such as an increase in oxygen demands secondary to increased metabolism in peripheral tissues (due to exercise, for example)
- Environmental stressors (changes in temperature, elevation, noise, etc.)
- Psychological stressors (increases in fear, anxiety, and such) (13, 74)

Additionally, an array of internal physiological conditions such as hydration, nutrient availability, hormonal sensitivity, and fatigue may alter the sympathetic response and influence heart rate and HRV (17, 34, 48, 79).

In the context of physical activity, the demand for greater force production and power output in the form of muscular work plays the largest role in the requirement for additional energy. In metabolically demanding sports, in which performance may be limited by aerobic metabolism, the production of this additional energy is driven by greater oxygen demand and thus higher heart rates. Given this, along with the highly variable nature of both internal and external influences across training and competition environments, heart rate during activity represents a summation of the body's integrated response to both the physical and mental loads placed upon it (70).

During periods of rest and reduced energy expenditure, a shift in ANS activity occurs, and the parasympathetic branch becomes the dominant influence in regulating heart rate (69). In contrast to the sympathetic branch of the ANS, the parasympathetic system plays the primary role in restoring homeostasis after periods of stress, as well as allocating energy to cellular repair, regeneration, and adaptation (78). Acting via acetylcholine release, input from the parasympathetic nervous system plays a primary role in heart rate modulation during rest, sleep, and other periods of reduced physical activity and mental stress (38).

This input, known as cardiac vagal tone, is largely responsible for reducing heart rate well below its intrinsic value at rest, and its withdrawal is the first component that increases heart rate above this level as energy demands increase (43). An increased level of cardiac vagal tone, in conjunction with morphological changes to the cardiovascular and neuromuscular systems, comprises two adaptations central to increased metabolic capability and has been linked to improved aerobic performance and reduced risk of injury under high workloads (64, 75, 86).

Together, the sympathetic and parasympathetic systems drive the adaptive machinery of the body that allows it to become better equipped to survive and perform across many environments. The relationship between these two branches of the ANS and their daily variations in response to acute and chronic loading plays a crucial role in general health, performance, and the risk of injury (77, 86). Monitoring changes in heart rate and HRV across various contexts represents the most common and proven method of gaining insight into this balance, with the aim of managing training load and optimizing athletic performance (13, 62, 64, 82).

HEART RATE AND HEART RATE VARIABILITY MONITORING

The growing prevalence of mobile phones, wearable devices, and modern signal transmission technology such as Bluetooth has made measuring and monitoring heart rate metrics more cost-effective, accessible, and practical than ever. Traditional watch-style devices, which connect to a chest strap and are primarily worn only during training sessions, have seen rising competition from newer devices that continuously measure and track heart rate throughout the day. The increase in mobile and tablet applications has also created greater opportunities for monitoring several athletes simultaneously through data hubs that can receive and process multiple signals at once.

Despite this rapid increase in the types of heart rate (HR) monitors, form factors, and apps, the sensors and methods used to detect HR generally fall into one of two categories: electrical (ECG) or optical (photoplethysmography) (60). Each type of sensor has its own strengths and limitations and may be better suited toward different kinds of measurements and uses.

Electrical Sensors

The first use of electrical signals to measure heart activity, known as **electrocardiography** (ECG or EKG), can be traced back to its invention by Dr. Willem Einthoven in 1895. This work earned Einthoven a Nobel Prize in the physiology and medicine category in 1924 (3). In subsequent decades, ECG became widely used throughout the medical field in cardiovascular disease research and prevention (87).

The sale of the Sport Tester PE 2000 by Polar Electro in 1983 marked the release of the first wireless ECG device and the beginning of its use in the fitness and sport industries (26).

Since the release of this first product, the accuracy, battery life, and ergonomics of chest strap-based sensors have improved, but the fundamentals of ECG used to detect heartbeats have remained largely unchanged. The primary advantage of ECG sensors over optical sensors is their accuracy across a variety of conditions (58). This is particularly true during exercise; research has consistently shown them to be more accurate at higher intensities and across more varied and dynamic movement patterns (30, 84). For this reason, ECG sensors are recommended and best suited for conditions that require the highest level of accuracy or for monitoring HR during high-intensity exercise.

Optical Sensors

The rise in the popularity of devices using optical sensors has been accompanied by improvements in their ease of use, the varying form factors that allow them to be worn on the wrist, and their integration with wearable devices that collect a variety of other health and fitness data (76). Unlike monitors that use electrical signals to monitor heart activity, devices with optical sensors use a newer method known as **photoplethysmography** (PPG) to detect changes in blood flow to determine HR (27).

Each time the heart beats, it sends a pulse of blood to tissues throughout the body. Photoplethysmography devices use an optical sensor consisting of a combination of light-emitting diode (LED) lights and a photo sensor to detect changes in light absorption as these pulses of blood perfuse tissues beneath the skin (27). Using this technique, modern PPG sensors are able to detect both HR and the beat-to-beat intervals necessary for HRV to a reasonable level of accuracy at rest and during low- to moderate-intensity training conditions (58). At higher HRs and during performance of rapid, acyclic movements, PPG sensors may be more prone to errors in measurement than electrical sensors, with significant differences existing between various PPG products on the market (58, 39).

Signal Transmission Technologies

With improvements in technology have come changes in the methods used to transmit HRs from the sensors that detect them to the receivers that display them. Today, these displays most often take the form of a watch, a mobile or tablet application, or another wearable device. Several pieces of commercial fitness equipment also have built-in displays capable of showing HR transmitted from various devices (e.g., treadmills, stationary bikes, rowing machines).

The oldest of these data transmission technologies is an analog 5-kHz radio signal patented and first used by Polar Electro (21). This technology relies on the receiving devices to process the radio signal to calculate and display HR. Today, the use of this technology is primarily limited to older devices and commercial cardiovascular equipment such as treadmills, rowers, and spin bikes. The 5-kHz devices are limited in transmission range and lack unique identifiers, making them impractical in group training environments.

The first of the two data transmission technologies that have largely replaced 5-kHz radio transmission is **ANT+**, an open source wireless data transmission protocol introduced in 2004 (24). The primary advantages of ANT+ are significantly improved range, often 30 to 50 meters or more depending on the device, and the ability to transmit a unique ID and connect to ANT+ hubs designed for group training environments (83). In addition, a wide variety of fitness devices and equipment such as speed sensors, power meters, and watches support the ANT+ protocol, significantly increasing its compatibility compared to the 5-kHz radio signal.

The most modern data transmission technology is **Bluetooth Low Energy**, which has also been incorporated across a variety of wearable devices. Like ANT+, it is an open-standard wireless communication protocol that allows for the transmission of various types of data between two devices (31). It is capable of significantly higher data transmission speeds than ANT+, and Bluetooth transmission has become the standard among mobile devices, tablets, headphones, fitness trackers, and more. Because of this, many HR monitoring devices now incorporate both Bluetooth and ANT+ to improve compatibility.

HEART RATE AND HEART RATE VARIABILITY MEASUREMENT

Heart rate and HRV represent easy-to-adopt measures providing powerful insights that can be used to guide understanding of the physiological demands placed on athletes, as well as their well-being status. The correct measurement and interpretation of these simple yet important measures are, however, critical in order to ensure their accuracy and ultimately their value.

Measuring Heart Rate

Because HR is relatively simple and noninvasive to monitor and record, it can be measured across multiple time frames and physiological conditions. In terms of fitness and performance, these measurements can be divided into two major categories: resting HR and HR during exercise (HRex). Heart rate measured at rest and during exercise may provide insight into different aspects of change in autonomic function, energy expenditure, fatigue, and fitness (1). A third category, the continuous monitoring of HR over 24 hours, has become more practical with the growth of fitness wearables. However, there is a lack of validating research in this area, so it is not discussed here.

The measurement of HR and HRV at rest has traditionally been used to reflect changes in both acute and chronic fatigue, as well as fitness (1). Since the sympathetic system is highly sensitive to a variety of stressors, resting measurements have been shown to be the most accurate when the conditions are standardized in terms of time of day, body position, nutritional intake, and environment (4). Lack of such standardization may account for inconsistent results in the literature and thus underscore the importance of monitoring during rest periods (13).

Heart rate recorded during exercise represents measurement during much greater dynamic and multidimensional physiological conditions, including rapid changes in intensity, body position, and psychological and physical environments, and is thus subject to greater variation and influences (13). The number of confounding variables makes data interpretation more challenging and may account for the lack of agreement in the literature on both submaximal and maximal testing results (13).

In addition to various fitness tests using HRex, many methods and calculations have been proposed to estimate both acute training load and changes in fitness and fatigue. The literature generally shows greater agreement as to the ability of HRex to reflect longitudinal improvements in fitness and performance, exhibited by lower relative HRex and greater HR recovery at a given level of power output and intensity, compared to its ability to serve as a clear marker of fatigue (13, 14).

Measuring Heart Rate Variability

Heart rate variability is widely acknowledged as a general marker of health, wellness, and fitness as its use has become more common through a number of wearables and mobile apps (25). Compared to HR, HRV measurement requires additional data processing and more specialized monitoring devices that are capable of measuring and transmitting beat-to-beat intervals with a high degree of accuracy (15). The use of chest strap monitors (ECG) has been widely validated in the literature, though a limited number of PPG sensors have also been shown to be generally accurate enough for HRV measurements (23, 35).

In order to differentiate changes in the ANS due to training from those caused by environmental noise and physiological conditions such as sound and light, body position, nutrition, and hydration, the best practice is to standardize these variables to the greatest extent possible within practical limitations. To achieve this, a range of measurement periods from as little as 30 seconds to up to 24 hours have been proposed and examined (22, 35).

Although overnight recordings may offer the greatest potential for standardization, the requirement for concomitant sleep wave measurement, varying body positions, the potential for sensor movement, lack of validation in the literature, and other practical limitations make this approach less viable (37). Current best practices in the field are most often shorter measurements, between 3 and 5 minutes, in line with commonly available mobile applications, recorded during a morning period upon waking (13). This time period may represent the best opportunity for standardization of environmental conditions and practicality.

Due to the sensitive nature of the sympathetic nervous system, best practices in HRV measurement include standardizing time of day, body position (most often supine or seated), breathing pattern, temperature, and prior nutritional intake, while limiting noise and other environmental stressors during the measurement process (4, 13, 72). While greater measurement frequency is generally recommended, this may not always be practical in the field, and literature has demonstrated that as few as three or four measurements per week are enough to provide meaningful insight (67).

Detection of Beat-to-Beat Intervals

The first step in calculating HRV is to accurately measure the precise time between successive heartbeats using either ECG or PPG sensors. Because ECG detects changes in the electrical activity of the heart and PPG uses changes in light to measure fluctuations in blood volume through the skin, they use different processing techniques to identify the signal peak and thus determine the time between successive heartbeats. Regardless of the type of device used, this time

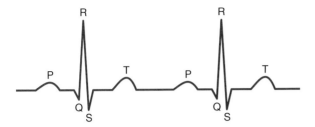

FIGURE 14.1 R-R interval.

is commonly referred to as the **R-R interval**, denoting the time between the peaks of two R waves in ECG-based measurements (see figure 14.1).

The literature has shown that both ECG and PPG devices are capable of detecting beat-to-beat intervals accurately (68), though comparisons between the two technologies have generally shown greater accuracy and consistency in ECG devices (84). This may be due to a higher level of difficulty in detecting signal peaks, increased potential for motion artifacts, and variations in PPG sensor quality among different manufacturers.

Filtering

A crucial and often overlooked step in the accurate calculation of HRV is filtering the R-R interval time series, often referred to as **artifact correction** (15). This process is necessary to remove ectopic beats (those arising outside the SA node), skipped beats, and other artifacts that may arise from movement or other signal issues. If left in the time series, even a single false beat can lead to a difference in HRV metrics of up to 50%, and thus proper filtering is essential for ensuring accuracy (13). This is especially true with the shorter-term measurements often employed in athletic settings, because this type of analysis is more sensitive to artifacts (15). Modern HRV mobile applications typically include automatic filtering algorithms, though more comprehensive computer-based solutions often include the ability to select from a range of filters and are thus more suitable for research and complex analysis (55).

Calculating Heart Rate Variability

A considerable number of analytical methods, including linear and nonlinear, have been proposed as a means of calculating HRV and different components of autonomic function (15). The two methods of calculation most often used today fall into the category of either **time-domain** (calculations that analyze the variability of time differences between R-R intervals)

or **power spectral analysis** (a more complex technique that analyzes the frequency at which R-R intervals change and breaks them into bands of low-frequency power [LFP], very low-frequency power [VLFP], and high-frequency power [HFP]). Of the two, time-domain measures are often considered more suitable for practical monitoring in athletic populations since they require shorter measurements (22), are less subject to respiratory influences, and day-to-day variations are likely lower, enabling a clearer separation between noise and meaningful change (12, 13). To further these efforts, statistical techniques such as data normalization are commonly used in the field. An example of this is log natural transform of RMSSD (root mean square of successive differences between normal heartbeats) (see table 14.1; 1, 15), one of the most widely reported and used HRV measures both in the literature and in common practice (64, 65, 67).

ANALYSIS AND INTERPRETATION OF HEART RATE AND HEART RATE VARIABILITY

The objective of every training program is to stimulate the body's adaptive machinery to produce positive changes in various physiological capacities, thereby enabling them to meet specific environmental demands with greater ease and efficiency. With respect to sport performance, these internal adaptations facilitate the potential for a higher level of skill execution and greater external power output (3).

To achieve this aim, training must repeatedly impart loads great enough to provide the level of biological stress necessary to stimulate adaptation. At the same time, if tissue or system loading is not offset by sufficient recovery, performance gains may suffer (54). In cases in which this loading chronically exceeds the body's biological ability to positively adapt to it, the potential for performance decrements, or even injuries, increases (19).

One of the primary challenges of every sport science practitioner is to design and manage training programs that achieve the appropriate level and pattern of loading for each athlete to continually improve fitness and preparedness over time. A vital part of these efforts is evaluating the acute and chronic effects of varying external loads on the body and its resulting internal responses. When used effectively, HR and HRV measures in sport can prove valuable in these efforts (particularly as part of a multivariate approach to contribute to an estimation of training load), provide

TABLE 14.1   Common Measures of Heart Rate Variability

Name	Domain	Description	Comments
SDNN (ms)	Time	Standard deviation of normal R-R (NN) intervals	Represents all cyclic variation over a reading and has limited statistical use since the measured variability increases with the recording duration
SDANN (ms)	Time	Standard deviation of average NN intervals for every 5-min cycle of a measurement	Used in longer HRV measures to estimate the variability due to cycles longer than 5 min
RMSSD (ms)	Time	Root mean square of successive differences in R-R intervals	Estimates the short-term, parasympathetic component of variability with useful statistical properties; one of the most commonly used measures in sport applications
pNN50 index (%)	Time	Percentage of consecutive NN intervals differing by more than 50 ms	Estimates the parasympathetic component of variability and correlates closely with RMSSD, though with less useful statistical utility
VLFP (ms^2)	Frequency	Absolute power of very low-frequency band (0.0033-0.04 Hz)	The physiological underpinnings are not as clearly defined as other frequency measures; questionable utility for variability measurements under 5 min
LFP (ms^2)	Frequency	Absolute power of low-frequency band (0.04-0.15 Hz)	Considered a measure of both sympathetic and parasympathetic modulation of HR and can be expressed in normalized units
HFP (ms^2)	Frequency	Absolute power of high-frequency band (0.15-0.4 Hz)	Considered a measure of parasympathetic modulation of HR (the component of variability linked to respiration) and can be expressed in normalized units
LF:HF	Frequency	Ratio of absolute power of low-frequency band to high-frequency band	Considered a measure of autonomic balance, where a high LF/HF ratio indicates sympathetic predominance
Total power (ms^2)	Frequency	The total HR power between 0.00066 and 0.34 Hz	Measures the variance of all NN intervals and is highly subject to body position and breathing rate

a gauge of changes in fatigue and readiness in response to loading and lifestyle factors, and track changes in fitness in response to chronic loading over time (7, 82).

MODELING TRAINING LOAD USING HEART RATE AND HEART RATE VARIABILITY

Years of research and practical experience in the fields of sport science and coaching have given rise to a wide range of tracking metrics, and associated models have been proposed to quantify the overall impact of a training session (8). The efforts to describe this impact with a single number, or a series of numbers, defined as the **training load**, have generally evolved into the use of either external metrics such as Global Positioning System (GPS) data, force-velocity measurements, number of repetitions, or training time—or internal measures such as specific blood and saliva markers,

HR, and HRV (80). Additionally, subjective markers such as rating of perceived exertion (RPE) and other psychometric tests and questionnaires have been proposed and used as part of a multivariate approach (8).

Within this framework, monitoring systems have extensively tracked HRex due to its relative ease of measurement in both individual and group training environments (1, 8, 13). As such, its use has been widely researched across a variety of team and individual sports. Heart rate variability during exercise has also been evaluated as a potentially useful metric (71), though the challenge of accurately measuring R-R intervals during activity, the additional time required for analysis, and the lack of literature demonstrating its utility in this regard makes it less suited for practical use than HR alone (13). In this respect, the effective use of HRex for estimating training load can be broadly considered within the scope of the two primary variables that define the impact of external loading and stress on the body: volume and intensity.

Given that HR increases above the intrinsic HR of 100 to 110 bpm are largely driven by the sympathetic nervous system and vary linearly with oxygen delivery during continuous activity, HR measures serve as a proxy for ANS activity and energy expenditure (1, 8).

When viewed over the course of a training session, HR expressed as a percentage of an individual's HRmax may provide a gauge of relative intensity, with higher HRs corresponding to greater sympathetic activity and anaerobic energy contributions (44). A model based on either three or five HR zones, most often built around a percentage of an individual's HRmax, is a commonly used method frequently incorporated into monitoring software. Different colors are used to represent different intensity levels and often used to help visualize the metabolic demands and energy expenditure of a training session (see figure 14.2). This approach may aid in targeting of specific intensity levels, that is, zones, in order to achieve a desired metabolic adaptation and change in fitness. In the field, a coach may use HR zone training on a practical level to program workouts composed of various amounts of time in each zone in an effort to achieve a specific training effect and overall load.

The use of HR zones as a means to quantify intensity is also incorporated into various models of the most widely researched method of using HRex to calculate training load, known as **TRIMP** (13). Since it was first proposed as a means of quantifying volume and intensity by Bannister in 1991, multiple variations of TRIMP using alternative calculations have been proposed, each with potential uses and limitations (see table 14.2; 5, 21, 49a, 51a, 52a, 72a, 76a). Today, various software solutions include the ability to automatically calculate TRIMP, and in many cases, additional proprietary training load indices. While this automation may appear practical, most of these proprietary metrics lack validation in the research, and thus their accuracy relative to more established TRIMP models cannot be determined.

MONITORING CHANGES IN FITNESS AND FATIGUE

As discussed previously, the use of HRV has been well researched across various sports, including running, cycling, canoeing, weightlifting, rowing, and team sports, as a means of assessing and monitoring the body's response to training and its corresponding impact on fitness and fatigue (18, 36, 49, 59, 66, 81). These efforts have produced mixed and often conflicting findings in data patterns, trends, and correlations to performance. As a result, interpretation and analysis of HR data is a widely debated topic (20, 50). This may be largely due to methodological considerations, population differences, and the potential for misinterpretation of the data (65). The purpose of this section is not to continue or contribute to this debate, but to review various strategies for analyzing and interpreting HRV data that are supported both within the literature and in the common practice of coaches and sport scientists in the field.

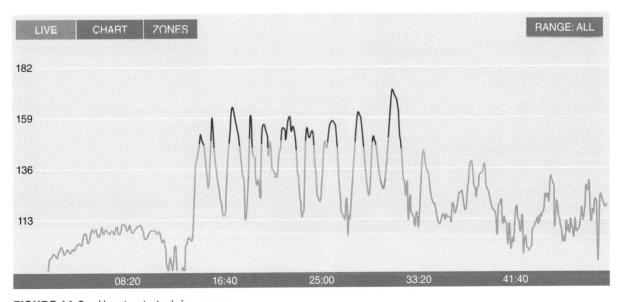

FIGURE 14.2 Heart-rate training zones.

TABLE 14.2 **Common Means of Quantifying Training Impulse**

Name	Researchers	Calculation	Comments
bTRIMP	Banister, 1991	bTRIMP = TD · ΔHR · 0.64 · $e^{1.92 \cdot \text{HR reserve}}$ (men) bTRIMP = TD · ΔHR · 0.86 · $e^{1.672 \cdot \text{HR reserve}}$ (women) TD = training duration (minutes) ΔHR = (HRex – HRrest) / (HRmax – HRrest)	While bTRIMP has been validated with some cardiovascular endurance sports, the reliance on mean HR limits the usefulness for describing internal training load in sports characterized by intermittent bouts of activity during competition or practice. This measure also fails to account for individual differences affecting training load beyond gender.
eTRIMP	Edwards, 1993	eTRIMP = %HRmax × Zone Coefficient <table><tr><td>*HR zones (%HRmax)*</td><td>*Coefficient*</td></tr><tr><td>50%-60%</td><td>1</td></tr><tr><td>60%-70%</td><td>2</td></tr><tr><td>70%-80%</td><td>3</td></tr><tr><td>80%-90%</td><td>4</td></tr><tr><td>90%-100%</td><td>5</td></tr></table>	Both the zone coefficients and HR zones are devoid of physiological or metabolic underpinnings, limiting their ability to describe TRIMP in an energetically meaningful way.
iTRIMP	Manzi, Iellamo, Impellizzeri, D'Ottavio, Castagna, 2009	iTRIMP = $\sum \Delta R \cdot t \cdot y$ y is a weighting factor based on an individual's HR–blood lactate (HR–BLa) relationship determined by plotting blood lactate levels over incremental increases above HRrest.	Each of an individual's HR values—instead of arbitrary HR zones—is incorporated into the TRIMP calculation, enabling it to model internal training load for sessions with a range of irregular HRs (as in many competitive events and practices). This measure is limited by the need to gather blood lactate levels, which may be impractical in a training setting.
TRIMP$_{\text{Lucia}}$	Lucia, Hoyos, Santalla, Earnest, Chicharo, 2003	Three zones were identified relative to ventilatory threshold (VT) and respiratory compensation point (RCP), such that: Zone 1 < VT < zone 2 < RCP < zone 3 TRIMP$_{\text{Lucia}} = (t_1) + 2(t_2) + 3(t_3)$ t is the time spent in a given zone.	This measure reflects the differing metabolic costs of training at varying intensities by measuring time in zones anchored to respiratory responses. It is limited by the need for lab testing to gather respiratory responses. The small number of zones overemphasizes differences in metabolic costs of relatively similar HRs in neighboring zones (e.g., 170 and 178 bpm).
TRIMP$_{\text{mod}}$	Stagno, Thatcher, Van Someren, 2007	TRIMP$_{\text{mod}}$ = TD · ΔHR · 0.1225 · $e^{3.9434 \cdot \Delta\text{HR}}$ TD = training duration (minutes) ΔHR = (HRex – HRrest) / (HRmax – HRrest) and was calculated across 5 zones. These zones were selected around the lactate threshold and onset of lactate accumulation.	Also referred to as "team TRIMP" since this measure relies upon the lactate values of an entire team to generate a weighting factor. It does not take into account low-threshold data and is limited by the need to measure blood lactate levels. The lactate zones themselves are arbitrary and the reliance on average HR gives an unrepresentative picture of activities with intermittent work periods.
TRIMP$_{\text{lac}}$	Seiler and Kjerland, 2006	Three zones were identified relative to blood lactate concentration such that: Zone 1 ≤ 2 < zone 2 < 4 ≤ zone 3 TRIMP$_{\text{lac}} = (t_1) + 2(t_2) + 3(t_3)$ t is the time spent in a given zone.	While this measure strongly correlates to session RPE in intermittent sport modalities, it is limited by the need to gather blood lactate levels, which may be impractical during training and unpleasant for athletes.

When considering the application of HRV metrics to the process of making training-related decisions, it is important to note that through changes in ANS activity, they reflect a summation of many different biological systems working together in response to various external stressors within the environment. This presents an opportunity to infer the response to training—as well as other key variables that directly modulate this response, such as sleep, nutritional status, psychological stress, and temperature—without time-consuming, expensive, invasive, or otherwise impractical methods. With this opportunity, however, comes the challenge of untangling the many factors underlying HR metrics and the complex nature of the body's stress response and corresponding changes in fitness and fatigue. In this regard, it can be useful to think of fitness and fatigue as different yet related responses of the body to various stimuli over time. Any interpretation of HR data needs to begin with the understanding that these responses are being gauged by indirect means. Because of this, the use of a multivariate approach is best practice when analyzing both HR and HRV data. Both of these metrics represent the collective output, or response, of the body, but they lack context of the stressors that stimulated this response. External metrics that describe the nature of external loading (such as force–velocity data, GPS data, running intensity and distance, measures of sets, reps, weight, and total tonnage), can help provide this context and are thus an integral part of turning HR metrics into actionable insight. Additional biomarkers and wearable-generated metrics that provide data on other modulating factors, such as sleep, nutrition, mental stress, and travel, can all contribute valuable information and improve the decision-making process that results from data analysis and interpretation (29).

Within this frame of reference, HRV data can be considered in the context of evaluating both acute and chronic changes within the body. In the short term, acute changes in these metrics have been shown to generally align well with variations in both training volume and intensity (13). Longer-term trends have proven more inconsistent in the literature and may reflect the accumulation of fatigue, changes in fitness and performance, or both. Trends have been shown to be highly variable within different individuals and sports and thus are likely dependent on the nature of the training being performed, the athlete's fitness levels and genetics, differences in monitoring methodologies, and other factors not yet fully understood (20, 50).

Evaluating Acute Responses

The acute response to any stressor is the mobilization of energy reserves via the sympathetic branch of the ANS. Following this stress exposure is a subsequent withdrawal of the sympathetic input and a concomitant increase in parasympathetic activation that drives the restoration of both homeostasis and energy stores over time. This process represents the fundamental stress–recovery–supercompensation curve that drives physiological adaptations depending on the nature of specific stressors as they are repeated over time. On a daily basis, variations in training load lead to large changes in the ANS that are reflected in both HR and HRV, though HRV has generally been thought to be the more sensitive measure of the two (13, 62, 65).

The primary training variables affecting the time course of this cycle and its reflection in both HR and HRV are volume and intensity. Of the two, intensity is thought to be a greater challenge to homeostasis during aerobically demanding exercise and thus is more influential for driving sympathetic activity and longer periods of increased HR (decreased HRV) at rest (13). High-intensity cardiovascular endurance exercise has been shown to require at least 48 hours for complete cardiac-autonomic recovery, compared to up to 24 hours for low intensity and up to 24 to 48 hours for moderate intensity (52, 77).

Given these responses, acute decreases in resting indices of HRV or increases in HRrest (or both), measured on a daily basis, may represent the body's initial response to this increased intensity and training load (62). As fitness increases and the body accommodates to a given level of loading, the time course of the stress–recovery–adaptation curve may decrease and a stronger parasympathetic response can often be seen in increased HRV (decreased HRrest) the day after loading (61). The same daily increase in response to loading is also frequently seen during periods of lower-intensity, higher-volume training, and in athletes with higher baseline levels of HRV, indicating greater aerobic capacity (13, 41). Within limits that are discussed in the subsequent section, these changes are generally thought to be indicative of positive adaptations, decreased risk of injury (86), and a sign that the athlete is accommodating to the training load (13).

It should also be noted that many common HRV mobile apps available today incorporate proprietary algorithms that automatically interpret changes in

HRV and HRrest to generate composite indices of recovery or fatigue or both (25). While such features increase the practicality of using these measures with a large group of athletes, the accuracy of these metrics may vary greatly between apps and devices, and there is a general lack of literature to establish their validity in relation to more established or direct measures.

In addition to resting HR measures, the use of HRex during periods of continuous, submaximal power output has also been proposed as a means of evaluating the acute physiological impact of changes in loading and fatigue. The results of this approach are unclear and controversial; some authors suggest that acute increases in HRex in response to the same power output reflect fatigue (10, 11), with others reporting weak or no associations between the two (14). An alternative approach, the use of **heart rate recovery** following exercise at fixed intensities, has also been suggested as a possible means of assessing acute changes in fatigue (46).

Heart rate recovery is a measure of how quickly HR decreases following periods of exertion and is driven first by the withdrawal of sympathetic input and then by subsequent reactivation of the parasympathetic system. Given this, measures of heart rate recovery over varying time periods, usually 60 seconds or less, may be indicative of ANS status, and thus reduced heart rate recovery may reflect acute increases in fatigue (47). Protocols using higher intensities between 85% and 90% of HRmax, followed by 60 seconds of recovery, have been reported as potentially more indicative of fatigue than protocols using lower intensities (46). When interpreting any type of HR recorded during exercise, it is important to note that environmental factors such as heat, hydration status, travel, and sleep, among others, may also play a significant role in modulating this response and should be considered in the analysis and extrapolation of the data (1, 13, 17, 20).

Evaluating Chronic Responses

As the body is exposed to chronic loading over time, changes in fitness, fatigue, and performance occur due to a variety of both physiological and morphological adaptations in the body. Many of these changes lead to either increased or decreased aerobic capacity and power output over the course of weeks or months that are either well correlated with, or in part caused by, differences in ANS function primarily reflected in varying trends in HR-derived metrics (4, 16, 57) (see tables 14.3 and 14.4; 47, 61, 77). Analyzing these

metrics over short, medium, and long time frames represents an effort to interpret the changes in both fitness and fatigue via patterns and trends in autonomic activity that may manifest themselves in both resting and exercise measures.

The challenge in these efforts is multifaceted given that fatigue and fitness may increase simultaneously (fitness–fatigue theory) (5). Further complicating matters are the highly varying and sometimes conflicting ANS responses tied to changes in performance that have been reported in the literature across different sports, individuals, training phases, loading patterns, and HR indices (40, 41, 42, 51, 65). An attempt to solve this challenge should include a multivariate approach that incorporates the analysis of HR metrics derived across both resting and exercise conditions, in conjunction with measures of external loading and changes in performance.

Although many HRV indices and HR measures exist, the most common metrics, in both the literature and in practical settings for evaluating trends in HR data monitoring during resting conditions, include both raw numbers and statistical measures such as lnRMSSD (often used in mobile HRV applications), HR, HRV coefficient of variation (RMSSD CV), and HRV normalized for HR (R-R interval) (13, 64, 65). During exercise conditions, HR response can be evaluated during both submaximal and maximal conditions, for example, via $\dot{V}O_2$max or lactate threshold testing. Within the context of various measures of loading and training phase, these parameters can help identify the chronic responses to training and separate meaningful change from noise to better inform training-related decisions (see tables 14.3 and 14.4; 73).

INNOVATIONS IN HEART RATE AND HEART RATE VARIABILITY MONITORING

Advancements in technology and data collection over the past decade have vastly increased the amount of data that can be measured and monitored relating to the external loading and the environment, as well as the varying internal responses that result. This has primarily occurred as a result of a greater number and more types of monitoring devices, providing increased availability at lower costs, along with a coinciding exponential growth in the number of mobile phone and desktop software applications and solutions capable of storing and (to varying degrees) analyzing this data (23, 25, 27, 50, 58, 68, 76). What has lagged behind

TABLE 14.3 Indicators of Increases in Fitness

Metric trends	Comments	Indicates
Increases in weekly averaged HRV with reductions in HRrest and CV (coefficient of variation) RMSSD	Often seen during low- to moderate-intensity loading with increasing volumes.	Positive training response. Loading is well tolerated.
Reduced HRex during continuous or intermittent high-intensity exercise	Averaged HR over previous 30 to 60 s is generally used for analysis.	Improvements in aerobic fitness and work capacity.
Increased 60-s heart rate recovery from 85% to 90% of HRmax	Recovery from higher intensities may be a more reliable indicator of meaningful change than lower intensities.	Increase in overall parasympathetic activity and reduced anaerobic energy expenditure for a given intensity.
Reduction in weekly averaged HRV with moderate increases in HRrest	May be connected to increased performance in the context of a tapering period with reduced loading. Most often seen as a positive only when following a period of prolonged increase in HRV.	Connected to performance when seen in the final stages of preparation.

TABLE 14.4 Indicators of Increases in Fatigue or Decreases in Fitness

Metric trends	Comments	Indicates
Reductions in weekly averaged HRV with increases in HRrest	Often seen during high-intensity loading and during the early stages of new training programs. Can also occur during tapering phase after prolonged increases in HRV as sympathetic activity increases in response to reduced volumes.	Likely indicates fatigue or maladaptation when measured over several weeks. May indicate improved readiness to perform when seen during short-term tapering periods. Decreased fitness when seen during periods of detraining.
Increase in CV RMSSD with reduced RMSSD or increasing HR	Often seen during periods of most intense loading phases as the ANS responds to high levels of stress.	Greater sympathetic activity. May reflect fatigue and lack of ability to cope well with training load.
Reduced RMSSD with reduced HR	Most likely to be seen in athletes with higher average RMSSD during periods of high-volume loading over several weeks.	Increased parasympathetic activity to the point of saturation. May indicate accumulated fatigue when trend is seen over several weeks.
Decreased heart rate recovery following high-intensity exercise with increases in HRrest	Most often seen during periods of detraining in conjunction with increases in HRrest.	Reduced parasympathetic activity and decreased aerobic fitness.

this exponential growth in the amount of monitoring, however, are well-validated models, automated systems, and educational resources that are necessary to help turn this additional information into actionable insights that can be used on a practical level to drive better training decisions (65, 66, 67).

Along these lines, following its use since the 1980s, the application of HR monitoring likely represents the most widely used and researched singular metric in the field of sport science. In spite of this, efforts to create uniform standards and best practices that are well validated and practical to implement across different group sizes and sports have largely fallen short (8).

Coaches and sport scientists in the field have been tasked with determining the most effective and time-efficient ways to implement HR monitoring and deciding where it fits into their training systems and load management models. With varying degrees of success, a wide range of monitoring systems and solutions have been tried and implemented across different teams and organizations, ranging from simple and low cost to complex and resource-intensive (8, 45).

Moving forward, the solution to the challenges of monitoring HR and other biometrics will most likely be found in the rapidly evolving field of big data solutions and models that are capable of far greater multivariate analysis than have been used in the past (53). The use of rapidly advancing machine learning techniques is already proving valuable in solving extremely complex probabilistic challenges and reshaping how strategic decisions are made in areas as diverse as poker and financial investments (28). As the volume of collectible data continues to grow, the application of this type of big data analysis and modeling, combined with collaborative efforts across research groups, organizations, and individuals, represents the next and most important steps forward. Sport analytics as a field is still in its relative infancy and is likely to continue to expand and evolve in scope, size, and utility in the coming years.

At the same time, rapid advancements in monitoring technology are also unlikely to slow down anytime soon. Improvements in sensor capabilities, including smaller size, greater accuracy, and an increased range of data that can be collected through noninvasive and passive means, will likely lead to devices that can deliver better and more integrated monitoring solutions. Such changes will require less effort from the end user, which is a key to compliance among athletes.

The end result of continued leaps forward in device technology, big data analysis, and collaborative efforts will ultimately be a much better and deeper understanding of the complex relationship between external stress and the body's internal response. This insight will facilitate better decision making and more effective loading and recovery strategies and interventions that are personalized based on a range of biomarkers and metrics, such that all athletes are able to achieve their maximal level of performance. In the coming decades, this personalization will ultimately become commonplace across the fields of both medicine and sport, leading to new levels of human performance, durability, and achievement.

CONCLUSION

As with many biological measures, both HR and HRV have the potential to be powerful tools in the arsenal of today's coaches and sport scientists, but they also have inherent limitations that need to be considered within the broader context of turning insight into application. Perhaps the greatest of these is the degree to which normal biological variation and factors such as inconsistencies in data collection, device error, methodological issues, and other unknown factors may obscure meaningful change (63). Each measure of HR function is subject to differences in these characteristics; and to compound matters, research has consistently demonstrated a high degree of inter-athlete variability in response to loading and external stressors (2, 9, 33).

The smallest worthwhile change (SWC) is an important concept that can be applied to HR monitoring (see chapter 18), but population-wide norms, even when established, may not be accurate or meaningful for a given individual (65). Given these limitations and others, HR metrics should best be viewed as a means to augment decision-making processes around load management and optimization. With respect to this aim, they are most effective when analyzed in combination with other biomarkers, direct measures of performance, subjective ratings, and the intuition and insight that come with experience in the field. As single markers of ANS function, they cannot be extrapolated to every area of fitness, health, or performance.

In addition, the use of HR metrics has been most well researched and supported in sports with high metabolic demands, such as cardiovascular endurance sports and various teams sports, with its utility less well understood in sports in which the generation of maximum force and power over very short periods of time is a key determinant of success. The effective use of HR metrics relies on leveraging their strengths, as well as the general ability to provide meaningful insight into markers of the biological response to acute and chronic loading, while recognizing their inherent limitations. Their use in driving training-related decisions should be focused around the key areas they are best suited to and as part of a broader monitoring strategy designed to meet the specific needs and demands of the coach, athlete, and organization as a whole.

RECOMMENDED READINGS

Atko, V. *Adaptation in Sports Training.* New York: Informa Healthcare, 2017.

Cardinale, M, Newton, R, Nosaka, K, eds. *Strength and Conditioning: Biological Principles and Practical Applications.* West Sussex, UK: John Wiley & Sons, 2011.

Freeman, JV, Dewey, FE, Hadley, DM, Myers, J, and Froelicher, VF. Autonomic nervous system interaction with the cardiovascular system during exercise. *Prog Cardiovasc Dis* 48:342-362, 2006.

Kamath, MV, Watanabe, M, Upton, A, eds. *Heart Rate Variability (HRV) Signal Analysis: Clinical Applications.* Boca Raton, FL: CRC Press, 2012.

Viru, AA. *Hormones Muscular Activity, Volume I: Hormonal Ensemble in Exercise.* Boca Raton, FL: CRC Press, 1985.

Viru, AA. *Hormones Muscular Activity, Volume II: Adaptive Effect of Hormones in Exercise.* Boca Raton, FL: CRC Press, 1985.

CHAPTER 15

Electroencephalography and Electroneuromyography

Roman N. Fomin, PhD

Cassandra C. Collins, BS

Modern sports place extremely high demands on an athlete's physiology. To meet these demands and perform optimally, athletes must undertake training programs that change the functioning of physiological systems within their bodies. This process of change is a form of adaptation: Just as an animal can change to become better suited to the demands of a new environment, so too can an athlete change to become better suited to the artificial environment of sport. Thus, the essence of sport training is to repeatedly place the body under the stress of a sport in order to optimize its performance.

Two of the primary physiological systems that underly sport performance are the **nervous system**, which stimulates movement, and the **muscular system**, which effects movement. The nervous system can be further divided into the **central nervous system** (CNS), which contains the brain and spinal cord, and the **peripheral nervous system** (PNS), which consists of the pathways that transmit information to and from the CNS. The main functional units of the nervous system are specialized cells called **neurons** that communicate by firing electrochemical signals. These electrochemical signals travel from upper **motor neurons** located in the **motor cortex** of the brain down the pathways of the PNS to the skeletal muscles, stimulating them to contract (see figure 15.1).

Together, the nervous system and skeletal muscles constitute the **neuromuscular system** of an athlete. The adaptations that occur in the neuromuscular system as a result of training determine the **functional state** of the athlete and thus readiness for performance.

Collecting information on the functional state of the motor system allows specialists to track the dynamics of systemic adaptive reactions, evaluate acute and cumulative training effects, and make more accurate training decisions for effective individualization and optimization of the training process. In short, monitoring the functional state of the neuromuscular system of athletes is a prerequisite for ensuring they are ready and able to perform at their best.

The two most important methods that sport scientists can use to monitor and evaluate neuromuscular changes in response to training loads are **electroencephalography** (EEG) and **electroneuromyography** (ENMG). Electroencephalography can be used to record and analyze the electrical activity of the brain during different functional states, including at rest and during motor activity. Electroneuromyography is a complex of electrophysiological methods for assessing the state of the neuromuscular system (mainly the peripheral part) by recording the bioelectric activity of nerves and muscles. Electroneuromyography can be used to evaluate both voluntary activity and activity of the neuromuscular system induced by stimulation.

ELECTROENCEPHALOGRAPHY OVERVIEW

The first step for athletes to optimize how their brain adaptively drives and manages the firing of the muscles is to gain visibility into the current state of their brain function. Electroencephalography was

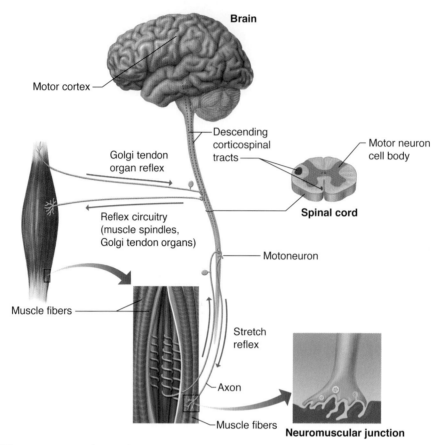

Brain

Motor cortex

Descending
corticospinal
tracts

Motor neuron
cell body

Golgi tendon
organ reflex

Spinal cord

Reflex circuitry
(muscle spindles,
Golgi tendon organs)

Motoneuron

Muscle fibers

Stretch
reflex

Axon

Muscle fibers

Neuromuscular junction

FIGURE 15.1   The neuromuscular system.

developed for this purpose and allows individuals to record and analyze the electrical activity of the brain in a safe and noninvasive manner.

Electroencephalography systems work by recording an amplified version of the electrical activity of many neurons in the brain firing synchronously. This synchronized neuronal activity results in a pulsing of brain activity that looks like waves. Like any wave, brainwaves can be described in terms of their frequency (oscillatory speed), amplitude (strength), and phase (point in the wave cycle). Neuroscientists name brainwaves according to set frequency ranges (i.e., alpha, beta, and theta), each of which is linked to different functions.

A typical EEG system consists of sensors called electrodes, a cap that the electrodes are placed in to ensure correct scalp placement, an amplifier, and a computer. Once placed in the cap, the electrodes make contact with the scalp and pick up the electrical impulses from the underlying brain area. The activity recorded from these electrodes is amplified and digitized to the computer, where athletes can visualize their brainwaves, or the data can be saved for later analysis (see figure 15.2).

The high temporal resolution of encephalography—the ability to record neural activity nearly in real time—is its primary advantage over other brain imaging technologies used by athletes today. While EEG records neural activity within a fraction of a second after its generation, technologies like magnetic resonance imaging (MRI) have up to a several-second recording lag. Magnetic resonance imaging does, however, have better spatial resolution, meaning that it can more precisely localize the origin of recorded brain activity. The development of low-cost, user-friendly, mobile EEG systems has rendered EEG a powerful and accessible performance tool for athletes and performance organizations alike to invest in.

Electroencephalography General Requirements

Electroencephalography systems use electrodes placed on the scalp to measure fluctuations in **voltage** (a difference in electrical potential between two points) in the underlying brain tissue. The voltage that EEG measures primarily reflects the summed charges of the

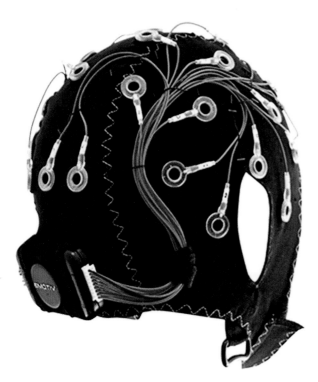

FIGURE 15.2 The Emotiv EPOC Flex wireless electroencephalography system.

excitatory postsynaptic potentials (EPSPs) created by the firing of many **pyramidal neurons**, the primary excitatory cells of the cerebral cortex.

The signal that EEG records is diluted by **volume conduction**, which is the passing of the electrical signal from its source in the brain tissue through the layers of the skull to reach the recording electrodes. Volume conduction is primarily responsible for the poor spatial resolution of EEG: EEG records a 2D version of a distant 3D signal, and thus the location of the signal cannot easily be inferred from the electrode recordings (24).

Electroencephalography Signal Recording

Electroencephalography **electrodes** are conductive sensors that make contact with the nonmetallic part of a circuit—the skin of the scalp. The sensors take the shape of small, metal discs (usually a sintered or electroplated Ag/AgCl material). Systems can use **dry electrodes** (electrodes that are placed directly on the scalp) or **wet electrodes** (electrodes that are connected to the scalp via a conductive medium such as gel or saline). Wet electrodes are more popular today because they reduce the contact **impedance** (resistance in an

AC circuit like the brain) of the electrode–skin interface. While volume conduction allows a neural signal to be carried as ions through conductive mediums in the brain, ions cannot easily pass through the skull, dead skin cells, hair, and air that separate the brain tissue from the electrode. Adding conductive gel reduces air pockets, allowing the signal to continue being conducted to the recording electrode (see figure 15.3; 18).

Since EEG measures voltage, the signal recorded at one electrode measures its voltage drop with a designated **reference** or comparison electrode. An EEG **channel** refers to this voltage difference recorded between two electrodes. Ideally, a reference electrode should be placed at as electrically neutral a location on the body as possible so the signal will not be significantly affected by electrical activity generated from muscle movement or other sources. Common choices include the mastoid (the bone behind the ear) or the earlobe. Often, instead of choosing a single reference location, a **common average reference** is used. In this case, the signal recorded at all electrodes is averaged, and the averaged signal is used as a common reference for each electrode.

The EEG systems used today typically use between 8 and 256 electrodes. Electrode placement is standardized according to the **10-20 system**. In order to cover all areas of the brain, the system divides the head into proportional distances from prominent skull landmarks such as the **nasion**, the point between the

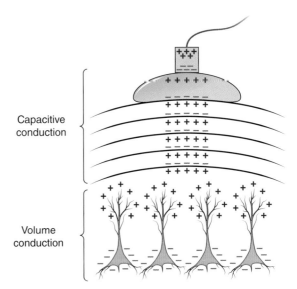

FIGURE 15.3 Gel aids volume conduction of the electrical signal from the brain to the electrode.

Reprinted by permission from A.F. Jackson and D.J. Bolger (2014, pg. 1061-1071).

eyes, and the **inion**, a small bump on the back of the skull. The distances between adjacent electrodes are either 10% or 20% of the total nasion-to-inion (front-back) or tragus-tragus (ear-ear) measurement of the skull (see figure 15.4; 20a).

Electrodes are labeled with letters according to their underlying brain target (i.e., F for frontal lobe) and numbers according to which side of the head they overlie (odd numbers denote the left side of the head, and even numbers signal the right side). Since the development of the 10-20 system, the **10-10 system** and the **10-5 systems** have been developed, which specify the placement of a higher density of electrodes—up to 300. Electrode placement according to these systems is accomplished with the use of EEG caps with holes labeled according to the given system to specify electrode placement. The caps come in various sizes to accommodate accurate placement on any head size.

Depending on study objectives and the capabilities of a given EEG system, a certain **montage** or group of electrodes is determined. In addition to the active recording electrodes, at least two electrodes are generally used to capture eye movements so eye movement can later be filtered out from the pure neural signal. A

VEOG (**vertical electrooculogram**) electrode placed below the eye aims to capture vertical eye movements like blinks. Similarly, a HEOG (**horizontal electrooculogram**) electrode placed just to the side of the eye aims to capture horizontal eye movements like saccades.

Electroencephalography Signal Amplification

Before the signal recorded at an electrode is transmitted to a computer, it is input into an amplifier where it is increased by a constant degree. The amplifier not only serves to increase the signal, but also filters out some interference from other electrical sources, including the tissue–electrode interface, power lines, and noise (31). A **high-pass filter** (typically set at 0.1-0.7 Hz) allows only frequencies higher than a specified number to be amplified, attenuating low-frequency undesirable bioelectric potentials from movements like breathing. In contrast, a **low-pass filter** can prevent high frequencies from interfering with the sampling rate (31).

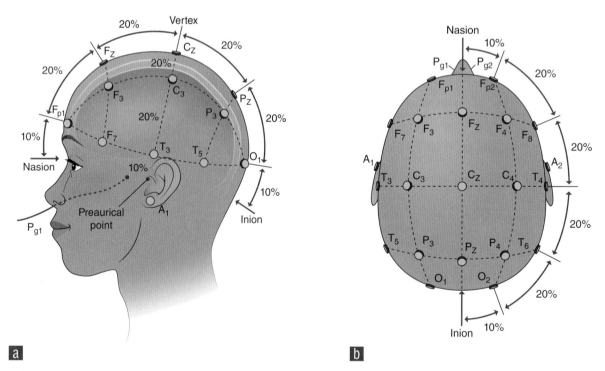

a   **b**

FIGURE 15.4   Electrode placement according to the 10-20 system: *(a)* nasion to inion (front-back) and *(b)* tragus to tragus (ear-ear).

Once the signal is amplified, it can be converted from analog to digital form. In order to convert the signal to digital format, measurements are taken at a certain **sampling rate**, or number of times per second. When purchasing an EEG system, it is important to know what the highest frequency of interest is (i.e., theta or gamma) since the minimum acceptable sampling rate should be 2.5 times this frequency.

In wireless EEG systems, the amplifier is typically attached to the EEG cap and the signal is transmitted to a computer via Bluetooth and a USB dongle; comparatively, in wired EEG systems the signal flows through a wire to the amplifier before being transmitted to a computer.

Electroencephalography Data Processing

After amplification, raw EEG data will still contain **artifact**—signals recorded in EEG data that were not produced by the brain (see figure 15.5; 21a). Artifacts must be removed before any meaningful analysis can be conducted. The most common sources of artifact in EEG data are as follows:

- **Electrooculogram** (EOG) artifacts are generated from eye movements like saccades and blinks. Electrooculogram artifacts tend to be higher amplitude and lower frequency than typical EEG signals and appear prominently in frontal channels recorded closest to the eyes.

- **Electrocardiogram** (ECG) artifacts are generated by the beating of the heart. These artifacts appear as a rhythmic pulsing superimposed on the EEG signal.

- **Electromyogram** (EMG) artifacts are generated by muscle movements like clenching the jaw or yawning. Movement often appears as a sudden, significant deviation in the signal with frequencies of about 100 Hz.

- Other physiological noise like sweating can result in a slow drift of the baseline EEG signal.

The easiest way to reduce noise in EEG data is by applying low- and high-pass filters. Eye movement is one of the largest sources of noise in EEG and can be corrected in various ways. Most modern EEG analysis programs have functionality to automatically identify and remove windows or **epochs** of EEG data that contain EOG artifact according to a given "blink" thresh-

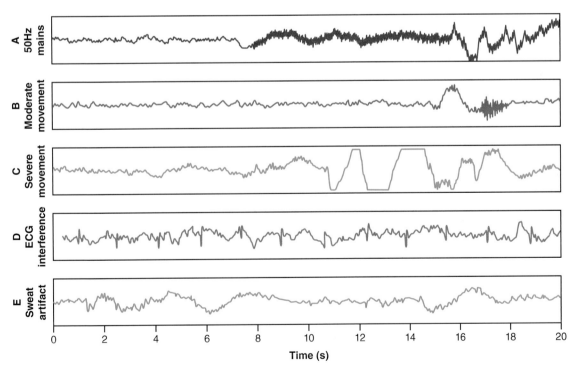

FIGURE 15.5 Examples of common artifacts in raw EEG data.

Reprinted by permission from S. Motamedi-Fakhr et al. (2014, pg. 21-33).

old. Unfortunately, this can result in the elimination of considerable data. For this reason, some specialists prefer to use other methods for removing artifact such as **independent component analysis** (ICA).

Independent component analysis is based on a technique called **blind source separation** (BSS) that uses linear decomposition to separate a signal into its components originating from different sources. Independent component analysis does this by identifying sources of variance in the data that are maximally statistically independent. Basically, it is as though ICA is working to pick out what a single individual is saying in a crowd of people talking at a party. Once ICA has identified the different components in a signal, it orders them by how much variance they account for in the data, placing the component that accounts for the most variance first.

Each component is typically evaluated for rejection based on its **scalp topography map**, which shows the distribution of activity across the brain, along with the component's time course data and its power spectrum. If two channels were used to track eye movements (an HEOG and a VEOG channel), at least two components should be rejected. Additional components can be rejected based on subjective judgment. Common reasons to consider a component for rejection include the following:

- If a component has a distribution that is strongly anterior in weight on the topography plot, it likely corresponds to EOG artifact generated by eye movement in the front of the head. This can be confirmed by looking for a high-amplitude, low-frequency "blink" event in the time course data.
- If all the signal or variance of a component appears to stem from just one electrode, the component likely reflects noise from muscle movement. Looking at the activity power spectrum can be useful to confirm this suspicion. The power spectrum for muscle activity may look like a quick drop and then rise in activity as opposed to the characteristic EEG distribution curve in which power density is inversely related to frequency (1 / frequency curve).

Electroencephalography Analysis During Sport Performance

When analyzing EEG data, specialists look at the frequency, amplitude, and phase relationships of brainwaves in the relevant brain areas for a given task. The electrophysiological data of EEG can then be correlated with behavioral metrics (e.g., accuracy, reaction time) to better understand the neural underpinnings of sport performance.

One of the most commonly analyzed EEG metrics is power. Specialists consider how the power of a given frequency of brainwaves (i.e., the alpha wave) changes in an area of the brain over time within a single athlete and between many athletes. In sports, the power of the **sensorimotor rhythm** (SMR) is often related to athletic performance. The SMR corresponds to the 12- to 15-Hz frequency range of brainwaves localized in the sensorimotor areas of the brain. Research suggests that athletes who exhibit more powerful SMR rhythms during sport performance achieve better outcomes (7, 8, 9). A more powerful SMR rhythm is believed to reflect more efficient sensorimotor processing and thus greater skill automaticity. Unsurprisingly, individuals experiencing "flow states" have been shown to demonstrate a higher-powered SMR (7, 9). See chapter 26 for further insights on flow states.

However, interpreting power changes is difficult because they can be ambiguous: An increase in power does not necessarily mean that more information is being exchanged in the brain. The reason is that EEG disproportionally represents synchronous activity in broad areas of the brain. Take the example of people chatting at a party. When many separate conversations are occurring at once, a great deal of information is being exchanged. Yet the average signal from the party would sound like a blurred, low murmur. In contrast, if everyone at the party starts chanting at once, less information is getting exchanged but the synchrony produces a much stronger signal. The same is true with EEG; a stronger signal may indicate more synchronous activity occurring but less information getting exchanged. Moreover, everyone's brain anatomy is different, meaning that for one individual an increase in power could mean the same thing regarding task performance as a decrease in power for another individual.

Two studies that analyzed the relationship between power in the **frontal midline theta (FMT) rhythm** and sport performance highlight the ambiguity of power changes. Frontal midline theta corresponds to the 4- to 7-Hz frequency range as recorded along the medial prefrontal areas of the brain. Frontal midline theta has been investigated as a marker of sustained attention. On the one hand, a study of elite basketball players revealed that FMT power was higher and more stable before successful free throws than unsuccessful shots (10). In contrast, a study of golfers found that lower-powered FMT values correlated with successful putting performance (19).

To avoid the ambiguity of power interpretations, sport scientists can look at measures of **functional connectivity**—how information is flowing between different areas of the brain. The most common EEG measure of functionality connectivity is **coherence**, a correlation coefficient measuring whether there is a constant amplitude ratio and phase shift between two recorded signals at each frequency band (29). A consistent relationship is the key for high coherence: Two signals can be highly coherent even if they have a **phase delay**—a time delay between a point in the phase of one signal and the same point in the comparison signal measured in angles—as long as the delay is consistent over time.

Electroencephalography studies reveal that elite athletes tend to exhibit highly stable coherence between brain rhythms in the visuospatial area of their parietal cortices and the rhythms in other areas of the cortex (12). This highlights the super visuomotor integration abilities that guide an elite athlete's preparation, execution, and control of motor movements (as discussed in detail in chapter 27).

Although true coherence can be a useful measure of functional connectivity, it can also arise or appear exaggerated due to random coherence created by volume conduction (29). With random coherence, the signal at multiple electrodes stemming from different cortical current sources becomes blurred together. The closer the electrodes are, the larger the potential that volume conduction is affecting their coherence. Using Laplacian coherence measures can help reduce interference from random coherence by emphasizing current sources at smaller spatial scales. However, Laplacian coherence must be used carefully, because it can also diminish the appearance of true coherence over a wide brain area (29).

Electroencephalography Analysis During Other Functional States

While it is useful to analyze the functional state of an athlete's brain during game-time performance, understanding and training how an athlete's brain works in other functional states can be an important avenue for performance enhancement.

Research in the past 20 years has increasingly shed light on the importance of optimizing brain rhythms when the brain is in **resting state** and not engaged in a goal-oriented task. Contrary to popular belief, the brain is not dormant when it is "at rest"; rather a series of **resting state networks** (RSNs) that compose a larger **default mode network** (DMN) are quite active. The DMN spans various areas of the brain, incorporating networks that deal with internal processing, self-referential thought, goal-directed stimulus selection, visual processing, speech production, and sensorimotor planning and execution (21).

Electroencephalography studies support the results of functional magnetic resonance imaging (fMRI) studies pointing to differences in the RSNs of athletes that reflect expertise (25). The amplitude of alpha brainwaves in the parietal and occipital RNS of karate athletes was found to be significantly higher for elite athletes than for amateur athletes or non-athletes. Likewise, the amplitude of parietal and occipital delta and alpha has been shown to be stronger in elite rhythmic gymnasts compared to non-athletes (2).

Interestingly, further research has revealed that while the brain rhythms of an active DMN can reflect athletic skill, so too can the ability to suppress the DMN when switching to engage the brain networks needed for a task (25, 27). Together, these results suggest that sport training leads to an optimization in both the neural synchronization and the task-preparatory suppression of resting state EEG rhythms.

Meditation is a powerful tool athletes can use to train their cortical rhythms, including the rhythms of the DMN. **Mindfulness meditation**, a practice that involves focusing one's attention on the present moment, has gained considerable traction with athletes. A few years of daily mindfulness practice (>894 hours) has been found to change the gamma rhythms of an individual's RSNs to indicate less internal and self-referential processing (i.e., mind wandering) and more of the environmental awareness that underlies focus during sport performance (6).

These neural changes may be the basis of the positive behavioral results athletes have benefited from after adopting mindfulness practices. Mindfulness practices have consistently been shown to decrease an athlete's performance anxieties and task-irrelevant thoughts in a sustained manner, as well as to increase their propensity to experience a flow state (5, 28, 32). Athletes can practice mindfulness and thus train their brain rhythms using apps like Headspace™ and Calm™ that offer guided meditations to help manage sleep, stress, and anxiety. Additionally, Muse is an innovative EEG headband that provides neurofeedback to aid in building focused-attention meditation practice (see chapter 27 to learn about how athletes are using neurofeedback to enhance their performance). The newest version of Muse even contains additional sensors to monitor heart rate, breathing, and body movement.

ELECTRONEUROMYOGRAPHY OVERVIEW

Electroneuromyography (ENMG) is a complex of electrophysiological methods for assessing the functional state of a human's neuromuscular system by recording and analyzing the bioelectrical activity of skeletal muscles and nerves at rest and during motor activity. Electroneuromyography is a general term that refers to a combination of all types of electrophysiological methods (invasive and noninvasive, voluntary, and evoked, clinical and practical, etc.) for recording and analyzing the bioelectrical activity of nerves and muscles (see figure 15.6). Comparatively, surface **electromyography** (EMG) is a specific term referring to the noninvasive surface EMG method (recorded by surface EMG sensors at rest or during voluntary muscular activity or both). These are the main types of ENMG used today:

- **Needle EMG** involves recording the electrical activity of individual motor units (MUs) and muscle fibers by introducing needle electrodes into the skeletal muscle. Due to its invasive and painful nature, needle EMG is mainly used for clinical purposes.

- **Surface EMG** (sEMG), the most widely used type of EMG in sport science, records the electrical activity of skeletal muscles using electrodes placed on the surface of the skin overlying the muscle of interest.

- **Stimulating EMG** records the electrical activity of skeletal muscles and peripheral nerves evoked by electrically or magnetically stimulating a separate part of the nervous system. It is successfully used to diagnose and treat diseases of the human motor system. Despite its great potential, this method is not yet widely used in sport science.

The following sections provide an overview of ENMG basics before delving into each of these types of EMG in more detail.

Electroneuromyography General Requirements

All modern ENMG systems include electrodes, a preamplifier, an amplifier, and a computer. Stimulating EMG systems also include a magnetic or electrical stimulator, and needle EMG systems use needles.

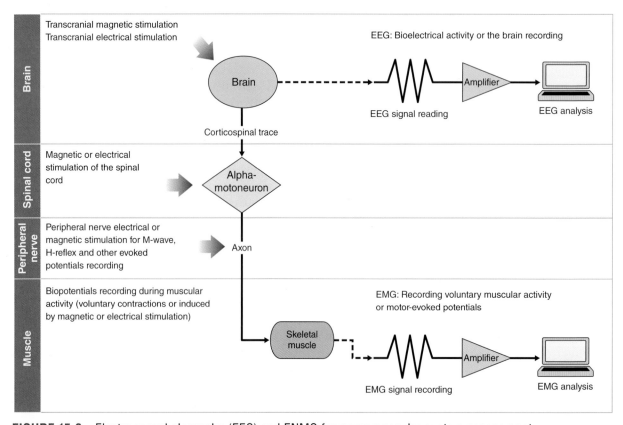

FIGURE 15.6   Electroencephalography (EEG) and ENMG for neuromuscular system assessment.

While EEG electrodes are placed on the scalp, ENMG electrodes are conductive pads placed on the skin of the body. Bioelectrical activity—voluntarily induced or evoked by a stimulator or needle—is registered by these electrodes and magnified by the preamplifier and the amplifier. A computer manages the technical characteristics of the stimulator and allows for the visualization and storage of the signal. Note that wireless sEMG systems developed in the second decade of the century allow sEMG signals to be transmitted without the use of connecting wires to a computer. However, for comprehensive ENMG study, wired systems are still used by many specialists.

Electroneuromyography studies must be carried out in a specially equipped room that maintains a constant comfortable temperature and humidity and adequate ventilation. The room should be located away from electromagnetic field generators (e.g., x-ray and physiotherapy devices), and the ENMG equipment must be grounded. All electrical safety requirements must be strictly followed.

Before application of the electrodes, the skin surface is degreased with alcohol and abraded, and any hair is shaved off. To improve the contact of the electrode with the skin, an electrode gel or electrode paste is used. When EMG is used to record more intense and complex intra-coordinated muscular activity such

as that seen in combat sports or rhythmic gymnastics, electrode pads must be fixed to the skin with special glue, adhesive plaster, adhesive, and rubber bands to study simpler muscular activity or resting state activity. Electrode pads that already have adhesive attached can be used. Each ENMG system comes with specific instructions for its safe use and operation.

Electroneuromyography Signal Recording

Depending on the desired functionality, three types of ENMG electrodes can be used: **recording, stimulating**, and **ground** electrodes or some combination of these (see table 15.1).

As their name suggests, **recording electrodes** are designed solely to register the bioelectric activity of MUs or muscles. **Surface recording electrodes** capture muscle activity at the skin's surface (cutaneous) while **needle recording electrodes** register biopotentials in the immediate vicinity of the source of potential generation (i.e., the MUs). Structurally, surface electrodes are usually discs, bars, or rectangular. Recording electrodes can be placed in different configurations on the muscles. When a **bipolar configuration** is used, two recording electrodes

TABLE 15.1   Electroneuromyography Electrode Characteristics by Type

	Recording electrode	Stimulating electrode	Grounding electrode
Shape	**Surface**	**Surface**	**Surface**
	Discs	Discs	Discs
	Cups	Bars	Rings
	Bars	Rings	
	Rings	**Needle**	
	Rectangular	Monopolar electrodes	
	Needle	Bipolar electrodes	
	Monopolar electrodes	Concentric electrodes	
	Bipolar electrodes		
	Coaxial bipolar electrodes		
	Single-fiber electrodes		
	Macroelectrodes		
	Multielectrodes		
	Fine-wire electrodes		
Type of recording or stimulation	Monopolar	Monopolar	Neutral reference (ground)
	Bipolar	Bipolar	
	Multipolar		

are placed equidistant or nearly equidistant over the studied muscle. For example, two disc electrodes may be built into a block with a fixed distance of 20 mm between their centers. Surface EMG primarily uses a bipolar electrode configuration. By contrast, stimulation EMG often uses both bipolar and monopolar configurations. When a **monopolar configuration** is used, the active electrode is located in the active zone of potential generation while the reference electrode is placed outside the potential generation zone. It should be noted that an increase in the area of electrodes and the distance between their centers lead to an increase in the amplitude of the recorded muscle potentials. To compare the data obtained in different laboratories, it is necessary to use standard electrodes with a fixed area and interelectrode distance.

Stimulating electrodes are usually designed to apply electrical stimulation to skeletal muscles and nerves. A stimulating electrode can take the shape of a disc, ring, or bar. Plate electrodes are convenient because they can work both for recording and for stimulation. Bar electrodes are used to stimulate deep nerve trunks. Ring electrodes are used to stimulate the sensitive fibers of finger nerves. Stimulating electrodes consist of two parts: the cathode (negatively charged) and anode (positively charged). During stimulation, electrical charges flow from one electrode to the other through tissues along the paths of least resistance.

Ground electrodes are designed to reduce noise from industrial currents. While stimulating electrodes are used to apply the current, ground electrodes serve to protect the patient and lab equipment from excess current and improve the recorded signal quality. By providing a conductive path for induced currents to flow through, ground electrodes can reroute noise into the ground rather than into the signal of interest. In the same way, ground electrodes can redirect excessive current from a patient's body or an exposed wire in lab equipment during a procedure like EMG.

Electroneuromyography Signal Amplification

The preamplifier and amplifier increase the low-amplitude signals of skeletal muscles (measured in microvolts) by several thousand times. This allows the sport scientist to visualize the EMG signal on a computer screen and conduct subsequent analysis.

The important technical parameters of the amplifier include input impedance and frequency bandwidth. As with EEG amplifiers, high- and low-pass filters control which frequency bands pass through the amplifier.

These are the main types of noises in the ENMG signal:

- **Electrical noise** comes from power lines, electrical equipment, and other electrical sources
- **Motion noise** is caused by movement of EMG electrodes on the skin during dynamic activities or wire movement
- **Physiological noise** is produced by electrical activity from the heart (electrocardiogram), respiratory signals, and other physiological signals
- **"Crosstalk" noise** comprises signals from neighboring muscles (14)

Solutions for ENMG noise reduction include ensuring that the skin is clean (i.e., wiped with an alcohol swab), accurately placing EMG electrodes on the target muscle, and ensuring good contact between the electrodes and the skin so the electrodes will not move. Applying these solutions for noise reduction will help maximize the ENMG **signal-to-noise ratio** (SNR)—the ratio between the EMG signal recorded during muscular contraction and the undesired electrical signal recorded during muscular rest. The higher the SNR, the higher the quality of the EMG signal.

For ENMG studies, **single-channel** (for stimulating a single nerve) and **multi-channel** (for stimulating two nerves) electrical stimulants are used to stimulate nerves or muscles with electrical current. Single, paired, or rhythmic stimuli of a rectangular shape are applied at a frequency varying from 0.1 to 100 Hz. The intensity of the electrical stimulation is regulated by current from 0.1 to 100 mA.

Electroneuromyography Signal Analysis

Equipping the ENMG system with a computer allows the amplifier and stimulator to be controlled from one keyboard, setting the appropriate technical characteristics for both: for example, sensitivity, bandwidth, and parameters of electrical stimuli. The presence of a computer with specialized programs significantly accelerates the EMG signal processing and analysis (see table 15.2).

TABLE 15.2   Electromyography Analysis, Key Metrics, and Interpretation

Analysis	Description	Metrics	Interpretation
Amplitude analysis	Calculates the main characteristics of the sEMG amplitude	Root mean square Mean absolute value Peak values Minimum and maximum values Slope values Moving average	Individual muscle force (isometric) Intermuscular relationships (compare relative contribution of different muscles)
Muscle activation	Defines muscular activation-deactivation (i.e., ON-OFF) timing and order	Activation time (ON-OFF) Activation order Delay time	Individual muscles ON-OFF time Muscle activation or deactivation order Coactivation
Integration	Describes the integrated input data series	Area under the curve	Total muscular activity Energy expenditure (EMG-cost)
Spectral analysis	Assesses different frequency components of the total frequency spectrum using fast Fourier transformation (FFT)	Median frequency Mean frequency Peak power Total power	Muscular fatigue (isometric)
Cross-correlation	Evaluates the time delay between 2 EMG signals	Measures similarity of two series (R_{xy})	Determine muscle fiber conduction velocity
Histogram	Calculates the number of occurrences for each interval over the entire data series	Histogram	Count number of threshold-driven EMG bursts Amplitude-driven event counter
Threshold	Determines the intervals where EMG signal and data series exceeds the specific threshold	EMG threshold values	EMG events recognition Muscle timing

Types of Electroneuromyography

Different types of ENMG can be used to monitor the naturally or artificially stimulated activity of an athlete's nerves and muscles. These are reviewed next.

Needle Electromyography

Needle EMG is an invasive and painful method for recording and analyzing the bioelectrical activity of individual MUs and muscle fibers by introducing needle electrodes directly into the belly of the muscle. Needle EMG is useful because it produces data on the electroactivity of individual muscle fibers and MUs, including their order of activation and deactivation and interaction with one another. The methodological features of needle EMG (the difficulty of handling the electrodes, its invasive nature, and the risk of injury or

infection) limit its practical use in sports compared to surface EMG or stimulation EMG. Nevertheless, for certain issues, needle EMG is the best and sometimes the only option. For example, it is only advisable to study the parameters of fatigued individual MUs with needle EMG.

Surface Electromyography

Surface EMG (sEMG) is a noninvasive and painless method for recording and analyzing the total bioelectric activity of skeletal muscles at rest and during movement using cutaneous (surface of the skin) electrodes located on the muscle. Due to its ease of use and painlessness, sEMG is the most widely used type of EMG in sport physiology, biomechanics, kinesiology, physiotherapy, sport training, and ergonomics. Surface EMG in sport science is used to study

- the degree of skeletal muscle activation during the execution of voluntary movements,
- the regulation of various muscles (e.g., synergists versus antagonists),
- the order in which muscles activate (i.e., turn "on" and "off") during movement,
- the interaction and coordination of muscles during movements, and
- the mechanisms of motor skill formation.

Surface Electromyography Equipment Modern sEMG systems have from 8 to 16 channels for recording sEMG signals. The lower-frequency range is set at 2 to 10 Hz and the upper at 10 kHz. The sensitivity of the amplifier is selected depending on the expected amplitude of the potentials. An example of the sEMG system is presented on the left of figure 15.7.

Surface EMG recording is conducted with bipolar electrodes that are **gelled** (with Al/AgCl, etc.) or **dry** (silver) and have a signal transmission range of about 20 m (21 yd). Modern sEMG systems use advanced high-quality sensor technology with small, and often fixed, interelectrode spacing. Each sensor has a built-in accelerometer, gyroscope, and 9-axis inertial measurement unit that allow it to discern movement activity time-synchronized with the sEMG signals. An example of a modern dry silver bipolar wireless sEMG sensor is presented in figure 15.8. This sensor consists of two parallel bars—each 1 cm long and 1 to 2 mm wide—that are spaced 1 cm apart.

Muscle selection for sEMG is determined by the objectives of the study and the technical capabilities of the EMG system (i.e., how many channels it has). Typically, sEMG of a complex movement records the activity of 8 to 16 muscles while sEMG of simple movements involves 2 to 6 muscles. Of the muscles selected, sEMG is recorded from the **leading** or main skeletal muscle for the sport-specific movement.

Accurate sensor placement will significantly increase the quality of sEMG signal and reduce crosstalk (13). The sEMG recording sensor should be placed between the muscle-tendon junction and the nearest innervation zone on the muscle belly's midline (see figure 15.8). To identify the innervation zone, use electrical stimulation or electrical surface mapping.

Surface Electromyography Procedure and Typical Patterns The amplitude and frequency of electrical potential recorded by sEMG reflects the magnitude of contraction of the recorded muscles. Surface EMG can be recorded while the athlete is in many different conditions (see figure 15.9):

- **Resting state sEMG** is typically recorded while an athlete is in supine position (lying down, face-up) with muscles completely relaxed. Recording this relaxed state is useful for measuring the ability of the subject to control muscle tension. See figure 15.9a.
- **Posture maintenance sEMG** is recorded while an athlete is maintaining a particular posture (i.e., lying down, sitting, or standing). In general,

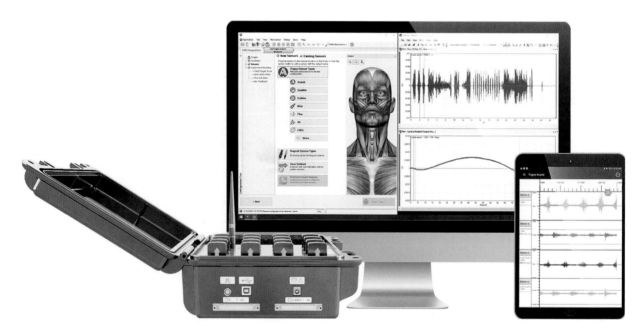

FIGURE 15.7 Surface EMG system produced by Delsys.

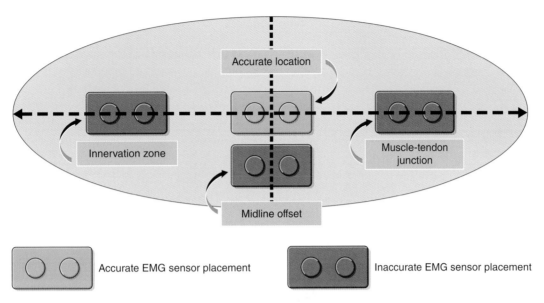

FIGURE 15.8   Surface EMG recording electrode placement on the muscle.

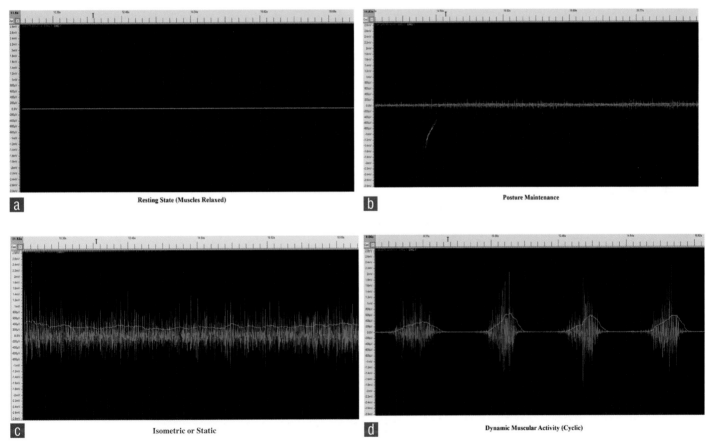

FIGURE 15.9   Electromyography patterns at different conditions: *(a)* resting state sEMG, *(b)* posture maintenance sEMG, *(c)* isometric or static sEMG, and *(d)* sEMG during cyclic motor activity.

posture maintenance sEMG records muscle activity with relatively small amplitude and moderate frequency. The largest amplitudes are recorded for the lower-extremity muscles, which bear the main load while maintaining vertical postures. Posture maintenance EMG is useful for identifying a sport-specific issue with muscle activity regulation since the key movements of each sport are associated with a particular posture (e.g., kayaking primarily involves sitting, swimming involves the prone position). See figure 15.9*b*.

- **Isometric or static sEMG** is recorded while an athlete maintains an isometric voluntary muscular contraction of a given degree—typically 25%, 50%, 75%, or 100% of the maximum amount of force an athlete can produce to contract that muscle or the **maximal voluntary contraction** (MVC). In some cases, static EMG is measured while the athlete is holding a standard load. Electromyography amplitude and frequency depend on the magnitude of the static effort, with the highest values observed at MVC. See figure 15.9*c*.

- Surface EMG during **cyclic** or **acyclic motor activity** (i.e., dynamic movement) is characterized by high-amplitude and high-frequency potentials generated at active phases of repeated motor actions. Examples of cyclic movements are running and cycling, while acyclic movements studied with sEMG include precision and rhythmic movements of fencing, gymnastics, and acrobatics. See figure 15.9*d*.

- Surface EMG can be recorded during a state of **fatigue** when skeletal muscles are experiencing a sharp decrease in performance, often evidenced by a visual tremor.

- Surface EMG at **reflex activity** records the electroactivity of the interneurons that carry information within the spinal cord (remember that many reflexes originate in the spinal cord rather than the brain motor cortex). Reflexes that can be assessed include "loading" and "unloading" reflexes, the tendon reflex, and the tonic vibration reflex. Special technical devices are used to elicit these reflexes.

Surface Electromyography Analysis   The first stage of sEMG analysis should be a qualitative assessment: The sport scientist conducts an analysis of the amplitude of the sEMG signal to establish the leading and supporting muscles for a sport-specific movement. Qualitative analysis of muscular electrical activity can then be supplemented by the quantitative analysis of sEMG using specialized platforms. Application of the

common EMG analysis methods presented in table 15.2 can provide valuable information for researchers.

MVC normalization is used to explore sEMG amplitude analysis in relation to MVC as a reference value. MVC normalization allows for comparison of the activity of the same athlete's muscle on different days or comparison of the same muscle between athletes. Typically, the MVC value is calculated before the EMG study at static efforts: Three trials are conducted (3-5 s each) with a 3-minute rest period separating each trial. The researcher selects the maximal value from these trials.

Despite its broad applications for sport science, sEMG still has several limitations (see table 15.3). The most significant challenge is the inability to accurately replicate the results of a past study. The optimal strategy for any EMG recording is to keep constant as many factors as possible. The approaches presented in table 15.3 can significantly help to standardize EMG research and reduce the observed variability of EMG results in repeated studies. See the "Recommended Readings" section for other sources of information.

Stimulation Electromyography

Stimulation EMG is a method of recording and analyzing the bioelectric activity of skeletal muscles and peripheral nerves by activating the nervous system with an electric or magnetic stimulus. Stimulation ENMG primarily generates two types of responses, as shown in figures 15.10 and 15.11—a motor response (M-wave) and a reflex response (H-reflex).

M-Wave   An **M-wave** is a **compound muscle action potential** (CMAP) evoked by the application of a single electrical or magnetic stimulus to a motor nerve (see figures 15.10 and 15.11). A typical comprehensive ENMG study begins with a CMAP recording. Since the M-wave is artificially evoked, it is not a natural physiological muscle response. In natural motor activity, active MUs work asynchronously; in contrast, artificial stimulation of a nerve causes a synchronous discharge of MUs that looks like a single wave—hence the name M-wave.

As with any type of ENMG study, the choice of muscle in which to stimulate an M-wave depends on the specific objectives of the study. As a rule, muscles are studied that underlie the execution of a basic motor action needed for the sport of interest. Typically, the most distally and superficially located muscles involved in the movement are stimulated (gastrocnemius, soleus, etc.).

TABLE 15.3   Surface Electromyography Limitations and Possible Solutions

Factors	Limitations	Solutions
EMG-signal recording factors	Variability in electrode placement (from one recording to the next and between subjects)	Locating the electrodes accurately on the muscle
	Variability of the degree of electrode–skin resistance	Always performing an impedance test
	Different interelectrode distance (if using a monopolar configuration)	Using stimulating electrodes with standard interelectrode distance
Movement control and muscular contraction regulation factors	Variability of the athlete's functional state before the EMG test (i.e., incomplete recovery, CNS or muscular fatigue or both, motivation)	Assessing at the same functional state (same time of the day, complete recovery, no fatigue, same motivation, same environment)
	Load and duration variability	Measuring applied load and standardize the protocol duration (volume and intensity control)
		Using audio and visual feedback for better regulation of the muscular contraction
	During static assessment—angle position variability	Standardizing the angle position using specific equipment (machines) or belts to achieve a sufficient fixation
	During dynamic assessment—range of motion(s) and velocity variability	Reducing range of motion and velocity variability using metronome, goniometers, and different training equipment (treadmills, isokinetic machines, etc.)

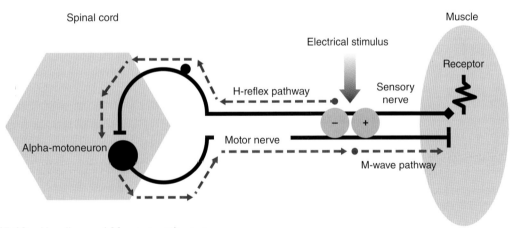

FIGURE 15.10   H-reflex and M-wave pathways.

An M-wave is recorded with surface electrodes since they record bioelectric activity of the target muscles as a whole, while needle electrodes record only isolated MUs or muscle fibers. The stimulating electrodes are placed in the area of the peripheral nerve projection, where they typically deliver a square-wave electrical stimulus that lasts 0.5 ms to 1 ms. A well-defined M-wave is obtained by progressively increasing the stimulus magnitude until 100% of the peripheral nerve fibers are activated.

The M-wave can be assessed by the following parameters:

- *Threshold*: the minimum value of electrical stimulation that creates an M-wave with minimal amplitude
- *Latency*: the time between the application of the stimulus and the muscle response
- *Amplitude*: the amount and synchronism of MU activity in the target muscle (typically measured as peak-to-peak amplitude)

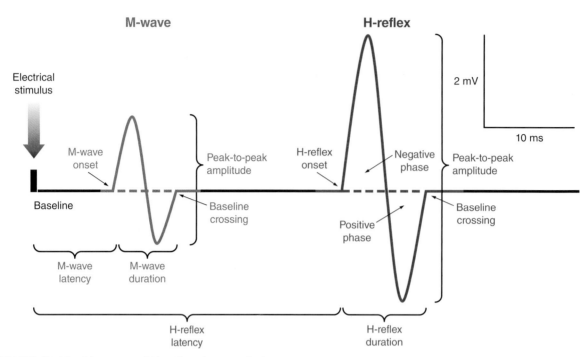

FIGURE 15.11   M-wave and H-reflex characteristics.

- *Duration*: the time from the moment of the initial deviation from isoline (baseline) until the moment of returning to isoline
- *Form*: biphasic or triphasic
- *Area*: calculated as the entire area under the M-wave curve

H-reflex   The **H-reflex** is the synchronized reflex response of MUs to the electrical stimulation of sensory and afferent nerve fibers (see figures 15.11 and 15.12). The H-reflex is an artificially induced analogue of the patellar tendon reflex and is one of the simplest reflexes carried out by a **monosynaptic reflex arc** (see figure 15.11). Monosynaptic reflex arcs involve two neurons—a sensory and a motor neuron—connected at one synapse. The H-reflex is widely used in sport as a powerful technique for measuring the **excitatory** and **inhibitory** mechanisms of spinal motor neurons (22, 34).

In adults, the H-reflex can typically be registered only in the muscles of the lower limbs (i.e., soleus, gastrocnemius) in response to tibial nerve stimulation of the **popliteal fossa**, a shallow depression at the back of the knee joint. The amplitude of the H-reflex depends on the subject's position: Subjects are usually asked to lie in supine position and relax their muscles as much as possible. Depending on study objectives, single, paired, or repeated stimuli may be used.

Just as with M-wave, sport scientists can analyze various aspects of H-reflex parameters (e.g., threshold, latency, amplitude [H-max/M-max ratio]), duration, form, and area to study short- and long-term neural adaptations in an athlete's neuromuscular system in a variety of sports (e.g., tennis, cycling, basketball, ballet) and activities (e.g., running, high-resistance training, interval training, stretching, resistance training) (1, 3, 4, 15, 17, 20, 23, 24, 26, 30, 33).

Assessment of Inhibitory Mechanisms

Inhibition is an active local neural process leading to the suppression or prevention of excitation. Like excitation processes, inhibition processes in the nervous system play a crucial role in regulating neural activity, muscular contractions, and coordination of motor activity.

Inhibition has three main functions:

1. *Regulation of excitation*: Inhibition can serve to suppress excessive excitation in the CNS or concentrate the excitation to a specific target area.

2. *Coordination*: Inhibitory processes suppress the activity of specific muscles and organs that should not participate in a particular motor action.

3. *Protection*: Inhibition protects neural centers from excessive overloading, or too much stimulation.

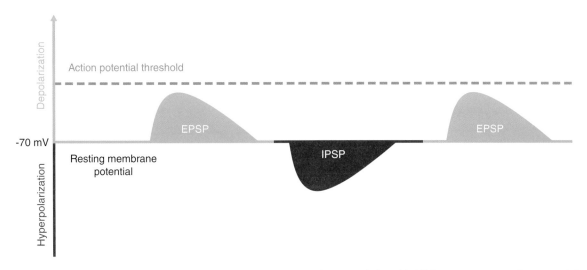

FIGURE 15.12 Relationship between excitatory postsynaptic potential and inhibitory postsynaptic potential.

Inhibition processes are always carried out by specific **inhibitory neurons**, which are activated by excitatory neurons (ironically, inhibition is prompted by excitation). Inhibition is brought about by inhibitory neurotransmitters (gamma-aminobutyric acid [GABA] is a common example) partially or completely suppressing the ability of a neural membrane to generate or conduct excitation. Neural impulses arising from the excitation of specific inhibitory neurons cause hyperpolarization of the postsynaptic membrane, generating an **inhibitory postsynaptic potential** (IPSP) (see figure 15.12).

An IPSP is a local inhibitory potential in the postsynaptic area that decreases (hyperpolarizes) a neuron's excitability, making it less likely to generate an action potential. In contrast, an **excitatory postsynaptic potential** (EPSP) is a local excitatory potential in a postsynaptic area that increases (depolarizes) the neuron excitability and creates better conditions for action potential generation. Excitatory postsynaptic potentials are prompted by excitatory neurotransmitters like glutamate.

Inhibition is commonly misconceived as fatigue: This is incorrect. While inhibition can occur at the same time as fatigue, inhibition is a separate process from fatigue that is caused by excitation and expressed as the suppression of excitation. The following types of inhibition are present in the spinal cord: **presynaptic**, **postsynaptic**, **autogenic (nonreciprocal)**, **recurrent**, and **reciprocal** (see figure 15.13). These inhibition mechanisms reflect the functional state of the neuromuscular system of the athlete in different conditions (i.e., resting state, fatigue, different training loads), and can be measured by specific ENMG methods.

Presynaptic Inhibition

Presynaptic inhibition occurs at the presynaptic terminal before a neural impulse reaches a synapse with a postsynaptic neuron. Presynaptic inhibition primarily functions to regulate all the afferent impulses traveling to neural centers in the spinal cord. The morphological basis of presynaptic inhibition is a special type of synapse called an **axo-axonal synapse**—a synapse where a nerve impulse travels between the axons of two nerve cells. Presynaptic inhibition works on the **"negative feedback"** principle, which regulates the flow of sensory information into the CNS (i.e., **"gates"** the flow). Presynaptic inhibition relies on GABA, the main inhibitory mediator of the CNS.

In sport science, presynaptic inhibition can be indirectly assessed by facilitation of the H-reflex at peripheral nerves. The higher the H-reflex facilitation, the lower the degree of presynaptic inhibition (16). Presynaptic inhibition can also be assessed by measuring the degree of H-reflex depression prompted by vibrostimulation of the Achilles: The higher the H-reflex depression, the higher the level of presynaptic inhibition.

Postsynaptic Inhibition

Postsynaptic inhibition can be direct or recurrent. **Direct postsynaptic inhibition** is an excitation of an inhibitory neuron prompting it to release inhibitory neurotransmitter (instead of an excitatory neurotransmitter) that causes hyperpolarization of the postsynaptic membrane and leads to a decrease in motor neuron excitability. **Recurrent postsynaptic inhibition** is a self-regulatory mechanism of the spinal

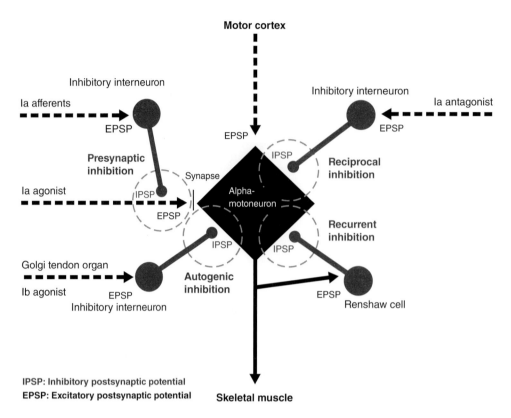

FIGURE 15.13   Neural inhibition mechanisms of the spinal cord.

alpha motor neuron (realized through the **Renshaw cell**, a specific inhibitory interneuron located in the spinal cord) to prevent excessive output and protect the motor neuron. Note that a motor neuron's axon has a recurrent collateral that is connected directly with the Renshaw cell. The Renshaw cell can directly inhibit the alpha motor neuron via the neurotransmitter glycine. Recurrent postsynaptic inhibition can be assessed by the H-reflex method.

Reciprocal Inhibition

Reciprocal inhibition is an agonist alpha motor neuron inhibition, evoked by activation of inhibitory interneurons after contraction of the antagonist muscle. Reciprocal inhibition is a basis for locomotion. Reciprocal inhibition is assessed by a paired stimulation technique (i.e., application of the fibular nerve conditioning stimulation and the tibial nerve testing stimulation).

Autogenic Inhibition

Autogenic inhibition (nonreciprocal) is a protective inhibitory mechanism that prevents muscles from damage. The primary mechanism of autogenic inhibition is neural volleys from the Golgi tendon organ of the activated muscle. The magnitude of the autogenic inhibition can be assessed by the "**silent period method**"—stimulating a peripheral nerve during a voluntary static muscular effort. The higher the voluntary muscular activation, the higher the magnitude of the autogenic inhibition.

In short, since excitatory and inhibitory processes work together to support sport performance, both are equally important for sport scientists to understand in order to build training programs that best adapt an athlete's physiology to a given sport. The spinal cord plays an especially large role in inhibition by regulating the descending and ascending motor neurons. The inhibition the spinal cord facilitates takes many forms, including presynaptic inhibition, postsynaptic and recurrent inhibition, autogenic inhibition via tendon receptors, and reciprocal inhibition. Despite the importance of inhibitory processes in sport performance, very little research has been done to better understand its functioning in athletes. To better identify the adaptive neuronal changes driven by inhibition, much more work is needed.

FUTURE DIRECTIONS FOR MONITORING THE NEUROMUSCULAR SYSTEM

As EEG and EMG systems continue to advance, athletes will have more effective tools at their disposal to monitor and even change the functioning of their neuromuscular systems in a real-time, sport-specific, integrated, and practical manner.

Future Directions for Electroencephalography

Currently, the usefulness of EEG for sport analysis is primarily limited by the following:

- Concerns about the spatial and temporal accuracy of signal recording arising from volume conduction and artifact contamination
- Variation in the literature results created by varying choice of study parameters and analysis methods
- Up-front cost of buying a traditional EEG system and specialized knowledge needed to record, analyze, and interpret data

Fortunately, with every year these limitations are lessened in degree by these developments:

- Better methods of correcting volume conduction and artifact contamination are being developed.
- Other brain-imaging technologies continue to get less expensive and better understood, allowing researchers to cross-reference the results from a battery of tools to obtain more accurate assessments of the performance of the brain (i.e., EEG, fNIRS, fMRI).
- More studies continue to be conducted, corroborating or undermining the claims of previous work and investigating whether the results of studies conducted with athletes in a single sport apply to other sports.
- New consumer products like the Muse headband are developed with integrated, easy-to-use EEG systems.

Despite the limitations of EEG, many elite athletes are already using EEG to conduct **neurofeedback training** to try to change their patterns of brainwaves to be more optimal for performance (see chapter 27 for more information about neurofeedback). However, in the future, **brain–computer interfaces** (BCIs) are likely to take performance technology one step further. Brain–computer interfaces collect and process data on signals from the CNS in real time and use this data to alter (enhance, restore, or direct) an action of the CNS. Brain–computer interfaces that collect EEG data tend to direct CNS output based on observed **event-related potentials** (ERPs), time-locked measured brain responses to specific stimuli. Brain–computer interfaces that use ERPs are already used for clinical applications such as allowing individuals with movement impairments to direct actions like typing by recording their brainwaves. This means that in the future, athletes could use BCIs consisting of a smartphone and a mobile EEG system to direct or enhance their sport performance using their brain rhythms.

Future Directions for Electromyography

Modern **textile EMG electrodes** embedded in athletic clothing can provide a practical alternative to traditional surface EMG, facilitating the collection of muscle excitation information in externally valid, field-based environments such as normal sport training facilities rather than scientific laboratories (11). Portable, cloud-based EMG technologies can provide unique new opportunities for the rapid processing and assessment of information about muscular activity, allowing coaches and athletes to practically apply this information to optimize management of the training process.

CONCLUSION

While technologies for monitoring and enhancing the performance of the neuromuscular system are still primarily used by specialists in lab settings, with each passing year these tools are rapidly being improved and adapted for use by the average athlete. These improvements include advances in the monitoring systems themselves (processing speed, reduction in size, increase in mobility, shift from local to cloud technology, etc.), advances in the research supporting applications for the systems, and the dramatic enhancement of predictive analytics supporting more athlete-specific individualization (i.e., helping athletes understand exactly how they should train for their specific sport). The result is that athletes have better tools at their disposal for monitoring the functioning of their neuromuscular system in a real-time manner with immediate, individualized physiological feedback.

However, many of these tools are still used individually rather than combined into an **integrated systemic approach** capable of monitoring all of an athlete's physiological systems in various functional states. In the next 10 years, it is imaginable that a battery of performance-monitoring tools (e.g., video analysis, EEG, ENMG, force sensors, etc.) could be combined into a single system to provide a comprehensive assessment of the degree of an athlete's adaptation for performance (see figure 15.14). This system would serve as an NCI—neuromuscular computer interface—allowing for data to be collected from various

types of CNS sensors with simultaneous, real-time recording and analysis to enhance an athlete's sport-specific preparation, performance, and recovery. Not only will the systems for monitoring and modulating athletes change, but so too will the environments that athletes train in.

As virtual and augmented reality technology advance, sport specialists, neuroscientists, and programmers can work together to create adaptive and realistic training environments for athletes. The input and output of the NCIs of the future could adapt the content of this virtual and augmented reality sport environment to provide an athlete with a completely customized training program for total optimization of that athlete's neuromuscular system.

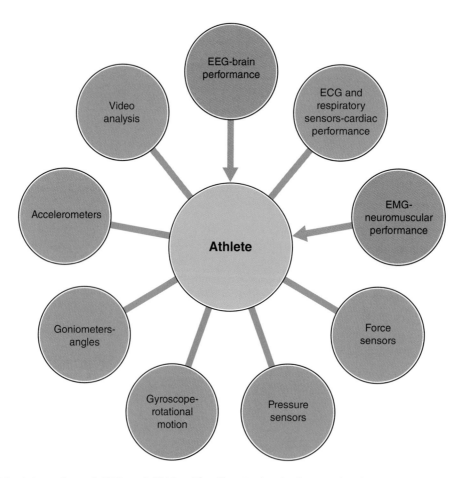

FIGURE 15.14 Integration of EEG and EMG with other technologies to simultaneously monitor an athlete's organism as a whole.

RECOMMENDED READINGS

Cohen, M. *Analyzing Neural Time Series Data: Theory and Practice*. Cambridge, MA: MIT Press, 2014.

Journal of Electromyography and Kinesiology, www.elsevier.com/locate/jelekin.

Kamen, G, and Gabriel, DA. *Essentials of Electromyography*. Champaign, IL: Human Kinetics, 2010.

Merletti, R, and Farina, D. *Surface Electromyography: Physiology, Engineering, and Applications*. Hoboken, NJ: John Wiley & Sons, 2016.

Schomer, DL, and Da Silva, FL. *Niedermeyer's Electroencephalography: Basic Principles, Clinical Applications, and Related Fields*. Philadelphia: Lippincott Williams & Wilkins, 2012.

CHAPTER 16

Biomarkers for Health and Performance

Xavier Schelling i del Alcázar, PhD

Julio Calleja-González, PhD

Nicolás Terrados, MD, PhD

The ability to accurately quantify the physiological state of the athlete or the impact of a training program on the body is crucial for understanding recovery needs and for allowing adequate rest before a second bout of exercise. This is an essential consideration that can allow sport scientists to develop more individualized programs, limiting the potential for health-related issues while maximizing the intensity of the workout to achieve meaningful performance improvements. This chapter reviews the primary considerations and principles of biomarker monitoring in sport and focuses on its application for the assessment of athlete health and performance.

INTERNAL REGULATION AND FEEDBACK SYSTEMS

In order to preserve life, all organisms require the ability to adapt to disturbances and stressors from the outside environment (25). In 1878, Claude Bernard pointed to "the fixity of the internal environment" as the condition of free and independent life (9). Later, in 1929, Walter B. Cannon developed the concept of internal regulation and coined the term **homeostasis**, which included the principle of dynamic stability (22).

The term homeostasis has undergone significant revision, with contemporary models differing significantly from the original formulation (homeokinesis [45], homeodynamics [36], and allostasis [80]). For the purpose of this section, homeostasis implies a dynamic process, not a steady state, whereby an organism attempts to maintain physiological stability through changing parameters of its internal milieu by matching them appropriately to environmental and contextual demands (60).

The biggest contribution to understanding the concept of internal regulation came from understanding how a **feedback loop** works (74). Feedback is defined as the information gained about a reaction to a product, which will allow the modification of the product. Therefore, feedback loops are the process whereby a change to the system results in an alarm that will then trigger a certain result. This result will either increase the change to the system (positive feedback) or reduce it (negative feedback) to bring the system back to dynamic stability (60). The magnitude of change of a variable relative to its baseline, and the recovery rate to such baseline, is known as the system's "gain" and its "gain time," respectively (81). The larger the gain and the gain time, the more efficient the physiological functions and signaling processes are (51). Biomarker monitoring consists of tracking these changes in the athlete's body over time, including both normative processes and pathogenic states (7), by analyzing the behavior of biological indicators such as measurable molecules in blood, urine, saliva, or any other human body sources (63).

The Complexity of Biological Systems

A hallmark of biological systems is their extraordinary complexity. The behavior of such systems is distinct from the behavior of their vast number of components (37), which interact with each other (directly and indirectly) to modulate the system's function (see figure 16.1; 43). A reductionist view involves reducing systems to their parts in an attempt to understand them (58). Biological systems, including the human body, often lack mechanical periodicity or linear dynamics and thus are referred to as **nonlinear systems** (66). Within nonlinear systems, output is often not proportional to input, and output for a given input value may not be constant over time (44). Exercise physiology itself contains innumerable nonproportionate phenomena, such as the all-or-none law in nerve cells and muscle fibers, or the ventilatory and lactate thresholds (thresholds are hallmarks of nonlinear dynamics) (44). In contrast to linear systems, breaking a nonlinear system down into its components and analyzing those parts under controlled conditions may not accurately reflect the complex behavior present nor capture the operating dynamic relationships (43). When implementing biomarker monitoring systems, the sport scientist must continuously consider the integrative, dynamic, and sometimes nonlinear nature of physiological processes (51).

The Athlete's Adaptation to the Environment

Understanding the athlete's adaptation (e.g., performance level or health status) to the environment (e.g., weather, training, nutrition, or sleep), can be conceptually seen as the relationship between environment (e.g., training) and outcome (e.g., performance) (88), but this in many cases is a rather complex and uncertain link, or what is called a **black box**. One might know some (or many) of the inputs in the box (e.g., training variables) and the outcome from the box (e.g., improved 20-m sprint time), but one cannot be completely certain (yet) of which specific physiological processes caused the improvement in performance (88). The reason is that several organ systems and their control mechanisms are involved in such adaptation (88), including different intracellular mechanisms that link the cellular function with the activity of the cellular genetic apparatus (55). For example, intensive cellular activity (e.g., due to a repeated sprint training session) increases the synthesis of proteins specially related to the functional manifestation. The synthesized proteins will be used as building material for renewing and increasing protein structures, or as enzyme proteins that catalyze the metabolic pathways that make the functional activity possible (e.g., anaerobic metabolic pathways) (88). As a result, the involved cellular structures enlarge, and the enzyme activities

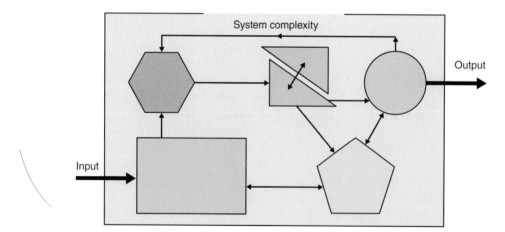

FIGURE 16.1 A system is composed of elements or parts (hexagon, pentagon, rectangle, triangles, and circle) that manifest their own behavior and can interact with each other (arrows). In addition, positive and negative feedback loops may be present among elements (circle output feeds back to the hexagon). The interaction and modulation of these elements under diverse conditions and at different times result in a dynamic system, which can respond to the input at a particular time under particular conditions with a specific output.

Adapted by permission from J.P. Higgins (2002, pg. 247-260).

are enhanced. Thus, the synthesis of these proteins ensures an adaptive effect (e.g., improved repeated sprint performance), and this process is known as **adaptive protein synthesis** (88).

The regulation of protein synthesis at all levels is accomplished via metabolites, hormones, and the nervous system (88). **Metabolic control** is the tool for adjusting metabolic processes in various tissues to sustain the requirements of the human body. The main principle of metabolic control is that the substrate/product ratio determines the activity of enzymes catalyzing the conversion of substrate into product (88). Hence, monitoring either a specific protein synthesis response (structures or enzymes), the level of a targeted metabolite (substrate or product), or a hormone as a proxy for the athlete's status and adaptation is the fundamental principle of biomarker monitoring, and is a way to unveil the processes involved in the athlete's adaptation black box.

BIOMARKERS IN SPORT

In a sporting context, **biomarkers** are often used to evaluate the impact of exercise on different biologic systems, organs, and tissues (63). Sport scientists can analyze metabolites and substrates found within the body to assess the main three areas relating to internal load monitoring in sport: fitness-related adaptations,

fatigue and recovery status, and health. Furthermore, to correctly interpret the biomarkers, sport scientists also have to account for the modulators that affect them (i.e., the environment and the athlete's cognitive and physical elements). Another consideration is the temporal factor inherent to any physiological response, which may be classified as acute (physiological response during exercise and immediately after it is finished), delayed (from 24-hour postexercise to a couple of days later), and chronic (which accounts for the physiological state lasting from several weeks to months) (26) (see figure 16.2).

Monitoring the acute effect of exercise on an athlete, or the associated fitness adaptations, is important to determine whether the athlete is properly responding to the training program, and whether the physiological adaptations are efficiently evolving toward the requirements of the sport (16). The magnitude of an acute physiological response is generally related to the stress level. Hence, the magnitude of the acute responses to a standard exercise bout is usually taken as a measure of the capacity of an individual to respond to physical stress (fitness). Examples of acute exercise responses include increased heart rate, pulmonary ventilation, sweating, core body temperature, catecholamine secretion and decreased vagal activity, gastrointestinal motility, and splanchnic perfusion (26). Over time, with proper adaptation to training,

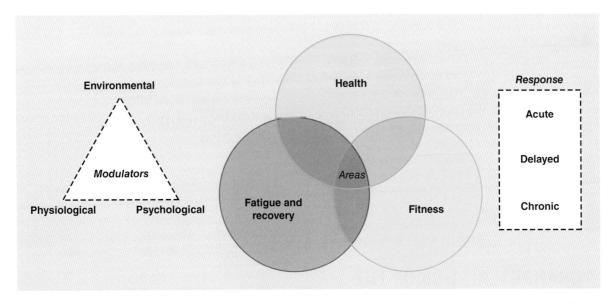

FIGURE 16.2 The three main areas of physiological monitoring in sport (health, fatigue and recovery, and fitness), the main modulators (environmental, physiological, and psychological), and the timing of the internal response (acute, delayed, or chronic). The three areas are interrelated, but the biomarker selection, the sampling protocol (frequency and timing), and the interpretation might be different based on the area, the temporal factor of the internal response, and the influence of each modulator.

physiological adaptations will allow for an increased capacity to exercise with less severe acute responses to the same absolute workload, for the same or better performance (26).

On the other hand, fatigue or the lack of recovery is a disabling symptom in which physical and cognitive functions are limited by interactions between performance fatigability and perceived fatigability (27). Monitoring fatigue and recovery status should allow for personalized training periodization (20), and can entail periods of short-term performance decrements that will eventually lead to an improvement in performance after recovery (functional overreaching), as well as help minimize or avoid long periods of performance stagnation (nonfunctional overreaching or overtraining) (40, 49, 56). Due to the inherent complexity of fatigue, there has been controversy in the literature regarding which parameters are most relevant for its monitoring (39, 63, 85), and no definitive marker has been identified (39, 85). As a consequence, the analysis of a combination of biomarkers has been suggested as the best practice for evaluating an athlete's fatigue and recovery state (19, 33, 48, 54, 63, 78).

Finally, comprehensive health monitoring can include a host of assessments, including hematology, immunology, inflammation level, oxidative stress, neuroendocrinology, liver and kidney function, gut microbiota composition, tendon parameters, cartilage, and bone parameters, and also nutritional needs, hydration status, or genetics. This area aims to identify contraindications for injury or illness and prevent the athlete from reaching pathogenic states, or, in case the pathology is already present, to know how to better intervene in each case based on the athlete's characteristics, individual response, and the environment (see also individualized medicine, personalized medicine, precision medicine [35]).

Unfortunately, research in these areas of sport science is relatively limited when compared to work in the general population, and much of what is known about monitoring internal response (especially as a fatigue and recovery indicator) comes from personal experience and anecdotal information, since many of these data remain protected and unpublished (39).

CHARACTERISTICS OF THE BIOMARKERS

A biomarker, as with any other type of data, in isolation does not translate into actionable information. Efficient and meaningful biomarker monitoring

requires proper contextualization, which is defined by specific principles, assumptions, and procedures.

Biomarker Monitoring Principles

Biomarker monitoring is performed for the purpose of evaluating the physiological responses to training and competition and to increase the effectiveness and efficiency of training and competition interventions. With respect to the use of biomarkers for monitoring purposes, consideration must be given to a variety of fundamental principles:

1. Information acquired must provide significantly greater insights than information obtained with the aid of simpler and less expensive monitoring tools.
2. Biomarker monitoring must be performed in the least invasive and disruptive manner possible.
3. Athletes should have access to their own biometric data when desired.
4. The obtained biomarkers must provide reliable, accurate, and valid information relative to the area or system being monitored.
5. Interpretation of results must consider the minimal clinically important difference to identify true sensitivity in athlete status.
6. Oversimplification of a physiological process may sometimes inaccurately reflect its complex behavior and hinder capturing the operating dynamic relationships, leading to faulty decisions based on such interpretation.
7. The information obtained should be understandable to key stakeholders and decision makers (coaches, medical and athletic performance staff, and the like), and when requested by the athletes themselves.
8. Biomarker monitoring is based on recording an athlete's responses throughout different stages of training and competition (e.g., off-season, preseason, regular season, playoffs, championships), and under the influence of the main elements of sport activities (training session, competition, traveling, and such).
9. Biomarker monitoring is a very specific process, depending on the sport event, the athlete's performance level, the athlete's characteristics (i.e., age, sex, body composition, or race), and the available resources (i.e., time, budget, or technology). Therefore, the selected biomarkers must effectively account for all these contextual factors.

Biomarker Assumptions and Conceptual Framework

The use of biomarkers in the analysis and monitoring of athlete health, well-being, and performance can be hugely beneficial and a means to gain valuable insights as to the body's ability to report to training interventions and competition. However, biological factors and biomarkers can be influenced by a host of physiological, psychological, and environmental conditions. Consequently, certain considerations are warranted when one is adopting such an approach, including the following:

1. Sport performance is influenced and limited by interactions between physiological and psychological factors. It may be modulated by challenges to homeostasis, alterations in neuromuscular function and in the capacity to provide an adequate activation signal to the involved muscles, and even disturbances in the psychological state.

2. Physiological adaptations (cellular, hormonal, and nervous) constitute the background for improved sport-specific performance.

3. Monitoring any physiological adaptations may have significance for determining the effectiveness of a training intervention.

4. Training periodization and programming may be evaluated using the physiological and functional changes determined from biomarkers.

5. Erroneous training management, producing undesired physiological adaptation or a hazardous drop in adaptability and body resources, may be detected with the aid of metabolic and hormonal analysis.

Biomarker Monitoring Procedures

When choosing the physiological source or specimen to analyze using biomarkers, it is important to consider the relevance of the biomarker according to the monitoring goal. For example, when investigating muscle metabolism, the value of the information obtained from each source decreases in the following order: (a) tissue biopsy, (b) arteriovenous difference, (c) venous blood, (d) capillary blood, (e) urine and saliva, (f) sweat. For direct information, biopsy collection is necessary (88). In addition, correct diagnostic and programming decisions rely on the accuracy and reliability of test results. Adequate athlete preparation, specimen collection, and specimen handling

are essential prerequisites for accurate test results. Indeed, the accuracy of test results is dependent on the integrity of specimens.

In all settings in which specimens are collected and prepared for testing, certified staff should follow current recommended sterile techniques, including precautions regarding the use of needles and other sterile equipment, as well as guidelines for the responsible disposal of all biological material (50).

Before the specimen collection, sport scientists should review the appropriate test description, including the specimen type, the required volume, a standardized procedure, the necessary equipment for collection, athlete preparation and instructions, and the storage and handling guidelines. Careful attention to routine procedures can eliminate most of the potential problems related to specimen collection. Some of the most common considerations regarding all types of specimen and biomarker collections are these (50):

- Provide the athlete, in advance, with appropriate collection instructions and information on fasting, diet, and medication restrictions when indicated.

- Examine specimen collection and transportation supplies before the collection time.

- Label the specimen correctly and provide all the required athlete information.

- Submit a quantity of specimen sufficient to perform the assay or analysis.

- Carefully tighten specimen container lids to avoid leakage and potential contamination.

- Maintain the specimen at the temperature indicated by the test requirements. When collecting specimens outdoors, a cooler with dry ice will help provide a moderate temperature until specimens are taken to the lab for processing.

According to the purpose of biomarker monitoring, there can be two main specimen collection procedures: to assess the athlete's basal state or to understand the athlete's response to specific interventions at specified times, as follows:

- *Basal state:* In general, specimens for determining the concentration of body constituents should be collected when the athlete is in a basal state (i.e., in the early morning after awakening, about 12 hours after the last ingestion of food, and without strenuous exercise having been performed in the last 24 hours). Reference intervals are most frequently based on specimens from this collection period.

- *Timed specimens:* There are two types of timed specimens. One is for a single specimen to be collected at a specific time (e.g., postprandial glucose); the other is for a test that may require multiple specimens to be collected at specific times (e.g., to test the effect of a certain intervention).

A complete testing cycle involves the following (41, 59):

1. Specimen collection (with different degrees of invasiveness)
2. Identification
3. Transportation (when the specimen is not analyzed on-site)
4. Preparation
5. Analysis
6. Reporting
7. Interpretation
8. Action

The identification of these steps and their implications may help to optimize the testing process, as well as rejection or acceptance based on procedures and time requirements (see figure 16.3). Finding the appropriate analytical quality and minimizing staff and athlete burden are critical for a successful implementation.

KEY METRICS FOR RELEVANT BIOMARKERS

An exhaustive review of the literature on every reported biomarker is beyond the scope of this chapter; therefore three summary tables present some of the most relevant biomarkers, clustered by different monitoring goals, as well as a brief description of the most often reported biomarkers in sport for each area of interest included in this section.

When considering the use of biomarkers, one must respect that the number of potential biomarkers in sport and medicine grows continuously due to technological and scientific advancement. Moreover, as discussed throughout this chapter, the interactive and systemic nature of any physiological process implies that several biomarkers are involved in more than one process and may behave in a nonlinear manner. Consequently, constant updates on available biomarkers and an integrative view of the athlete's internal response comprise the best practice for biomarker selection.

Biomarkers have been grouped as indicators of muscle status (muscle adenosine triphosphate [ATP] metabolism, muscle damage, and endocrine response), immune system and inflammation, oxidative stress, nutrition and hydration, and others (liver metabolism; kidney parameters; hormonal profile; tendon, cartilage, and bone parameters; autonomic nervous system and neuroendocrine parameters; and genetics).

Muscle Status

Muscle status refers to the fatigue and recovery state of the muscle, and its assessment should focus on specific aspects (see table 16.1): metabolic homeostasis (e.g., anabolic-catabolic balance, protein and amino acid deficiencies, substrate availability), muscle damage, endocrine regulation of muscle repair, adaptations, and excitability (52). The latter aspect is not a topic of discussion for this chapter.

Muscle Metabolism

The ability of an athlete to perform physical work is intrinsically linked to the metabolic pathways sustaining ATP requirements for the given muscular performance (83). During moderate to severe dynamic exercise, **ammonia** production and branched-chain amino acid (BCAA) oxidation rise, showing an exponential relationship with aerobic power (72). Ammonia is produced from the deamination of amino acids in the liver, muscle, and the kidneys; and an elevated level in blood has been suggested to be

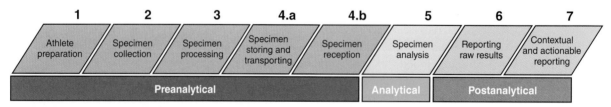

FIGURE 16.3 Description of the different phases involved in biomarker monitoring: preanalytical (collection to preparation), analytical (analysis), and postanalytical (reporting to action).

TABLE 16.1   Muscle Status, Inflammation, Immune System, and Oxidative Stress Biomarkers

Group criteria	Subgroup	Biomarker
Muscle status	Muscle metabolism	Lactate Ammonia Inorganic phosphate Oxipurines (hypoxanthine, xanthine) Free amino acids (tryptophan, glutamine, glutamate) Branch-chained amino acids (leucine)
	Muscle damage	Myoglobin Creatine kinase Enolase Myosin heavy chains Aldolase Lactate dehydrogenase Aspartate aminotransferase Alanine aminotransferase 3-Methylhistidine Blood urea nitrogen Myocardial markers (N-terminal proB-type natriuretic peptide, troponins cTnT, cTnI)
	Endocrine response	Testosterone Free testosterone Dehydroepiandrosterone Interleukin-like growth factor 1 Sex-hormone binding globulin (SHBG) Luteinizing hormone Cortisol Growth hormone Free testosterone-to-cortisol ratio
Inflammation		Blood differential Complete blood count Leukocytes C-reactive protein Tumor necrosis factor Interleukin-6 Interleukin-1 Interleukin-1β Interleukin-8 Interleukin-10 Interleukin-12p40 Leukemia inhibitory factor Monocyte chemotactic protein-1 Soluble intercellular adhesion molecule-1 Serum platelet granules
Immune system		Secretory immunoglobulin A Cluster of differentiation 3 (CD3) CD4 CD8+ CD4/CD8+ Natural killer Alpha-amylase Lactoferrin Lysozyme

(continued)

TABLE 16.1 Muscle Status, Inflammation, Immune System, and Oxidative Stress Biomarkers *(continued)*

Group criteria	Subgroup	Biomarker
Oxidative stress	Lipid peroxidation	Acid reactive substances Isoprostanes 8-Isoprostane
	Protein peroxidation	Protein carbonyls
	Antioxidant capacity	Glutathion Glutathion peroxidase Catalase Total antioxidant capacity Superoxide dismutase Uric acid
	Balance	Reduced glutathione/glutathione disulphide (GSH/GSSG)

an indicator of an abnormality in ATP and nitrogen homeostasis (5). LA is the product of the anaerobic breakdown of carbohydrates (8). Venous **blood lactate** concentration is a well-known muscle metabolism marker, and its change in blood is broadly used as a training load indicator or for training intensity organization (or both) (see figure 16.4; 2, 38, 53, 57, 73).

During the evaluation of exercise intensity when muscles are primarily using mitochondrial fat oxidation (which has been reported to occur at an intensity between 47% and 75% of $\dot{V}O_2$max, varying between trained and untrained individuals), LA values do not change; but as soon as muscles start using extramitochondrial pathways (i.e., glycolysis), venous blood lactate concentration increases. Figure 16.4 shows LA values from a top-level athlete, with very low LA and respiratory quotient (RQ) values indicating mitochondrial fat oxidation. A change to higher LA and RQ values reflects an increase of the glycolysis. Moreover, analysis of LA is used in clinical exercise testing for exercise programming (exercise using lipolysis or glycolysis) and assessments of the effects of therapy and physical training (38).

Muscle Damage

Muscle fatigue is not always accompanied by muscle damage; therefore it has been recommended that different biomarkers be used for each condition (17, 65). Damage to the extracellular matrix (e.g., due to contusions or eccentric contractions) may increase permeability of the sarcolemmal membrane, increasing the efflux of certain products such as creatine kinase and myoglobin (17). **Myoglobin** concentration in blood can vary widely in both pathological and physi-

ological conditions, but it has been extensively used as an indicator of exercise-induced muscle damage (82)—although muscle cell apoptosis may also be triggered by increased oxidative stress (65). **Creatine kinase** (CK) is an enzyme found in the heart, brain, skeletal muscle, and other tissues. Strenuous exercise, contusions, muscle inflammation, myopathies such as muscular dystrophy, and rhabdomyolysis significantly increase blood CK (65). This sensitivity is well established and makes CK, and its isoform 3, a popular blood-borne marker of muscle strain in sport (17).

Endocrine Response

Proper hormonal signaling is essential for the expected physiological adaptations to training and competition. **Testosterone** promotes protein synthesis, red blood cell production, glycogen replenishment, and a reduction in protein breakdown. Conversely, **cortisol**, besides its beneficial acute effects on substrate availability or protein turnover, works antagonistically to testosterone, inhibiting protein synthesis by interfering with the binding of testosterone to its androgen receptor and by blocking anabolic signaling through testosterone-independent mechanisms. When chronically elevated, cortisol is catabolic and immunosuppressive (52). Consequently, the **free testosterone-to-cortisol ratio** (FTCR) has been widely used for studying and preventing overtraining in different sports (see figure 16.5; 75). The use of FTCR for flagging overtraining was originally based on two criteria: an absolute value lower than 0.35×10^{-3}, or a decrease of the ratio of 30% or more in comparison to the previous value (4, 28, 75). **Insulin like growth factor 1** (IGF-1) is a messenger produced in the liver

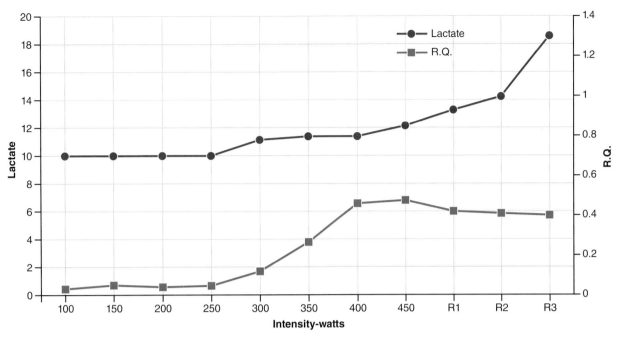

FIGURE 16.4   Blood lactate concentration and respiratory quotient during an incremental test (unpublished data from authors' laboratory).

that transmits the effects of human growth hormone to peripheral tissues and mimics the pro-anabolic and blood glucose–lowering effects of insulin. A decrease in IGF-1 accompanied by an increase in the respective binding protein (IGF-BP3) has been proposed to indicate a state of glucose austerity after depletion of carbohydrate stores due to endurance training (79).

Immune System and Inflammation

The hypothesis of a U-shaped relationship between physical activity and resilience to disease suggests that although regular moderate doses of physical activity have beneficial effects on health, excessive amounts or intensities of physical activity have negative consequences (90). The types of immunological assessments most commonly reported, especially in human exercise studies, involve analyses of blood-borne circulating immune proteins (e.g., interleukin-6, interleukin-1β, C-reactive protein, interleukin-8, tumor necrosis factor alpha), circulating blood leukocytes (e.g., CD4+ T cells, CD8+ T cells, B cells, neutrophils, monocytes), and salivary and plasma antibody or immunoglobulin (Ig) concentrations (90). **Interleukin-6** (IL-6) belongs to a group of cytokines that act as both pro-inflammatory (monocytes, mac-

rophages) and anti-inflammatory (myocytes) cytokines (33). Interleukin-6 is usually determined in the serum and is probably the most frequently studied cytokine (18). Interleukin-6 has been reported to be influenced by exercise training and is thought to be an important mediator of the acute response to exercise (18, 79). Its increase is related to exercise duration, intensity, the muscles engaged in mechanical work, and endurance capacity (33). **Tumor necrosis factor alpha** (TNFα) is a pro-inflammatory cytokine that is predominantly produced by macrophages and able to induce apoptosis, inflammation, cell proliferation, and cell differentiation. It is a part of the cytokine system, which modulates organo-neogenesis (18), including muscle regeneration and recovery (65). The production of **immunoglobulin A** (IgA), specifically secretory IgA (SIgA), is the major effector function of the mucosal immune system; SIgA together with innate mucosal defenses such as **α-amylase, lactoferrin**, and **lysozyme** provides the first line of defense against pathogens present at mucosal surfaces. Acute bouts of moderate exercise have little impact on mucosal immunity, but very prolonged exercise and periods of intensified training can result in decreased saliva secretion of SIgA (90). Nevertheless, careful interpretation of immune system and inflammatory response biomarkers is required, because not all changes in these parameters translate to tissue inflammation

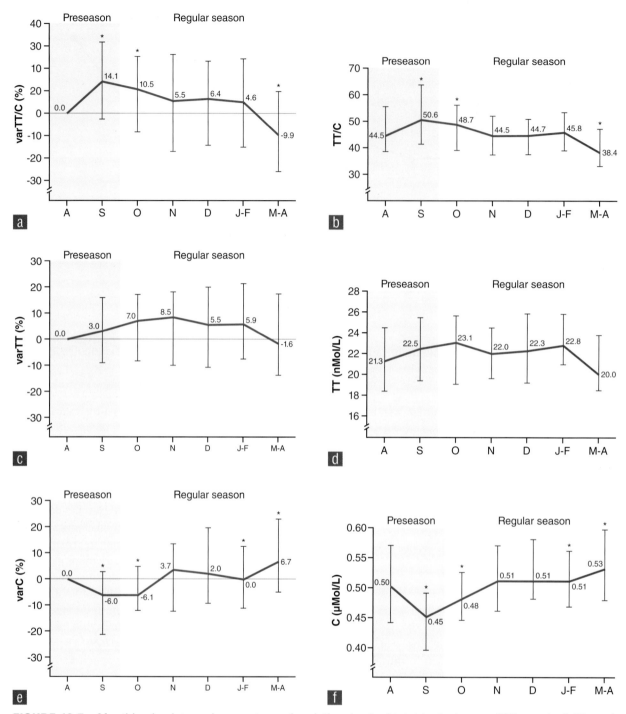

FIGURE 16.5 Monthly absolute and percentage of variation (var) of total testosterone (TT), cortisol (C), and testosterone-to-cortisol ratio (TT/C) throughout the season. Pooled data from four consecutive seasons in professional Spanish basketball players. Values are shown as median (red line) and interquartile range (vertical intervals).

*Significant differences (p-value, Cliff's Δ or Cohen's d, Δ or d interpretation): *(a)* S versus M-A (0.000, 0.40$^\Delta$, moderate), O versus M-A (0.001, 0.36$^\Delta$, moderate); *(b)* S versus M-A (0.000, 0.66^d, moderate), O versus M-A (0.001, 0.19^d, small); *(e)* S versus J-F (0.002, 0.30$^\Delta$, small), S versus M-A (0.000, 0.40$^\Delta$, moderate), O versus M-A (0.001, 0.34$^\Delta$, moderate); *(f)* S versus J-F (0.002, 0.42$^\Delta$, moderate), S versus M-A (0.000, 0.15$^\Delta$, small), O versus M-A (0.001, 0.38$^\Delta$, moderate).

A = August; S = September; N = November; D = December; J-F = January-February; M-A = March-April.

Reprinted by permission from X. Schelling, J. Calleja-Gonzalez, L. Torres-Ronda, and N. Terrados (2015, pg. 373).

and immune suppression resulting in a higher risk of infections (90). Instead, it has been suggested that a reduction in the volume and function of lymphocytes (and other immune cells) in peripheral blood might represent a heightened state of immune surveillance and immune regulation driven by a preferential mobilization of cells to peripheral tissues (21). Likewise, the acute elevations in IL-6 and IL1-β found after exercise may be more important for the metabolic, rather than the immunological, responses to exercise (90). Consequently, individualized longitudinal measurements, comprehensive immunity and inflammation biomarker panels, and an integrative analysis that also considers other factors involved in immune suppression must also be employed.

Oxidative Stress

Free radicals (FR) are reactive compounds that are naturally produced in the human body. They can exert positive effects (e.g., on the immune system) or negative effects (e.g., lipids, proteins, or DNA oxidation). To limit these harmful effects, an organism requires complex protection provided by the antioxidant system. This system consists of antioxidant enzymes, which include **superoxide dismutase** (SOD), **catalase** (CAT), and **glutathione peroxidase** (GPX), and nonenzymatic antioxidants, including a variety of FR dissipaters such as **vitamin A**, **vitamin C**, **vitamin E**, **flavonoids**, and thiols (including **glutathione** [GSH], **ubiquinone Q10**, **uric acid**, **bilirubin**, **ferritin**). Micronutrients such as **iron**, **copper**, **zinc**, **selenium**, and **manganese** act as enzymatic cofactors. The antioxidant system efficiency depends on nutritional derivatives (vitamins and minerals) and on endogenous antioxidant enzyme production, which can be modified by exercise, training, nutrition, and aging. Moreover, antioxidant system efficiency is important in sport physiology because exercise increases the production of FR (30, 64). But once again, no single measurement of oxidative stress or of antioxidant status is going to be sufficient. Indeed, the interpretation of the values coming from a single marker could be a source of error. Therefore, a battery of measurements, including **total antioxidant capacity** (TAC), isolated antioxidants, and markers of FR-induced damage on lipids, proteins, and DNA, seems to be the best way to assess oxidative stress (31, 70).

Nutritional and Hydration Status

A mismatch between the dietary intake of macronutrients (carbohydrates, proteins, and lipids), micronutrients (vitamins and minerals) and fluid and the needs of training and competition can be a cause of poor performance and ultimately of issues relating to health and well-being (see table 16.2) (61, 84).

Some of the most frequently researched **micronutrients** in sport are **iron** and its metabolic indicators such as ferritin, transferrin, transferrin saturation, total iron binding capacity, and hemoglobin. Iron deficiency, with or without anemia, can impair muscle function and limit work capacity, leading to compromised training adaptation and athletic performance (84). **Vitamin D** regulates calcium and phosphorus absorption and metabolism and plays a key role in maintaining bone health. A growing number of studies have documented the relationship between vitamin D status and injury prevention, rehabilitation, improved neuromuscular function, reduced inflammation, and decreased risk of stress fracture (84). **Calcium** is especially important for growth, maintenance, and repair of bone tissue, regulation of muscle contraction, nerve conduction, and normal blood clotting. The risk of low bone mineral density and stress fractures is increased by low energy availability, and in the case of female athletes, menstrual dysfunction, with low dietary calcium intake contributing further to the risk (84).

As for the assessment of **macronutrient** requirements, research has very well documented the critical role that **carbohydrate** availability plays in exercise capacity. This is emphasized during prolonged moderate- to high-intensity exercise, in which the reliance on endogenous carbohydrate stores becomes increasingly important relative to lower-intensity exercise. Studies in humans clearly demonstrate that fatigue during a prolonged exercise bout coincides with low muscle glycogen content, and the ingestion of carbohydrate is causally related to the maintenance of performance in humans via the attenuation of glycogenolysis, the maintenance of euglycemia or carbohydrate oxidation, or both (1). Metabolism biomarkers such as blood **glucose** or **hemoglobin A1c** levels, an indicator of the average amount of glucose in the blood over the last 1 to 3 months, have been extensively used to assess the basal or timed mobilization and availability of

TABLE 16.2 Nutritional and Hydration Status Subgroup Biomarkers

Subgroup	Biomarker
Micronutrient metabolism	Vitamin D (25-hydroxycolecalciferol)
	Vitamin K (group)
	Vitamin E
	Vitamin B (group)
	Calcium
	Phosphate
	Magnesium
	Sodium
	Potassium
	Zinc
	Chromium
	Manganese
	Iron profile (iron II+III, ferritin, transferrin, transferrin saturation, total iron binding capacity, hemoglobin)
Macronutrient metabolism	Glucose
	Hemoglobin A1c
	Triglycerides
	Free fatty acids
	Cholesterol
	Lipids
	Omega-6:omega-3 ratio
	Total protein
	Albumin
	Globulin
	Blood urea nitrogen
	Free amino acids
	Branched-chain amino acids (leucine)
Hydration status	Blood urea nitrogen (BUN)/creatinine$_{blood}$
	Arginine vasopressin
	Copeptin
	Urine specific gravity
	Osmolality
Food absorption and allergies	Immunoglobulin E
	Gut microbiota

carbohydrates (23). Dietary **protein** interacts with exercise, providing both a trigger and a substrate for the synthesis of contractile and metabolic proteins, as well as enhancing structural changes in non-muscle tissues such as tendons and bones. Proteins also play a central role in biological processes such as catalysis, transportation, immunology, and messaging (84). Nitrogen balance markers, which reflect protein breakdown, for determining protein intake effect or as a proxy for exercise strain include plasma **ammonia**, **urea**, and **creatinine** (71). Additionally, **leucine** is likely the most influential amino acid with regard to skeletal muscle protein synthesis. Leucine directly and indirectly stimulates the mammalian target of rapamycin (mTOR), a key regulator of translation within the cell (34). Its potential ergogenic effect on athlete performance justifies the increased attention in sport to ensure the optimal availability of this amino acid. **Lipids** are a necessary component of a healthy diet, providing energy, essential elements of cell membranes, and facilitation of the absorption of lipid-soluble vitamins. Fat, in the form of plasma free fatty acids, intramuscular triglycerides, and adipose tissue, provides a fuel substrate that is both relatively plentiful and increased in availability to the muscle as a result of endurance training (84). Common biomarkers of the lipid profile are **total cholesterol, low-density lipoprotein cholesterol** (LDL), **high-density lipoprotein cholesterol** (HDL), and **triglycerides**. In addition to these, it is not uncommon to also analyze the levels of specific fatty acids such as **omega-3** and **omega-6**, and their balance (**omega-6:omega-3 ratio**). Excessive amounts of omega-6 polyunsaturated fatty acids (PUFA) and a very high omega-6:omega-3 ratio promote inflammation and autoimmune diseases, as well as cardiovascular pathology and cancer, whereas increased levels of omega-3 PUFA (a low omega-6:omega-3 ratio) exert suppressive effects (77).

Being properly **hydrated** contributes to optimal health and exercise performance. In addition to the usual daily water losses from respiration and gastrointestinal and renal sources, athletes also need to replace sweat losses (84). Assuming an athlete is in energy balance, daily hydration status may be estimated by monitoring early morning body mass (measured upon waking and after voiding), or before and after training or competing, since acute changes in bodyweight generally reflect shifts in body water. **Urinary specific gravity** and urine or saliva **osmolality** can also be used as a proxy for hydration status via measuring the concentration of the solutes in these fluids (84).

Other areas of interest in biomarker monitoring (see table 16.3) include gut health parameters (i.e., microbiota), cartilage parameters (e.g., cartilage oligomeric matrix protein), tendon parameters (e.g., hydroxyproline), bone parameters (e.g., osteocalcin, pyridinoline), genes related to sport performance (e.g., alpha-actin 3 protein gene, angiotensin-converting enzyme gene), genes related to tissue regeneration (e.g., myostatin gene), genes related to pathology (e.g., collagen type I alpha 1 gene, collagen type V alpha 1 gene), and gene-expression biomarkers related to adaptation to exercise (microRNA [29]).

ANALYSIS AND INTERPRETATION OF BIOMARKER DATA

In order to provide actionable insights based on the collected biomarkers, a proper analysis and interpretation of the raw data is required. This considers things such as the dynamic nature of biomarker normal values (i.e., dynamic stability), the individual response of athletes to the same stressors (i.e., interathlete variation), and the minimal change required to affect the functionality of a biological system (i.e., minimal clinically important difference).

Reference Values and Interindividual Variation

Reference values for biomarkers, specifically those adapted to athletes, are still lacking (39, 52). Consequently, it is a common practice to use the reagent manufacturer's reference values as a standard, which can be misleading because highly trained athletes can have biomarker levels that would be reported as potentially pathological in the general population (63).

On the other hand, since about the turn of the century it has been reported in several studies, and replicated by different groups, that adaptation to the environment (and to exercise) varies on an individual basis (15), with some subjects exhibiting no meaningful or negative changes postintervention (11, 14, 86). These subjects have been conventionally labeled as nonresponders (15, 86). It has, however, been proposed that this term be replaced by the term "low sensitivity" since there may be no one who is truly a nonresponder to every exercise adaptation (11, 67).

Nevertheless, this heterogeneity has been demonstrated in the responsiveness to regular physical activity also (46). In some cases, the pretraining level of a phenotype has a considerable impact on the individual adaptations (14). Pooled data from different studies suggest that around 10% of subjects demonstrate an adverse response to training, exhibiting an increased disease risk, while 7% of subjects exhibit an adverse response in at least two variables (13). These individual variations have to be accounted for when one is analyzing internal loads or physiological response. Therefore, it is advisable to individualize reference values as much as possible, considering previous observations in the athlete, and controlling all subjects regularly in order to establish their own reference scale (46, 63).

Minimal Clinically Important Difference

Practitioners need to ensure that a given physiological measurement of fitness, fatigue and recovery, or health can be reliably, accurately, and quickly interpreted, considering its validity as a predictor or proxy for the monitored area (3, 85). To do so, the interpretation of a biomarker result must start with knowledge of the

TABLE 16.3 Other Subgroup Biomarkers

Subgroup		Biomarker
Liver parameters		Amino transferases Bilirubin
Kidney parameters		Creatinine Urea Blood urea nitrogen Cystatin C
Hormonal profile		Total testosterone Free testosterone Cortisol Somatomedin Parathyroid hormone Thyroid-stimulating hormone Triiodothyronine Thyroxine
Autonomic nervous system and neuroendocrine parameters		Catecholamines Glucocorticoids Brain-derived neurotrophic factor 5-Hydroxytryptamine interaction
Bone parameters		Bone formation markers (bone alkaline phosphate, osteocalcin, carboxyterminal propeptide of type I procollagen) Bone resorption markers (pyridinoline, deoxypyridinoline, carboxyterminal cross-linked telopeptide of type I procollagen, carboxyterminal cross-linking telopeptide of type I collagen, amino-terminal cross-linking telopeptide of type I collagen)
Cartilage parameters		Cartilage oligomeric matrix protein Sulfate glycosaminoglycans
Tendon parameters		Hydroxyproline Hydroxylysine
Genes	Athletic performance	Alpha-actin 3 protein gene (ACTN-3 577R, 577X) Angiotensin-converting enzyme gene (ACE D and I alleles)
	Tissue regeneration and growth	Insulin-like growth factor 1 gene (IGF-1 rs7136446) Myostatin gene (MSTN or growth and differentiation factor-8, GDF-8) Growth and differentiation factor-5 (GDF-5 rs143383)
	Tendon and ligament pathology	Collagen type I alpha 1 gene (COL1A1 Sp1 TT) Collagen type V alpha 1 gene (COL5A1 rs12722) Matrix metallopeptidase 3 gene (MMP3 rs679620) Tenascin C gene (TNC)
	Gene expression	Micro RNAs

minimum amount of change that is not the result of measurement error (i.e., minimum detectable change or MDC), as well as the minimum amount of change that has been established as practically important (i.e., minimal clinically important difference or MCID) (24).

The magnitude of the selected MCID is critical in order for the process of biomarker monitoring to be useful and informative in the field (85). There are two main approaches for quantifying a MCID: the anchor approach, in which the change in the biomarker is associated with the change in another external variable, the anchor (85); or the statistical approach, in which the MCID can be based, for instance, on the standard error of measurement (SEM) (94) or on the between-subjects standard deviation for the measured biomarker (10). Also, changes in biomarkers have been often interpreted through standardized scales, for example, as a given range of the within- subject or between-subjects standard deviation (see figure 16.6). Different thresholds have been proposed for trivial, small, medium, large, and very large changes (6). For injury or illness analysis, binary or survival outcome metrics such as odds, risk, or hazard ratios can be considered in a similar fashion (85). Nevertheless, the validity and reliability of the chosen method should be periodically reviewed through prognostic-longitudinal type studies (32, 42).

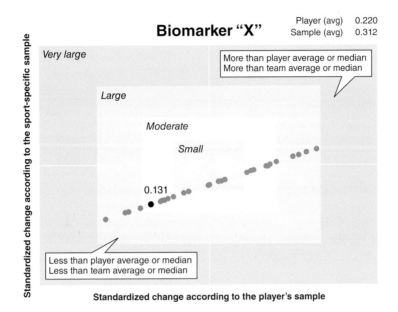

Biomarker panel for a given monitoring goal

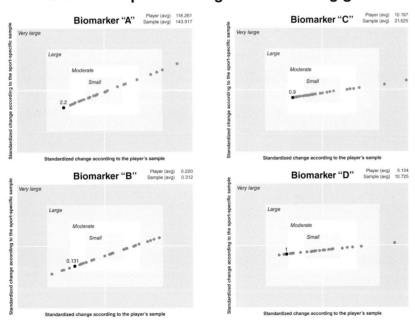

FIGURE 16.6 A practical example of biomarker change visualization.

In order to explore the meaningfulness of a biomarker variation, it is important to properly contextualize it, considering the individual variations and the expected variations within a specific population. Hence, the sport scientist could visualize together the standardized change of a biomarker according to the athlete historical records and to a specific sample (e.g., sport-specific or team records). Figure 16.6 shows an example of such contextual visualization for a Spanish professional basketball player (authors' unpublished data) where the sport scientist can see all the records for a given athlete (gray dots) with the black dot being the last record with the raw value as the label. To build a chart such as this, the sport scientist needs to check for normality in the raw data first, and to transform it when indicated. Then, for each record the sport scientist calculates two standardized values (effect sizes): the athlete's historical records (horizontal axis) and the team's historical records (vertical axis). The resultant quadrant chart will show when a value is meaningfully above or below the norm. The values used to define the effect size thresholds in the charts are small <0.6, moderate 0.6 to 1.2; large >1.2 to 2, and very large >2. As mentioned throughout this chapter, analysis of a combination of biomarkers has been suggested as the best practice to assess any monitoring area (e.g., muscle status, inflammation, immune system, oxidative stress). In this instance, the four smaller quadrant charts in the figure represent a biomarker panel for an integrative interpretation of multiple muscle damage biomarkers (e.g., creatine kinase, myoglobin, aldolase, and lactate dehydrogenase).

In some cases, the nonstationarity and nonlinearity of signals generated by living organisms challenge traditional mechanistic approaches based on conventional linear statistical methodologies (37). Moreover, it has been suggested that it is the dynamics of the physiological processes (systems) rather than their structure (components) that gives the essential information for their functioning (44). Hence, different concepts and techniques from statistical physics, which deals with fields with an inherently stochastic nature, have been applied to a wide range of biomedical problems, from molecular to organismic levels, to try to understand the "hidden information" in physiologic time series (37).

Biomarker Monitoring Laws and Ethics

The exponential increase in the collection of various types of athletes' biometric data in professional sport, including all biomarkers, has led to some concerns regarding biodata ownership, privacy, and security (47, 62). Most (if not all) biomarkers collected by a sporting organization in the United States fall within the parameters of the Health Insurance Portability and Accountability Act of 1996 (HIPAA), according to the definitions relating to health information. Under HIPAA, most of the medical staff employed by professional sport teams would be considered health care providers subject to the privacy and security requirements of HIPAA (62). Similar legal acts for data protection can be found worldwide.

Besides the legal issues around biodata ownership, privacy, and security, there is an increasing concern around genetic testing (93). Consequently, in 2008 the United States passed the Genetic Information Nondiscrimination Act (GINA), which prohibits employers and other covered entities (which include hospitals, physicians, and other caregivers, as well as researchers who have access to health care information) from requesting genetic information on employees (i.e., athletes) or their family members.

On the other hand, from an ethical point of view, the use of genetic testing for talent identification in sport has been heavily questioned. In a review in 2013, Pitsiladis and coauthors concluded, "Current genetic testing has zero predictive power on talent identification and should not be used by sporting organizations, athletes, coaches or parents" (69). Furthermore, in a position statement from the Australian Institute of Sport in 2017, the authors pointed out that the use of genetic phenotypes as an absolute predictor of athletic prowess or sport selection is unscientific and unethical (89). Given the multifactorial nature of human athletic performance, information gained from genetic testing should never be used for inclusion or exclusion in talent identification (89). Hence, careful attention to these types of regulations and ethical considerations must be paid when one is implementing biomarker monitoring.

EVOLUTION OF BIOMARKER DATA

Technology is improving so rapidly in today's world of sport science that thinking forward is limited to a few years as opposed to decades (11). The exponential growth in technology and information since the turn of the century has opened up new ways to understand the body and how people interact with the environment, but it is a recurrent challenge to translate the new and abundant information into actionable knowledge.

The informational revolution has mainly occurred because of the reduction in the size of devices and components, routinely developed using nanotechnology; the increase in data processing speed enabling data reporting in real time; and the reduction of costs allowing the widespread use of technology (87). These factors can have two main implications in biomedicine and exercise physiology specifically in the near future (76):

- An enormous volume of data, the ability to gather information from thousands of people, more frequently throughout the day, and every day, in a noninvasive, nondisruptive way (e.g., smart fabrics, smart watches and phones, breath analyzers, monitoring 24 hours a day, 7 days a week)

- An increase in data quality, the ability to dig deeper in areas such as genomics, transcriptomics, proteomics, or metabolomics, and to synchronize different sources of data (e.g., physiological, physical, psychological, and environmental)

To date, most of the studies on biomarkers and athletic performance and fatigue and recovery have focused on a limited number of variants in small, and often heterogeneous, cohorts, resulting inevitably in spurious and conflicting results (91). Sport science should not be restricted to the current and common practice of focusing on potential biomarkers, typically defined by author preferences or from biases in the published literature, and the reliance on small, statistically underpowered observational studies (12). Sport science in general, and exercise physiology in particular, need to shift to an unbiased exploration of biomarkers using all the power of genomics, epigenomics, transcriptomics, proteomics, and metabolomics and their interaction with the environment (e.g., nutrition, sleep, mood, training workloads) (76), in combination with large observational and experi-

mental study designs with the emphasis firmly on replication (12), and attending to the stochastic and nonlinear mechanisms involved in physiologic control and complex signaling networks (37). Therefore, large, collaborative initiatives, such as those seen in systems biology research centers (92), precision and personalized medicine initiatives (35), or research consortiums (68), can be joined by sporting organizations to share data sets and to take advantage of cutting-edge methodologies for meaningful progress to be made in the area of exercise physiology and sport science (91).

CONCLUSION

A biomarker is a biological indicator, such as a measurable molecule in blood, urine, saliva, or any other human body source, that reflects underlying changes of a physiological process over time. The fundamental principle of biomarker monitoring in sport is assessing specific protein synthesis responses, or the levels of targeted metabolites or hormones as a proxy for the athlete's fitness, fatigue and recovery, or health status. The main areas in biomarker research in sport include muscle status, immune system and inflammation, oxidative stress, nutrition and hydration, tendon, cartilage, and bone parameters, hormonal profile, and genetics. Nevertheless, the inherent complexity of all physiological processes requires a comprehensive biomarker panel for reliably assessing an athlete's state, and includes other aspects such as nutrition, sleep, workloads, or mood state. In addition, a proper biomarker monitoring plan requires the sport scientist to be up-to-date on the newest available biomarkers and techniques, to ensure that the information provided will be greater than the information obtained with the aid of simpler and less expensive monitoring tools. The sport scientist also needs to consider the staff's and athlete's burden due to the specimen collection procedures, and to consider all legal and ethical aspects around biodata ownership, privacy, and security. The next step in sport science is to explore old and new biomarkers using all the power of genomics, epigenomics, transcriptomics, proteomics, and metabolomics, as well as their interaction with the environment (e.g., nutrition, sleep, mood, workloads), in combination with large observational and experimental study designs, attending to the stochastic and nonlinear mechanisms involved in physiological control and complex signaling networks.

RECOMMENDED READINGS

Bouchard, C, Rankinen, T, and Timmons, JA. Genomics and genetics in the biology of adaptation to exercise. *Compr Physiol* 1:1603-1648, 2011.

Higgins, JP. Nonlinear systems in medicine. *Yale J Biol Med* 75:247-260, 2002.

Meeusen, R, Duclos, M, Foster, C, Fry, A, Gleeson, M, Nieman, D, Raglin, J, Rietjens, G, Steinacker, J, and Urhausen, A. Prevention, diagnosis, and treatment of the overtraining syndrome: joint consensus statement of the European College of Sport Science and the American College of Sports Medicine. *Med Sci Sports Exerc* 45:186-205, 2013.

Pitsiladis, Y, Wang, G, Wolfarth, B, Scott, R, Fuku, N, Mikami, E, He, Z, Fiuza-Luces, C, Eynon, N, and Lucia, A. Genomics of elite sporting performance: what little we know and necessary advances. *Br J Sports Med* 47:550-555, 2013.

Viru, A, and Viru, M. *Biochemical Monitoring of Sport Training*. Champaign, IL: Human Kinetics, 2001.

CHAPTER 17

Perception of Effort and Subjective Monitoring

Shaun J. McLaren, PhD

Aaron J. Coutts, PhD

Franco M. Impellizzeri, PhD

Athlete monitoring is considered an important aspect of the training process, which aims to maximize sport performance and health. The underlying concept of the training process is that performance potential can be improved when an athlete's biological systems are overloaded in order to induce adaptive responses. However, stressing the human body's systems has some inherent risk relating to the balance between the stimulus and the recovery necessary to allow positive adaptations (i.e., **training adaptation**). This places importance on both the measurement and the management of the training stimulus—typically referred to as **training load**—and the associated responses (75, 76). Coaches and practitioners (e.g., sport science, strength and conditioning, medical) typically agree on the benefits of this process and its theoretical basis, in that evaluating the effectiveness of a training program, managing the training stimulus, detecting fatigue, tracking changes in performance capacity, programming adequate recovery, and managing injury risk are highlighted as important justifications for **athlete monitoring systems** (4, 147, 150, 163).

Load is a generic term that may assume different meanings based on the context. For example, in mechanics, load is viewed as the physical stress on a mechanical system or component. However, within an athlete monitoring context, training and competition loads commonly imply a psychophysiological load that is the product of frequency, intensity, and volume. It can be divided into internal and external components:

External load is the athlete's performance outputs (e.g., movement and activity counts during a session such as meters run, weight lifted or thrown), and **internal load** is the relative, within-exercise biochemical (physiological and psychological) and biomechanical responses to external load (75, 76, 159). External load is the means by which an internal load is induced, but individual characteristics such as age, physical fitness, and genetics influence this relationship (see figure 17.1; 75).

The response to training and competition loads manifests as changes to the body's cardiorespiratory, metabolic, neuromuscular, musculoskeletal, and endocrine systems. These changes can be both negative and positive—ranging from tissue overload, failure, and overtraining to functional tissue adaptation, respectively (159)—and can last on an acute, chronic, or permanent basis. Whatever the underlying reference theory (e.g., homeostasis and general adaption syndrome [41] or allostasis [83]), exercise-induced biological and mechanical stress are antecedents of any adaptation (160). This means that internal training and competition loads, in combination with the aforementioned individual characteristics, are the primary determinants of the training response (see figure 17.1). More information on the training process can be found in chapter 2.

The quantification of load and subsequent response is challenging. While this is considered an essential component of athlete monitoring, there is no estab-

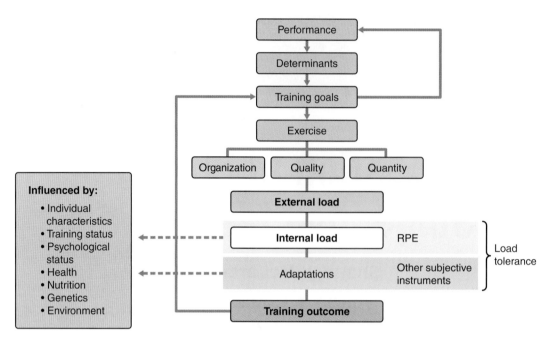

FIGURE 17.1   The training process and the role of subjective monitoring tools.

Adapted by permission from R.M. Impellizzeri, S.M. Marcora, and A.J. Coutts (2019, pg. 270-273).

lished gold standard, and many misconceptions exist (75). Internal load, external load, and the training response are construct terms, meaning that they cannot be directly measured and must instead be quantified by surrogate indicators (proxies). Selecting load and response proxies as part of athlete monitoring systems should be based on theoretical, technical, and contextual considerations. This includes reliability, validity, sensitivity to change, specificity to the sport or athlete demands, the ability to provide immediate feedback, time efficiency, ease of administration, cost-effectiveness, and scalability to large groups of athletes (37, 133, 137, 147, 150).

The selection of load and response proxies should also depend on the information required by the coach to adjust the training plan. For example, the coach may want to use separate measures of volume and intensity for any specific exercise typology (nature of the stimulus), or a global measure combining both (see figure 17.2). The **training impulse** (TRIMP) metric proposed by Banister (7) is an example of an attempt to combine volume (expressed in minutes) and intensity (based on heart rate reserve and adjusted by an exponential coefficient) in a single measure.

Subjective feedback provided by athletes has historically been used to optimize and adapt training. As such, it is not a surprise that the perception of effort (i.e., intensity) and response constructs such

as recovery and fatigue are ranked among the most common tools used by coaches for monitoring training (4, 147, 150, 163). The main difference between the historic use of subjective feedback and advancements since about the turn of the century is that these perceptions were not quantified using numeric tools, but instead were acquired in a qualitative manner. Asking athletes, for example, how they feel in order to better understand if they are coping with training, and to appraise whether volume and intensity are optimum, has long been a common strategy for many coaches. Even when athletes are not directly asked for such feedback, coaches often try to understand athlete training loads and the associated responses by interpreting their physiognomy, body language, and other mannerisms. However, this approximation can entail substantial errors, with coaches typically estimating intensity lower than that experienced by players (27, 85, 95, 161). While the qualitative athlete–coach interaction still—and will always—have value, there are now means to quantify the subjective experiences of athlete training and competition loads, as well as the responses to these loads. When selected and implemented correctly, these psychometric methods can provide standardized, valid, and reliable quantification of the training process.

The aim of this chapter is to provide an overview of perception of effort and its use as an indicator of

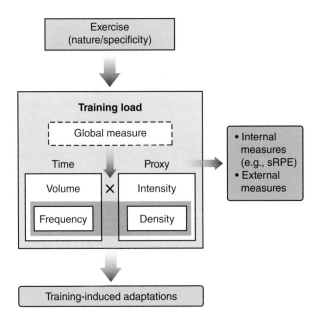

FIGURE 17.2 The construct of training load and its components (specificity, volume, frequency, intensity, and density).

exercise intensity and internal load, as well as to briefly describe and evaluate subjective measures of athlete response that have long been featured as part of monitoring systems. An important aim is to critically appraise the psychometric methods of subjective tools in athlete monitoring, which, in the view of the authors of this chapter, form the foundation for successful application.

MEASUREMENT OF EXERCISE INTENSITY AND INTERNAL LOAD USING PERCEIVED EXERTION

Perception is the elaboration of elementary experiences provided by the sensory system (58, 106). It is the active process of detailing and organizing sensorial information within the brain to give a meaning (15, 106). **Perception of effort** (also called **sense of effort** or **perceived exertion**) has been associated with several definitions, yet the authors of this chapter feel the most appropriate is the "conscious sensation of how hard and strenuous a physical task is" (101). The authors deleted the word "heavy" from this definition (apparent in the original reference, see [101]) because in an athlete monitoring context, it may easily be interpreted as the heaviness of an object being lifted (e.g., resistance training), rather than the actual perceived exertion associated with the task (63).

The terms effort and exertion are often used interchangeably (78, 123), although this is not a consensus view (1). The semantic differentiation between effort and exertion might have relevance from a scientific point of view, but in practice this is not a real concern for athlete monitoring. The reason is that evidence suggests athletes cannot differentiate between the two terms (78). Effort should, however, be clearly differentiated from other exercise-induced perceptual sensations, such as fatigue, pain, discomfort, force, pleasure, and enjoyment. These other feelings are different conceptual constructs with distinct neurophysiological pathways (63) and applications to the training process. However, it is not always intuitive or easy for athletes to disassociate these sensations from effort, because they are often strongly related. A key challenge for those quantifying perceived exertion in athlete monitoring is ensuring that athletes have a good awareness of what effort is, and is not, through an understanding of these other perceptions.

Rating of Perceived Exertion

Perceived exertion depends mainly on how hard or easy it feels to either breathe (e.g., breathlessness, respiration frequency) or contract the working limbs (e.g., muscle strain) during physical tasks (15, 65, 148). Indeed, this feeling grows with the intensity of a stimulus (23) and has been quantitatively linked to markers of respiration, circulation, and physical output during exercise (11, 15, 32, 134). It is therefore a temporal phenomenon that is instantaneous to any given point during athlete training or competition. This has an important role in the self-regulation of behavior (e.g., autoregulation of external load and pacing) and can be quantified using a **rating of perceived exertion** (RPE). Here, a numeric value is assigned to the magnitude of effort perceived at a given time point, ranging from a minimum to a maximum.

The use of RPE within athlete monitoring is usually entirely retrospective, however. That is, RPE are typically provided following training or competition, and are given as a cognitive appraisal or reflection of the effort experienced throughout the session. When athletes recall their RPE for the entire training session or competition, it represents a component of the so-called **session RPE** (sRPE) (54). The terms RPE and sRPE are sometimes used almost interchangeably, but it is important to stress that sRPE is the correct term for a post-hoc appraisal of effort experienced during a period of training or competition, and simply represents an application of RPE.

In theory, sRPE should serve as a measure of internal training and competition intensity, although the effects of exercise duration on sRPE are not yet conclusive. Nonetheless, when multiplied by the volume of exercise (i.e., duration), **sRPE training load (sRPE-TL)** can be quantified to express internal load as a single impulse-type metric. Conceptually, this can be thought of as the area under the curve of an athlete's perception over time (see figure 17.3). The sRPE-TL can be summated for a given cumulative time frame of the athlete's training schedule, such as a day, week, microcycle, or mesocycle. This poses both a limitation and a benefit of sRPE as a load proxy: It does not accurately reflect the structure-specific nature of different exercise modalities, but it can provide a global measure that is useful for understanding how the athlete perceived and tolerated the total load, determined by the combinations of different types of training modalities and competition.

Ratings of perceived exertion are not the perception of effort itself—they are numeric values assigned to the perception. According to Borg and Borg (16, 21), individuals can describe and communicate their perceptual intensities reasonably well using various linguistic terms. Perceptual intensities can also be quantified using numbers, but an additional step is to associate these numbers with qualitative intensity ratings. This process is best achieved by using standardized verbal expressions on a scale. The construction and use of rating scales represents a major development in the measurement of perceived exertion, and the application of these scales to quantify sRPE in athlete monitoring is almost universal. However, this process requires a conscious interpretation and subsequent communication of a perception and therefore has the potential to cause a mismatch between the numeric rating and the actual sensation. Rating perceived exertion with as much validity as possible is therefore

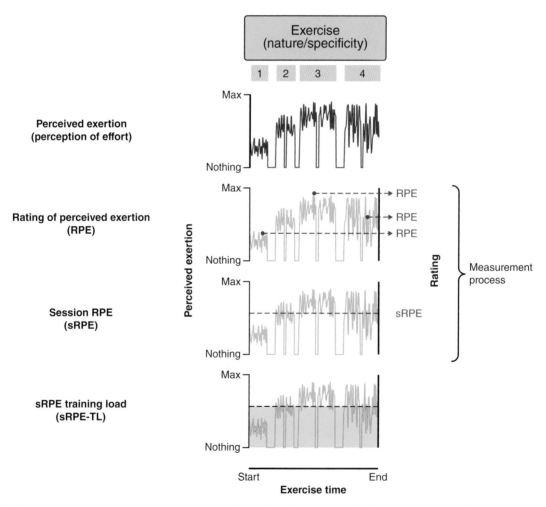

FIGURE 17.3 Conceptual overview of perceived exertion during sport training and competition.

crucial to mitigate error between the actual perception and the quantitative response given by athletes.

Category Scaling

A **category scale** consists of verbal labels assigned to a number on an interval scale. This was the method used for developing Borg's 6-20 RPE scale (12, 14), constructed to give data that increase linearly with stimulus intensity, such as heart rate and oxygen consumption, during an incremental test (15, 32, 64, 134). This is also consistent with Borg's range model (10, 11), which asserts that the subjective intensity ranges from minimal to maximal and is equal between individuals. The RPE scale has advantages as an instrument that is easy to understand and simple to use, providing data that are easy to interpret (23). An issue with this scale, however, is that it does not account for changes in the response that are not proportionate to the stimulus (13). Indeed, the stimulus (S)–response (R) relationship of perceived exertion is best described as nonlinear because the same change in a stimulus (e.g., absolute running speed) causes greater changes in the response (e.g., perceived exertion) at higher intensities. This is known as exponential growth or a **ratio function** (16). A further issue is that the 6-20 RPE scale is a closed scale with a risk of some truncation at the end values (23). This means that the end of the scale is capped, and it is not possible for athletes to give a rating beyond their current or historical perceived maximum.

Category Ratio Scaling

To address limitations of category scaling methods, **category ratio** (CR) scales were developed to combine the properties (and benefits) of category scales with ratio methods. A CR scale therefore includes discrete categories of absolute effort, but the difference between categories is numerically exponential. For example, Borg's CR 10 scale (deciMax; CR10®) has anchored categories of easy (2 arbitrary units [au]), moderate (3 au), and hard (5 au), but the numeric difference between moderate and hard (2 au) is twice that of the difference between easy and moderate (1 au). Consequently, the responses provided are nonlinear ratio data that are consistent with Borg's range model. This means that CR-derived values of RPE (and sRPE) can be used for absolute and relative comparisons of intensity within and between individuals (16, 73). Additional features such as the so-called fixed star

help avoid ceiling effects associated with the RPE 6-20 scale by allowing athletes to assign values higher than maximum in case they should perceive such effort (16, 63). It should be acknowledged that CR scaling does not allow for perfect ratio data, but is a scale that comes close to possessing ratio properties. For this reason, the term semi-ratio is also used (16). Nevertheless, it has been suggested that this is acceptable for treating the data statistically and mathematically as belonging to a ratio scale (11, 16).

Borg's CR10® scale has arguably been the gold standard method for providing RPE, owing to the aforementioned properties of CR scaling. It can often be misinterpreted as a simple 0 to 10 category scale, however. This becomes problematic because athletes may tend to report integer values, which distorts the ratio properties of the scale and causes deviations in the scale's S–R functions (22). The Category-Ratio 100 scale (centiMax; CR100®) has received attention in the quantification of sRPE. The CR100® scale (ranging from 0-120) is a fine-grained version of the CR10® scale (ranging from 0-11) and was developed to overcome the aforementioned issues and increase the possibility of detecting smaller changes in effort perception (16). Research in soccer players (50) has shown less clustering of ratings around the verbal anchors when comparing CR100® sRPE with CR10® sRPE. This suggests that the CR100® scale provides a more accurate measure of exercise intensity and is the optimal method for rating perceived exertion.

The selection and placement of the CR scale's verbal anchors was developed through quantitative analysis. The choice of adjectives and adverbs is based on semantic concepts such as interpretation (intensity behind the expression) and precision (degree of variation indicating how much individuals agree). These descriptors, working as multiplicative constants, and their placement and spacing were chosen to correspond with their numeric values from a series of iterative trials (10, 16, 20). Accordingly, even though RPE and sRPE have been used for resistance training, the verbal anchors on the CR scales were originally developed for cardiovascular-type exercises. Therefore, the congruency of the verbal descriptor with the context of resistance training should be examined. Nonetheless, practitioners and coaches using CR scales to quantify sRPE should understand that the scaling of psychophysiological constructs is complex, and the development of these scales came not simply from adding verbal descriptors on a numbered line based on intuition or aesthetic appearance.

Scale Customization

Unfortunately, it is not uncommon to encounter modified RPE scales that employ additional features such as the use of color, facial expressions, or images (see figure 17.4). These scales are prevalent not only in amateur or recreational settings, but within elite sporting organizations (8). Importantly, these scales are not validated to the degree of psychometric rigor of the CR scales and often lack key principles: precise operational definitions of the construct measured, generalizability to a broad population, selection of the appropriate subjects for the development, external validation and creation of norms, choice of the scale type, the range model (minimum to a maximum), the size of the subjective dynamic range, and avoiding or limiting end effect (open end and fixed star).

Modifications to appropriate scales may introduce considerable bias in the rating process. Here, bias likely arises when individuals' rating is influenced by their perception of the scale feature (e.g., their perception of the color red or a happy face), rather than the feeling of effort. Any additional cues (symbols or colors) added to the scale should be congruent with the values of the verbal anchors. Even scales populated with a border around each effort category are subject to the same pitfalls because this likely forces a categorical or discrete response (e.g., ordinal data), whereas effort perception is best viewed as a semicontinuous ratio variable if it is rated using the recommended method of CR scaling. In this regard, ratio level data are best represented as positions along a continuous number line—rather than members of discrete categories—for which non-integer responses should be possible.

When a scale is modified, coaches and practitioners should be aware that replacement of the verbal anchor positioning or terminology can change the functional relation between the reference construct and the data. This means that once a scale has been modified, it is now a different scale, not even a variation. Modification of the measurement properties makes quantitative comparison difficult (16), and the interpretation of sRPE data from training and competition may be inaccurate. To put this simply, if these scales are used to measure sRPE, then one may not be measuring sRPE at all.

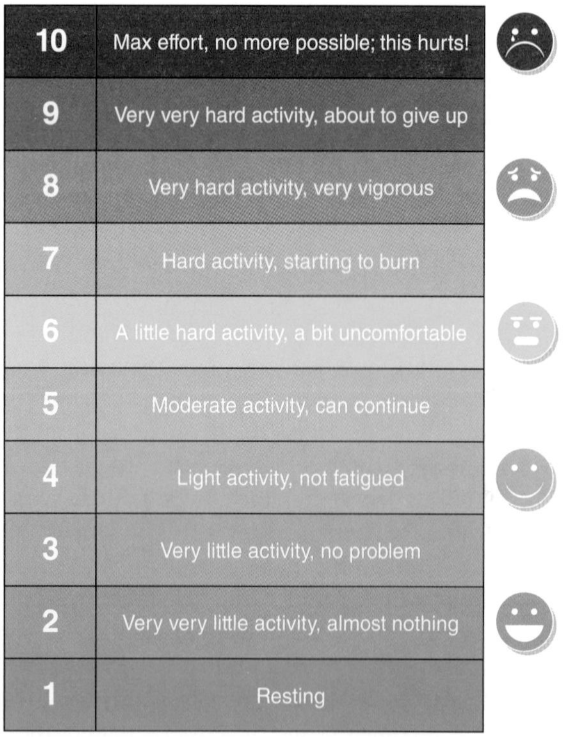

MEASUREMENT PROPERTIES OF RPE AND SRPE

Any athlete monitoring measure must possess acceptable measurement properties so that it can be applied with both accuracy and confidence in the data generated. Without entering into too much technicality, this section briefly presents the key measurement properties that subjective measures should be judged by as shown in table 17.1 (114, 154). This applies to sRPE as measures of training intensity, sRPE-TL as a measure of load, and also to subjective training response measures discussed later in this chapter. This section discusses the most pertinent measurement properties of sRPE and sRPE-TL.

Validity

Validity is a broad concept (5), and the validation process depends on the type of validity assessed (74, 114). The CR and 6-20 RPE scales are unquestionably valid for measuring perceived exertion because they were developed using psychophysical methodology. Of course, this does not mean that they do not have limitations (e.g., the CR scales are not a perfect form of ratio scaling). Since perceptions must be rated and communicated (a process that has the potential to be

10	Max effort, no more possible; this hurts!
9	Very very hard activity, about to give up
8	Very hard activity, very vigorous
7	Hard activity, starting to burn
6	A little hard activity, a bit uncomfortable
5	Moderate activity, can continue
4	Light activity, not fatigued
3	Very little activity, no problem
2	Very very little activity, almost nothing
1	Resting

FIGURE 17.4 Example of a customized RPE scale that violates many optimal psychometric principles. These scales should be avoided in athlete monitoring.

TABLE 17.1   An Overview of the Key Measurement Properties for Subjective Monitoring Tools in Athlete Monitoring

Measurement property	Description
Reliability domain	The extent to which subjective scores for athletes who have not changed are the same for repeated measurement under several conditions
Internal consistency	The degree of interrelatedness among the items
Reliability	The proportion of the total variance in the measurements that is attributable to true difference among athletes
Measurement error	The systematic and random error of an athlete's subjective measure that is not attributed to true changes in the target constructs
Validity	The degree to which subjective outcomes and their tools (scales, instrument, etc.) measure the constructs they are intended to measure
Content validity	The degree to which the content of a subjective outcome or its measurement tool is an adequate reflection of the construct to be measured
Face validity	The degree to which the items of a subjective outcome or its measurement tool indeed appear to be an adequate reflection of the construct to be measured
Construct validity	The degree to which a subjective outcome is consistent with hypotheses (for instance, with regard to internal relationships, relationships to scores of other instruments, or differences between relevant groups) based on the assumption that the measurement tool provides a valid assessment of the target construct
Structural validity	The degree to which the scores of a subjective measurement are an adequate reflection of the dimensionality of the construct to be measured
Cross-cultural validity	The degree to which the performance of the items on a translated or culturally adapted measurement tool is an adequate reflection of the performance of the items on the original version of the measurement tool
Responsiveness domain	The ability of subjective outcomes and their tools to detect change over time in the construct to be measured

Adapted from Mokkink et al. (2016).

influenced by measurement error and conscious bias), an empirical evaluation of validity is also necessary.

Exercise intensity is a theoretical and holistic concept, meaning there is no gold standard criterion measure against which RPE validity can be examined. There are, however, variables considered valid indicators of exercise intensity that should be theoretically associated with RPE, including heart rate, oxygen uptake, blood lactate concentration, and muscle electrical activity. The results of several meta-analyses confirm that in various exercise modalities such as running, cycling, swimming, and resistance exercise, RPE is strongly associated with these other cardiopulmonary, metabolic, and neuromuscular measures of internal exercise intensity (see table 17.2) (32, 88). From a practical perspective, these data suggest that a change in RPE is strongly associated with a change in the other proxies of exercise intensity, suggesting that they are convergent of a similar construct. In this regard, correlation coefficients ≥0.50 are considered acceptable to provide evidence

for construct validity (153). It is important to note that while these associations provide evidence for RPE construct validity, they should not be interpreted as causal (e.g., one cannot conclude that perceived exertion is generated by heart rate, blood lactate, etc.). These associations simply imply that RPE is related to other constructs of exercise intensity.

Although other measures of internal exercise intensity can be difficult to obtain in the applied setting, similar evidence of construct validity exists when RPE are applied to quantify sRPE in sport, including continuous running and cycling, swimming, and combat sport training (61). Evidence also suggests that the combination of multiple exercise intensity indicators, such as session average heart rate and postexercise blood lactate concentration, explains more of the variance in sRPE than single measures in isolation (39). As a measure of internal load, sRPE-TL is strongly associated with TRIMP during a range of non-resistance training modes in sports such as soccer, rugby league, basketball, Australian football,

TABLE 17.2 Results of Several Meta-Analyses Examining the Convergent Validity of RPE in Exercise and Athlete Training

Meta-analysis	Exercise and training type	Other intensity or load construct	Pooled relationship (r; 95% confidence interval) with RPE
Chen, Fan, Moe (32)	Treadmill and track running, cycle ergometry, and swimming	Heart rate; % $\dot{V}O_2$max; Ventilation; Respiration rate; Blood lactate concentration	
Lea, Hulbert, O'Driscoll, Scales, Wiles (88)	Resistance training	Muscle electrical activity; External volume load	
McLaren, Macpherson, Coutts, Hurst, Spears, Weston (108)[b]	Team-sport field training	Total distance; High-speed distance; Accelerometer load	

[a]Determined by resistance load (kg) and its interaction with one or more of these: sets, repetitions, repetition time, and rest time between sets.

[b]Session RPE-TL (session RPE × session duration [min]).

Canadian football, interval training, cycling, rowing, swimming, Taekwondo, gymnastics (TeamGym), diving, sprint kayak, karate, water polo, tennis, and fencing (61). Further evidence for construct validity can be established from the sRPE-TL relationships with external training load. This is the case because, according to training theory, a valid construct of internal load should be associated with external load since it is the means by which load is induced (see figure 17.1 on page 232) (75, 76). This has indeed been evidenced during field-based team-sport training and also resistance training (see table 17.2) (88, 108).

A final validity context can be exemplified in the relationship between sRPE-TL and changes in training outcomes, such as fitness or performance. This is again supported by the training process framework (75, 76), because such changes are determined by internal load. However, given the complex dose–response relation between training load and performance (28, 125), it is unlikely that any single measure can reflect a high portion of the variance in performance changes. This also holds true for a

simple relation examined with basic linear models, because changes in training outcomes exist within complex systems (9, 94). Nevertheless, sRPE-TL, as well as other internal load indicators such as TRIMP, has shown some associations with changes in training outcomes such as fitness and performance (54, 77). Importantly, these associations appear stronger than those with external load, a finding supported by training theory (75, 76) and one that further highlights the importance of internal load quantification.

Unlike positive changes in the training outcome, such as fitness and performance, sRPE-TL does not appear to be associated with negative consequences of the training process such as noncontact muscular injuries (91). Some believe that this is evidence for dismissing sRPE as a useful load monitoring tool (117, 118), but such claims are nonsensical. By definition, sRPE is a general measure of exercise intensity and the associated psychophysiological stress. Injuries undoubtedly occur because at some point within exercise, a mechanical load exceeds the critical limits of biomaterials (e.g., soft tissue). The true etiology of an injury is complex. It is dependent on the ever-evolving and nonlinear interactions among multiple dynamic factors. To assume that there is an association between sRPE and injury is not only illogical, but misleading, and it reinforces an overreliance on using single proxies of training load to manage injury risk. This is an oversimplification of a complex problem. When applied correctly, sRPE should be used to guide the training process based on principles of progression and overload, in conjunction with the coach's or practitioner's professional knowledge and experience. These are all parts of the ever-complex injury prevention puzzle.

Reliability

Reliability relates to the degree of consistency and reproducibility in a measure (see chapters 8 and 18). In the context of athlete monitoring, establishing the reliability of an internal load proxy can often be difficult because internal load is itself inherently sensitive and therefore has the potential to be unstable. This fact is supported by the poor test–retest reliability of several physiological markers such blood lactate concentration and oxygen uptake (45, 116). When the internal response to exercise appears reproducible, however, evidence suggests that sRPE are a reliable measure of subjective exercise intensity. This has direct transfer to sRPE-TL, given that duration is constant in retest designs. In a study examining the reproducibility of the internal intensity responses to constant-load running and cycling at different intensities (40%-90% maximal oxygen uptake), Herman and colleagues (66) reported nearly perfect relationships and low standard (typical) **errors of measurement**—an estimate of within-athlete variability—between two training days for sRPE (retest correlation coefficient $r = 0.88$, standard [typical] error of measurement = 1.2 au, percentage of maximal oxygen uptake [0.98, 3.2%], average heart rate [0.96, 3.7% point of maximum]). These findings appear consistent with studies conducted in the applied environment. Moderate to very high intraclass correlation coefficients (ICCs; 0.55-0.99) (97) and typical errors of ~0.1 to 1.5 au (deciMax) for sRPE have been reported for resistance training (43), rugby league (56) and basketball (98) skills training, steady-state interval cycling (162), controlled intermittent running (140), and fencing footwork training (156).

INFLUENCE OF PSYCHOLOGICAL FACTORS IN ATHLETE MONITORING

Because perceived exertion is a cognitive task involving neural and biological processes in the brain, the influence of psychological factors is highly likely (99, 102). These factors may ultimately result in conscious bias during the rating process. The nature of the interaction of these factors with perceived exertion is dynamic and complex, however. It is also dependent on the manner in which RPE are applied. For example, the psychobiological framework of cardiovascular endurance performance is an effort-based decision-making model grounded in motivational intensity theory (98, 122). In the context of athlete monitoring, in which RPE are used as a postexercise cognitive appraisal (i.e., sRPE), potentially important psychological influences may include affect phenomena (core affect, such as pleasure and displeasure, tension and relaxation, energy and tiredness, mood and emotions) (49, 90) dispositional traits (characteristics, abilities, or feelings such as extraversion, resistance, endurance, behavioral activation, behavioral inhibition, etc.) and situational factors (e.g., self-efficacy). The reason it is important to understand and acknowledge these potential influencers is so that coaches and practitioners can formulate strategies to control or account for them when sRPE are applied in athlete monitoring.

Affect phenomena, dispositional traits such as extraversion, behavioral activation, psychological resistance (i.e., to pressure, criticism, and stress), psychological endurance (i.e., persistence and determination), leadership, and self-efficacy (before and during exercise) have demonstrated negative associations with RPE. This suggests that more positive affect phenomena, higher exercise self-efficacy, and more positive dispositional traits are associated with lower perceived exertion (36, 62, 107, 124). However, these associations are evident only for low or submaximal exercise intensities, such as those performed below the ventilatory threshold (36, 62). Such a finding is consentient with Rejeski's model of perceived exertion (131, 132), which states that psychological factors should mediate perceived exertion at low or submaximal exercise intensities. Whether this also holds true for sRPE is yet to be determined.

The potential for complex psychological factors to evoke under- or overestimated RPE, beyond that of the true exercise-induced internal load, can be seen as a limitation of sRPE. However, this can also present as a benefit in athlete monitoring, depending on whether the coach desires a quantification of exercise load or intensity in the context of the athlete's current physiological and psychological state. For example, mental fatigue can increase exercise RPE (42) but it also impairs physical and technical performance in athletes (103, 144). A more legitimate concern is the issue of athletes being unable to disassociate sRPE from exercise-induced sensations or feelings that are often strongly associated with perceived exertion. To help overcome this problem, sport scientists and practitioners should look to standardize the data collection environment and be mindful of situations in which other exercise-induced feelings may influence sRPE responses.

VARIATIONS OF SUBJECTIVE MEASURES IN ATHLETE MONITORING

When Foster and colleagues (53, 54) proposed the sRPE method, they reasoned that there must also exist other identifiable and quantitative characteristics of a training program that could be calculated to further understand training periodization and the demands placed on the athlete. To this end, indices of training monotony and strain were proposed. **Training monotony** refers to the day-to-day variability in an athlete's weekly training load and is given as the average daily load divided by the standard deviation (both including zero values for rest days; table 17.3). A higher value would represent less variability and therefore greater monotony, and vice versa. **Training strain** is then the product of weekly training load and training monotony, designed to combine both indices as an overall value (see table 17.3). While these concepts are mathematically logical and have some physiological rationale, there is little evidence linking them with incidence of overtraining and other negative consequences of the training process. However, if coaches or practitioners believe that monotony and strain provide an accurate representation of the athlete's tolerance to training and are useful for load planning or adjustment, they may wish to include the metrics within athlete monitoring as an adjunct to sRPE.

Another variation of RPE within athlete monitoring

is **differential RPE** (dRPE). This involves an athlete providing separate ratings for the perceived central or respiratory exertion (e.g., breathlessness) and peripheral or local exertion (e.g., leg muscle). In the context of athlete monitoring, this may prove useful as a means of overcoming the limitations associated with a single, gestalt measure of exercise intensity (72, 164). Emerging evidence suggests that dRPE demonstrate face, content, and construct validity (convergent and discriminant) in team-sport athletes (106, 108, 162). From a practical perspective, simply asking athletes to separate their global sRPE into dRPE can provide sport scientists with a more detailed quantification of internal training load (109), in particular pertaining to respiratory and muscular exertion, which incur differing amounts of recovery time to baseline and have different adaptation pathways (128, 159).

ASSESSMENT OF TRAINING AND COMPETITION RESPONSE USING SUBJECTIVE MEASURES

Compared to perceived exertion, the response to training and competition is a broader concept with multiple domains. As previously mentioned, these responses are typically acute or chronic changes to key systems—including cardiorespiratory, metabolic, endocrine, neuromuscular, and musculoskeletal—as well as overall functional output (i.e., physical performance). Ultimately, the efficacy of the training process is athlete-centered, and the goal is to determine how individuals are coping with demands to avoid excessive fatigue through optimization of the stimulus. This is a holistic issue involving constructs and dimensions that are not objectively measurable, which is why biomarkers can have limited utility and often fail to accurately reflect how the athlete is tolerating the load (i.e., distinguish between acute and chronic changes induced by training) (137).

The challenges of quantifying response are not novel to sport science. Many of these fundamental issues have long been present in health care settings, which is why **patient reported outcome measures** (PROMs)—questionnaires measuring the patients' views of their health status—are popular clinical tools. Following the same logic, the use of questionnaires for assessing the subjective responses to training and competition has become common in sport science (137, 139). Historically, the interest in subjective responses was related to overtraining and specifically

TABLE 17.3 Calculating Load, Monotony, and Strain Using the sRPE Method (Example From a Rugby League Athlete During the In-Season Phase)

Day	Session	Duration (min)	sRPE[a] (au)	sRPE-TL (au)	Daily load (au)
Monday	Off-feet recovery	30	1.3	39	39
Tuesday	Field training (intensive, noncontact)	75	6.0	450	625
	Resistance training (upper-body strength focus)	50	3.5	175	
Wednesday	Field training (extensive, contact)	60	7.5	450	675
	Resistance training (lower-body strength focus)	50	4.5	225	
Thursday	Rest	-	-	0	0
Friday	Field training (captain's run)	30	2.0	60	78
	Resistance training (whole-body power focus)	25	0.7	18	
Saturday	League game	70	9.5	665	665
Sunday	Rest	-	-	0	0
	Weekly total	*390*			*2,082*
	Monotony (au)[b]				*0.89*
	Strain (au)[c]				*1,844*

[a]Collected via the CR100® scale and converted to deciMax units: (CR100 rating 4 10)

[b]Monotony = Average daily load ÷ Standard deviation daily load

[c]Strain = weekly load × monotony

as diagnostic confirmation or to detect early symptoms for preventing or avoiding its progression (e.g., from nonfunctional overreaching to overtraining) (115). Interest in subjective responses in athlete monitoring has increased as a way to optimize training adaptations, hence physical performance (38), thus also reducing the risk of overtraining (80, 139).

The goal of using subjective measures in quantifying an athlete's response to training and competition is to measure one or a combination of constructs such as recovery, fatigue, and pain or soreness. In this regard, questionnaires—typically referred to as **instruments**—are often employed. Instruments themselves are composed of items (individual questions) that are thought to be a relevant component of the target construct (see figure 17.5). Usually the summation of item responses gives a total score for the construct. Some of the most common instruments used to measure the subjective training response are outlined in table 17.4 (137, 139).

Without entering into too much technicality, PROMs are common and well established (29). They

belong to a research area called **clinimetrics**, which is based on psychometric principles and methods (47, 105). Sport science does not currently have these advanced instruments or item banks because interest in them as a routine athlete monitoring tool is still

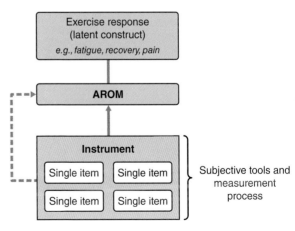

FIGURE 17.5 Conceptual overview of athlete reported outcome measures (AROMs) in athlete monitoring.

TABLE 17.4 Common Athlete Reported Outcome Measure Instruments in Sport Science

Instrument	Abbreviation	Primary constructs assessed
Perceived Recovery Status Scale (87)	PRS	Recovery
Recovery Stress Questionnaire for Athletes (79)	RESTQ-S	Recovery, stress
Acute Recovery and Stress Scale (68)	ARSS	Recovery, stress
Short Recovery and Stress Scale (69)	SRSS	Recovery, stress
Recovery-Cue (81)	-	Recovery, stress
Daily Analyses of Life's Demands of Athletes (136)	DALDA	Stress
Perceived Stress Scale (35)	PSS	Stress
Training Distress Scale (59)	TDS	Physical symptoms
Athlete Burnout Questionnaire (129)	ABQ	Physical and psychological symptoms
Multi-Component Training Distress Scale (96)	MTDS	Mood, physical symptoms, stress
Mood questionnaire (33)	Mood	Mood, physical symptoms
Profile of Mood States (111)	POMS	Mood
Short form (141)	POMS-SF	Mood
Modified (60)	POMS-M	Mood
Adolescents (152)	POMS-A	Mood
Brunel Mood Scale (151)	BRUMS	Mood
Training Distress Scale (130)	POMS-TDS	Mood
State-Trait Anxiety Inventory (146)	STAI	Anxiety
Competitive State Anxiety Inventory-2 (104)	CSAI-2	Anxiety
State-Trait Personality Inventory (145)	STPI	Emotional disposition
Emotional Recovery Questionnaire (93)	EmRecQ	Emotions
Overtraining questionnaire of the Société Française de Médecine du Sport (89)	SFMS	Behavioral symptoms

Based on Saw, Main, and Gastin (2016).

developing. However, to avoid reinventing the wheel (squared), the authors of this chapter advise coaches and practitioners rely on the established literature and methodology available in other areas, where these instruments have been commonplace for decades. To this end, the chapter refers to subjective measurement of the response to training and competition (mainly symptoms and physical signs) as **athlete reported outcome measures** (AROMs). For this reason, the authors rely more on clinimetrics terminology and methodology than on psychometric methods when referring to AROMs in the context of athlete monitoring. That is, the psychometric instruments discussed in this section are not examined with respect to their role of exploring psychological aspects associated with training, but as attributes (symptoms) influenced by training (47). More psychologically oriented AROMs, or any other psychological instruments, are not a matter of expertise for coaching and sport science staff. This necessitates experts (i.e., psychologists) for correct interpretation and also implementation.

Since AROMs cover a wide range of concepts and constructs, it is beyond the scope of this chapter to discuss the psychophysiological theory of each domain in isolation, or the many different measurement options (31, 121, 149, 165). Instead, the focus is on the general concepts behind instrument selection, validity, and reliability, as well as the challenge of developing an AROM system based on individual needs.

Instrument Selection

An important concern of AROMs is whether the data obtained are appropriate, meaningful, and useful for a specific purpose. Handling single- and multi-item questionnaires may seem a straightforward task, but— and as with measuring perceived exertion—there is a wide scope for error and misuse. For these reasons, the phases of instrument development present as a unique consideration and provide subjective assurance that items measure the specific dimension of interest. Since there are few specific guidelines for developing AROM systems in sport science (137), established recommendations available in clinimetrics, such as the **COnsensus-based Standards for the Selection of Health Measurement INstruments** (COSMIN) (114, 154) must be consulted.

Saw and colleagues (137) have presented an interesting and useful framework of the steps to establish the purpose, stakeholder engagement, and feasibility of implementing AROMs in a sport context (see figure 17.6; 137). For selecting the most appropriate instruments and items, the authors of this chapter refer to and adapt the guidelines of a joint initiative between the COSMIN and the **Core Outcome Measures in Effectiveness Trials** (COMET) (126, 127). This initiative aims to provide guidance on what and how to select measurement instruments. As such, this model can be extended and is therefore useful for AROMs and any measure, including performance-based options. This framework is shown in figure 17.7 (126, 127), and the following sections briefly provide a practical elaboration of the four steps for selecting the most appropriate AROMs and measurement instruments.

Step 1: Conceptual Consideration

The first step encompasses the definition of and agreement on the construct, outcome, or domain one wants to measure, a task that should include both coaches and practitioners. This is probably the most insufficiently considered but fundamental step when one is deciding what measures to use. It is an error to implement something that is simply available and try to provide a meaning once the data are collected. Exploration of further information provided by data already collected can be useful and is a legitimate strategy, but it should not be the norm. Post hoc justification is prone to bias and forced explanations to give sense to numbers. This may be even more problematic with the use of AROMs since they can be relatively easy to collect, especially with single items.

Coaches and practitioners should decide what information is needed and why it can help optimize the training process or athlete management. This is exemplified by a hypothetical thought process in figure 17.8.

Step 2: Finding Existing Outcome Measurement Instruments

Once one has defined what to measure (and why), one should find the established AROMs for measuring the target constructs. This is a much more objective process compared to conceptual consideration and can be achieved by searching in three main sources: systematic reviews; original articles; and other sources such as online databases, textbooks, and guidelines. If no instruments are available, it is possible to consider the development of a new instrument (137). However, the authors of this chapter warn against this unless absolutely necessary. If that is the case, then proper methods must be used. Developing an instrument is a long process requiring time, expertise, and several validation studies.

Further consideration should be given to the type of scaling used. For example, since it may be desirable to differentiate between normal responses induced by training and responses that are perceived as higher or lower than normal (or planned or accounted for or both), a relative bipolar scale might be more appropriate than an absolute unipolar scale. A **unipolar scale** focuses on presence or absence (in fatigue or recovery, for example) in absolute terms, whereas **bipolar scales** focus on relative deviations from normal in two opposing directions: negatively or worse and positively or better. This conceptual consideration also helps further refine the target constructs. See, for example, the single items of fatigue and recovery under sport science validation in figure 17.9, which have been adapted from occupational medicine (158), to theoretically satisfy the hypothetical necessities outlined in figure 17.8.

Step 3: Quality Assessment of Outcome Measurement Instruments

Once an AROM is identified, it is important to examine and understand whether the instrument is properly developed and validated (risk of study bias) and if it possesses acceptable psychometric properties. Acceptable psychometric properties are those previously discussed (see table 17.1), whose quality should be adequate to support the use of the AROM in the target athlete population and within the context of its application (e.g., discriminative or longitudinal, individual or group level). This also implies that the AROM should have been developed specifically for the population of interest (e.g., athletes) to ensure content validity. Alternatively, it should have been

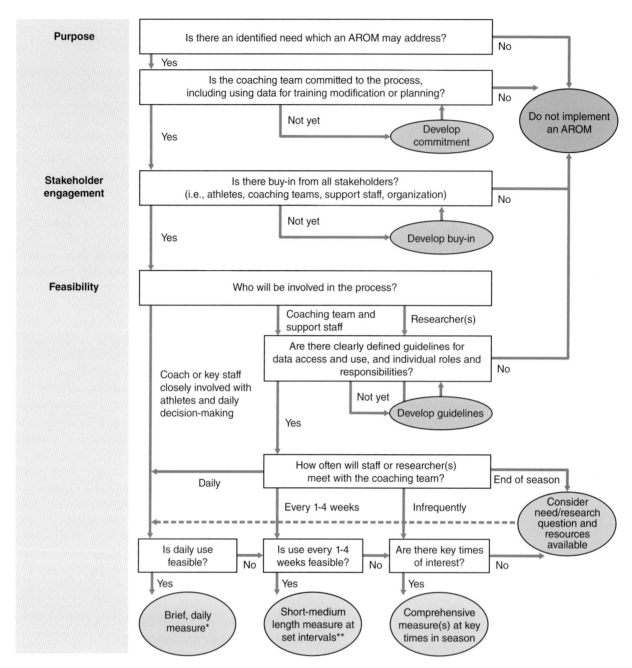

FIGURE 17.6 Steps to establish the purpose, stakeholder engagement, and feasibility of implementing AROMs in a sport context.

*Consider supplementing with a more comprehensive measure at set intervals or at key times in the season.

**Suggested intervals include weekly, fortnightly, or once per microcycle. Consider supplementing with a brief daily measure during intense training phases, or a more comprehensive measure at key times in season.

Reprinted by permission from A.E. Saw et al. (2017).

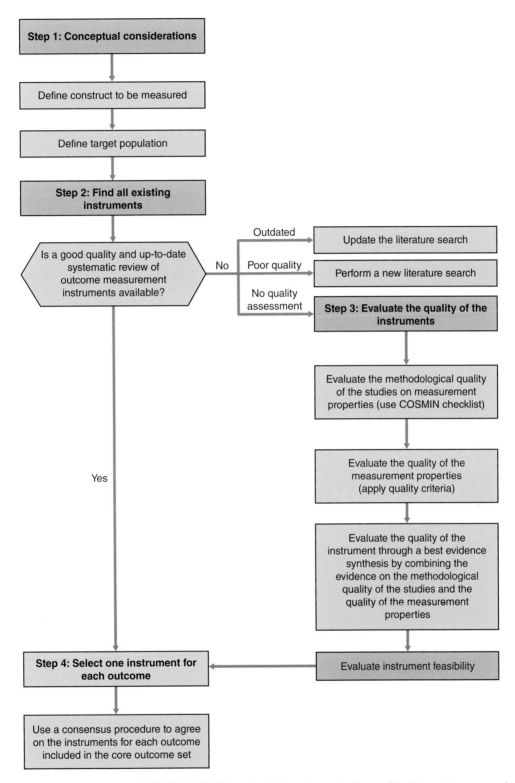

FIGURE 17.7 Flowchart of the COSMIN–COMET methodology for selecting subjective outcomes and measurement instruments, adapted, and applied to AROMs in a sport context.

Reprinted by permission from C. Prinsen et al. (2016, pg. 19).

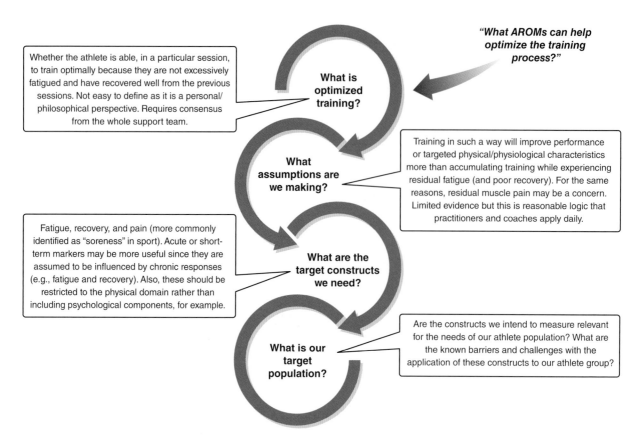

"What AROMs can help optimize the training process?"

What is optimized training?

Whether the athlete is able, in a particular session, to train optimally because they are not excessively fatigued and have recovered well from the previous sessions. Not easy to define as it is a personal/philosophical perspective. Requires consensus from the whole support team.

What assumptions are we making?

Training in such a way will improve performance or targeted physical/physiological characteristics more than accumulating training while experiencing residual fatigue (and poor recovery). For the same reasons, residual muscle pain may be a concern. Limited evidence but this is reasonable logic that practitioners and coaches apply daily.

What are the target constructs we need?

Fatigue, recovery, and pain (more commonly identified as "soreness" in sport). Acute or short-term markers may be more useful since they are assumed to be influenced by chronic responses (e.g., fatigue and recovery). Also, these should be restricted to the physical domain rather than including psychological components, for example.

What is our target population?

Are the constructs we intend to measure relevant for the needs of our athlete population? What are the known barriers and challenges with the application of these constructs to our athlete group?

FIGURE 17.8 A hypothetical thought process of conceptual considerations for selecting an AROM.

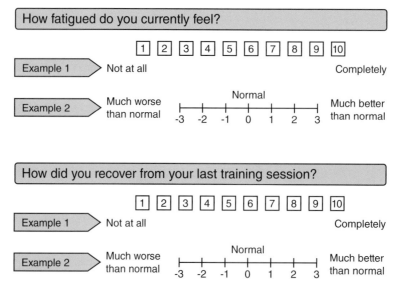

FIGURE 17.9 Example of single-item AROMs adapted from an occupational context (158). In this case, fatigue and recovery are the target construct. Responses are shown for absolute (unipolar scale) and relative (compared to normal; bipolar scale) options.

cross-validated in the target athlete population. The next section summarizes the measurement properties that need to be examined for selecting an instrument or items, as well as some validated tools.

Step 4: Generic Recommendations for Selecting Instruments of a Core Outcome Set

The last step is the selection (or recommendation) of the instrument. In theory, if there are no quality studies examining the measurement properties or if these properties are deemed inadequate, then the instrument should not be used or recommended. Clearly, one cannot expect—especially in this early stage of AROM development in sport science—to have several instruments adequately satisfying all the mentioned criteria. Still, while some weaknesses are acceptable, the instrument must have some minimal evidence of validity and reliability. Otherwise, the data may be misleading to decision making in practice. An instrument that is not valid, for example, may indicate stability in a target construct when it is actually changing, or vice versa (121, 165). Therefore, any limitation or weakness of the instrument should be considered when one interpreting the measures.

Existing Instruments for Measuring AROMs

The literature offers few instruments specifically developed for athletes. Fortunately, some of the most popular do appear to be supported by evidence (i.e., with several validation studies).

Multi-Item and Multidimensional Instruments

The **Recovery Stress Questionnaire for Athletes** (RESTQ-S) (79) and its derivatives, **Acute Recovery and Stress Scale** (ARSS) (68) and the **Short Recovery and Stress Scale** (SRSS) (69), are among the few AROM instruments developed and validated (to some degree of satisfaction) specifically in athletes. The original RESTQ-S (79) consists of 77 items (19 scales with 4 items each plus 1 warm-up item) that athletes answer retrospectively using a Likert-type scale. The RESTQ-S includes seven general stress components (general stress, emotional stress, social stress, conflicts or pressure, fatigue, lack of energy, physical complaints), five general recovery

components (success, social recovery, physical recovery, general well-being, sleep quality), three sport-specific stress components (disturbed breaks, emotional exhaustion, injury), and four sport-specific recovery components (being in shape, personal accomplishment, self-efficacy, self-regulation). Each of these subscales is measured using four items that should reflect the specific domain. These RESTQ-S subscales are further combined to reflect two higher-order constructs: recovery and stress (79).

The ARSS includes eight components (4 items each, 32 in total) reflecting the dimension of recovery composed of physical performance capability, mental performance capability, emotional balance, overall recovery, and the stress dimension (including muscular stress, lack of activation, negative emotional state, and overall stress) (68). The SRSS instead measures the same dimensions of the RESTQ-S and ARSS but is much shorter (using eight items that combine to provide a measure of recovery and stress [69]), making it easier to implement. Although there are usually concerns in psychometrics about using single items, the SRSS developers provided evidence for construct validity on the single items used and evidence that they can be combined to provide a measure of recovery and stress. This evidence of validity is not, for example, available for other popular single items commonly used in sport (see next section). Another instrument providing some evidence of validity and specifically developed for athletes is the **Multi-Component Training Distress Scale** (MTDS, 22 items) (96), measuring depression (5 items), vigor (4 items), physical symptoms (3 items), sleep disturbance (3 items), stress (4 items), and fatigue (3 items).

For coaches and practitioners interested in measuring any of the aforementioned constructs, instruments such as the RESTQ-S, ARSS, SRSS, and MTDS appear to be appropriate tools, even if an examination of their measurement properties according to COSMIN guidelines has not yet been conducted. Other instruments commonly used in sport science (see table 17.4) (139) do not appear to possess the same evidence of validity or to measure appropriate target constructs related to the training process in athletic populations. With that being said, readers should remember that, within sport science, AROMs should be implemented to quantify physical symptoms of the training response as opposed to psychological aspects (where psychology experts should be consulted). Coaches and practitioners might therefore consider restricting domains of the RESTQ-S, ARSS, SRSS, and MTDS to physical symptoms only.

Single-Item Instruments

The use of single items (i.e., individual questions that collectively form instruments) has historically attracted the interest of researchers and practitioners in several fields (medicine, marketing, etc.) because they are simple, are easy to use, and facilitate a high completion rate (26, 44, 48, 143). Single items also possess good face validity, because it is immediately clear to athletes which construct is being measured, and they probably evoke less boredom, fatigue, and frustration associated with instruments (158). Based on psychometric theory, however, multi-item instruments are considered necessary to appropriately reflect concepts that cannot be measured directly (121). Therefore, single items seem to be acceptable alternatives but might be limited to some constructs, and users must accept the risk of lowering sensitivity in construct validity following changes (i.e., simplicity at the cost of detail). Therefore, with the use of single items, these limitations should be considered and acknowledged.

If the response construct of interest is multidimensional and complex, it presents a challenge for single-items, and multi-item AROMs would be advisable. Alternatively, if the construct or domain is relatively simple, unambiguous, and reasonably unidimensional, the use of single items seems to be acceptable. The item should be formulated so that the construct of interest is clear. Failure to meet these requirements would cause lack of content validity (construct too broad to be assessed with one item) as well as poor construct validity and higher measurement error. Unfortunately, most of the single items used in sport science fail to meet these minimum criteria.

Among all the constructs assessed using a single item in sport settings, only a few can be reasonably considered relatively simple and unidimensional (or concrete) and thus assessed with one question: fatigue, muscle pain (soreness), and possibly recovery. Nevertheless, the construct validity of these items should be examined and demonstrated by assessing, for example, their convergence with reference questionnaires that are considered valid measures of the construct of interest. An example of construct validation is the study by Van Hooff and colleagues (158) examining the convergent and discriminant validity (using POMS as the reference) for a single item measuring fatigue in an occupational context (e.g., figure 17.9). This validation would also need an instrument validated in the population of interest as a reference (i.e., athletes).

Wellness

Among the most commonly used AROMs are so-called wellness items (sometimes also referred as well-being, welfare, daily subjective questions, Hooper index, etc.) (30, 40, 86, 113, 120). The lack of consistency in a definition of the construct that is supposed to be measured by these items (e.g., wellness, well-being, welfare) suggests the absence of a reference framework, making it difficult to ascertain what the domains of interest are and why. Several single items have been used to measure different dimensions of this undefined and generic domain in research and practice (e.g., fatigue, recovery, sleeping, stress, mood, enjoyment, irritability, health causes of stress and happiness, desire to train, energy level, general health, etc.) (2, 40, 57, 70, 135). Yet these items and their combination into a single score (2, 30) have never been validated. Furthermore, most of those items do not satisfy the basic requirements for their use. Constructs like stress, mood, and desire to train are inherently multidimensional and complex and so cannot be measured using single items. Even quality of sleep is an ambiguous construct that is not easily interpreted (e.g., quality of actual sleep achieved versus difficulty falling asleep). To the best of our knowledge, no single items of wellness have been sufficiently validated to a level that warrants recommending them.

Warnings about using nonvalidated instruments for monitoring training can be tracked back to the 1990s (71). Unfortunately, this is probably even more common nowadays and some of these items are even included in athlete management systems (as are customized scales for sRPE). Since these items are already widespread, it is probably pragmatic simply to suggest considering the aforementioned limitations when applying them in athlete monitoring. Furthermore, it is important to suggest once again that coaches and practitioners restrict the use of single-item AROMs to unidimensional constructs that can be appropriately measured in such a way (e.g., fatigue [112], pain [15]).

Evaluation of Measurement Properties of AROMs

Readers can refer back to table 17.1 for the key measurement properties that AROMs should be judged by. As with sRPE, the most important considerations are those relating to validity and reliability. However, in comparison to sRPE, quantifying AROMs presents very different validity and reliability challenges that are worthy of discussion.

Validity Assessment

Difficulties arise when one is attempting to assess the validity of AROMs because they measure athlete-centered latent constructs and are the only means by which a quantification can be made. Applying this principle to the validation of AROMs, an instrument developed to measure components like stress and recovery measured by the RESTQ-S and derivatives (ARSS and SRSS), these should be compared to already validated and accepted measures of stress and recovery. In the absence of reference instruments, other measures of similar constructs can be used. Indeed, the construct validity of the RESTQ-S has been examined, for example, by assessing the correlation between the 19 subscales and POMS, and strong correlations were reported (80). Because the two measures converge, this is evidence of construct validity.

Construct validity can also be assessed by comparing the AROM with an instrument supposedly measuring a different construct. In this case, the rationale is that the two measures diverge. The fatigue domain of the RESTQ-S is negatively related to vigor measured using the POMS ($r = -0.45$) (119). Alternatively, validity can be examined by the ability of the AROM to differentiate between groups assumed to possess different levels of the target construct. The MTDS, for example, showed higher scores in the athletes classified at higher risk of overtraining using the **Athlete Burnout Questionnaire** (129) compared to those at low risk (96).

An earlier section in this chapter supported the validity of the RPE and sRPE through the association with objective measures of exercise intensity. Unlike these associations, however, it is quite challenging to provide evidence of construct validity of most AROMs through associations with biomarkers of stress. Indeed, AROMs generally do not correlate with specific objective markers such as physiological stress, immune function, inflammation and muscle damage, or endocrine and erythrocyte levels (139). That being said, Saw and colleagues (139) found AROMs to reflect acute and chronic training loads with superior sensitivity and consistency compared to objective measures in a review of 56 studies. Their evidence suggests that some AROMs are typically impaired with an acute increase in training load and

in prolonged periods of training, whereas reductions in load have the opposite effect (139). If an assumption can be made that higher training and competition loads are a proxy for poor recovery, greater fatigue, and so on, then these findings may be reasonably interpreted as some evidence for responsiveness and validity (at least generally and conceptually). However, this should be formally tested with respect to a reference framework and clear *a priori* definitions.

Structural validity is important when one is deciding whether single items can be combined (e.g., score summed) to create a scale or subscale. This can be examined in an explorative or confirmatory approach. This is crucial, as the assumption that a single item reflects a common construct must be verified. For this reason, combining the scores of single items and attributing a meaning to the summation (e.g., summated wellness scores) should be avoided. This approach is even more concerning if the higher-order latent construct and its dimensions are not defined. For wellness items this is a severe and common flaw. Indeed, there is no clarity about what higher-order construct these wellness items are supposed to measure and therefore whether the single items really reflect this (undefined) construct. Even more problematic is the absence of studies showing whether these items really measure what they are supposed to measure. Again, due to these limitations, the authors of this chapter warn against using these items.

Reliability Assessment

When measuring latent constructs using instruments composed of multiple items, an additional aspect of AROMs is the internal consistency of instrument items. This refers to the degree to which individual items accurately reflect the target construct (and therefore, earn their place in the total score). Internal consistency can be assessed using Cronbach's alpha (α), a metric similar to a correlation coefficient according to which values greater than or equal to 0.70 are considered acceptable (121). As an example, the α values for the RESTQ-S have been reported to be between 0.67 and 0.89, and this purportedly increases with familiarity (79). Similarly, for the MTDS, internal consistency of the items within subscales ranges from 0.72 to 0.86 (96).

Regarding the test–retest reliability of AROMs, it is beyond the scope of this chapter to identify and summarize the known reliability estimates given the vast range of existing AROMs applied in sports (see table 17.4). But conceptually, the value of such an exercise is questionable given the aforementioned validity concerns. Even with AROMs developed specifically for athletes and demonstrating enough validity to warrant consideration in monitoring systems (e.g., RESTQ-Sport, ARSS, SRSS, MTDS), there is a lack of studies reporting measurement error. Rather than letting this issue present as a barrier to implementation, the authors of this chapter recommend that coaches and practitioners using the RESTQ-S, ARSS, SRSS, or MTDS assess the test–retest reliability of scores within their own contexts (athletes, training program, etc.) until they can refer to published evidence.

COLLECTION OF sRPE AND AROMS IN THE APPLIED ENVIRONMENT

Because sRPE and AROMs are subjective in nature, there is of course a potential for several sources of conscious bias to compromise the accuracy of data (6, 138). In this regard, readers are referred to the extent to which observed ratings and scores do not meaningfully capture their intended constructs (3, 63). These biases likely exist due to cognitive and situational factors, which are not mutually exclusive (6, 138). However, when these biases are understood in terms of their origins and likely situations, coaches and practitioners can implement various strategies to control or mitigate their influence in athlete monitoring. Table 17.5 summarizes the main sources of cognitive and situational factors that may involve conscious bias in sRPE and AROMs. Also provided are sample scenarios within the applied environment and some practical approaches to control for the undesirable effects.

Session RPE is a postexercise cognitive appraisal, and therefore the time delay between exercise termination and reporting presents as a unique and potentially important cognitive factor (142). A 30-minute delay was initially recommended so that "particularly difficult or particularly easy segments toward the end of the exercise bout would not dominate the subject's rating" (54). While this theory is logical, there is limited data to support the so-called latency effect (34, 51, 67, 84, 92, 157). Furthermore, the 30-minute postexercise window can be impractical, particularly when dealing with large groups of athletes who have other responsibilities after the training session (e.g., in the professional setting: recovery, nutrition, technical meetings, additional training, media) (50). Evidence also suggests that there is no substantial difference between ratings collected immediately postexercise (≤30 min) and those reappraised up to 24 to 48 hours later (44, 111, 123). Team-sport athletes have also demonstrated the ability to accurately recall their sRPE (as opposed to reappraising) 48 hours after the initial appraisal (50)—which may be required if initial ratings are lost or misplaced. Session RPE therefore appears robust to response shift and recall bias, which provides more flexible data collection options.

With regard to the timing of AROM, there are no restrictions as to the time of day at which athletes complete reports; this depends entirely on situational constraints and how the data are to be used. If coaches and practitioners are implementing AROMs to determine how athletes are coping with training or to adjust training programming or both, then providing reports in the morning makes the most sense. Indeed, this is common practice since identification of red flags may warrant adjustment of an athlete's planned training load, intensity, volume, or type for that day (155). However, some athletes feel unable to give an accurate appraisal of their AROMs early in the morning and would prefer to report after training or at the end of the day (138). Posttraining reports may therefore be used to evaluate the acute training responses (e.g., fatigue) to specific sessions or days, but this would remove the utility of AROMs as a readiness-to-train assessment. Ultimately and importantly, the influence of situational, psychosocial, and cognitive factors likely differs between time windows. Furthermore, the response set used, for instance, "right now," "today," or "in the past week" is also of relevance, with longer periods of recall more susceptible to error (138). Collectively, this would suggest that well-defined and *a priori* consensus and subsequent consistency in the data collection process are key to mitigating conscious bias.

LIMITATIONS AND MISCONCEPTIONS OF sRPE AND AROM

Some believe that sRPE and AROMs are not valid tools to quantify aspects of the training process because of their subjective nature (25, 117, 118). This presumably refers to the fact that perception is a cognitive process that has the potential to be mediated by nonphysiological factors, or indeed for athletes to lie about their responses (117). As presented throughout this chapter, properly obtained ratings and responses are psychometrically valid measures of their intended

TABLE 17.5 Strategies to Counteract Sources of Bias When Collecting sRPE and AROM in Athlete Monitoring

Source of bias	Description	Sample scenarios	Strategies to mitigate*
Cognitive factors	Inaccuracies arising from the mental processes underlying sRPE and AROMs; this includes the interpretation of concepts and questions, information retrieval, decision making, and response generation	• Miscomprehension of the latent constructs that are being assessed (e.g., confusion between exertion and fatigue) • Recall error: providing responses based on the wrong time of target appraisal (e.g., perception of recovery right now versus yesterday evening) • Confusion as to what information to retrieve in order to answer the question (e.g., what the feeling of effort or exertion is mainly based upon) • Using scales incorrectly (e.g., using CR10 as though it were a simple 0-10 scale)	Ensure that athletes have a clear understanding of each construct, the procedures to be followed, and the scales or instruments to be used. This can be achieved by using the following strategies: • Giving thorough and concise operational definitions of the target constructs (e.g., exertion, fatigue, recovery) and other constructs that may distort these perceptions (e.g., discomfort) • Stating the target time of appraisal within each question (e.g., "Right now [emphasized], how well recovered do you feel?") and ensuring that the time of recall is minimized and always consistent • Providing reference points as to what information should be sought to appraise each construct (e.g., following soccer training, sRPE mainly depends on how hard or easy it felt to breathe and drive the legs) • Giving an overview of the scales before use and explaining any features (including their rationale) that might not be obvious (e.g., fixed star, open end); training exercises such as anchoring, as well as the blackness test, may be worthwhile to ensure competency
Situational factors	Inaccuracies arising from deliberate deception in responses, usually the result of external influences and for the purpose of social or personal desirability	• Deliberate deception involved in responses to give coaches and practitioners the impression that the athlete is coping with training and in a fit state, as a means of gaining selection, for example • Deliberate deception involved in responses to provide the individual with personal gain, such as reducing time-on-task or to have training modified (e.g., reduction of intensity or volume) • Refusal to respond (or respond accurately) due to a perceived lack of confidentiality, anonymity, or privacy	Aim to increase overall buy-in and motivation to respond accurately, as well as increasing confidence regarding data protection. The following are ways to achieve this: • Ensuring that athletes understand the purpose of athlete monitoring and the training process (links with performance and health) • Making the data collection process simple, easy to administer, and complete, accessible, and flexible; processes should also be kept consistent where possible and administered at the earliest possible (or reasonable) stage in an athlete's career • Promoting an autonomy-supportive culture in all aspects of the performance program • Giving athletes casual and infrequent feedback on their data and using this opportunity to gain their feedback on the monitoring processes • Aligning all monitoring and data collection processes with General Data Protection Regulation (2018) and any additional data protection guidelines in place in the organization

*Can be provided through formal education, verbal reminders, responding to athlete questions, or via app-based help buttons.

constructs, and these constructs are empirically valid proxies of training and competition intensity and the resultant responses. Perceived exertion is, by definition, an internal measure because it is centrally generated in association with demands of the body's systems and tissues during physical tasks. This logic also holds for AROMs such as fatigue, recovery, and pain. The fact that athletes are able to lie about their responses is a feasibility issue, which is separate from validity. But this is evident in many forms of subjective data acquisition within the applied environment, such as lying to a team's physiotherapist or physician about a medical issue. If athletes are willing to lie as a perceived means of improving their selection availability, then the issues may manifest from within the culture of the team, group, or performance environment as opposed to a subjective measure.

The potential for measurement error and conscious bias does present as a limitation with sRPE and AROM. This is of course a legitimate drawback with any subjective instrument. The design of a data collection system—from athlete instruction to measurement and environmental factors—should therefore aim to mitigate measurement error and conscious bias (6). As previously discussed, this may include providing athlete (re-)education on the definitions of perceived exertion and AROM constructs; conveying their purpose within athlete monitoring; collecting AROM via validated instruments and at the same time of day; collecting sRPE at the appropriate postexercise time and using professional judgment to mitigate any potential end-exercise effects or situational factors; using the nonmodified CR10® or CR100® scales; and showing the scale to athletes in private, away from others, and having them gauge their rating by using the verbal anchors and subsequently pointing to the scale.

DEVELOPMENT OF A SUBJECTIVE MONITORING SYSTEM

When sRPE and AROMs are accurately obtained, they can be used as intended and in the same manner as other processes of load and response—which is managing the athlete training process through the programming of training principles (see chapter 2). This chapter has alluded to many of these practical applications throughout, such as the measurement of sRPE via appropriate scales, the calculation of sRPE-TL and other associated metrics (e.g., monotony, strain), and a framework for selection of AROMs and strategies to mitigate conscious bias. There is clearly potential to discuss the analytical and decision-making processes, but that is beyond the scope of this chapter. It is more important to summarize practical strategies that ensure validity in sRPE and AROM so that coaches and practitioners can be confident about the data they analyze and subsequently interpret.

Education and Instructions

Formal education should convey to athletes what latent constructs are proposed for measurement and why they are being quantified as part of the monitoring system. This helps mitigate misconceptions and may reduce subsequent risks of cognitive and situational bias. Instructions should inform athletes how to appraise the constructs of interest, such as the scaling process or instrument overview. This helps reduce measurement issues and the associated compromise to measurement properties of the data. Importantly, education and instructions should be clear, concise, and consistent to uphold measurement validity.

The authors of this chapter believe that the education process is best conducted orally, in a formal manner with visual prompts, and carried out infrequently within the calendar (e.g., start of the preseason phase or new macrocycle). A short (<5 min) presentation might be optimal, with athletes able to ask questions at the end. The presentation may include the following:

- An overview of the purpose and value of collecting sRPE and AROMs within monitoring
- Definition of each construct:
  - Perceived exertion (and its separation from other exercise-related feelings)
  - Fatigue, recovery, pain (soreness), and so on
- An overview of the scaling tools:
  - CR10® or CR100® scales for sRPE
  - Validated instruments and items for AROMs
- An overview of the rating and recording process:
  - When and where data should be provided
  - How data should be provided (i.e., cognitive appraisal considerations)

Thereafter, practitioners may need only to remind athletes of the key points and specific instructions, which can be done verbally and on an individual basis. This is particularly feasible during the data collection process, which provides a natural avenue for both athletes and practitioners to ask questions. For example, athletes could be asked questions such as "What do you think about when providing your sRPE?"

Data Collection Procedures for sRPE

Practitioners and coaches may find complete instructions on RPE collection in Borg Perception (https://borgperception.se). It should be noted, however, that these instructions are bound to the Borg CR-Scales®, which are a copyrighted product (22). For proper administration, a formal license agreement should be signed by those administering the scales. The license agreement may be either a short-term contract or a long-term subscription renewed yearly. A summary of the most important aspects of these instructions in relation to sRPE is presented in table 17.6.

There are also several training tasks that athletes can complete to help ensure their understanding of sRPE and their competency using the CR scales. Anchoring refers to the process of familiarizing athletes with the entire range of sensations on the CR scales (123). Memory anchoring is perhaps the most pragmatic option and involves athletes recalling a past training session or competition for each effort category on the scale. In exercise anchoring, these levels of exertion are purposefully programmed. This might be achieved, for example, by having an athlete perform a graded endurance test to volitional exhaustion ($\dot{V}O_2$max, Yo-Yo intermittent recovery test, etc.) or an incrementally loaded 1RM test, or both, and having the athlete provide RPE for each completed stage (110).

Additionally, since the CR scales can be used to measure other perceptions such as brightness, Borg's blackness test can be administered as a training tool (18, 19). Here, athletes are shown different grayscale tones, ranging from white (i.e., minimum) to black (i.e., maximum), and are asked to rate blackness via the CR scales (24). The levels of blackness are closely linked to the verbal anchors on the CR scales (e.g.,

TABLE 17.6 Recommendations for Collecting sRPE in Athlete Monitoring

Points	Instructions to athletes or strategy
When collecting data from groups, the risk of conscious bias increases due to lack of concentration and verbal contamination.	Approach athletes in isolation or take them aside to ensure concentration and appropriate engagement and so that any dialogue cannot be heard by other athletes.
In some postsession situations, the influence of conscious bias or psychological factors cannot be avoided (e.g., in group transport, athletes must be within close proximity of one another, or, following a competition defeat, a negative affective response likely persists for several hours).	Postpone data collection for up to 24 hours and collect at a time when sources of conscious bias or the influence of affect phenomena associated with the session are reduced.
Give athletes examples of what perceived exertion is as a means of guiding cognitive decision making. They should be instructed that sRPE depends on how performing training or competition felt, not what they actually performed during this session.	"Your sRPE is the conscious awareness of how difficult the session felt. Think about how easy or hard it was to breathe and how easy or hard it was to drive your (legs, arms). Try not to think about what you did, but how it felt."
Athletes should understand that their rating refers to the feeling experienced during the exercise and not at the point of data collection (at rest).	"Your ratings should reflect the whole session on average; try not to think about any specific time point during (training, competition)."
Try to ask the question using clear and neutral terminology. "How was your workout?" (e.g., Foster and colleagues [54]) may be too vague, and "How hard was your session?" may bias away from or toward the "hard" anchor.	"What was your session RPE for that (training session, match, race, etc.)?" "How easy or hard was that (training session, match, race, etc.)?"
Measuring sRPE with the CR scales is the gold standard method because of their complex psychometric properties. Without visual prompting, athletes will likely refer to a scale in their head or use absolute magnitude estimation, which is far less valid for quantifying sRPE and makes between-athletes comparisons almost redundant.	Show athletes the scale (CR10® or CR100®).
Encourage athletes to make their decision based on the verbal anchors. The words are for them, the numbers are for the practitioners! Having athletes point to the scale encourages not only this, but also the recording of more precise numeric values and mitigation of verbal contamination effects in those yet to provide ratings.	"Read the verbal expressions and then point to the location on the scale that best represents your sRPE."

50% blackness would represent *hard*; 5 au or 50 au on the CR10® and CR100® scales, respectively) (19), such that answers can be scored for accuracy and level of precision. This can be a useful habituation exercise and may quantitatively assess an athlete's ability to use the CR scale independent from the feeling of effort (95).

Data Collection Procedures for AROMs

It is difficult to offer specific instructions and procedures for AROMs, given that these may differ depending on the construct of interest, its measurement (items and instruments), and the time of day at which ratings are provided. These are, however, available with properly validated instruments and items, which is another reason for the recommendation to select these tools over nonvalidated or customized alternatives.

It is commonplace for AROMs to be administered digitally, which can increase the flexibility and accessibility for athletes as well as speeding up data processing for coaches and practitioners. Another benefit of administering AROMs via a digital medium is the increased opportunity for athletes to complete their reports in private to reduce peer influence and social bias. In addition, this option limits time-on-task and the associated perception of a time burden: "the more clicks, the less compliant" (138). This is also true for the frequency of data input, which should occur often enough to inform coach and practitioner decision making but not so often that athletes perceive it to be an annoyance or not worthwhile. While frequency is highly specific to the needs of different individuals, two or three times per week seems a reasonable recommendation for assessing both acute and chronic responses to training and competition.

CONCLUSION

The need to understand athletes' training and competition demands alongside how well they are coping with these demands is fundamental to managing the training process. Internal load and the associated response to this load are athlete-centered constructs, in which psychophysiological feedback has a unique role. Monitoring the training process with subjective measures is a common practice, and validated methodologies are available. Whether and how to use these tools is a decision that should be based on the information required by coaches and practitioners, as well as feasibility within the context of application. These methods have clear strengths and limitations, as do all athlete monitoring tools. It is the authors' view that successful implementation and utility of subjective monitoring is founded upon principles of strong conceptual understanding and rigor in the measurement process. When methods are modified (such as scales, questionnaires, and data collection procedures), are not properly validated, and are not developed within a clear conceptual framework, limitations are inevitable, and any potential benefit of implementation all but disappears. When used correctly, subjective measures of load (e.g., sRPE) and the training response (e.g., AROMs) can be extremely powerful assets to those responsible for athlete management and the training process.

RECOMMENDED READINGS

Borg, G. *Borg's Perceived Exertion and Pain Scales*. Champaign, IL: Human Kinetics, 1998.

Foster, C, Florhaug, JA, Franklin, J, Gottschall, L, Hrovatin, LA, Parker, S, Doleshal, P, and Dodge, C. A new approach to monitoring exercise training. *J Strength Cond Res* 5:109-115, 2001.

McLaren, SJ, Macpherson, TW, Coutts, AJ, Hurst, C, Spears, IR, and Weston, M. The relationships between internal and external measures of training load and intensity in team sports: a meta-analysis. *Sports Med* 48:641-658, 2018.

Prinsen, C, Vohra, S, Rose, MR, Boers, M, Tugwell, P, Clarke, M, Williamson, PR, and Terwee, CB. Guideline for selecting outcome measurement instruments for outcomes included in a Core Outcome Set. 2016. https://cosmin.nl/wp-content/uploads/COSMIN-guideline-selecting-outcome-measurement-COS.pdf. Accessed August 27, 2020.

Saw, AE, Kellmann, M, Main, LC, and Gastin, PB. Athlete self-report measures in research and practice: considerations for the discerning reader and fastidious practitioner. *Int J Sports Physiol Perform* 12:S2127-S2135, 2017.

PART V

Data Analysis
and Delivery

CHAPTER 18

Statistical Modeling

Mladen Jovanović, MS
Lorena Torres Ronda, PhD
Duncan N. French, PhD

The world of sport is complex, with high levels of uncertainty. To better understand this complexity and help predict the behavior of that world, mathematical models and data analytics have become more apparent in sport science (57, 73). Some of these mathematical models involve **statistics**, which aim to simplify the complex and uncertain realities of sport in the hope of describing it, understanding it, predicting its behavior, and helping to make decisions that guide strategic interventions (25, 46, 48, 61). The variety of statistical models that can be adopted in a sporting context is large (51, 52), as they move beyond subjective–objective dichotomy and to qualities such as transparency, consensus, impartiality, correspondence to observable reality, awareness of multiple perspectives, awareness of context dependence, and investigation of stability (20). Indeed, statistical models must be acted upon based on cumulative knowledge, rather than solely relying on single studies or even single lines of research (3). This chapter discusses the primary statistical and mathematical models in the first part and statistical inferences later that are applicable to the sport scientist.

DATA TYPES

Data can be classified on one of four scales—nominal, ordinal, interval, or ratio:

- A **nominal scale**, also referred to as **categorical**, is defined as a scale used for labeling variables into distinct classes and does not involve a quantitative value or order. Examples include sex (e.g., male, female), treatment group (e.g., control, treatment, placebo), and location (e.g., New York, Boston).

- An **ordinal scale** is like a nominal scale but with implied order between levels and with unknown difference between each one. For example, ordinal scale data include **Likert** scales (e.g., muscle soreness from 0-10, a rating of perceived exertion [RPE] scale ranging from 0-10). With ordinal scales, the order is known but the difference between the levels is unknown.

- An **interval scale** is a numeric scale in which both the order and the exact differences between the values are known and quantifiable. The most common example of an interval scale is temperature. With a temperature scale (Celsius or Fahrenheit), the difference between 50° and 60° is the same as the difference between 80° and 90°, which is 10°. The problem with an interval scale is the lack of a true zero. Without true zero it is impossible to compute ratios.

- A **ratio scale** is an interval scale, but with the true zero. The Kelvin temperature scale is the most common example. With the Kelvin temperature scale, the ratio can be computed. For example, it can be said that 500 K is twice as warm as 250 K.

STATISTICAL MODELING

Within statistical modeling there are different classes of tasks, including **description**, which is used to summarize and describe data; **prediction**, which is the process of applying a statistical model to data for the purpose of predicting new or future observations; and **causal inference**, which is the process of drawing a conclusion about a causal connection (see figure 18.1).

Description

Description provides a quantitative summary of acquired data. These quantitative summaries are termed **descriptive statistics** and are usually broken down into two main categories: **measures of central tendency** and **measures of spread**, or **dispersion**. Descriptive statistics involve all quantitative summaries that are used to describe data without making predictive or causal claims. For example, **linear regression** between two variables can be used as a descriptive tool if the aim is to measure linear association; but in some instances, it can also be used in predictive and causal analyses. Elsewhere, **effect sizes** such as change, percent change, or Cohen's *d* (discussed in more detail later) represent descriptive statistics used to compare two or more groups, but are also commonly used in causal tasks to estimate the average causal effect of a treatment.

To provide further explanation of descriptive statistics, the most common descriptive tasks in sport science are given as examples, including comparisons of means (i.e., comparing two independent groups, comparing two dependent groups) and measuring the association between two variables.

Comparing Independent Groups

Suppose that height measurements are carried out on 100 people (N = 100), with N = 50 females and N = 50 males. Males and females represent independent groups. Figure 18.2 depicts common techniques used to visualize such independent group observations.

Sample descriptive statistics for each group can be found in table 18.1 (page 260). **Mean** (or **average**) and **mode** are measures of **central tendency**. The **median** is the middle number of a series of numbers and can be useful for data with a non-normal distribution. **Standard deviation** (SD), **median absolute difference** (MAD), **interquartile range** (IQR), **min**, **max**, and **range** are all common measures of **spread** or **dispersion**. Percent **coefficient of variation** (%CV) is also a measure of dispersion, but is standardized, which allows for comparison of variables that are on different scales. **Skewness** (**skew**) is usually described as a measure of **asymmetry**, or the distortion in a symmetrical normal distribution curve. Skewness can be quantified as the extent to which distribution varies from normal (a perfectly symmetrical data set will have a skewness of 0), with a negative skew having a longer or fatter tail to the left, and a positive skew showing a longer or fatter tail to the right. If the skewness is between −1 and −0.5 (negatively skewed) or 0.5 and 1 (positively skewed), the data are considered moderately skewed. If skewness is less than −1 (negatively skewed)

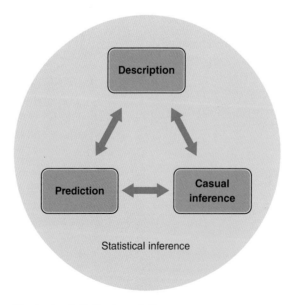

FIGURE 18.1 Three classes of tasks in statistical modeling.

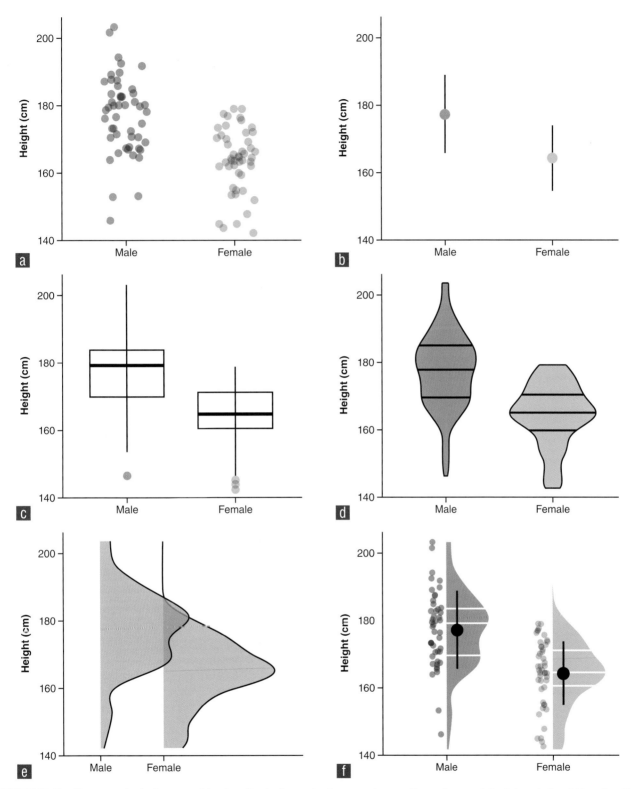

FIGURE 18.2   Common technique used to visualize independent group observations. A complete data set should be visualized rather than represented only by descriptive summaries, such as means *(a)* Simple scatterplot; *(b)* Mean and standard deviation as error bars; *(c)* Box plot. Horizontal line represents median, or 50th percentile, whereas boxes represent 25th and 75th percentile. Vertical lines represent min and max (although they can extend up to 1.5 × IQR [interquartile range] with points outside of that interval plotted as outliers); *(d)* Violin plots represent double-sided density plots with 25th, 50th, and 75th percentile lines; *(e)* Density plots indicate sample distribution; *(f)* Raincloud plots that combine kernel density plots as "clouds" with accompanying 25th, 50th, and 75th percentile lines, mean ± standard deviation error bars, and jittered points as rain.

TABLE 18.1   Common Descriptive Statistics or Estimators

Sex	N	Mean (cm)	SD (cm)	%CV	Median (cm)	MAD (cm)	IQR (cm)	Mode (cm)	Min (cm)	Max (cm)	Range (cm)	Skew	Kurtosis
Male	50	177.20	11.52	6.50	179.14	12.17	14.01	180.91	146.07	203.28	57.21	−0.24	0.24
Female	50	164.18	9.38	5.71	164.60	8.48	10.46	164.37	142.28	179.03	36.75	−0.59	−0.27

or greater than 1 (positively skewed), the data are considered highly skewed. **Kurtosis** measures the tail heaviness of the distribution and reflects the presence of outliers. High kurtosis in a data set is represented by fatter, longer tails in the direction of the skewness, whereas low kurtosis is indicated by light tails and thus a lack of outliers.

Mean as the Simplest Statistical Model   Sample **mean** can be considered the simplest statistical model. With this estimator, all of the data points are represented by a single quantitative summary. But how does one choose an estimate that represents the sample best? An estimate that has the minimal error represents the optimal metric. Error is defined using a loss function that penalizes difference between a model estimate or prediction and observations. One such loss function is **root mean square error** (RMSE). RMSE represents a measure of the model fit, or, in lay terms, how well a statistical model fits the observed data. A lower RMSE represents lower error and thus a better fit. For example, using body height data from the female group, it is possible to search for a body height estimate that minimizes the RMSE (see figure 18.3). That body height estimate would be considered the best representation of the sample, and thus the simplest statistical model.

As a result of this search, the body height estimate that minimizes the error is 164.18 cm, and the accompanying RMSE is equal to 9.38 cm. As shown in table 18.1, this optimal body height estimate is equal to the sample mean. Standard deviation of the sample is equal to RMSE. From a statistical modeling perspective, the sample mean can then be considered the sample estimate that minimizes the SD, and the sample SD can be seen as a measure of the model fit.

This search for the estimate that minimizes the loss function can be expanded to other statistical models. For example, linear regression can be seen as a search for the line that minimizes RMSE. This approach of estimating model parameters belongs to the family of ordinary least squares (OLS) methods. The example

given here involves only one parameter that needs to be optimized, in this case the height estimate, but real-life problems can involve numerous parameters. The simple search through parameter state-space would take forever when it comes to problems involving more than only a few parameters. Algorithms that solve this computational problem are numerous (e.g., Bayesian inference). The take-home message here is that even simple descriptive statistics can be seen as statistical models.

Effect Sizes   Besides having to describe groups, sport scientists are often interested in comparing them. In order to achieve this, a collection of estimators termed **effect size** statistics can be used. Briefly, in a narrow sense, effect size refers to a family of standardized measures, such as Cohen's *d*, while in a broad sense it refers to any measure of interest, standardized or not. The approach to effect size statistics here involves a broad sense of the definition, in which all group comparisons are considered effect size statistics. In order to estimate effect sizes, one group or variable must be identified as the baseline or control. The most common effect size statistics can be found in table 18.2, where female height is considered control and compared to male height.

The difference, or **mean difference**, is calculated by subtracting group means. **Percent coefficient of variation of the difference** (%CVdiff) is the standard deviation of the difference divided by mean difference. **Percent difference** (%), or mean percent difference, is calculated by dividing mean difference by the mean of the control group, in this case the female group, multiplied by 100. **Mean ratio**, as the name suggests, is a simple ratio between the two means. **Cohen's *d*** represents the standardized effect size, and for this reason, Cohen's *d* is often written as **ES** (short for effect size). Cohen's *d* for independent groups is calculated by dividing mean difference by pooled standard deviation.

Why Cohen's *d* could be used instead of other effect size estimators can be demonstrated by a simple

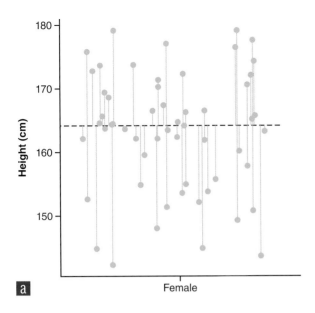

a
Female

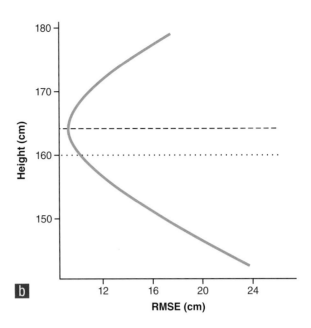

b
RMSE (cm)

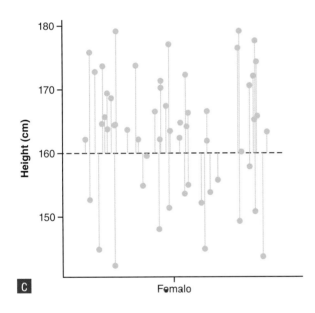

c
Female

FIGURE 18.3   Sample mean as the simplest statistical model. *(a)* Dashed line represents an estimate, in this case the mean of the sample. Vertical lines represent residuals between estimate and observed values. *(b)* Each estimate has a RMSE (root mean square error) value. Central tendency estimate with the lowest RMSE value is the sample mean. *(c)* Similar to *(a)*, this panel depicts residuals for a central tendency estimate with higher RMSE.

TABLE 18.2   Effect Size Statistics for Estimating Differences Between Two Independent Groups

Difference (cm)	SDdiff (cm)[a]	%CVdiff[b]	% Difference	Ratio	Cohen's *d*	Common language effect size	Overlap
13.02	14.86	114.12	7.93	1.08	1.24	0.81	0.54

[a]SDdiff: standard deviation of the difference divided by mean difference.
[b]%CVdiff: percent coefficient of variation of the difference.

example (10). In this study, the authors examined the relationship between performance in the Yo-Yo intermittent recovery test level 1 (Yo-YoIR1) and the 30-15 Intermittent Fitness Test (30-15IFT) and compared the sensitivity of both tests to training. The study used one group with two dependent samples (i.e., pretraining and posttraining). It was then possible to adopt the rationale that comparing estimated effect sizes could be used to establish the difference between two independent groups (i.e., Yo-YoIR1 and 30-15IFT). Table 18.3 presents pretraining results and the effect sizes estimated with percent change and Cohen's d (10).

Since Yo-YoIR1 and 30-15IFT use different scales (i.e., total meters covered and velocity reached, respectively), percent change estimator is not a good choice to compare the effect sizes between the two tests. Instead, Cohen's d is a standardized estimator, so it should be used in comparing tests or measures that have different scales.

After estimating effect sizes, the question that naturally follows is that of **magnitude** (i.e., how big is the size of the effect?). Since Cohen's d is a standardized estimator, it allows for the establishment of magnitude thresholds. Based on the original work by Cohen (13), Hopkins (32, 37) suggested the following magnitudes of effect (see table 18.4). According to table 18.4, the difference in mean height between males and females would be considered large, as well as the changes in Yo-YoIR1, whereas in 30-15IFT it would be considered moderate.

Cohen's d, as well as associated magnitudes of effect, is commonly hard to interpret by nonstatistically trained professionals (e.g., coaches). Consequently, McGraw and Wong (49) suggested a common language effect size (CLES) estimator, which could be more intuitive to understand. The CLES represents the probability that an observation sampled at random from one group will be greater than an observation sampled at random from another group. For example, if a male and female are taken at random from the two sample groups and this was repeated 100 times, how many times would the male be taller than the female (see figure 18.4)?

By simply counting based on 100 random paired samples, males are taller in 84 cases, or 84%. Using probability, that is equal to 0.84. In other words, if someone randomly selects a male and a female from the two groups and bets that the male is taller, the bet would be correct 84% of the time.

The CLES can be estimated using what is called a **brute-force** computational method or an **algebraic** method. The brute-force method involves generating all possible pairwise combinations from the two groups (in the previous example, that is equal to $50 \times 50 = 2,500$ cases), and then simply counting the cases in which males are taller than females. This method can be very computationally intensive. In comparison, the algebraic method assumes normal distribution of the observations in the groups and estimates the **standard deviation of the difference** (note that standard deviation of all pairwise differences estimated with the brute-force method would be very similar to algebraically derived standard deviation of the difference):

$$\text{SD}_{difference} = \sqrt{SD^2_{males} + SD^2_{females}}$$

Algebraically, CLES is then derived assuming normal distribution (where the mean of the distribution is equal to mean difference between the groups, and standard deviation of the distribution is equal to standard deviation of the difference) by calculating probability of the different scores higher than zero (see

TABLE 18.3 Training Intervention Effect Sizes for Yo-YoIR1 and 30-15IFT

Test	Pretraining	% Change	Cohen's d
Yo-YoIR1	1,031 ± 257 m	35%	1.2
30-15IFT	17.4 ± 1.1 km/h	7%	1.1

Data from Buchheit and Rabbani (2014).

TABLE 18.4 Magnitudes of Effect

Magnitude of effect	Trivial	Small	Moderate	Large	Very large	Nearly perfect
Cohen's d	0-0.2	0.2-0.6	0.6-1.2	1.2-2.0	2.0-4.0	>4.0

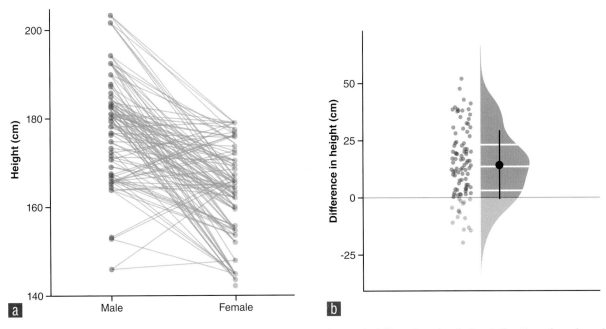

FIGURE 18.4   Drawing 100 pairs at random to estimate the probability of males being taller than females. *(a)* Scatterplot of 100 pairs drawn at random from two samples. Since paired males and females are being compared, lines can be drawn between each of the 100 draws. Blue lines indicate taller males, while orange lines indicate taller females. *(b)* Distribution of difference between males and females for each of the 100 pairs drawn.

figure 18.4*b* for a visual representation). Table 18.2 presents the algebraically computed CLES estimate.

The CLES equivalent is used as a performance metric in class prediction tasks, termed **area under the curve** (AUC), where 0.5 is a predictive performance equal to a random guess, and 1 is perfect predictive separation between two classes (38, 43). **Overlap** (OVL) represents the overlap between the two sample distributions. Provided that samples are equal, the OVL is equal to 1. Provided that there is a complete separation between the two samples, the OVL is equal to 0 (see figure 18.5*a*). Overlap can be estimated with brute-force computational methods (which does not make assumptions regarding sample distribution) and with algebraic methods that make normality assumptions.

Since Cohen's *d*, CLES, and OVL are mathematically related, it is possible to convert one to another (assuming normal distribution of the samples and equal SD between the two groups for the OVL estimation). Figure 18.5*b* depicts the relationship between the Cohen's *d*, CLES, and OVL. Figure 18.5*c* depicts the relationship between the CLES and OVL.

Table 18.5 presents Cohen's *d* magnitudes of effect with accompanying estimated CLES and OCL thresholds.

The Smallest Effect Size of Interest   The **smallest effect size of interest** (SESOI) is the minimum important effect size that has a practical or clinical significance (66). There is no single way to approach definition and estimation of SESOI, but it is usually based on either the known **measurement error** (ME) (e.g., the minimum detectable effect size) or the effect size that is large enough to be practically meaningful (e.g., the smallest worthwhile change) (5, 11, 31, 35, 39, 45, 70, 72). In this chapter, statistical models and estimators that use SESOI are referred to as **magnitude-based**.

To look into magnitude-based estimators, consider ±2.5 cm to be height SESOI, or the difference that would be practically significant. In other words, individuals with a height difference within ±2.5 cm would be considered practically equivalent (from the minimal important effect perspective), or it might be hard to detect this difference with a quick glance (from the minimum detectable effect perspective).

The simplest magnitude-based statistic is **mean difference divided by SESOI range** (difference to SESOI). This estimator, similar to other standardized estimators (e.g., %CVdiff, Cohen's *d*) allows comparison of variables in different scales, but it also gives more insight into differences from a practical

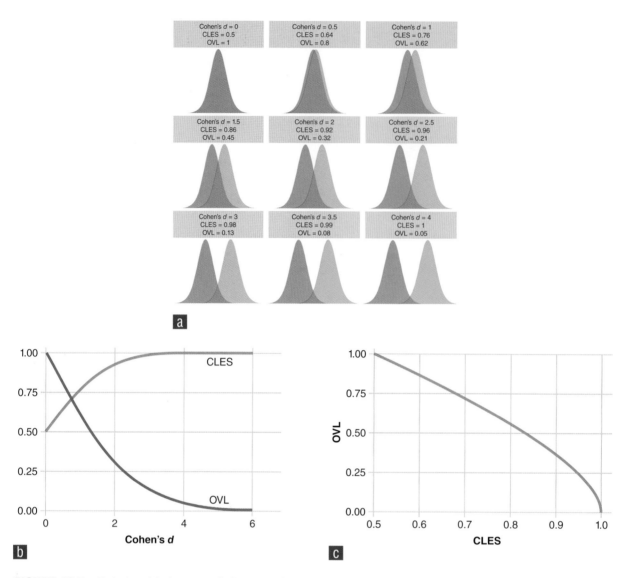

FIGURE 18.5 Relationship between Cohen's *d*, CLES, and OVL. *(a)* Visual display of the samples with varying degrees of separation, and calculated Cohen's *d*, CLES, and OVL. *(b)* Relationship between the CLES and OVL to Cohen's *d*. *(c)* Relationship between CLES and OVL.

TABLE 18.5 Magnitudes of Effect for CLES and OVL Estimated Using Cohen's *d*

Magnitude of effect	Trivial	Small	Moderate	Large	Very large	Nearly perfect
Cohen's *d*	0-0.2	0.2-0.6	0.6-1.2	1.2-2.0	2.0-4.0	>4.0
CLES	0.50-0.56	0.56-0.66	0.66-0.80	0.80-0.92	0.92-1.00	1.00
OVL	1.0-0.92	0.92-0.76	0.76-0.55	0.55-0.32	0.32-0.05	0.00

significance perspective. A second magnitude-based statistic is **standard deviation of the difference divided by SESOI range** (SDdiff to SESOI). This estimator, similar to %CVdiff, would show how variable the differences are compared to SESOI. Similarly, the CLES estimator can become magnitude-based by using SESOI. Rather than being interested in the probability of a random male being taller than a random female (out of the two sample groups), it might be more interesting to estimate how probable lower, trivial, and higher differences (often defined as harmful, trivial, and beneficial) defined by SESOI are.

Using brute-force computational methods and drawing all pairwise combinations from the two groups (i.e., 50 × 50 = 2,500 cases), and using ±2.5 cm SESOI as a trivial difference, probabilities of lower, trivial, and higher difference can be estimated by calculating the proportion of cases within each magnitude band (see figure 18.6). On the figure, the distribution over SESOI (blue) indicates the probability of randomly selected males being taller than randomly selected females, with a height difference of at least SESOI magnitude. The distribution under SESOI (orange) indicates probability of randomly selected females being taller than randomly selected males, with a height difference of at least SESOI magnitude. The gray area indicates the probability of randomly

selecting a male and female with a height difference within the SESOI band.

Table 18.6 shows the estimated probabilities of observing lower, trivial, and higher differences in height between a randomly selected male and female using the brute-force computational method and the algebraic method. These estimates answer a particular question: If a random male and random female are compared from the sample, how probable are lower or trivial or higher magnitudes of difference in height? Asking such a magnitude-based question regarding random individual difference represents a form of prediction questioning and a predictive task. In this chapter, such questions are answered using **magnitude-based prediction** approaches.

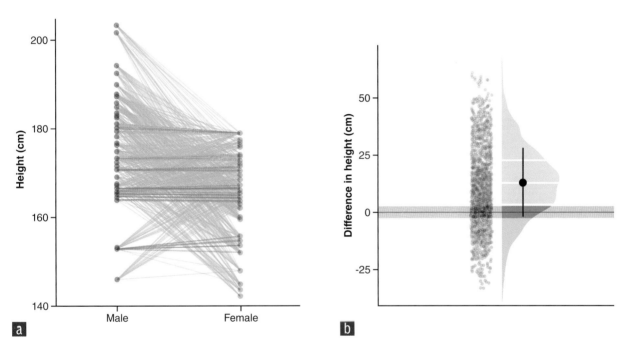

FIGURE 18.6   Pairwise comparison of males and females to estimate probability of lower, trivial, and higher magnitude of difference. *(a)* Scatterplot of all pairwise combinations (50 × 50 = 2,500), drawn randomly out of two samples. Since paired males and females are being compared, lines can be drawn between each 2,500 draws. Blue lines indicate that males are taller than females higher than SESOI; gray lines indicate pairs with a height difference less than or equal to SESOI, while orange lines indicate females taller than males higher than SESOI. *(b)* Distribution of the differences between males and females for all 2,500 pairwise combinations; shaded band indicates SESOI.

TABLE 18.6   Estimated Probability of Observing Lower, Trivial, and Higher Differences in Height

Method	Lower	Trivial	Higher
Brute force	0.13	0.09	0.77
Algebraic	0.15	0.09	0.76

It is common to represent means as a systematic component or fixed effect (e.g., mean difference), and variability around the mean (i.e., $SD_{difference}$) as a stochastic component or **random effect**. It is unfortunate that common statistical modeling and analysis, particularly in sport science, takes the stance of approaching and treating between-individual variation as **random error**. The approach suggested in this chapter complements group-based or average-based statistics with magnitude-based predictions that aim to help answer individual-based questions common to sport practitioners. Table 18.7 presents magnitude-based estimators that can complement common effect size statistics (see table 18.2) when one is comparing two independent groups.

Comparing Dependent Groups

To better understand dependent samples, or paired-sample analysis, it is helpful to consider a simple pretest (pre) and posttest (post) experimental design, a training intervention for a group of males (N = 10) who undertook bench press training. The training intervention required participants to perform the bench press two times a week for 16 weeks. The 1RM load was assessed before (pre) and after (post) the training intervention. The two samples are dependent because they are from the same participants. Table 18.8 contains individual pre and post scores, as well as the change (kg) in the bench press 1RM. As the table shows, some of the participants showed an increase in the weight, and some did not.

Describing Groups as Independent

Table 18.9 contains descriptive statistics applied to pre, post, and change scores in the bench press 1RM for the intervention group. Figure 18.7 visualizes the scores using three raincloud plots.

TABLE 18.7 Magnitude-Based Effect Sizes for Estimating Differences Between Two Independent Groups

SESOI lower (cm)	SESOI upper (cm)	Difference to SESOI	SDdiff to SESOI	Lower	Trivial	Higher
-2.5	2.5	2.6	2.97	0.15	0.09	0.76

TABLE 18.8 Individual Pre and Post Scores, and the Change in Bench Press 1RM

Athlete	Pre (kg)	Post (kg)	Change (kg)
Athlete 01	102.86	107.37	4.52
Athlete 02	103.88	106.58	2.71
Athlete 03	96.19	92.13	−4.07
Athlete 04	101.01	109.06	8.05
Athlete 05	103.02	127.07	24.06
Athlete 06	88.60	82.72	−5.87
Athlete 07	107.51	104.67	−2.84
Athlete 08	99.01	127.63	28.62
Athlete 09	104.39	127.14	22.75
Athlete 10	93.75	129.98	36.23

TABLE 18.9 Descriptive Analysis of Pretest, Posttest, and Changes as Independent Samples

Test	N	Mean (kg)	SD (kg)	% CV	Median (kg)	MAD (kg)	IQR (kg)	Mode (kg)	Min (kg)	Max (kg)	Range (kg)	Skew	Kurtosis
Pretest	10	100.02	5.71	5.71	101.93	3.99	6.76	102.85	88.60	107.51	18.91	−0.64	−0.87
Posttest	10	111.44	16.28	14.61	108.22	25.91	21.98	127.90	82.72	129.98	47.26	−0.30	−1.39
Change		*11.41*	*15.19*	*133.12*	*6.28*	*16.68*	*25.19*	*−0.11*	*−5.87*	*36.23*	*42.10*	*0.32*	*−1.68*

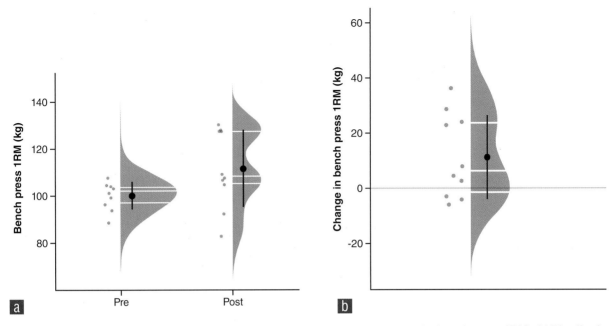

FIGURE 18.7   Raincloud plots of the pretest, posttest, and change scores in the bench press 1RM. *(a)* Distribution of the pretest and posttest scores. *(b)* Distribution of the change score.

Effect Size Estimators for Difference and Change

Table 18.10 contains the most common effect size estimators used when describing the change in pre and post paired data. The terminology used in this chapter differentiates between the **difference**, which is used for independent groups, and the **change**, which is used in paired or dependent groups.

The **mean change** (or simply change) is calculated by the change score. The standard deviation of the change (SDchange) is a standard deviation of the change values. It represents a measure of dispersion of the change scores. The percent coefficient of variation of the change (%CVchange) is the standard deviation of the change divided by mean change, multiplied by 100. **Percent change**, or **mean percent change**, is calculated by taking a mean of the ratio between the change and the pretest, multiplied by 100. **Mean ratio**

represents the mean of the post to pre ratios. Cohen's *d* represents standardized effect size of the change. In the paired design, Cohen's *d* is calculated by dividing the mean change by the standard deviation of the pretest scores. The CLES, for the paired samples, represents the probability of observing a positive change; OVL, for independent groups, represents the overlap between the pre and post scores.

Magnitude-based effect size estimators involve the use of SESOI and are presented in table 18.11. Similar to magnitude-based effect size estimators with independent groups, magnitude-based effect size estimators with paired samples involve change to SESOI and SDchange to SESOI, as well as proportions of lower, trivial, and higher change scores. Figure 18.8 depicts how proportions of lower, trivial, and higher change scores are estimated. As with two independent groups,

TABLE 18.10   Effect Size Statistics for Estimating Change in Two Dependent Groups

Change (kg)	SDchange (kg)	%CVchange	% Change	Ratio	Cohen's *d*	CLES	OVL
11.41	15.19	133.12	11.42	1.11	2.0	0.77	0.64

TABLE 18.11   Magnitude-Based Effect Size Statistics for Estimating the Change Between Two Dependent Groups

SESOI (kg)	Change to SESOI	SDchange to SESOI	Lower	Trivial	Higher
±5	1.14	1.52	0.14	0.20	0.66

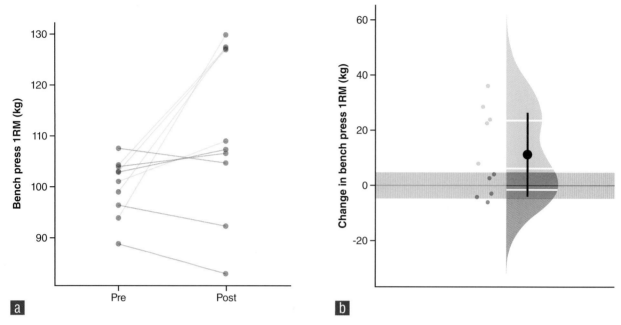

FIGURE 18.8 Visual analysis of the dependent group scores using SESOI. *(a)* Scatterplot of pretest and posttest scores. Green lines indicate changes higher than SESOI upper, gray lines indicate change within the SESOI band, and the red line indicates a negative change lower than SESOI. *(b)* Distribution of the change scores. Green area represents proportion of change scores higher than SESOI upper; red area represents proportion of negative change scores lower than SESOI lower; and gray area indicates trivial change, which is within the SESOI band.

these proportions can be estimated using the brute-force method (i.e., simply counting the change scores within lower, trivial, and higher zones) or the algebraic method, where SDchange is used and an assumption of normally distributed change scores is made.

Using the data shown in tables 18.8 through 18.11, it might be tempting to claim that the training intervention is causing changes in the bench press 1RM, but one should be cautious about drawing that conclusion. It is important to keep in mind that the effect size estimators are used only descriptively, without any causal connotation. In order to make causal claims, further criteria need to be taken into account (see the "Causal Inference" section).

Associations Between Two Variables

So far, single variable descriptive statistics have been dealt with. However, sport scientists are often interested in the relationship or association between two variables. One of these variables takes the role of the **dependent variable** (outcome or target variable) and the other of the **independent variable** (or predictor variable). For example, assume that female soccer players (N = 30) were tested using two tests: Yo-YoIR1 and maximum aerobic speed (MAS) test.

Figure 18.9 depicts the association between these two tests using a scatterplot.

Pearson product-moment correlation coefficient (Pearson's *r*) is a measure of the strength of the linear relationship between two variables. Pearson's *r* is a

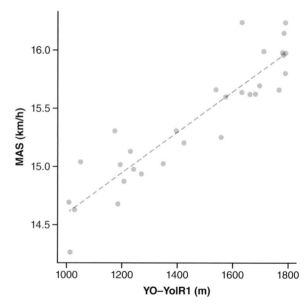

FIGURE 18.9 Scatterplot between two variables. Dashed line represents linear regression line.

standardized measure that can take values ranging from −1 to +1, where 0 indicates no relationship, and −1 and +1 indicate a perfect relationship. Negative Pearson's *r* values represent negative association (i.e., as one variable increases, the other decreases), while positive Pearson's *r* values represent a positive association (i.e., as one variable increases, so does the other one). **R-squared** (R^2) represents the variance explained, or how much the model explains the variance in the target variable. In this example the model is linear regression. *R*-squared is the standardized measure of association that can take values ranging from zero (no association, or no variance explained) to 1 (perfect association, or all variance explained). *R*-squared, as its name suggests, represents Pearson's *r* squared. **Maximal information coefficient** (MIC) is a novel measure of the strength of the linear or nonlinear association between two variables and belongs to the **maximal information-based nonparametric exploration** (MINE) class of statistics (1, 62). The MIC is a standardized measure of association that can take values ranging from zero (no association) to 1 (perfect association). As opposed to Pearson's *r*, MIC can detect nonlinear association between two variables. The statistical model, or the machinery underlying Pearson *r* and *R*-squared, is linear regression. Similar to a sample mean, linear regression can be seen as an optimization algorithm that tries to find the line passing through the data with minimal error.

Although measures of association between two variables, such as Pearson's *r* and *R*-squared, are symmetrical (meaning that it does not matter which variable is predictor or target), one cannot reverse the linear regression equation to get Yo-YoIR1 from MAS.

Prediction

Predictive modeling is defined as "the process of applying a statistical model or data mining algorithms to data for the purpose of predicting new or future observations" (69). Usually, a predictive statistical model is treated as a black box and implies that the focus is not on underlying mechanisms and relationships between predictor variables, but rather on the predictive performance of the model (9, 69, 75).

Linear regression (as previously discussed) can be used to help answer prediction questions (e.g., "If I know someone's Yo-YoIR1 score, what would that person's MAS score be?"), rather than those considering association (e.g., "How is Yo-YoIR1 related to MAS?"). This section introduces essential concepts of predictive analysis that are needed to

answer such questions. Firstly, some overarching provisos relating to prediction must be considered.

Overfitting

Imagine that the true relationship between back squat (BS) relative 1RM and vertical jump height during a bodyweight squat jump is known. This true relationship is referred to as a **data generating process** (DGP) (12), and one of the aims of causal inference tasks is to uncover parameters and mechanisms of DGP from the acquired sample. With predictive tasks, this aim is of no direct interest, but rather a reliable prediction regarding new or unseen observations. The DGP is usually unknown; but with simulations, such as this one, DGP can be known, and it is used to generate the sample data. Simulation is thus an excellent teaching tool since one can play with the problem and understand how the statistical analysis works—because the true DGP is known and can be compared with estimates (12, 33, 65). The DGP is assumed to consist of **systematic component** *f(X)* and **stochastic component** ε.

The systematic component is assumed to be fixed in the population (constant from sample to sample) and captures the true relationship *f(X)* among variables in the population (e.g., this can also be termed the **signal**), while the stochastic component represents random noise or random error, which varies from sample to sample. Random error is assumed to be normally distributed with a mean of zero and standard deviation that represents an estimated parameter (with either RMSE or RSE). Thus, RMSE or RSE are estimates of ε.

The objective of causal inference or explanatory modeling is to estimate the *f(X)* (estimate is indicated with the hat symbol: $\hat{f}(X)$), or to understand the underlying DGP. With predictive analysis, the goal is to find the best estimate of *Y* or $\hat{y}$. The underlying DGP is treated as a black box.

To demonstrate the concept of overfitting, two samples (N = 35 observations) from the DGP with relative BS ranging from 0.8 to 2.5 are generated. These samples are training and testing samples (see figure 18.10). The training sample is used to train the prediction model, while the testing sample will be used as a "holdout" sample for evaluating the model performance on the unseen data.

The model used to predict squat jump from BS is **polynomial linear regression**. Note that first degree polynomial functions represent simple linear regression. Increasing polynomial degrees increases the flexibility of the polynomial regression model,

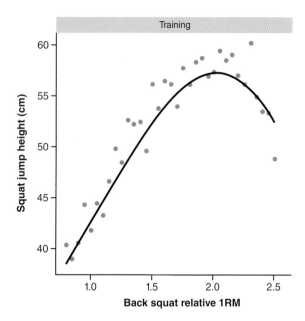 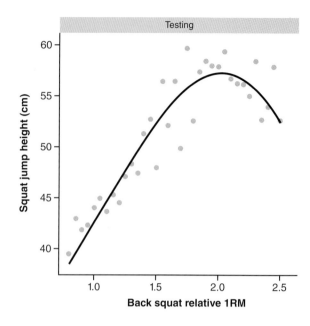

FIGURE 18.10 Two samples simulated from the known DGP. Black line represents the systematic component of the DGP and is equal for both training and testing samples. Observations vary in the two samples due to the stochastic component in the DGP.

thus can represent a **tuning parameter** that can be selected based on the model performance. Indeed, if the flexibility of a model is increased, the error within the model is progressively minimized. However, increasing order can be performed infinitely, and therefore it is more appropriate to adopt a fixed modeling approach using the systematic component of the DGP. In other words, the focus will be on finding the polynomial degree that minimized model error (or alternatively maximized model fit). Statistically, model fit can then be evaluated using the **similarity factor** (*f2*), which is the logarithmic reciprocal square root transformation of the sum of squared error, and represents a measurement of the similarity in the percent dissolution between two polynomial curves (see figure 18.10).

Cross-Validation

In order to evaluate the predictive performance of a model, sport scientists usually remove some percentage of data and use it as a testing or holdout sample. Unfortunately, this is not always possible (although it is recommended, particularly to evaluate final model performance, especially when there are multiple models and there is much model tuning). One solution to this problem is cross-validation (38, 43, 75). There are numerous variations of cross-validation, but the simplest one is **n-fold cross-validation** (see

figure 18.11). N-fold cross-validation involves splitting the data into 5 to 10 equal "folds" and using 1-fold as a testing or hold-out sample while performing model training on the other folds. This is repeated over N-iterations (in this case 5-10), and the model performance is averaged to establish the cross-validated model performance.

With predictive analysis and machine learning, different models' tuning parameters are evaluated (as well as multiple different models) to estimate the one that gives the best predictive performance. It is thus important to use techniques such as cross-validation to avoid overfitting or overly optimistic model selection.

Interpretability

As explained earlier, predictive models prioritize predictive performance over explanation of the underlying DGP mechanism (which is treated as a black box). However, sometimes it may be valuable to know which predictor is the most important, how predictions change when a particular predictor changes, or why a model made a particular prediction for a case of interest (43, 53, 63). **Model interpretability** can be defined as "the degree to which a human can understand the cause of a decision" (50, 53). Some models are more inherently interpretable (e.g., linear regression), and some are indeed very complex and

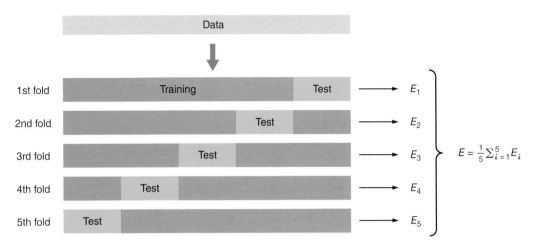

FIGURE 18.11   Cross-validation.

hard to interpret (e.g., neural networks). There are, however, model-agnostic techniques that can help increase model interpretability (53, 54), though they are beyond the scope of this chapter.

Magnitude-Based Prediction Estimators

As with the magnitude-based estimators used to address association between two variables as discussed earlier, one can use target variable SESOI to get magnitude-based estimates of predictive performance. Rather than using RMSE as an estimate of the model fit in training data, one can instead use cross-validated RMSE (cvRMSE) and SESOI.

Continuing with the squat jump and relative squat 1RM example, one can assume that the SESOI in the squat jump is ±1 cm. For the sake of this example, one can feature engineer (43, 44) the relative squat 1RM variable to include 20-degree polynomials. This way, 20 predictor variables have been created. In order to avoid overfitting, an elastic-net model (18) is used, as well as repeated cross-validation involving three splits repeated 10 times. Predictive model performance is evaluated by using cross-validated RMSE, together with magnitude-based performance estimators.

Elastic-net models represent a regression method that linearly combines the *L1* and *L2* penalties of the lasso and ridge methods, or alpha and lambda tuning parameters (18, 38, 43). A total of nine combinations of tuning parameters is evaluated using repeated cross-validation, and the model with minimal cvRMSE is selected as the best one. Performance metrics of the best model are further reported. Table 18.12 presents cross-validated best model performance metrics together with model performance on the cross-validated data set.

Using *a priori* known SESOI provides a practical anchor to evaluate predictive model performance. Reported SESOI to cvRMSE (1.11), as well as cvEquivalence (0.41), indicates very poor predictive performance of the model. Therefore, in practical terms, using relative squat 1RM does not produce practically meaningful predictions given SESOI of ±1 cm and the model, as well as the data sample used.

Model performance can also be visualized by using the training data set (see figure 18.12). The gray band in figure 18.12, *a* and *b*, represents SESOI, and as can be observed visually, model residuals are much wider than SESOI, therefore indicating poor practical predictive performance.

Predictive tasks focus on providing the best predictions on novel or unseen data without concern for the underlying DGP. Predictive model performance can be evaluated by using magnitude-based approaches to give insights into the practical significance of the predictions. These magnitude-based prediction estimators can be used to complement explanatory or causal inference tasks, rather than relying solely on the group-based and average-based estimators.

Causal Inference

Two broad classes of inferential question focus on "what if" and "why," **Forward causal inference** is the "what if" scenario ("What would happen to the unit or group with or without treatment X?"), and **reverse causal inference** is the "why" scenario ("What causes Y, and why?") (19). Forward causation is a more

TABLE 18.12   Common Predictive Metrics and Magnitude-Based Predictive Metrics*

SESOI (cm)	cvRMSE (cm)	SESOI to cvRMSE	cvEquivalence	RMSE (cm)	SESOI to RMSE	Equivalence
±1	1.79	1.11	0.41	1.53	1.3	0.48

*Metrics starting with "cv" indicate cross-validated performance metrics. Metrics without "cv" indicate performance metrics on the training data set, which is often more optimistic.

Equivalence represents a proportion of residuals inside the SESOI band. In other words, the proportion of trivial differences between observed and predicted scores.

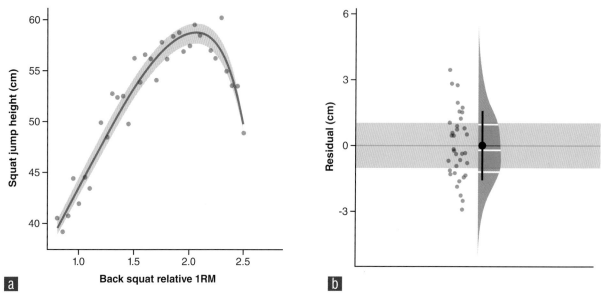

a

b

FIGURE 18.12 Model performance on the training data set. *(a)* Model with the lowest cvRMSE is selected. SESOI is depicted as a gray band around the model prediction (blue line). *(b)* Residuals scatterplot. Residuals outside of the SESOI (gray band) indicate prediction where error is practically significant. Equivalence represents proportion of residuals inside the SESOI band.

clearly defined problem, where the goal is to quantify the causal effect of a treatment or intervention. Questions of forward causation are most directly studied using randomization (19) and are answered from the causality-as-intervention and counterfactual perspectives. Reverse causation is more complex and is more related to explaining the causal chains using the **system-variable** approach. In this chapter the main focus is on forward causation. The challenge is to find a parameter θ that characterizes the causal inference of X on Y and find a way to estimate θ. The data can come from a controlled, randomized experiment or an observational study. In this chapter, causal inference is approached from the **counterfactual theory** or **potential outcomes** perspective (4, 19, 25, 40, 61) that defines causes in terms of how things would have been different had

the cause not occurred, as well as from the **causality-as-intervention** perspective (19), which necessitates clearly defined interventions (21, 23, 27).

Correlation Is Not Causation

Does playing basketball (X) make you taller (Y)? This is an example of a causal question, an attempt to establish a correlation between these two phenomena. But correlations (cause-and-effect questions) can lead to wrong assumptions. A popular example has been used elsewhere (58, 59, 60, 61). Figure 18.13 shows the correlative relationship between a variable A (e.g., exercise) and a variable B (e.g., cholesterol) (which looks like a causal relationship but is not). If one just looks at the correlative relationship between variables A and B, the relationship appears to be causal. But this correlation actually happens because

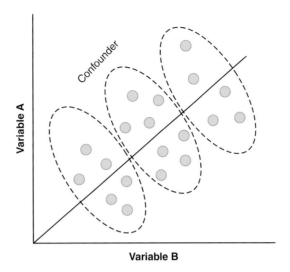

FIGURE 18.13 Why the logic of association is inefficient. An example of the relationship between variable A (cholesterol) and variable B (exercise).

both variables share a common cause or confounder, which, in this example, could be age. The dashed ovals represent groups of ascending ages.

Using the descriptive estimators introduced in the "Description" section, one can quickly calculate the group means and SDs, as well as their difference (see table 18.13). However, does this mean the difference between basketball and control represents an average causal effect? No, unfortunately it does not.

Potential Outcomes or Counterfactuals

To explain why this is the case, an alternate counterfactual reality needs to be imagined. What is needed are two potential outcomes: $Height_0$, which represents the height of the person if that person does not play basketball, and $Height_1$, which represents the height of the person if that person plays basketball (see table 18.14). As can be guessed, the basketball group has known $Height_1$, but unknown $Height_0$, and vice versa for the control group.

Unfortunately, these potential outcomes are unknown, as well as the individual causal effects. It is unknown what might have happened to individual outcomes in a counterfactual world (i.e., alternate reality). A good control group serves as a proxy to reveal what might have happened "on average" to the treated group in the counterfactual world where they are not treated. Since the basketball data is simulated, the exact DGP is known (the true systematic or fixed causal effect of playing basketball on height is exactly zero), which again demonstrates the use of simulations

as a great learning tool, in this case for understanding the underlying causal mechanisms. Individual causal effect in this case is the difference between two potential outcomes: $Height_1$ and $Height_0$.

The observed mean group difference (11.26 cm) is due to average causal effect (−0.27 cm) and selection bias (11.52 cm). In other words, observed mean group difference can be explained solely by selection bias. This is indeed true, since the DGP that generated the sample data involved zero systematic causal effect of playing basketball on height.

On top of the selection bias involved in the example presented, other **confounders** might be involved, such as age, sex, race, experience, and others, some of which can be measured and some of which might be unknown. These are also referred to as the **third variable** (or **omitted variable**) that confounds the causal relationship between the treatment and the outcome. In the example presented, all subjects from the basketball group might be older males, whereas all the subjects from the control group might be younger females, and this could explain the group differences rather than a causal effect of playing basketball. According to Hernán (22) and Hernán and Robins (26), three types of biases are involved in causal inference: (a) confounding, (b) selection, and (c) measurement bias. **Confounding** is the bias that arises when treatment and outcome share causes. This happens because treatment was not randomly assigned (22, 26). For example, athletes who are taller might be choosing to play basketball due to success and enjoyment in

TABLE 18.13 Descriptive Analysis of the Groups

	Mean (cm)	SD (cm)
Basketball	198.50	5.20
Control	187.24	7.20
Difference	11.26	8.88

TABLE 18.14 Counterfactuals of Potential Outcomes That Are Unknown

Athlete	Treatment	Height$_0$ (cm)	Height$_1$ (cm)	Height (cm)	Causal effect (cm)
Athlete 07	Basketball	???	205	205	???
Athlete 01	Basketball	???	203	203	???
Athlete 05	Basketball	???	199	199	???
Athlete 03	Basketball	???	194	194	???
Athlete 09	Basketball	???	193	193	???
Athlete 08	Control	198	???	198	???
Athlete 06	Control	189	???	189	???
Athlete 02	Control	187	???	187	???
Athlete 10	Control	185	???	185	???
Athlete 04	Control	178	???	178	???

contrast to their shorter peers. On the other hand, it might be some hidden confounder that motivates tall athletes to choose basketball. Known and measured confounders from observational studies can be taken into account to create ceteris paribus conditions when one is estimating causal effects (4, 22, 26, 47, 64, 70).

STATISTICAL INFERENCE

Generalizing from a small sample to a larger population is known as making **inferences**. **Population** refers to all the members of a specific group (i.e., everyone in a well-defined group), whereas **sample** refers to a part or subset of that population.

The difference between the true population parameter and a sample estimate is due to the **sampling error**. When one is performing simulations, the true population parameters are known, but in real life there is uncertainty about the true parameters, and this uncertainty needs to be quantified in some way. This is the goal of **statistical inference**: that is, to generalize about a population from a given sample while taking into account uncertainties of the estimates.

Statistical Inference and Probabilities

The theory of statistical inference rests on describing uncertainties by using **probability**. Since there are two kinds of uncertainty, there are two kinds of probabilities. Aleatory uncertainties are described using **long-frequency** definitions of probability. For example, it can happen that when rolling a six-sided die you toss a 6 four times in a row, but in the long run (meaning here infinite number of times), the probability of tossing a 6 is equal to 1/6, or a probability of 0.166, or 16.6% (assuming fair dice, of course). Probability viewed from this perspective represents a long-frequency distribution, or the number of occurrences of the event of interest divided by number of total events. It is a number between 0 and 1. 0 means the event of interest will never happen while 1 means it will always happen.

There are two major schools of statistical inference, **frequentist** (i.e., leaning on long-frequency interpretation of probability) and **Bayesian** (leaning on degree-of-belief interpretation of probability) (16, 17, 20).

Frequentist Perspective

Using simulations is an outstanding teaching tool (12, 33) and very useful for understanding the frequentist inference. In frequentist inference, probabilities are calculated and revolve around sampling distributions.

Figure 18.14 shows a hypothetical population in which the true mean height is 177.8 cm and the standard deviation is 10.16 cm (On the left side [a], we have a scenario where N = 5 athletes are randomly sampled for the population, while on the right side [b] we have N = 20 athletes randomly sampled). Individuals are represented as blue dots (see figure 18.14, c and d), and the estimated mean height is represented by the orange dots. Then, this sampling is repeated 50 times as well as the mean for every sample calculated, and the distribution of the sampled means drawn (see figure 18.14, e and f). This distribution is called **sampling distribution of the sample mean**, and the standard deviation of this distribution is referred to as **standard error** or **sampling error**. Since the estimate of interest is the mean, the standard deviation of the sampling distribution of the mean is called **standard error of the mean** (SEM). In figure 18.14, e and f, the mean of the sampling means is designated by a black dot, and error bars represent SEM.

As represented in figure 18.13f, the larger the sample, the smaller the standard error, which is visually seen as narrower sampling distribution.

Sampling

Although the sampling distribution of the mean looks like a normal distribution, it actually belongs to the Student's t-distribution, which has fatter tails for smaller samples (see figure 18.15). Besides mean and standard deviation, Student's t-distribution also has **degrees of freedom** (DF), which is equal to N – 1 for the sample mean. Normal distribution is equal to Student's t-distribution when the degrees of freedom are infinitely large.

Since Student's t-distribution is fatter on the tails, critical values that cover 90%, 95%, and 99% of distribution mass are different from those commonly used for the normal distribution. Table 18.15 contains critical values for different degrees of freedom. For example, 90% of the sampling distribution will be inside the $\bar{x} \pm 1.64 \times$ SEM interval for the normal distribution, but for Student's t with DF = 5, 90% of the sampling distribution will be inside the $\bar{x} \pm 2.02 \times$ SEM interval.

Confidence Intervals and Estimation

The uncertainty of an estimated parameter can be represented with **confidence intervals** (CI). This implies that when sampling is repeated an infinite number of times, a 95% CI will capture a true parameter value 95% of the time. Assuming that in a sample (N = 20) the mean height is 177.8 cm (and SD is 10.16 cm), the calculated 95% CIs will capture true population parameter 95% of the time. Confidence intervals can use different levels of confidence (e.g., 90%, 95%, 99% [17]) They are a great solution for visualizing uncertainties around estimates (see figure 18.16 on page 278).

NULL-HYPOTHESIS SIGNIFICANCE TESTING

There are two approaches to statistical inference: (a) **hypothesis testing** and (b) **estimation** (14, 42). **Null-hypothesis significance testing** (NHST) is still one of the most common approaches to statistical inference, if not the most common, although it is heavily criticized (see references 14, 42). In order to make inferences about a population, one uses a sample of the population. When using NHST, the sample parameter is going to be tested against a null hypothesis (H_0), which often takes the "no effect" value. For example, imagine that you know the true population mean height of a country, but in one particular region, the mean height of the sample differs from the population mean; NHST tests how likely you are to observe the sample mean given the null hypothesis (i.e., mean height of a country).

Figure 18.17 (page 279) shows the population mean height as the null hypothesis, and the estimated probabilities of observing a sample mean of 180 cm (N = 5), 182.5 cm (N = 10), and 185 cm (N = 20). A one-sided approach is used for estimating probability of observing these sample mean heights. A one-sided approach is used when the direction of the effect is certain. The two-sided approach is depicted also; this calculates the probability for the effect of the unknown direction.

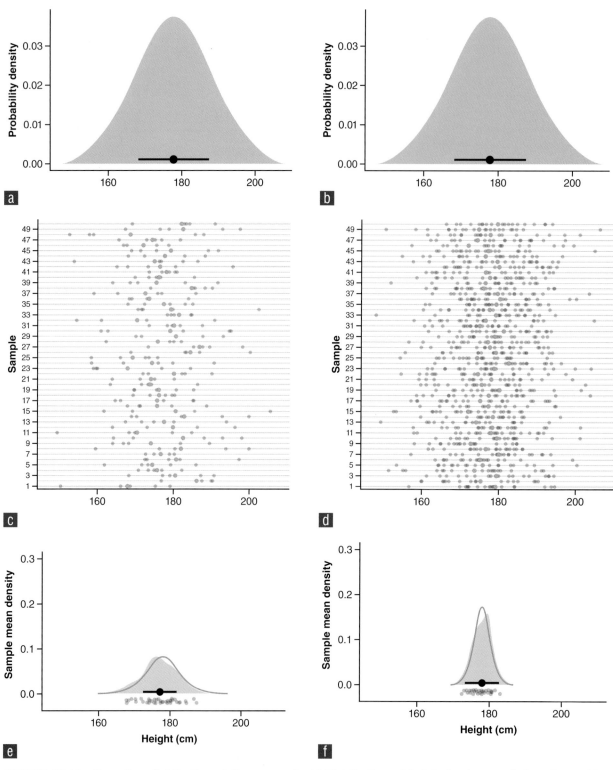

FIGURE 18.14 Sampling distribution of the mean. *(a, b)* Distribution of height in the population. From this population samples are drawn. Fifty samples are taken with N = 5 *(c)* and N = 20 *(d)* observations. Each observation is indicated by a blue dot. Calculated mean, as a parameter of interest, is indicated by an orange dot. *(e, f)* Distribution of collected sample means from *(c)* and *(d)*. This distribution of the sample means is narrower, indicating higher precision when higher N is used. The black dot indicates the mean of the sample means, with error bars indicating SD of the sample means. Orange lines represent hypothetical distribution of the sample means when number of samples is infinitely large.

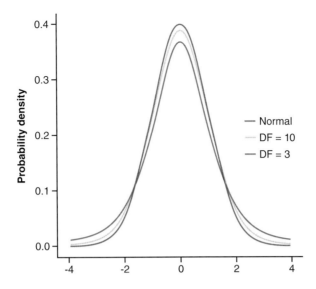

FIGURE 18.15   Example of Student's t-distribution.

DF = degrees of freedom.

TABLE 18.15   Critical Values for Student's t-Distribution With Different Degrees of Freedom

	50%	90%	95%	99%	99.9%
DF = 5	0.73	2.02	2.57	4.03	6.87
DF = 10	0.70	1.81	2.23	3.17	4.59
DF = 20	0.69	1.72	2.09	2.85	3.85
DF = 30	0.68	1.70	2.04	2.75	3.65
DF = 50	0.68	1.68	2.01	2.68	3.50
(Normal)	0.97	1.64	1.96	2.58	3.29

In this example, that would be a sample mean height difference of ±2.2, ±4.7, ±7.2 cm or larger.

The calculated probability of observing a sample mean (or larger) is called the **p-value**. It is easy to interpret p-values as probability of the null hypothesis ($p[H\{O\}|Data]$), but that is incorrect. P-values are correctly interpreted as a probability of obtaining data assuming the null hypothesis is correct (given a null hypothesis). Figure 18.17 shows how different sample sizes will produce different p-values for the same mean difference. This happens because sampling distribution of the mean will be narrower (i.e., smaller SEM) as the sample size increases, and the p-value will be smaller as the sample size increases. It is thus important to realize that p-values do not reveal anything about the magnitude of the effect. In the case of sample mean, a *t*-test is performed by using the calculated *t* value and appropriate Student's t-distribution (see figure 18.14; table 18.16). Once the

p-value is estimated, one can reject the null hypothesis or not.

Out of sheer convenience, alpha is set to 0.1 (10% error), 0.05 (5% error), or 0.01 (1% error). If a p-value is smaller than alpha, the null hypothesis can be rejected, and it will be stated that the effect does have statistical significance. Keep in mind that this does not imply the magnitude of the effect, only that the sample data come from a different population as assumed by the null hypothesis (see table 18.16). For example, in a sample of 20 participants where the mean height is 185 cm, using the known population mean (177.8 cm) and SD (10.16 cm), the *t*-test yields *t* = 3.17. Can the null hypothesis be rejected using a two-sided test and alpha = 0.05? We must check that DF = 20 (which is not exact, but it will serve the purpose), and 95% of sample distribution (with alpha = 0.05) will be within ±2.08. Since *t* was 3.17, which is higher than 2.08, the null hypothesis can therefore be rejected (see figure 18.16*b*).

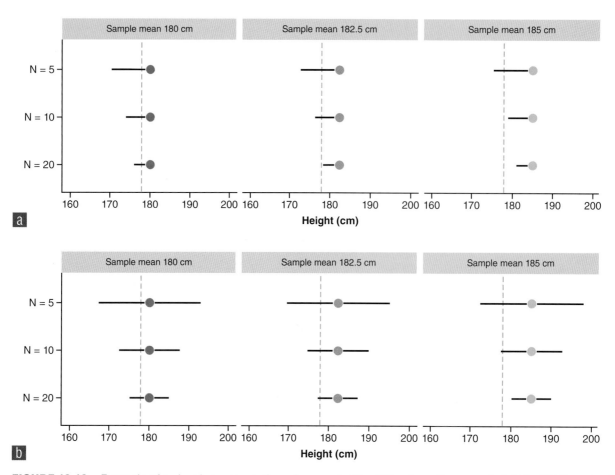

FIGURE 18.16 Example of a visual representation of a sample (N = 20), where the mean height is 177.8 cm (and SD is 10.16 cm), and confident intervals are calculated at 95%.

- **Type I error**, also called alpha (α), refers to making the error of rejecting the null hypothesis when the null hypothesis is true.
- **Type II error**, also called beta (β), refers to making the error of rejecting the alternate hypothesis when it is true.

Type I and Type II errors are inversely related; the more willingness to make Type I errors, the less likeliness to make Type II errors, and vice versa (see table 18.16). It is important to keep in mind that with NHST any hypothesis is either rejected or not.

Statistical Power

Assuming that the alternate hypothesis is true, the probability of rejecting the null hypothesis is equal to 1 − β. This represents the **statistical power** and depends on the magnitude of the effect one aims to detect (or not reject). Figure 18.18 (page 280) gives

examples of one-sided and two-sided statistical power calculations and the null hypothesis for difference in sample mean height (alpha of 0.05), for ±2.5, ±5, and ±7.5 cm (+2.5, +5, and +7.5 cm for one-sided test) in N = 5, N = 10, and N = 20.

The higher the magnitude of the effect, the more likely one is to detect the difference in height means (by rejecting the null hypothesis). Statistical power is mostly used when planning studies to estimate the sample size needed to detect effects of magnitude of interest—for example, if one wants to know what sample size is needed to detect a 2.5-cm difference (with 80% power, alpha 0.05) and is expecting a sample SD of 10 cm.

Minimum Effect Tests

Rather than using null hypothesis of no effect, sport scientists can also perform one-sided NHSTs by using SESOI thresholds to infer practical significance. These

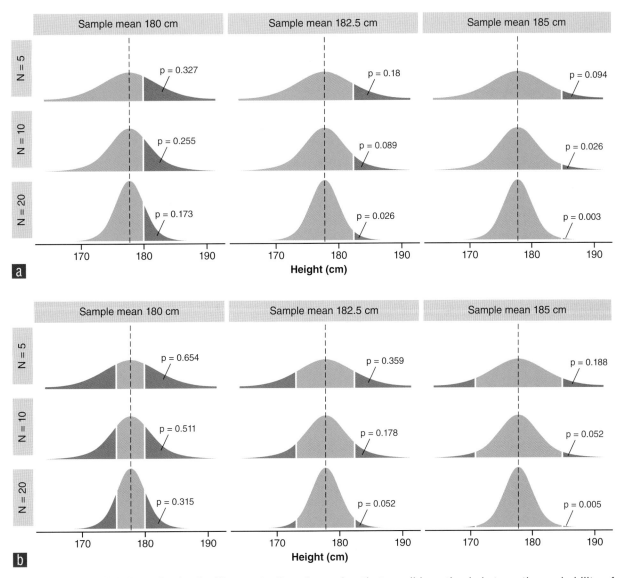

FIGURE 18.17   Null-hypothesis significance testing. Assuming that a null hypothesis is true, the probability of observing a sample parameter of a given magnitude or larger is estimated by calculating proportions of sampling distribution that are over sample parameter value. The larger the sample size, the smaller the width of the sampling distribution. *(a)* One-sided approach is used when one is certain about the direction of the effect. *(b)* Two-sided approach is used when the expected direction of the effect is unknown.

are called **minimum effect tests** (METs) and can distinguish between six different conclusions: lower, not higher, trivial, not lower, higher, and equivocal effect (6, 68) (see figure 18.19).

Note that in an example in which 95% CIs cross the null hypothesis, NHST will yield p > 0.05. This means that the null hypothesis is not rejected and the results are not statistically significant. Confidence intervals can be thus used to visually inspect and conclude whether or not the null hypothesis would be rejected if NHST is performed.

MAGNITUDE-BASED INFERENCE

Batterham as well as Hopkins and colleagues (7, 37) proposed a novel approach to making meaningful inferences about magnitudes, called **magnitude-based inference** (MBI). This approach has been criticized (6, 8, 15, 36, 55, 67, 68, 74) for interpreting CIs as Bayesian credible intervals and for not controlling for Type I and Type II errors.

Clinical MBI considers that one would use a treatment (e.g., program, training, intervention) if the effect

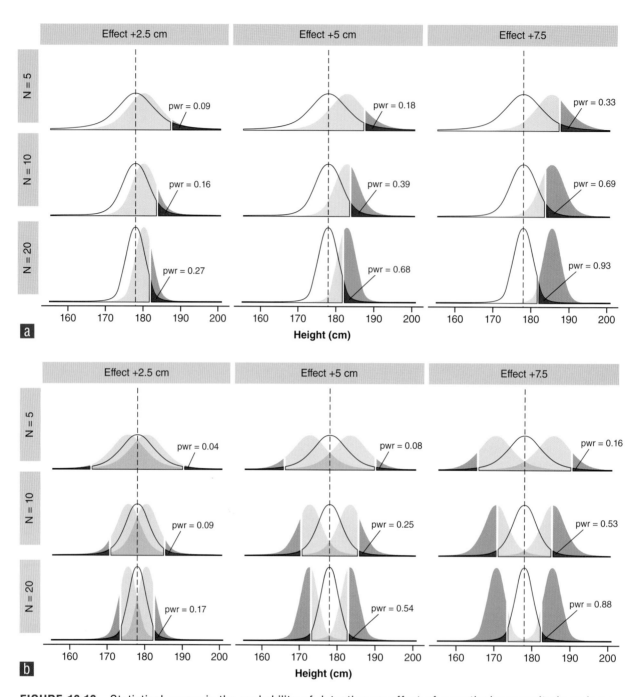

FIGURE 18.18 Statistical power is the probability of detecting an effect of a particular magnitude or larger. Statistical power is shown in dark blue and represents the probability of rejecting the null hypothesis given that the alternative hypothesis is true. (a) One-sided approach. (b) Two-sided approach.

TABLE 18.16 Type I and Type II Errors

	True H_0	True H_a
Rejected H_0	Type I	
Rejected H_a		Type II

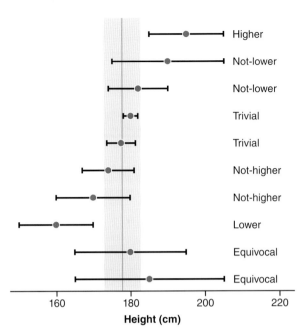

FIGURE 18.19 Inference about magnitudes of effect. Representation of SESOI between six magnitude-based conclusions.

is possibly beneficial and most unlikely harmful. Probabilities are interpreted with regard to whether the true effect is beneficial, trivial, or harmful, and have to do with acceptable uncertainty or adequate precision. For clear effects, the sport scientist describes the likelihood of the effect being beneficial, trivial, or harmful using the scale provided in table 18.17.

In **nonclinical MBI**, the inference is about whether the effect could be substantially positive or negative, rather than beneficial or harmful effects.

As mentioned earlier, CIs do not convey any probability distribution information about the true parameter. Although CIs, Bayesian credible intervals (with flat or noninformative prior distribution), and bootstrap CIs tend to converge to approximately the same values for very simple tests (such as *t*-test for the

sample mean), interpreting CIs established using the frequentist approach as Bayesian credible intervals is not a valid approach to statistical inference (68) (see figure 18.20).

Using MBI as a simple descriptive approach to interpret CIs can be rationalized, but making inferences from estimated probabilities is not recommended (11). If frequentist approaches are used for magnitude-based statistical inference, METs should be used instead.

There are numerous difficulties with frequentist inference (41, 42). The results are not intuitive and are usually erroneously interpreted from the Bayesian perspective. Error rates need to be controlled and adjusted when multiple comparisons are made. Various assumptions, that is, assumptions of normality, noncollinearity, and others, need to be made and tested; and for more complex models, such as hierarchical models, p-values and CIs are only approximated (41, 42).

MEASUREMENT STUDIES

Measurement studies include validity and reliability analysis. The **validity** of a measurement is a measure of its one-off association with another measure; it gives information about how well a measurement is supposed to measure. There are two types of validity measurements: **concurrent validity**, which compares the measurement against a gold standard, and **convergent validity**, which compares the measurement to another measure that ought to have some relationship. On the other hand, the **reliability** of a measure is the association with itself in repeated trials in order to show how reproducible the measurement is.

Measurement error (ME) is involved in all measurements; it occurs when an **observed score** is different from the true score (TS) (2, 56, 70) due to an error in the measurement. This results in

TABLE 18.17   Scale of Effect Probabilities

0.5%, most unlikely	✗ The effect is unlikely beneficial
0.5%-5%, very unlikely	
5%-25%, unlikely	
25%-75%, possibly	✓ The effect is possibly or likely or very likely or most likely beneficial
75%-95%, likely	
95%-99.5%, very likely	
>99.5%, most likely	

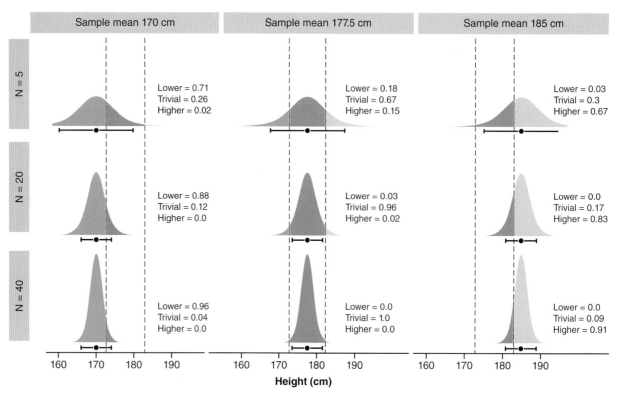

FIGURE 18.20 Bayesian interpretation of the confidence intervals used in MBI.

measurement bias that affects descriptive analysis, causal inferences (22, 24, 26), and predictive performances (43). In mathematical notation, the observed score (OS) comprises the hypothetical **true score** and measurement error (ME); that is, $OS = TS + ME$ (2, 71).

In the sport science domain, since the measured objects are usually humans, measurement error comprises that of the instrumentation as well as biological noise (71). **Instrumentation noise** is assumed to be error caused solely by the measurement apparatus (71). **Biological noise**, on the other hand, is defined as an error in the observed scores caused by biological processes including, but not limited to, circadian rhythm, nutritional intake, sleep, and motivation (71). Both instrumentation and biological noises consist of two types of errors: systematic error and random error (see figure 18.21).

Systematic error represents a constant (and stable) error across measurements; it is commonly referred to as **bias**. With measurement instruments that have a linear response, systematic error can be further divided into (a) proportional and (b) fixed (30, 33, 34). **Random error** (ε) represents the unknown (and unpredictable) error, which varies between measurements. Random errors are often represented and modeled using a **Gaussian normal distribution** (mean

and SD). For example, a group of five athletes are measured using a novel bodyweight scale, performing five trials separated by 1 minute. The assumption is that there should not be any changes in the measurements across these trials (i.e., athletes are not allowed to use the bathroom, consume water or food, exercise, or change their clothing; and no biological noise is involved—no fluctuations in bodyweight due to motivation or fatigue). The TS of the athletes is known, and also the instrumentation noise of the novel bodyweight scale, which tends to have proportional bias equal to factor 1.01 (i.e., an athlete weighing 100 kg [which is that athlete's TS], will have OS equal to 101 kg due to proportional bias, while an athlete weighing 50 kg will have OS equal to 50.5 kg) (see table 18.18).

The objective of the analysis is to estimate DGP parameters of the measurement error (the proportional bias, fixed bias, and the SD of the random error). Unfortunately, since TS is unknown, proportional bias and fixed bias cannot be estimated. To overcome this problem, OS is usually compared to a **gold standard** measure that can serve as a proxy to TS. What is left to be estimated is the SD of the random error, which is often referred to as the **typical error** (TE) of the test. In the same example as before, TE is estimated using individual SD of the OS in the five trials (see table 18.19). The mean of athletes' typical errors is equal

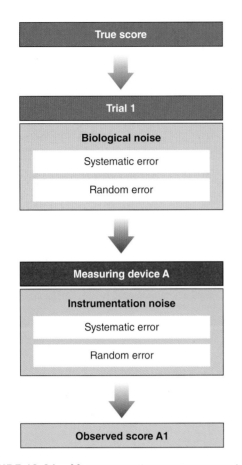

FIGURE 18.21   Measurement error components.

to 0.51 kg, which is quite close to the DGP random error parameter of 0.5 kg. The difference between the estimated and the true value of the random error SD is due to the sampling error. Unfortunately, this method of estimating TE is not always practically feasible. Typical error is usually estimated with two trials (OS1 and OS2) by using SD of the difference scores across athletes (30, 71). The estimated TE is a very useful metric in sport science since it can be used for (a) estimating the likelihood of the individual's true change after an intervention, (b) estimating the reliability of the test (28, 29, 31, 33, 34, 37), and (c) defining SESOI.

INTERPRETING INDIVIDUAL CHANGES USING SESOI AND TE

The bench press example (see table 18.8) can showcase interpretation of the individual changes by using smallest effect size of interest and TE. The measurement error in a 1RM bench press test is estimated using a TE estimator and is equal to 2.5 kg. Practically, this means that due to the biological variation and noise, as well as instrumentation error, 1RM in the bench press would tend to vary normally distributed with TE equal to 2.5 kg, given, of course, no real change in strength. Since the measurement error is involved in both pretest and posttest, due to error propagation, the expected TE for the change score is thus equal to $\sqrt{2} \times TE$ (3.54 kg). For

TABLE 18.18   Simulated Five Trials From Known True Score and Measurement Error

Athlete	TS (kg)	OS 1 (kg)	OS 2 (kg)	OS 3 (kg)	OS 4 (kg)	OS 5 (kg)
Athlete 01	77.93	79.03	79.96	79.37	79.47	78.61
Athlete 02	76.11	77.55	77.48	77.05	77.83	77.83
Athlete 03	77.04	78.11	79.03	79.14	78.65	78.18
Athlete 04	54.96	56.79	56.24	55.52	56.58	55.58
Athlete 05	84.03	86.67	85.92	85.37	85.53	86.84

TABLE 18.19   Individual Mean and SD From Five Trials

Athlete	Mean	SD
Athlete 01	79.29	0.50
Athlete 02	77.55	0.32
Athlete 03	78.62	0.47
Athlete 04	56.14	0.58
Athlete 05	86.06	0.66

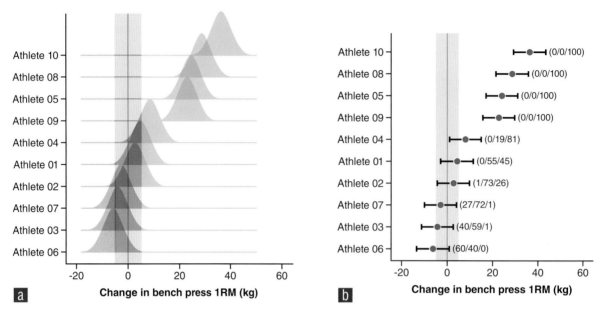

FIGURE 18.22 Analysis of individual change scores using SESOI and TE. *(a)* Uncertainty around TSs can be depicted using normal distribution whose SD is equal to TE. The probability that the observed change is lower, trivial, or higher can be estimated using the surface within lower, trivial, and higher magnitude bands. *(b)* 95% confidence intervals around change scores are calculated using $\pm 1.96 \times \sqrt{2} \times TE$. Numbers in parentheses represent the proportion of the surface area in the lower, trivial, and higher magnitude bands. These are interpreted as probabilities of the TS being in the lower, trivial, or higher magnitude band.

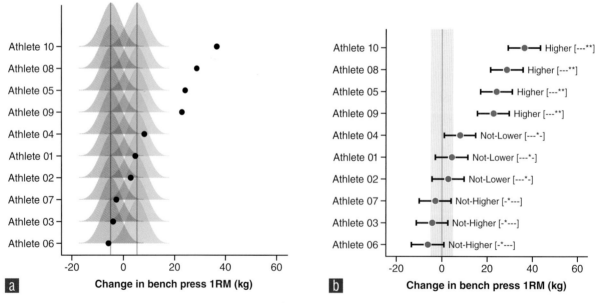

FIGURE 18.23 METs approach to interpreting individual change scores. *(a)* Since true change scores are unknown, only the probability of seeing observed scores or higher can be tested, given the known TE and assumed TS. In order to do this, minimal effect tests are performed, assuming two TS null hypotheses: one at the lower SESOI threshold (red) and one at the upper SESOI threshold (green). Typical error can be interpreted as SD of the error distribution. Black dots indicate observed individual change. The focus is on estimating the probability of observing this change, given two hypotheses. *(b)* The 95% CI around change scores are calculated using $\pm 1.96 \times \sqrt{2} \times TE$ and depicted using error bars. Final inference using five METs is reported. The METs significance (assuming alpha = 0.05), indicated by an asterisk, is reported in the brackets for each of the five tests performed.

example, ±5 kg can be considered minimal important change, which will be used as SESOI. Since both TE and SESOI are known, the objective of the analysis is to estimate the probability that an individual change in score is practically significant (i.e., lower, trivial, or higher compared to SESOI). Technical error specifies how much of an observed score randomly varies around the TS.

Figure 18.22a shows how individual observed scores change **probabilistically** using the known TE, with error bars representing 95% CI. The numbers in parentheses in figure 18.22b represent estimated probabilities of the true change score being lower, trivial, and higher compared to SESOI. To be more certain of individual changes, TE needs to be smaller, compared to SESOI. The ratio between SESOI and TE can thus represent an estimate of the test sensitivity to detect practically meaningful changes. Bench press 1RM change of +/- 11.93 kg is the smallest change in which we have 95% confidence it is over SESOI.

As explained in the "Statistical Inference" section, this method of individual analysis interprets the TE and associated CI from the Bayesian statistics perspective. This is not the correct interpretation, since the individual's TSs are not known, only the observed scores. A typical error shows the variance of the observed scores around the TS, not vice versa (i.e., Bayesian inverse probability). Thus, visual representation from figure 18.20 is not statistically valid. Since in this case the TSs are not known, the focus is on the probabilities of seeing the observed score given the assumption about where the TS is assumed to be. For this reason, the question is as follows: How likely is the observed score, given the known TE and assumed null hypothesis (i.e., TS, that is assumed to be zero as null hypothesis)? This demands an answer and interpretation of TE from the frequentist perspective. Thus, the correct interpretation of the individual changes involves the use of minimum effect tests (METs). This approach to interpreting individual changes is depicted in figure 18.23.

CONCLUSION

In their daily practices, sport scientists should start any statistical analysis by asking the questions that they are trying to answer using the data. These questions of interest should not only guide the approach to statistical analysis, but also guide data collection and finally interpretations of the analysis and modeling results. In order to answer these questions with data, the sport scientist must keep in mind that small-world models are always a representation of the large world. There is no entirely objective approach to performing this analysis, rather a pluralism of approaches (51, 52). The value of these models for the small-world representations should be judged by qualities, as suggested by Gelman and Hennig (20), including "transparency, consensus, impartiality, correspondence to observable reality, awareness of multiple perspectives, awareness of context dependence, and investigation of stability." Finally, the importance of cumulative knowledge rather than reliance solely on single studies or even single lines of research should be recognized (3).

RECOMMENDED READINGS

Jovanović, M. *bmbstats: Bootstrap Magnitude-Based Statistics for Sports Scientists*. Mladen Jovanović, 2020.

Gelman, A, Hill, J, and Vehtari, A. *Regression and Other Stories*. Cambridge University Press, 2020.

McElreath, R. *Statistical Rethinking: A Bayesian Course With Examples in R and Stan*. 2nd ed. Boca Raton: Taylor and Francis, CRC Press, 2020.

James, G, Witten, D, Hastie, T, and Tibshirani, R. *An Introduction to Statistical Learning: With Applications in R*. New York: Springer, 2017.

Kuhn, M and Johnson, K. *Applied Predictive Modeling*. New York: Springer, 2018.

Injury Risk Modeling

Johann Windt, PhD
Tim Gabbett, BHSc (Hons), PhD

Maximizing athlete availability and readiness to perform is a crucial responsibility of the sport scientist. For elite sporting clubs, injuries and therefore missed playing time impose a notable financial burden on the organization (28, 38). Moreover, athlete availability increases the chances of success in both individual (70) and team-sport environments (25, 37, 39). Therefore, sport scientists should carefully consider how to screen, monitor, and model athlete data in a way that allows them to inform decisions regarding the health and performance of athletes under their supervision.

As an overarching principle, sport scientists should aim to align their theory, data collection, and data analysis, ultimately informing their interpretation and reporting (21, 93) (see figure 19.1). To monitor any process and outcome in sport, one must begin with a **theoretical framework** that informs the monitoring process. Theory provides sport scientists the insight to decide what data to collect (and at what frequency). Finally, the sport scientist can implement an appropriate **analytical approach**. This chapter addresses **injury risk modeling** within the context of this framework. Throughout, the chapter differentiates the implications of the injury risk model for the sport scientist in both a research and an applied context.

INJURY RISK THEORY

The classic model that has informed injury prevention research and practice since the early 1990s is the 1992 sequence of prevention model by Dr. van Mechelen and colleagues (53). The model can be summarized as follows:

1. What injuries are occurring? Establish the extent of the problem through injury surveillance and epidemiological work.

2. Why are these injuries happening? Identify relevant risk factors through etiological research.

3. Develop and implement strategies that address causal factors. Design preventive strategies that address modifiable risk factors identified in step 2.

4. See if the intervention worked. Reevaluate the injury problem as in step 1 to determine whether the preventive strategy was effective.

Understanding What Injuries Occur

The model having originated in the sports medicine research arena, the sport scientist can learn a lot from it to apply in practice. The starting point, highlighted by step one of the model, is to understand the context of the epidemiology; which injuries impose the biggest burden within the sport and within the specific athlete

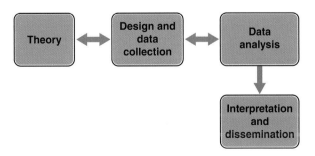

FIGURE 19.1 A framework for aligning theory, data collection, data analysis, and subsequent reporting in sport science.

demographic that the sport scientist works with. This problem is best defined through **injury burden**, the cross-product of injury incidence (how frequently injuries occur) and injury severity (how many days are missed due to the injury) (5):

$$Injury\ burden \left(\frac{days\ missed}{1,000\ hours} \right) =$$

$$frequency \left(\frac{injuries}{1,000\ hours} \right) * severity \left(\frac{days\ missed}{injuries} \right)$$

Published epidemiological literature will provide a foundation for the sport scientist entering into a new sporting context, like identifying that hamstring injuries may impose the biggest burden within professional men's soccer (5), while knee and shoulder problems pose the greatest challenge in junior handball (1). However, sport scientists should not stop with published epidemiological literature and should engage with the sports medicine department within their environment to ensure that athlete health is monitored and documented consistently. Implementing injury surveillance enables sport scientists to understand the burden of different injuries within their specific team and to provide baseline data to evaluate future interventions. Once these injuries have been identified, the sport scientist needs to understand their etiology. That is, why do these injuries occur?

Understanding Why These Injuries Occur

Sport injuries occur, fundamentally, when the physical forces on a given tissue exceed the tissue's capacity and physical breakdown occurs (32). The reasons for this breakdown are multifactorial, workload-dependent, tissue-specific, and complex. Working to better understand each of these principles will underpin the sport scientist's measurement and analytical choices.

Multifactorial Nature of Sport Injuries

Sport injuries are multifactorial. This concept, central to sport injury causation, was presented by Dr. Meeuwisse in 1994 (54), and highlights that factors internal (e.g., age, flexibility, previous injury) and external (e.g., opponent behavior, playing surface, protective equipment) to the athlete play an important role in determining an athlete's predisposition and susceptibility to injury. Finally, an inciting event occurs at the point of injury. As described

in subsequent reviews that built on this original multifactorial model, these concepts have important implications for how data should be collected and analyzed (6, 7).

Workload Dependence of Injuries

Athlete workloads and subsequent adaptation are fundamental sport science principles (14, 15, 82). The concepts of training load modeling and external and internal workload are covered in greater detail in chapter 2 and part IV of this text. Much of the traditional workload research dealt with performance modeling (8, 9) or designing workouts like interval training schemes (31). Since 2000 (especially since 2010), there has been an exponential rise in research examining the workload–injury association (27, 43). Interested readers are referred to systematic reviews (13, 24, 27, 43, 93), methodological reviews (93), and consensus statements (83) that discuss workload–injury research in greater detail; the key concepts and considerations are summarized here.

Total athlete workloads were associated with injury in early research in basketball (2), rugby league players (44), baseball pitchers (49, 66), and cricket players (68). Most of these studies were performed at the team level, identifying that more players on a team were injured during time periods when the team experienced higher training loads. The challenges to these findings in isolation were that all athletes were grouped together, preventing any differentiation between athletes who might be at different injury risks, and the only logical preventive strategy was to minimize workloads.

Changes in load have been the primary focus of workload–injury investigations since about 2010. The rate of workload progression, like week-to-week changes in workloads, can be quantified in several ways (65, 74). However, the most common measures of workload progression have been some sort of variation of the **acute:chronic workload ratio** (ACWR). The ACWR compares the amount of training performed recently (usually a week) to the amount of training performed over a longer period (usually a month) (88). All in all, the majority of research that has investigated the rate of progression in training load has shown that injury risk increased as the rate of progression increased (24, 27, 33, 43, 83).

Although research at the team level identified higher injury rates with higher workloads, and athletes may have a theoretical workload ceiling that they can tolerate (42), training allows athletes to prepare for competition demands and develop more robust physical qualities. Therefore, at the individual level it may not be surprising that higher chronic (longer-term) workloads have been identified as protective in several contexts. Runners with a higher weekly training volume (>30 km/week) entering a marathon were half as likely to be injured as those with <30 km/week of training (69). Gaelic football players with higher chronic workloads were more robust to given increases in workload (51), and in some cases, athletes with greater preseason training volumes have been shown to have a lower risk of injury in-season (60, 96).

The **workload–injury model** (see figure 19.2; 94) built on foundational injury etiology models (6, 54, 55) by explicitly incorporating the workload effects (discussed earlier) on subsequent injury risk (94). Athletes enter into activity with a risk profile, including their previous injury history and a collection of internal risk factors. Some of these factors (e.g., aerobic capacity, strength) are modifiable and change over the course of a season. Other factors are nonmodifiable (e.g., sex, age, anthropometrics). With a given risk profile,

athletes engage in training or competition, which is the application of a given workload. This applied workload is the vehicle through which athletes are exposed to external risk factors (e.g., opponent behavior, environmental conditions).

After the training or competition session has concluded, athletes may or may not have experienced an injury through a given inciting event and reenter the cycle. However, their risk profile is now altered for subsequent activities because the act of training or competing affects their modifiable internal characteristics, in accordance with the volume and intensity of the workload applied and the athlete's tolerance to the load. Some of these changes may be negative, like decreased neuromuscular control in a fatigued athlete following a match. Conversely, the athlete's risk profile improves over time through adaptation to the applied workloads as physical qualities develop. In summary, the workload–injury etiology model describes three ways in which workloads relate to

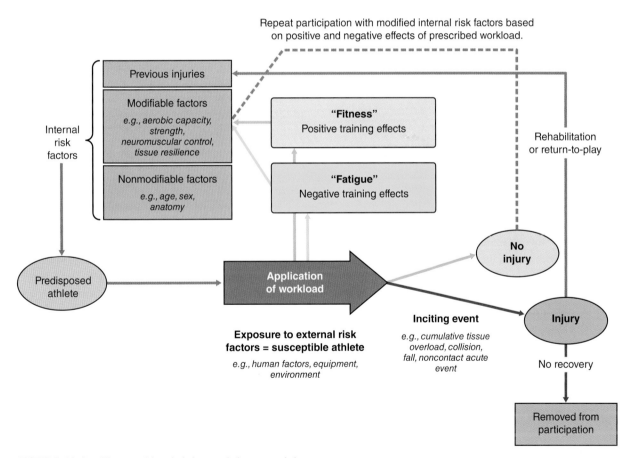

FIGURE 19.2   The workload–injury etiology model.

Reprinted by permission from J. Windt and T.J. Gabbett, (2016, pg. 428-435).

sport injury risk:

1. Workloads are the vehicle by means of which athletes are exposed to external risk factors, so the greater the exposure or workload, the higher the overall potential for injury will be.

2. Workloads can improve athletes' risk profiles through positive adaptations and well-developed physical qualities that lower subsequent injury risk. This may help to explain some findings showing that higher chronic workloads are associated with a reduced injury risk (51, 69).

3. Workloads that increase athlete fatigue and negatively alter an athlete's modifiable risk factors may increase subsequent injury risk. This may help to explain the continued finding that rapid spikes in workload increase subsequent injury risk (27, 43).

Debugging Acute:Chronic Workload Ratios and Workload Progression Calculations The ACWR describes the size of an athlete's recent workload (i.e., acute load) in relation to the workload the athlete has performed over a longer period (i.e., chronic load). It approximates the workload an athlete has performed relative to the workload for which that athlete has been prepared. Several iterations of the ACWR have been proposed—such as differentiating between coupled (in which the most recent week is included in the chronic calculation) and uncoupled (in which the most recent week is not part of the chronic load calculation) (47), or using rolling averages or exponentially weighted moving averages (92). The progression in workload can be quantified in these and many other ways, some of which are defined and illustrated conceptually in table 19.1.

An example will serve to illustrate the concept, demonstrate the calculations, and visualize the measures—two runners in the final 2 months leading into a half marathon (see figure 19.3). Athlete 1 is a former college soccer player who is now working an office job and runs only occasionally. One month before the race, Athlete 1 decides to run the half marathon and ramps up training rapidly in preparation for the event. Athlete 2 is a recreational marathon runner who plans to run the same half marathon as a part of training for an upcoming marathon.

Examining the loading patterns of these two athletes clearly demonstrates several points. First, all measures of workload progression indicate that Athlete 1 is entering the half marathon event with a load that has been increasing in recent training (ACWR$_{Coupled}$: 1.9, ACWR$_{Uncoupled}$: 2.7; week-to-week

change: +37 km: refer to table 19.1 for calculation differences). In contrast, all measures of progression indicate that Athlete 2 is entering the marathon in more of a tapered state, with recent training less than that athlete's chronic training base (ACWRs <1.0 on the day before the half marathon, week-to-week change −22 km). In this case, and in many other circumstances, different calculations will show similar landscapes, predominantly whether workloads are increasing or decreasing. Further, the sport scientist may choose to use different values for acute and chronic loads or even use the differences between these values (e.g., absolute or percentage) instead of ratios. However, all these measures will provide different values, so it is important for sport scientists to choose one and remain consistent with it, such that they become very familiar with the measures they are using and what constitutes a meaningful change in those metrics.

The second observation a sport scientist may make from this fictional example is that Athlete 2 is also better prepared for running the half marathon from a loading perspective, because this athlete enters it with a substantially higher chronic training load. Several of Athlete 2's training runs have exceeded the half-marathon distance, so the training has been better preparation for the specific demands of the race through progressive overload and a slight taper before the race. Combining the chronic load and workload progression would allow a sport scientist to infer that with regard to workload, with all other factors being equal, Athlete 2 is likely to enter the race fresh and prepared while Athlete 1 may enter it fatigued and underprepared.

The Acute:Chronic Workload Ratio Debate and Scientific Progress There has been much discussion and debate in the scientific literature for and against various aspects of the workload–injury association, including the ACWR. Researchers have directly criticized it (16, 48, 56, 57), suggested modifying it (18, 47, 88, 92), and supported its use (23, 40, 75, 95). Criticisms of the ACWR include these:

- It is challenging to implement continual workload monitoring in some professional team contexts (e.g., football [soccer] or basketball). This criticism is not exclusive to the ACWR but can be considered similar for all monitoring that relies on complete data for longitudinal calculations.

- Using rolling averages may not be as sensitive to load changes compared to other strategies (e.g., exponentially weighted moving averages

TABLE 19.1   Definitions, Equations, and Visual Representations of the Coupled ACWR, Uncoupled ACWR, Week-to-Week Change ACWR, and Exponentially Weighted ACWR

Measure	Equation	Technical definition	Visual representation (95)
Coupled traditional ACWR	$$\dfrac{A}{0.25 \bullet \left(A + W2 + W3 + W4\right)}$$	The ratio between the most recent week of work with the average of the most recent 4 weeks	
Uncoupled traditional ACWR	$$\dfrac{A}{0.333 \bullet \left(W2 + W3 + W4\right)}$$	The ratio of the most recent week of work with the average of the 3 preceding weeks	
Week-to-week change ACWR	A ÷ W2 (relative change) *or* A − W2 (absolute change)	The ratio or absolute difference between the last week versus the preceding week	

Visual representation — Coupled traditional ACWR:

	Sun	Mon	Tue	Wed	Thu	Fri	Sat
Month 1	31	1	2	3	4	5	6
	7	8	9	10	11	12	13
	14	15	16	17	18	19	20
	21	22	23	24	25	26	27
Month 2	28	29	30	1	2	3	4
	5	6	7	8	9	10	11 Current day
	12	13	14	15	16	17	18
	19	20	21	22	23	24	25
	26	27	28	29	30	31	1

Visual representation — Uncoupled traditional ACWR:

	Sun	Mon	Tue	Wed	Thu	Fri	Sat
Month 1	31	1	2	3	4	5	6
	7	8	9	10	11	12	13
	14	15	16	17	18	19	20
	21	22	23	24	25	26	27
Month 2	28	29	30	1	2	3	4
	5	6	7	8	9	10	11 Current day
	12	13	14	15	16	17	18
	19	20	21	22	23	24	25
	26	27	28	29	30	31	1

Visual representation — Week-to-week change ACWR:

	Sun	Mon	Tue	Wed	Thu	Fri	Sat
Month 1	31	1	2	3	4	5	6
	7	8	9	10	11	12	13
	14	15	16	17	18	19	20
	21	22	23	24	25	26	27
Month 2	28	29	30	1	2	3	4
	5	6	7	8	9	10	11 Current day
	12	13	14	15	16	17	18
	19	20	21	22	23	24	25
	26	27	28	29	30	31	1

(continued)

TABLE 19.1 Definitions, Equations, and Visual Representations of the Coupled ACWR, Uncoupled ACWR, Week-to-Week Change ACWR, and Exponentially Weighted ACWR *(continued)*

| Exponentially weighted moving average ACWR | $$EWMA_{Today} = \delta_a$$ $$+ ((1 - \delta_a) \times EWMA_{Yesterday})$$ $$\delta_a = \frac{2}{N + 1}$$ Where δ_a is a value between 0 and 1 that represents the degree of decay. Higher values discount older values more rapidly. N is the chosen time decay, usually 7 and 28 days to parallel the traditional ACWR, though other values can be chosen as well. | The ratio between an exponentially weighted average of loads in the last 7 days compared to an exponentially weighted average of loads over the last 28 days | |

(calendar visual representation)

A (acute), W2, W3, and W4 correspond to each of the last 4 weeks, respectively.

Figures in visual representation column reprinted by permission from J. Windt and T.J. Gabbett (2019, pg. 990).

[EWMA]) (56, 57). Exponentially weighted approaches are influenced more by recent values, such that yesterday's load affects the calculation more than the load 4 days ago (for example, see table 19.1). Notably, the sport scientist should also be aware of the challenges unique to the EWMA approach, like the initial value problem and the time it takes for different initial value models to converge (i.e., ~50 days) (88).

- Ratios carry certain assumptions and involve several mathematical challenges worth considering (48).

- "Mathematical coupling" occurs (in the traditional 1:4 rolling average ACWR approach) because the most recent training week is included in both the acute and chronic loads, which induces a correlation between the acute and chronic workloads and decreases between-athletes variability (47).

- The ACWR has other mathematical limitations as a predictive tool.

Among the most notable features of scientific inquiry is the progression of knowledge through discovery, debate, reflection, and refinement. The workload–injury field is no exception, and the sport science community has benefited and continues to benefit from these ongoing discussions. The principles behind the workload–injury research field reflect basic principles of training; namely, failing to prepare athletes for the demands of a sport or competition and doing too much too soon will predispose an individual to a heightened risk of injury.

On one hand, the ACWR has presented a means for sport scientists to think about progression and sparked discussion about how workload monitoring may inform performance- and health-based decisions. On the other hand, there are several challenges and prospects for improvement that sport scientists should be aware of (88). Indeed, it may become clear that other methods of quantification are more appropriate in certain sporting contexts (17, 76), and sport scientists are encouraged to continually reflect on how monitoring can be used to inform health and performance decisions.

Looking forward, research thus far has almost exclusively used observational studies, with the next step including randomized trials with load education, modification, or intervention or more than one of these (27, 33). Several recommendations and considerations for methods to calculate and analyze the ACWR (e.g., methods, nested case–control studies, splines versus discretized bins) have also been suggested to continue improving the research field and address previous challenges like unmeasured confounding and sparse data bias (88).

Tissue-Specific Adaptation

Returning to the injury definition, the point at which physical forces on a tissue exceed the tissue's capacity to handle the applied forces, the sport scientist would

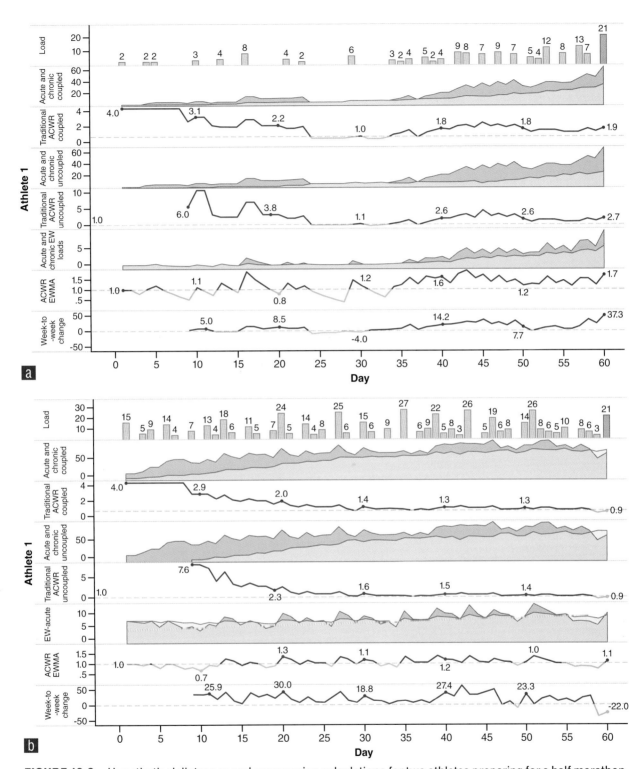

FIGURE 19.3 Hypothetical distances and progression calculations for two athletes preparing for a half marathon.

be wise to consider all the aforementioned factors as elements that contribute to the load on the tissue or factors that relate to the tissue's capacity. Generally speaking, factors fall into three categories (62):

1. *Factors that load the tissue:* These are the workload variables of interest. These will vary depending on the sport and tissue. Examples include throws for a baseball pitcher's or a handball player's shoulder (58, 66), swings for a volleyball player's shoulder or jumps for a volleyball player's knees (4), or high-velocity running loads for hamstring injuries (51).

2. *Factors that modify the distribution and magnitude of the load during activity:* For example, poor scapular kinematics can alter the distribution of load on the athlete's shoulder during each throw.

3. *Factors that affect the overall tissue capacity:* Examples include eccentric hamstring strength and age for hamstring injuries (67) or an athlete's dietary intake (e.g., collagen synthesis with gelatin supplementation) (79).

A study of 679 handball players demonstrated this tissue-specific approach and how internal risk factors can modify the effect of a workload spike. In this 31-week study, the risk of injury was approximately two times higher when the weekly throwing load increased by 60% compared with the preceding four weeks (i.e., an uncoupled ACWR of 1:4 weeks). When the weekly throwing load increased by 20% to 60% compared with the preceding four weeks, the injury rate was approximately four or five times higher for those athletes with weak external rotation strength (hazard ratio = 4.0, 95% confidence interval [CI] = 1.1-15.2) or those with scapular dyskinesis (hazard ratio 4.8, 95% CI = 1.3-18.3) (58). In this instance, poor shoulder rotation strength was a variable representing tissue capacity, while scapular dyskinesis was a factor that influenced the distribution of throwing load on the tissue (62). As another example of this type of framework, this approach has also been described as a framework for understanding running injuries (11).

Sport scientists should consider what factors would influence tissue loading, load modification, and load capacity for the most common injuries within the given sport. Furthermore, they should also consider the load–adaptation timeline for different tissues to consider what rates of workload progression would be most advantageous or most detrimental. For example, a given training session may impose a different load from a physiological and biomechanical perspective,

and the affected tissues may adapt at different rates (85). On a more detailed level, one can also think of the loading on specific muscles, tendons, or bones at a specific tissue level.

Complex Systems Approach

Complex systems approaches are a final consideration for sport scientists when thinking about injury etiology, as a growing body of scientists are calling for a move away from reductionism toward these complex approaches (12, 41). Even multivariable approaches that account for several risk factors and workload variables are still reductionistic in the sense that they assume that the whole is equal to the sum of the component parts. As described by Bittencourt and colleagues (12), complex systems are characterized by

- an open system that allows for an emergent outcome (i.e., injury) through many different paths (i.e., risk factor, workload, and inciting event combinations),
- nonlinear relationships between variables,
- a recursive loop in which the system output returns as the subsequent input,
- self-organization, and
- uncertainty.

The fundamental thinking shift brought about by a complex systems approach injury etiology is a migration from risk factors to risk profiles (i.e., regularities) that consist of a collection of risk factors from all relevant variables (i.e., **web of determinants**), which interact to increase the likelihood of an emergent pattern (i.e., injury). This theoretical framework may inform how the sport scientist thinks about injury etiology, but these models may be challenging to implement in practice, since they require a more advanced skill set in statistical modeling, as well as a sample size of injuries and athletes greater than most sport scientists will have in their sporting environment.

INJURY RISK DATA COLLECTION

The theoretical foundation underlying injury risk subsequently informs the next step in the framework (see figure 19.1 on page 287), in which data is collected. During this phase, researchers and sport scientists must decide on what they are going to monitor or measure and how frequently, and then implement data collection within their environment.

Choosing the Right Measures

Measures must be carefully chosen by sport scientists as they consider the theoretical injury burden within their context. Every measure that is adopted may place an additional burden on athletes or practitioners (or both) since each data stream will require collecting, cleaning, analyzing, and reporting. From an applied perspective, practitioners should adopt only measures that they are confident can be implemented in their environment and will inform their decision making in the daily training environment.

From a research perspective, more data collection can also create more challenges than solutions, given the problems with underpowered studies and a lack of replicability in several research fields (22, 59, 64). Researchers should consider the power of their analyses both when recruiting participants and when running their statistical models. To recruit more participants, many have advocated larger multisite studies (26). From a modeling perspective, it is also important to remember that for every variable included in a model, more injuries (i.e., cases) are needed (26, 63). This is also known as the **events per variable** (EPV) requirement. A common suggestion is to include approximately 10 events (i.e., injuries) per variable in a statistical model. With all this said, more collection is not always better, and technology or measurements should be adopted by researchers and practitioners only with a clear goal in mind.

From an injury risk perspective, understanding the epidemiology of a specific sport (e.g., prevalence, incidence) helps in filtering down which injuries should be prioritized. As an oversimplified example, performing regular handheld dynamometry testing for external and internal shoulder rotation strength would make little sense in a sport like soccer in which shoulder injuries are of minimal importance.

Thinking at the tissue level can help sport scientists understand which measures to prioritize. Tissue and tissue capacity are critical (86), so screening measures should be those that are linked to the tissue capacity relevant to the high-burden injuries.

Monitoring Frequency

If the sport scientist decides to analyze workload progression through some sort of ACWR or week-to-week change, the workload metrics of interest must be measured for all training and competition participa-

tion. If the workload cannot be measured in certain circumstances (e.g., wearable microsensors are not allowed to be worn in games) or technological difficulties cause load to be missing, the workloads will have to be estimated or imputed from other available data.

Workloads are not the only component of injury risk models that may change dynamically over time. Since athletes can (and should be expected to) adapt from their training regimes, modifiable risk factors should be evaluated at time intervals that correspond with the rate at which the sport scientist expects them to change. The failure to do so is a major limitation to several screening studies that measure only at baseline. For example, Nordic hamstring strength measured at preseason may not reflect hamstring strength throughout the season, since this is a trainable physical attribute (45). Thus, the at-risk athletes at the time of testing may no longer belong to this group when they experience an injury.

Finally, variables that are considered important but stable (e.g., age, sex, previous injury history) can be measured only once at baseline as part of an athlete intake and subsequently considered in modeling approaches.

Implementing Monitoring Tools

Workload–injury research and applied monitoring depend on longitudinal measurement success. Therefore, athlete and practitioner buy-in is paramount for success, and addressing the barriers to implementation is crucial. Qualitative interviews with elite athletes have identified that both exaggerated interventions and a lack of feedback or intervention from monitoring systems are major athlete barriers (10, 61).

Analyzing the Data: Association Versus Prediction

Once sport scientists understand the epidemiology and etiology of the most important injuries within their environment (theory), and decide which workload and athlete characteristic data they want to collect and how frequently (data collection), they are left with a data set of intensive longitudinal data to analyze (87).

Sport scientists should be careful not to confuse association with prediction (3, 52, 73, 80). Just the fact that a risk factor may increase a group's injury risk (e.g., low eccentric hamstring muscle strength) (67) does not mean all athletes who have low eccentric hamstring muscle strength will experience a hamstring strain. The challenges of screening data for prediction were discussed in detail by Bahr (3).

In the same way, workload variables in isolation have been associated with injuries, but they are limited in their ability to predict injury in an athlete on a given day (30). The sport scientist should be cognizant that the probability of injury on a single day in an athlete is quite low (e.g., 0.78% per training day). The relative risks increase with rapid workload progressions, and the probability of injury in a longer time period (e.g., a week) is higher, but it should be evident that a high workload progression (e.g., >1.5 ACWR) does not mean an athlete will become injured. Further, this should be contextualized with other available information to inform decision making. For example, age (both younger and older athletes), poor lower-body strength, and poor aerobic fitness have been shown to increase injury risk in response to rapid changes in workload (50).

Nonetheless, several injury prediction attempts have been made in the literature, with somewhat more promising findings when accounting for multiple variables (20, 72). As one example, Gupta and colleagues (35) found that the odds of injury were 42 times higher in athletes with at least two at-risk factors compared with athletes with none or with one (relative risk of 4.29 [90% CI: 1.84-10.18]). Factors included exposure, squat scores, concussion history, position category, average PlayerLoad™, movement efficiency, and the coefficient of variation for average PlayerLoad™. The sensitivity (88%) and specificity (85%) of their model were also high, although these were in-sample predictions.

Quantifying Uncertainty

As discussed in greater detail in other sections of this book, quantifying measurement error (noise) and understanding a minimally important difference in each variable of interest (signal) are crucial when one is analyzing monitoring data (71, 84).

Determining Academic Analytical Approaches

The intensive longitudinal data that athlete monitoring produces presents several challenges from an analyti-

cal perspective. First, repeated measurements from several athletes mean that the data are clustered and each observation should not be treated as independent. The analytical choice should distinguish within-athlete changes from between-athletes differences. Second, data are likely to be unbalanced, with unequal numbers of observations from different athletes as some leave or join a team at different times of the year. Third, some factors (e.g., workload, wellness) may change regularly, while others remain stable (e.g., sex, age), and the analysis approach should be able to account for these time-dependent changes.

Robust modeling of injury risk that controls for several risk factors requires large data sets with many injuries (63, 64, 73). These types of data sets are uncommon in applied sport settings and sometimes even in larger research centers. In academia, this has contributed to calls for data sharing between research centers that move researchers closer to these types of data sets (26).

In the research arena, the analytical approaches used to evaluate the workload–injury association should be able to account for the theoretical components discussed earlier, namely, the longitudinal, multifactorial, and repeated measurement nature of these data (93). The appropriateness of analytical approaches has improved, which provides an opportunity for sport scientists looking to publish their work by enhancing the analytical approaches used previously.

Sport injury researchers have begun to implement machine learning approaches to explore and analyze the data (19, 42, 72). Dimensionality reduction has also been used to consolidate the amount of data coming from wearable microsensors (90) and to choose between several derived workload variables (91). These reduced data sets (e.g., the components from a principal component analysis) can then be used to evaluate individual training sessions and how training is progressing longitudinally.

Determining Applied Analytical Approaches

For sport scientists working in applied sport settings, the limitations of data set size for robust statistical modeling are important to note, and the uncertainty around injury risk stratification needs to be acknowledged. Certain academic approaches (e.g., time-to-event modeling) (63, 64, 73) are unlikely to be performed in most applied environments for these reasons. Instead, the collective findings from the academic literature should be considered alongside the sport scientist's theoretical framework and experience to inform how to analyze and interpret monitoring and screening data.

Comparative Modeling

One of the most important questions for any sport scientist to ask when analyzing or reporting data is "compared to what?" Simple attempts to answer this question can yield valuable insight. When analyzing athlete workloads, are some athletes or positions substantially underloaded compared to others or to themselves, potentially leaving them unprepared for competition demands? Are athletes training in a way that prepares them for the various aspects of competition? For example, compared to game demands, team-sport athletes may build a large total volume in training, but their high-speed running loads, collisions, and acceleration and deceleration workloads may also be important to consider in the context of average and maximum match demands, and offer a distinct type of load (90).

Summation of High-Risk Scenarios

Sport scientists must identify increased-risk conditions and establish flagging systems that stratify athletes at risk by the number of risk factors present (35). These at-risk conditions will vary depending on the sport and the injuries of interest, but it is often at the intersection of several factors that injury risk increases (e.g., low hamstring strength and short fascicle length, or low hamstring strength and previous hamstring injuries, poor external rotation strength and throwing load increases). Workload scenarios (e.g., low chronic workloads or rapid workload progressions) may be quantified for several different parameters (e.g., high-speed load, total distance). Those athletes with several risk factors identified may require additional attention by way of workload modification or additional training to correct other modifiable risk factors.

Within-Subject Analyses

Single-subject analysis has also been promoted by some in the sport science field (77, 78). These analyses focus on within-athlete changes through normalized scores like z-scores ([value of interest − average value]

/ standard deviation). Statistical process control is one more formal approach that is often used to identify outliers through a control chart, where entries outside a threshold (e.g., 2 standard deviations) are flagged (77, 78). These types of control charts can be implemented with various ACWR iterations, different workload variables, or other longitudinal measures (e.g., athlete self-reported wellness measures).

Identifying Unexpected Findings From Predicted Values

More sophisticated modeling strategies can also be employed in applied practice with enough data from a given athlete, and subsequently be used to identify unexpected values. Acknowledging that there are some limitations and challenges in rating of perceived exertion (RPE) collection, such as diverse influences on athletes' reported values (e.g., winning or losing a match) (36), RPE can be predicted for each athlete using traditional regression approaches or more sophisticated machine learning models (19). A drastic departure from the expected RPE value could indicate an adverse response to training. This same approach to identifying adverse or unexpected internal load responses can be used to compare heart rate loads from a given external load (46).

An Applied Heuristic Load Monitoring Model

While selecting from these different analyses can inform the sport scientist's data analysis work, consistently returning to a framework and heuristic for workload-based decisions can be helpful. The athlete monitoring cycle has been proposed elsewhere and may serve as a starting point (see figure 19.4; 34). The monitoring cycle begins with quantifying the load athletes have performed, in this case quantifying the external loads that are most relevant for the sport and injuries of interest. Screening variables and modifiable internal risk factors can be measured as well, understanding that they contribute to load tolerance. Once the athletes' external load is quantified, their internal workload can be measured, with both external and internal loads compared to the planned loads to inform future training steps. Finally, athletes' perceptual well-being and markers of readiness may influence training decisions and modification when necessary, through both increasing or decreasing loads.

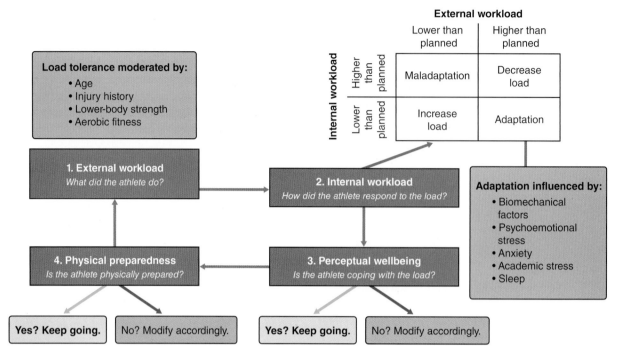

FIGURE 19.4 The athlete monitoring cycle.

Adapted by permission from T.J. Gabbett et al. (2017, pg. 1451-1452).

INJURY RISK DELIVERY, DISSEMINATION, AND DECISION MAKING

Returning to the foundational sequence of prevention model, injury surveillance, and etiological inquiry inform the design of preventive measures (step 3) that can be evaluated (step 4). Theory-driven data collection and analysis can inform the sport scientist's understanding of injury risk, but this information will not prevent any injuries if some sort of preventive action is not taken. Therefore, the relevant information must be delivered in an understandable way to coaches and other organization staff who can make better-informed performance and training decisions. Not surprisingly, communication between the sport science staff, medical staff, and coaching staff is essential, with higher injury burden associated with poor communication (29).

In the opinion of the authors of this chapter, sport scientists must keep at least four things in mind. First, their role is to work alongside other members of the integrated support team operating in a collaborative decision-making environment. Within this environment, their expertise and ability to analyze and report data may inform various decisions across different departments (89). Second, they need to report the information in a way that supports these decisions as seamlessly as possible, providing a decision support system that honestly treats the uncertainty in the data while still conveying a simple message (71). Given the importance of data reporting, readers are referred to chapter 21 for a more thorough discussion. Third, workload monitoring is important for performance preparation, not simply injury risk management. The sport scientist should think about training not just to prevent injury, but to have the athletes ready and prepared to perform their best. Finally, the same set of information can also result in different decisions based on risk-modifying variables (81). The willingness to play an athlete who is deemed at higher risk may be much higher during a vital playoff game that the athlete is eager to participate in than an exhibition or preseason match.

CONCLUSION

Sport scientists should think through their theoretical framework when deciding what to measure, how often to measure it, and how to analyze the resultant data. When considering this in an injury risk context, sport

Chapter 19 Injury Risk Model | 299

scientists should identify the most common injuries within the team, organization, or sport by reviewing the epidemiological literature within their sporting population and by analyzing internal injury surveillance records. Once sport scientists have identified the injuries that present the greatest burden in their sport (5), they should review the known risk factors for these injuries and determine which measures of training and competition workload are the most relevant for that tissue or injury type. When feasible, workload should be monitored continuously, and modifiable risk factors should be measured in parallel with how frequently they change. Workload measures may also be analyzed and contextualized in a way that allows the sport scientist to understand how training reflects the average and highest demands of competition, the training base of each athlete, and the rate of progression for the athlete.

The underlying principles within this chapter apply not only to modeling injury risk, but other outcomes as well. In all instances, data analysis is not about implementing statistics blindly, but rather a thoughtful endeavor that embraces subject matter expertise with analytical decisions.

RECOMMENDED READINGS

Bahr, R. Why screening tests to predict injury do not work—and probably never will…: a critical review. *Br J Sports Med* 50:776-780, 2016.

Ruddy, JD, Cormack, SJ, Whiteley, R, Williams, MD, Timmins, RG, and Opar, DA. Modeling the risk of team sport injuries: a narrative review of different statistical approaches. *Front Physiol* 10, 829, 2019.

Vanrenterghem, J, Nedergaard, NJ, Robinson, MA, and Drust, B. Training load monitoring in team sports: a novel framework separating physiological and biomechanical load-adaptation pathways. *Sports Med* 47:2135-2142, 2017.

Windt, J, Ardern, CL, Gabbett, TJ, Khan, KM, Cook, CE, Sporer, BC, and Zumbo, BD. Getting the most out of intensive longitudinal data: a methodological review of workload–injury studies. *BMJ Open* 8:e022626, 2018.

Windt, J, and Gabbett, TJ. How do training and competition workloads relate to injury? The workload—injury aetiology model. *Br J Sports Med* 51:428-435, 2016.

CHAPTER 20

Data Mining and Nonlinear Data Analysis

Sam Robertson, PhD

Performance analysis in sport has been used for many decades as a means to quantify the performances of athletes and teams via systematic observation (50). The methods of data collection and processing for performance analysis have changed substantially, predominantly due to concomitant improvements in computing and technology. These improvements have meant that a number of different types of data previously confined to collection in laboratories, using cumbersome equipment, can now be obtained within training or competition environments. As is the case in many industries, these computing and technology developments have revolutionized sport science, in particular performance analysis.

PERFORMANCE ANALYSIS

As a direct function of these developments, three main considerations relating to data have emerged for the contemporary sport scientist. First, sport is now generating both a greater volume and new types of data at rapid rates. This is creating new insights into previously unknown or immeasurable phenomena in sporting settings, with the rate of progress showing no signs of abating. In fact, global data volume is growing at roughly 50% per year, equating to a 40-fold increase in the next decade (46a). However, this also means that sporting organizations need to be prepared for handling these volumes of data with respect to their infrastructure. In sporting environments, sport science data is often the most voluminous, varied, and complex. Data types range from unstructured match videos (of varying quality and perspectives), to third party–provided player and team statistics, as well as self-reported qualitative text responses from athletes, scouts, and coaches.

A second consideration is that generally speaking, both the quality and fidelity of data are continually improving. Although this is an overwhelmingly positive development, it has also created conundrums for the sport scientist. Some data types, for instance, those obtained from inertial measurement units, are available to the practitioner at frequencies beyond what is realistically required in order to be useful in practice. Thus, the sport scientist requires some foresight with respect to where advancements in technology lie in the future, not least importantly when developing appropriate infrastructure by which to store, access, and analyze data. Improved data quality, along with increased volume, also has implications for the long-term relevance of currently developed models. New insights into complex problems gleaned solely from access to new and better data have the potential to render currently accepted models and resulting practices redundant. This higher quality and volume of information that practitioners will have at their disposal will in turn make it difficult to compare and contrast with previously undertaken research and practice (60).

Third, new and improved ways of handling data are being developed. These relate to the processing, storing, and querying of data, as well as, of course, the analysis. These developments are largely due to advancements in computer science, which has achieved new frontiers not only with respect to how data is processed but also with respect to how meaningful patterns in complex data can be identified. These three considerations together suggest that data mining represents one of the most useful tools that sport scientists have at their disposal.

DATA MINING

Sometimes considered as pertaining to a suite of analytical techniques and their resulting outputs, **data mining** is actually a much broader discipline, entailing methods of processing, storing, reporting, querying, and ultimately visualizing data. Simply speaking, data mining consists of searching for patterns and solving data-related problems in a database (73). Thus, it emphasizes learning in a manner similar to the way humans do. The data-mining process can be broken down into four stages (see table 20.1).

While all four stages of the process are important, due to the specific relevance of stages 3 and 4 to the sport scientist, these are elaborated upon further in this section, along with a discussion about the advancements of deep learning.

Machine Learning

One of the many advantages of data mining is the variety of methods and techniques available to the end user in order to obtain the generalizations and inferences referred to in stage 3 of table 20.1. One of these methods is **machine learning**, which relates to computer systems that learn from data without being explicitly instructed or programmed to do so (32). Sometimes the term machine learning is used interchangeably with the term data mining, but machine learning can be differentiated due to its emphasis on developing accurate and predictive models, whereas data mining emphasizes the discovery of new information and insights in databases.

A typical framework for machine learning, adapted for sport science, is presented in figure 20.1. The second row of the figure shows the various machine-learning tasks. Fundamentally, machine-learning tasks are often differentiated as to whether they are supervised or unsupervised, although semi-supervised tasks and reinforcement-learning tasks also exist.

Supervised tasks relate to those that rely on labeled data, specifically data that consists of paired inputs and outputs. For example, for each action or set of actions, a resultant output or event is also included. Labeled data sets can then be used for the purposes of training an algorithm, thereby leading to the modeling of relationships and interdependencies between an output variable (be it continuous or categorical) and its corresponding set of inputs. Consequently, supervised tasks are commonly used for prediction problems. In contrast, **unsupervised tasks** consist of unlabeled data, whereby an output variable is either unknown or not required. Consequently, they tend to be more useful for descriptive purposes, or uncovering new patterns in previously unexplored data sets. Semi-supervised tasks differ also, in that they consist of some combination of labeled and unlabeled data. **Reinforcement tasks** entail a machine being exposed to a given environment in order for it to train itself through an iterative process of trial and error (31).

Under each of these tasks, various families of methods exist by which the task can be carried out. These families are sometimes considered differently in the literature, but they are often grouped into five types. For supervised tasks, relationship modeling and classification methods are typically used. For unsupervised tasks, clustering and association methods are the most commonly applied (50). Semi-supervised and reinforcement tasks may employ combinations of these other approaches, although the latter will also tend to use a fifth method, which is control (55). Within each of these individual methods, various techniques also exist, each of which has its respective benefits depending on the intended application.

TABLE 20.1 Stages of the Data-Mining Process

Stage	Description
Stage 1: Data storage	Physically and systematically storing data in a set location with a view to its being recalled at a point in time. Computing memory is also an important consideration in this process.
Stage 2: Abstraction and representation	Translating these stored data into formats and representations that can be used for analysis and for deriving insights.
Stage 3: Generalization and inference	Use of such data to create new knowledge and recommendations that can be used to inform action.
Stage 4: Evaluation	Feedback mechanisms provide a set of quality characteristics relating to the generalizations and inferences that can be then used to inform refinements and improvements.

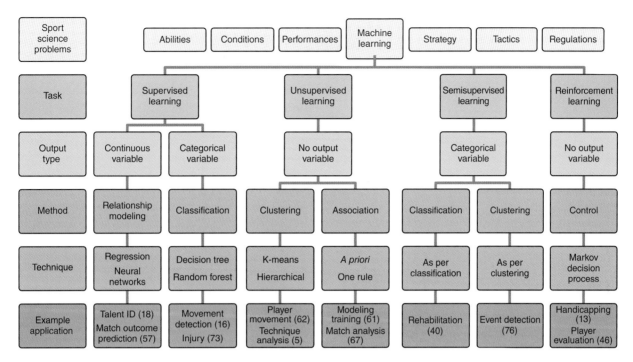

FIGURE 20.1   Sport science machine-learning framework.

Of the previously mentioned methods, **relationship modeling** is perhaps the most commonly observed. It works by fitting a function or model that best describes relationships between a set of variables and a specific outcome of interest (dependent variables). **Regression analysis** is the best-known type of relationship modeling, with multiple variations available. **Neural networks** have been developed as a more sophisticated form of relationship modeling (although they may also be used for classification) (21). Named according to its resemblance to the human brain's nervous system, their main advantage over traditional regression approaches is that they are able to account for nonlinear interactions between both input and output variables, while also learning without being explicitly programmed. These models work by incorporating multiple nodes, which are capable of transmitting information between other nodes they are connected to. Outputs of each neuron are then represented as a nonlinear function, with the exact weighting updated as learning progresses. Neurons may be assembled into a varying number of layers, depending on the level of complexity required.

The other form of supervised learning, **classification**, aims to predict a given discrete class output (i.e., category or group) using a set of input variables (2). Unlike unsupervised methods, where no prior knowledge exists pertaining to class membership, in classification this information is known. Information used to classify in sport science may include match outcome, athlete playing position, gender, or weight class. Common machine-learning classification techniques include

- support vector machines, which have been used to distinguish various sport-specific movements from inertial measurement unit data (17, 74) or to identify talented athletes from fitness test results (69);
- decision trees, used to model illness incidence (70) and explain win–loss match outcome in team sports (57, 59); and
- random forest, which has been observed in applications such as team selection (54) and tactical analysis in football (56).

Clustering represents a method of unsupervised learning that aims to summarize key features of data into groups using just the features of the data and no output information (unlike what occurs in classification) (50). The result of a cluster analysis is the formation of a number of groups, which in some cases are defined by the end user. Instances or items are grouped together based on their level of similarity as defined by these features, or the extent to which they are dissimilar from other groups. Common techniques under this method include

- *k*-means, used to develop distinctive team profiles based on performance indicators (62) or to identify different center-of-pressure patterns (5);
- hierarchical clustering, applied to examine relationships between motivation and performance in athletes (27) and identify cognitive structures of athlete technique (72); and
- self-organizing map, used to diagnose the presence of fatigue in gait patterns (33) or visualize changes in game style and collective movement in team sports (42, 48).

Association rule mining aims to extract meaningful and typically frequently occurring patterns in data (1). A number of types of rule mining exist. Simple association rule mining aims to discover commonly occurring associations with different states, whereas sequential rule mining also emphasizes the time course or sequencing of such events. Fuzziness is also often incorporated into some rule-mining techniques. This method differs from the Boolean logic often used by other machine-learning methods, in that it allows for some ambiguity in inputs and outputs, rather than forcing yes or no or true or false decisions. Commonly used rule-mining techniques include

- *A priori*, used to identify constraint patterns in training environments (61) and preferred patterns of play in team sport (11);
- FURIA, used to measure similarities in biomedical data sets (23) and as a framework for monitoring rehabilitation progress from knee injury (63); and
- FP growth, used to detect growth hormone abuse (53) and nutritional monitoring in athletes (45).

Evaluation of Machine Learning Models

Model performance can be evaluated in a variety of ways in machine learning; these differ depending on the type of method used. In relationship modeling, for instance, absolute measures such as root mean square error or mean absolute error are popular, whereas relative measures such as the coefficient of determination, often referred to as R^2, seek to delineate the variance in the output variable that is explained by the predictor variables. Information criterion measures can also be used to provide the goodness of fit of a model (9, 71) and thus can be used for model selection.

In classification problems, the confusion matrix is regularly used. This serves to provide a comprehensive evaluation of the matrixes performance under various settings. In table 20.2 a simple yes or no scenario is presented via a confusion matrix.

This scenario can be considered a performance analysis problem whereby the model aims to predict whether a team will win a given match. In the scenario, "yes" would indicate that the team is predicted to win the match; "no" will mean that the team is predicted to lose. The table shows that there are a total of 165 matches in the sample, with the model predicting "yes" 110 times and "no" on 55 occasions. However, the table shows that in actuality the team went on to win the game 105 times and lost on 60 occasions. Multiple pieces of information can be obtained from the table; some of this is descriptive, whereas other information relates to the performance of the model itself. For instance, true positives (TP) relate to instances in which the model predicted the team to win the game, and the team did in fact go on to win the game. True negatives (TN) refer to instances when the model predicted the team to lose and the team also lost. False positives (FP) refer to the model predicting a win but the team went on to lose (an upset loss), whereas a false negative (FN) is seen when the model expected a loss and the team went on to win (an upset win). Performance of the model can then be described via various rates extracted from this descriptive information. For instance, model accuracy is determined by obtaining (TP + TN) / total = (100 + 50) / 165 = 0.91. The misclassification or error rate is calculated by obtaining (FP + FN) / total = (10 + 5) / 165 = 0.09. The model sensitivity is determined by TP / actual Yes = 100 / 105 = 0.95, whereas its specificity is calculated as TN / actual No = 50 / 60 = 0.83. Precision answers a question: When the model predicts

TABLE 20.2 Sample Confusion Matrix

n = 165	Predicted: No	Predicted: Yes	Sum
Actual: No	True negative = 50	False positive = 10	60
Actual: Yes	False negative = 5	True positive = 100	105
Sum	55	110	

"yes", how often is it correct? It can be calculated as TP / predicted "yes" = 100 / 110 = 0.91. Prevalence, on the other hand, details how often this occurs in the data sample and is calculated as actual "yes" / total instances = 105 / 165 = 0.64. Unsupervised methods have a variety of different types of evaluation metrics available that differ substantially based on the technique used. Examples include error metrics between cluster centroids or a range of different indexes (3). For instance, larger distances between cluster centroids may indicate greater heterogeneity between groups. This process is considered more equivocal than in supervised problems, particularly when no ground truth is available.

Similar to statistics, machine-learning models also require both testing and evaluation. This process ensures that the results are generalizable to new data and scenarios. One of the most common ways in which these models are evaluated is through validation. A variety of different validation approaches exist, including the following:

- **Split-sample validation** splits the available data into a training set and a test set. Agreement does not exist as to what constitutes the ideal percentage split between training and testing (39); however, values such as 66% / 33% and 80% / 20% are commonly noted. The model is built using only the training set, with resulting performance then recorded. Once the model is built, the performance of the trained model can be compared on the test set. Substantial differences between train and test model performance can indicate over- or underfitting; this is described in greater detail later. This method of validation is typically used on larger data sets, in which sufficient instances exist for both training and testing.

- **k-fold validation** divides the data set into k number of parts or "folds." Typically, 10 folds are used; however, using 5 is also common. The model is run on k–1 of these parts, with a single part removed to test the model. The process is then repeated k times. Depending on the k selected and the sample size of the data set, model performance can vary substantially.

- **Leave-one-out validation** equates the number of folds used to the number of instances in the data set. This form of validation is advantageous in that it is able to use all points within a data set; however it can be computationally prohibitive with larger data sets. Its near equivalent in statistics is the method of jack-knifing.

Overfitting is one of the major issues experienced by machine learning, particularly when the sample size is small. Overfitting refers to a model that maps its training data so well that the model performs comparatively much more poorly when run on new data (20) (see figure 20.2). Machine learning tends to be more prone to overfitting than linear analysis approaches. This is the case because these tend to be more flexible in their ability to map complex data and can therefore often derive more specific solutions to a given problem. This is in contrast to underfitting, which often results when a model is too simple relative to the inputted data. Many linear statistical approaches fall victim to underfitting when implemented on data sets that contain complex relationships (57).

An example of overfitting with respect to sport science can be seen in talent identification, whereby a model to predict future performance of an athlete is constructed based on historical data collected from previous successful performers. An underfit solution may use a single value or linear function as shown in figure 20.2 to classify these "successful" or "unsuccessful" athletes. For instance, it might stipulate that in order for an athlete to succeed at a given sport, the athlete must have a minimum height or body mass. An overfit solution to the same problem could entail a scenario in which a multitude of prerequisites are enforced, such as reaching certain benchmarks on physical or technical tests, which may map a certain population or sport very well but not extend to new cohorts. Fortunately, a number of features have been built into many machine-learning techniques to reduce or avoid overfitting; these include complexity parameters (44) and pruning methods (49).

Deep Learning Methods

Deep learning is an advancement in machine learning that deals with finding and making sense of intricate structures within high-dimensional unstructured data (16). Unstructured data refers to information that is not arranged in an organized manner and can include data types such as images and vision. Consequently, deep learning has allowed for advancements in areas such as natural language, including sentiment analysis (8) and language translation (34, 68). Machine-learning techniques such as those discussed earlier are limited comparatively in their capacity to handle data in their raw format and have been outperformed by deep-learning techniques on a range of problems including image (41) and speech (29) recognition.

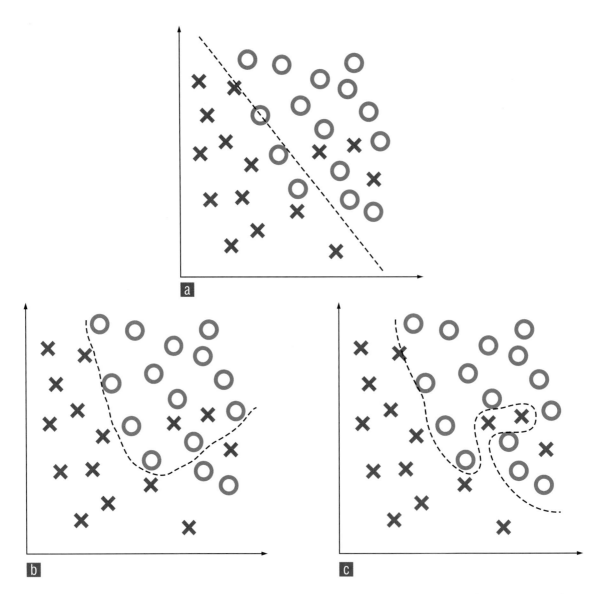

FIGURE 20.2 Overfitting data using machine learning: *(a)* underfitting, *(b)* appropriate fit, and *(c)* overfitting.

Deep-learning methods operate by learning representations. One of the most well-known deep-learning techniques is the convolutional neural network. At an initial level the raw input is taken and transformed into a higher-level, more abstract representation. Following multiple transformations, incredibly complex models can be constructed. Analysis of an image is a common example. The image can be considered as an array of pixels. In an initial network layer, fine-grained detail such as edges at certain locations in the image are represented. A second network layer may identify motifs by identifying patterns in these edges, whereas a third will assemble these motifs into objects more familiar to the human viewer. Further layers follow and identify combinations of these objects. An important

consideration with deep learning is that this process does not require human involvement; it is informed via the algorithm's inherent learning procedure.

DATA MINING IN SPORT SCIENCE

Increasingly, data-mining analysis methodologies are applying machine-learning techniques to obtain improved insights into large data sets. One reason for the increased uptake in such techniques in sport science is their ability to be used across a breadth of applications. This has seen use of machine learning extend to areas as diverse as training load (6), models for the development of talent (18), automated recognition of sport-specific player movements (17), and scaling match demands based on anthropometric and sex differences (52). On the field, player tracking data combined with match event data has been used to understand passing networks (14), the definition and visualization of pressure (4, 67), modeling within-team relative phase couplings (65), and probabilistic movement models and zones of control (10). In summary, data-mining methods can be used for just about any problem sport scientists come across.

Decision Support Systems

Fundamentally, most of the applications listed here emphasize altering the decision-making processes or outcomes of individuals or organizations. Since competitive sport can consist of chaotic, dynamic environments, humans often require the assistance of external aids. **Decision support systems** represent one of the most common ways in which data mining and machine learning is incorporated into the operational structures of sporting organizations. These systems provide objective evidence for decision making in such environments (66), typically using historical data to produce a recommendation or assessment based on output generated by a machine-learning algorithm (37). They also tend to incorporate back-end databases where information can be not only accessed and queried, but also reformatted for multiple purposes (25).

The advantages of decision support systems in comparison to human decision making have been well established for a variety of tasks. The psychologist Paul Meehl was one of the early advocates of such systems, quoted in 1954 as saying, "A considerable fraction of (human) clinical time is being irrationally expended in the attempt to do . . . prognostic jobs that could be done more efficiently . . . through the systematic cultivation of complex statistical methods" (47a). More work has further confirmed such commentary. One example includes a meta-analysis of 136 studies, which compared decision support system models against human judgments showing that humans outperformed the models in just 6% to 16% of cases (28). Research on sporting scenarios has shown similar results on drafting and trading in both the National Basketball Association (NBA) (47) and the National Football League (NFL) (39). In the NFL, the limitations of human raters in using information volume to the same extent as analytical models have also been shown in the task of evaluating players (51). A good system may even facilitate easy querying across different areas of a sporting organization, for instance,

exploration of relationships between performance data and membership, marketing, or social media content.

It is therefore unsurprising that decision support systems are becoming increasingly common in performance sport and have been reported in the literature for purposes such as player performance evaluation (12), competition planning (50), and athlete monitoring (58). However, despite these considerable successes, they have experienced limited uptake in certain environments (58). A number of challenges must be overcome in order for decision support systems to experience adoption and sustained use by sporting organizations. These include

- willingness of users to accept and act on recommendations,
- structured integration of the system into the organization's workflow and network infrastructure,
- overcoming users' fear of losing control of the decision-making process to machines, or of their role being replaced, and
- facilitating regular and reliable use by practitioners (7, 15).

Thus, a good decision support system will display the following characteristics:

- It is highly accurate in addressing a problem, particularly in a manner that is meaningfully improved over existing practice.
- It provides the user with multiple formats in which to consider the data and analysis output.
- It provides a feasible solution for organization, with respect to utility, user feedback, cost, and training time for staff.
- It provides insights into the quality of inputted data.
- It allows for parsimonious solutions to be outputted, thus removing data redundancies.
- It allows for the identification of sources of various biases in specific recommendations.

A good decision support system should also possess the ability to communicate findings via different visualizations. This is particularly important, as irrespective of model complexity in sporting environments, the output will nonetheless end up in a human decision maker's hands who is then required to interpret and act upon the information. To this end, visualizations are often more useful than detailed written reports because they offload cognitive work to automatic perceptual processing (36). Consequently, an appropriately designed visualization can improve time efficiency, since it may require only recognition from the end user, as opposed to the searching and conscious processing associated with written reports. As a result, recommendations outputted from visualizations may also be interpreted and acted upon more quickly than those obtained via written reports (43).

Of course, visualizations cannot always be used to replace raw data and written reports. They also have the potential to be misleading; this can occur even unintentionally as part of the analysis. Fortunately, many machine-learning techniques can display interchangeability and flexibility with respect to how their output can be presented. Concepts such as informational and computational equivalence are important to consider in this respect. The former can be explained by an example of two visualizations or reports in which all information contained in one is inferable from the other, and vice versa (43). Although difficult to achieve, some of the best visualizations for fast operational decision making can allow the user to obtain as much relevant insight as a written report or data table. Computational equivalence relates to the processing and computational demands required in order to generate two reports containing the same level of information. In sport science, it is becoming increasingly important now given the emergence of vision and other large data types that require additional computing power.

Visualizations should also be able to illustrate uncertainty in predictions or recommendations. It is also well established that they can help to facilitate this compared to written reports (38). This is more important than often realized, since when people do not understand uncertainty in a recommendation, they do not tend to trust the recommendation. Consider the weather forecast as an example. With so many open-access, easy-to-use visualization software options available, this is a valuable, yet easy area for the sport scientist to upgrade skills in.

Outperformance of Human Decision Making

While the benefits of decision support systems are indeed multiple, fundamentally their main purpose is to improve decision making beyond levels currently seen in an organization. In addition to the characteristics listed earlier, decision support systems are likely to further improve their performance compared to humans in the future. This is so because they can consider more voluminous and complex information than a human can when addressing a problem while also reliably maintaining large records of historical data. Thus, the greater the number of potential options that exist, the greater the complexity of data or level of disagreement among stakeholders as to what constitutes best practice, and the more advantageous decision support systems become (7, 30). This was recognized in the late 1990s by Fogel and colleagues (22), who observed,

> By their very nature, complex adaptive systems are difficult to analyze and their behavior is difficult to predict. It is hoped that intricate computer simulations will provide useful tools for accurately forecasting the behavior of systems governed by the interactions of hundreds, or possibly thousands, of purposive agents acting to achieve goals in chaotic, dynamic environments.

The theory of bounded rationality also provides a means by which to further this understanding. The theory holds that the decision making of individuals is influenced by the information to which they have access, their cognitive limitations, and the finite time they have in which to act (35, 64). Bounded rationality posits that in complex situations, individuals who intend to make rational decisions are bound to make satisfactory choices, rather than maximizing or optimizing ones (24, 26). For data mining in sport science, this has a profound influence. It helps to explain why in complex problems, multiple viewpoints may exist both within and between organizations. This could simply be due to how these organizations, or individuals within organizations, consider different types and volumes of information when faced with certain decisions. This in turn has implications for the manner in which interdisciplinary high-performance staff teams are constructed, since individuals from different disciplines typically have undergone varied training and exposure to multiple theories. It also helps to illustrate that because no individual ever considers all relevant information on a specific problem, an optimal solution will never be arrived at. Further, what represents an appropriate solution today may no longer be accurate or sufficient in the future, particularly as technology improves and data volume grows. However, applications of data-mining and accompanying decision support systems should bring the industry at least somewhat closer to this unattainable optimal solution. Although potentially a sobering thought, an awareness of this scenario should engender humility in contemporary sport scientists. They should recognize that they will never have access to all of the relevant information on most problems that they face. Acknowledging this can render them more likely to adopt a growth mentality with respect to their knowledge base, as well as potentially develop an open mind with respect to networking and developing new skill sets. Such an awareness is crucial for the development of all scientists, and future training and formal education of sport scientists should emphasize the enhancement of such qualities.

Improvement of Efficiency

The onset of data mining also has clear implications for how humans can integrate with the functions of machines in order to improve not only outcomes, but also their work efficiency. As discussed earlier, the predominant research covering human and machine integration has tended to emphasize human limitations. In order to increase the uptake of data mining in the practical setting, the sport scientist may be required to develop adroit strategies by which to drive adoption. Rather than solely focusing on human limitations, developing an understanding of both where and why humans and machines differ in their processing of various problems is of particular value and can serve to alleviate any potential angst about machines taking over. Given that most humans do not like their limitations to be constantly highlighted, in the early stages of adoption, decision support systems should be seen as a supplementary resource in order

for stakeholders to first see them as an opportunity rather than as a threat to their own judgments.

Another pertinent question relates to which processes and operations within the sporting environment should be selected first for decision support. This question can be answered by defining each process based on its respective characteristics, thereby defining its decision support readiness (see figure 20.3).

Common characteristics, some of which may constrain the given process, can include its frequency (e.g., daily), its relative importance to the organization (measured qualitatively or, for example, based on financial implications), its complexity (computationally or based on stakeholder feedback), and the time required or afforded in which to undertake the given process. Others exist and can also be considered depending on the requirements or emphasis of the organization. Processes that experience the strongest influence of constraints can be considered those most suitable for adoption as decision support systems.

The resulting concomitant gains in efficiency create the possibility for many tasks undertaken by sport scientists to be either offloaded completely or have their efficiency dramatically improved. Some of this saved time can be spent on identifying and implementing new and innovative initiatives. Sport scientists often have one of the few roles in sporting environments with the word "science" in their title, but for too long their ability to contemplate new initiatives in the field has been overwhelmed by a perceived need to become expert users of technology. Thus, the ramifications of decision support adoption

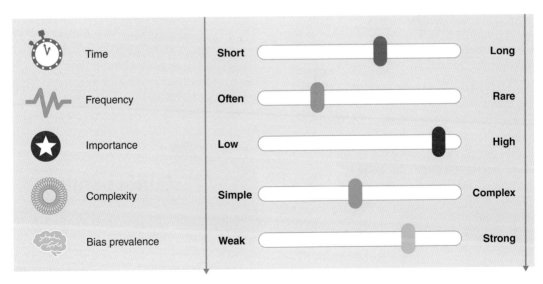

FIGURE 20.3 Decision support readiness model.

are nontrivial; such systems have the potential to fundamentally shift the typical role structure of the contemporary sport scientist.

In summary, it is important to note that although staff working in sport are expected to be experts in their given domain, very rarely does their expertise include formal training in decision making. Thus, decision support adoption provides a means by which complex decisions and processes can be offloaded to semi- or even full automation. From both a decision accuracy and operational efficiency standpoint, this will do both these individuals and the organization a favor.

Computational Thinking

In sport, an advantage of trialing different methods or techniques on a problem is that they may differ in their respective solution, thus providing the user with multiple options for action. Although most of the time the end user will simply want the most accurate or high-performing solution to a problem, on some occasions it is equally important that the solution be both viable and feasible for implementation in the given environment. This is often connected to the extent to which the nature of the output corresponds with the specific operational processes of the work environment. This can be referred to as the operational compatibility of the solution.

"**Computational thinking** is the thought processes involved in formulating a problem and expressing its solution in such a way that a computer—human or machine—can effectively carry out" (72a). It encourages logical organization of data, abstractions and pattern recognition, reformulation of problems, process efficiency, and automation. In doing so, one of its major benefits is that the method typically provides a multitude of solutions to the same problem. Given that computation has joined both theory and experimentation as the recognized third pillar of science (7a), a key challenge for sporting organizations is recruiting individuals and teams of individuals who are skilled in computational thinking, irrespective of whether they possess formal training in the area.

Computational thinking provides an intellectual framework for addressing the problems faced in a given environment. Previously, humans have tended to ask how computers can help them undertake science, whereas now they are starting to ask what science can learn from computers. Conceptualizing, and ultimately addressing problems in a manner similar to the way a computer or machine does, is a human skill

that is in dire need of development in the sport science workforce. If growth continues as expected with respect to data emanating from technologies, then this is only going to become more important in the future.

The aforementioned analytical developments represent an epistemological challenge for not just sport science, but science in general. If data growth continues at the rate described earlier in this chapter, it is clear that current approaches of querying structured databases will no longer be suitable in order to achieve new discovery and learning (3a). When this is combined with the ability of deep learning and computing to use large quantities of data, induction is consequently a reasonable position to take on many questions as a scientific method for knowledge discovery. Thus, it may shift scientific inquiry away from its traditional emphasis on theory development and toward a position of continual model updating and iteration. In particular, for complex phenomena without clearly defined causal structure, theory application will be both entirely inappropriate and infeasible. In problems relating to human performance, in which much data is still to be obtained, this will also move humans further away from existing working models that seek to adequately explain it.

This line of thinking may take some getting used to in the scientific community, however. Modern data mining has been criticized for reversing the standard theory—leading to data collection—to a data-collection-first approach (i.e., data fishing expedition). However, if for complex phenomena the models designed in the future are going to be recursive, this begs the question—why theorize at all? Further, if in the age of big data, "patterns emerge before reasons for them become apparent," then the data-collection-first approach may in fact present a way forward (19). Irrespective of what lies ahead for scientific inquiry, machine and deep learning are likely to continue to see improvements over existing approaches when deployed on complex tasks, because they require less human involvement and thus are well placed to handle any anticipated growth in data volume and types.

CONCLUSION

Data mining should form part of the contemporary sport scientist's toolkit. In order for the sport scientist to advance the direction of research as well as thrive in applied environments, at a minimum, a working understanding of data mining along with machine learning and decision support systems is now required.

This chapter has summarized the basics of data mining and machine learning, as well as providing examples of how these areas can directly benefit the individuals and organizations working within sport environments. Implemented appropriately, data mining and machine learning have the potential not only to improve the accuracy and efficiency of decision making, but fundamentally change the way in which those in the sport industry conceptualize, implement, and evaluate new ideas in sport science.

RECOMMENDED READINGS

Cun, Y Le, Bengio, Y, and Hinton, G. Deep learning. *Nature* 521:436-444, 2015.

Grove, WM, Zald, DH, Lebow, BS, Snitz, BE, and Nelson, C. Clinical versus mechanical prediction: a meta-analysis. *Psychol Assess* 12:19-30, 2000.

Robertson, S, Bartlett, JD, and Gastin, PB. Red, amber, or green? Athlete monitoring in team sport: the need for decision-support systems. *Int J Sports Physiol Perform* 12:S273-S279, 2017.

Sprague Jr, RH. A framework for the development of decision support systems. *MIS Q* 4:1-26, 1980.

Wing, J. Computational thinking benefits society. 2014. http://socialissues.cs.toronto.edu/index.html%3Fp=279.html. Accessed September 20, 2020.

CHAPTER 21

Data Delivery and Reporting

Tyler A. Bosch, PhD
Jacqueline Tran, PhD

This chapter focuses on the effective delivery of data insights to audiences in performance sport. While this objective may seem simple, the process for delivering meaningful insights to others deserves as much thought, care, and methodology as gathering, organizing, and analyzing data. Communication is an essential part of this process, and there are multiple ways to effectively communicate data across an organization. One of the most important aspects of this process is to define the questions one is trying to answer or the problems one is trying to solve. This not only sets expectations for the communication process but also helps define these aspects:

1. The data that is needed
2. The time required to complete the analyses
3. Other variables one may need to consider
4. The methods that one uses (statistical, visual, and what context is needed)

The questions need to be well defined in order to be useful, as broad questions can result in ambiguous answers. Delivering data insights through visualizations and reporting is fundamentally about **communication**. The quality and effectiveness of this communication require coordination and alignment between the characteristics of the **recipient**, the capabilities of the **messenger**, and the clarity and accuracy of the **message**. The primary goal is to be understood exactly as intended. While the person designing visualizations will have preferences and personal style, it is important to remember that clarity and meaningfulness for the audience are the main priorities. The aims of this chapter are (a) to encourage sport scientists to design data visualizations by thinking of the audience first (i.e., the recipients); (b) to identify key skills and ways of thinking that are useful for sport scientists (i.e., the messengers) who use data visualizations to communicate with others in performance-sport settings; (c) and to put these principles and skills into action by showing and deconstructing real-world data visualization examples that are relevant to sport (i.e., the messages).

DATA VISUALIZATION DESIGN WITH THE AUDIENCE IN MIND

When people think of individuals and the groups they belong to, it is easy to jump to conclusions (i.e., use heuristics to make rapid judgments) about someone's capability to interpret a visualization based on that person's group membership. However, the reality is that performance-sport programs are made up of people with a range of backgrounds, experiences, and skills. It is unlikely that all athletes or coaches need assistance to understand data visualizations, or that those with science training will understand the visualizations without any assistance or support. Therefore, it is important to do the work to understand the individuals in the audience, and then tailor the approach to support them.

At the heart of good design is inclusive thinking about the users of a design and how they will interact with it. In the context of this chapter, users are the audience who will receive, review, and interact with the data visualization (i.e., athletes, coaches, performance-team members). One can take inspiration from the universal design framework, according to which universal design is "the design of products and environments to be usable to the greatest extent possible by people of all ages and abilities" (22). That means getting to know the audience, designing with empathy for their capabilities and characteristics, and reflecting on biases, choices, and potential blind spots. The universal design framework includes seven principles that reflect the original motivations for universal design of physical spaces, products, and services (21) (see table 21.1; 2). Table 21.1 presents suggestions for how these principles might be understood and best adapted for communicating data insights within performance sport.

The role of sport scientists is not simply to fulfill a report-producing function, but to use science to enhance human performance. This can apply to the work they do in enhancing the performance of coaches and other staff, just as it does to the athletes they support. Every report, every presentation, every visualization that sport scientists produce may also be an opportunity to educate and upskill. As part of designing for inclusion when preparing data visualizations, sport scientists also have opportunities to think about how to scaffold learning for an audience, particularly if it is an audience that they engage with repeatedly over time. Supporting and improving the data literacy of an audience can create opportunities for deeper engagement between those receiving the information and the sport scientist. In return, this engagement provides opportunities for sport scientists to improve their professional skills and competencies by seeking out feedback and then adapting their practices based on the audience's experiences. Sport scientists can ask specific questions to gather useful feedback to improve their data visualizations and tailor these visualizations to the needs of the audience. Instead of asking vague questions such as "What did you think of the chart?" it is preferable to ask for details, for example, "What is the key message you notice from the chart? And how did you judge that?"

FUNDAMENTALS OF HUMAN VISUAL PERCEPTION

What is it that makes data visualization such a powerful medium for communication? Humans have evolved to possess a means for quickly making sense of the world around them based on what they can see. They view objects and surfaces, as well as their relative position and motion, and form images in the mind's eye about what that view represents (4). When people engage their visual perception, a raft of rapid, pre-attentive processes take place before they have conscious awareness that they are looking at something (7, 10). By understanding the fundamentals of pre-attentive perception and visual cognition, sport scientists can use appropriate visual features (e.g., size, shape, depth, clustering) that will help the audience to quickly and accurately understand the key messages in a data visualization.

Pre-Attentive Attributes

Pre-attentive attributes are the first things the end user will focus on subconsciously. These visual properties are processed within 200 ms of exposure to the visual. Using these appropriately can be a valuable tool within the toolbox, but inappropriate use can mislead the audience. Table 21.2 describes the four visual properties, as well as recommendations for use in reporting. Throughout this chapter, examples of different visual styles are provided.

Gestalt Principles

Observations from psychology research conducted in the 20th century remain valuable to the contemporary understanding and application of data visualization. The **gestalt principles** (1, 23) describe how humans make inferences about how visual information is organized and related to one another (see table 21.3; 7, 23). These principles are useful as a framework for matching meaning to visual form. For instance, objects that have the same color will be perceived as belonging to the same group (the similarity principle). Sport scientists apply this principle when they use colors to distinguish data that belongs to players on different teams.

TYPES OF DATA VISUALIZATIONS

Many options can be used for visualizing data; some options serve to better represent the data being presented than others. However, one of the most important aspects of visualization and reporting is connecting with the end user. Design of visuals should make it easy for the user to connect with the data and the message. Figure 21.1 (page 318) presents some of

TABLE 21.1 Principles of Universal Design and How They Might Apply in Designing Data Insights for Performance-Sport Audiences

Principle and definition	Examples of application in performance sport
Equitable use: The design is useful and marketable to people with diverse abilities.	Individuals on a performance team—athletes, coaches, performance support staff, management or executive staff—will use their own contexts, experiences, tools, and capabilities to make sense of your work. Design the analyses and reports to be accessible to audiences of different skills, abilities, backgrounds, and perspectives.
Flexibility in use: The design accommodates a wide range of individual preferences and abilities.	Consider providing multiple platforms for audiences to access a visualization. For example, some individuals prefer to interpret plots printed on paper, while others like to explore interactive charts. You could design a static version of the visualizations for printing purposes, and a dynamic or interactive version to be accessed on a device or online.
Simple and intuitive use: Use of the design is easy to understand, regardless of the user's experience, knowledge, language skills, or current concentration level.	A simple data visualization can have layers; it can be sophisticated, but most importantly, the central meanings and key messages are distilled, clearly articulated, and prominent.
Perceptible information: The design communicates necessary information effectively to the user, regardless of ambient conditions or the user's sensory abilities.	When planning and designing a data visualization, consider and account for these aspects: (a) The characteristics of the audience: Are there people who have a certain form of color blindness? How do gestalt principles affect human visual perception? (b) The circumstances people may be in when they receive your work: How much time will the audience have to view and interpret the visualization? What environment will they be in? For example, will they be on the field while coaching, or interpreting the visualization after training in a quiet room?
Tolerance for error: The design minimizes hazards and the adverse consequences of accidental or unintended actions.	Adverse consequences may arise from a data visualization if the audience makes inaccurate judgments from the data displayed (which may then lead to ineffective decisions). These are ways to minimize such a risk: • Visualizing uncertainty in the measures and estimates, to show the data for what it is and avoid conveying false precision to the audience. • Ensuring that sensitive or confidential data is adequately protected, and constraints are in place to prevent the misuse of data (or uses other than those agreed upon by the people from whom data was collected). Be extra careful when sharing a plot along with its source data! • Clearly articulating the interpretations of the data and working with the audience to build shared understanding about what kinds of judgments are and are not reasonably supported by the data displayed.
Low physical effort: The design can be used efficiently and comfortably and with a minimum of fatigue.	In the context of data visualizations, design plots that require little mental or cognitive effort for the audience to see and understand the key message. By thoughtfully designing with human pre-attentive processes in mind, color, form, spacing, and movement can be used to quickly convey meaning. When working with a particular audience repeatedly over time, consistency of visual styling can also be beneficial.
Size and space for approach and use: Appropriate size and space is provided for approach, reach, manipulation, and use regardless of user's body size, posture, or mobility.	Create visualizations that enable flexibility in their sizing and spacing. Use white space or negative space to avoid visual clutter and make clearer comparisons between measures or groups.

the most common visual types for reporting of data, which are as follows:

- *Bar plot:* This type of visual is probably the most common of all, and bar plots can be used with a variety of data types. However, they are best used when the data represents an accumulation. Think of the bar as a glass being filled; as liquid (i.e.,

data) is poured in, it can either fill it partially or completely full. Counts and sums of variables are appropriate uses of bar plots. However, caution is warranted when using bar charts as an average of a group because the group average represents a single value and not the accumulation of values. See figure 21.1a (page 318).

- *Line plot:* This type of visual is also common and

TABLE 21.2   Attributes of Pre-Attentive Processing

Pre-attentive attribute	Visualization design recommendations
Color *(intensity, hue)*	• Use visually distinct colors to highlight important points of interest. Note that visual distinctiveness depends on the overall color palette; bright green text is not distinctive on top of a bright green background. • Use colors to convey meaning. For example, a color gradient could be used to visually highlight increasing or decreasing values in a continuous variable.
Form *(orientation, line length, line width, size, shape, curvature, enclosure, added marks)*	• Create axis labels that are easy to read and interpret. Abbreviations may be useful, although abbreviations that are nonstandard can be confusing. With long axis labels, flipping the orientation of the axes may be preferable to rotating labels. • As a standard approach, start axes at 0 for numeric variables plotted in bar charts (i.e., avoid using truncated axes). • Use line types, widths, and colors that appropriately represent the data. For example, use a continuous line when plotting observed data and a dashed line for showing model estimates. • Use sizing and shapes to visually identify specific features and ensure that the shapes are consistently applied. For instance, use one shape per measure to distinguish between measures (e.g., one shape for lactate, another shape for heart rate). • Ordering is useful for visually showing structure that is inherent within the data, such as ascending and descending order or time and date order. Note that people from different cultures may have different interpretations of visual order.
Spatial positioning	• Set axis ranges that accurately reflect the data. If differences are small between data points, using a small axis range may inappropriately exaggerate the differences. • Display data from different measures in side-by-side plots. Combining two different measures on the same plot (i.e., with primary and secondary axes) can imply a relationship where none may exist. • Consider adding reference lines to aid visual interpretation. • Consider whether visual elements can be removed without removing critical meaning. For example, adequate negative space between multiple charts reduces the need for borders.
Movement	• Use movement and animation in visuals purposefully (i.e., showing movement in spatiotemporal tracking data).

TABLE 21.3   Gestalt Principles of Visual Perception

Gestalt principle	Definition
Proximity	When objects appear visually close to one another, humans tend to perceive the objects as belonging to a group.
Similarity	When objects look similar to one another (e.g., in size, color, shape), humans tend to perceive them as belonging to a group or displaying a pattern.
Common fate	Elements that move in the same way tend to be perceived as being grouped together.
Symmetry and parallelism	Lines and curves that are symmetrical or parallel to one another tend to be perceived as being grouped together.
Continuity	The human eye will typically follow the smoothest (simplest) path when viewing lines, regardless of how the lines were actually drawn.
Closure	When an object is incomplete or not completely enclosed, humans will tend to ignore the gaps and perceive a closed shape. Elements that form a closed figure tend to be perceived as being grouped together. Humans tend to perceive visual connection between sets of elements that do not actually touch each other in a composition but appear to form a closed (bounded) object.

may be used in conjunction with other plots to represent a third variable on a different axis, or to represent a rolling average of the data. Line plots are used frequently in time series data to show change over time in a specific variable of interest. With use of line charts, missing data requires a plan; if one day's or multiple days' worth of data are missing, thought must be given to how to handle connecting the lines between with missing data points. By leaving the lines connected, a linear relationship between those time points could be inferred, which may not be accurate since the data is missing. See figure 21.1*b*.

- *Point plot:* A point plot is another common plot usually used in time series data but can also be useful to show the variation in a measurement between members of a group. Instead of using a bar plot for an average, all the points from the group could be used, which allows the user to understand the variability of the data. This is really important since the mean of a measurement does not represent anyone on the team, and knowing which players fall where adds important information. See figure 21.1*c*.

- *Density plot:* Density plots show the distribution of the data; these types of plots take a while to fully understand, but they can be extremely useful when comparing days of training or players or other categorical variables. Density plots can quickly show where most of the values fall for any numeric measurement and the degree of overlap between measured groups. Density plots also provide a way to calculate the probability of a value falling within a specific range. This can provide some context as to how often a measure like that occurs. Density plots should be used only with a large sample; otherwise there will be spikes in the data. See figure 21.1*d*.

- *Violin plot:* Violin plots are a great way to demonstrate the range and density of a measurement. The wider the violin plot is at a given point, the more data points fall in that area. This is an excellent way to show individual norms and how a specific day of training falls within the total distribution of data. The density portion of the violin plot can add a lot of context. See figure 21.1*e*.

- *Box plot:* Box plots are similar to violin plots since they show the range and middle 50% of where the data falls. However, without an understanding of the density of the data (or where most of the data falls) can result in interpretations being inaccurate, especially if the data is heavily skewed. See figure 21.1*f*.

- *Radar chart:* Radar charts may be among the most polarizing types of charts. One key consideration with radar plots is the scaling of the data and whether everything has an appropriate scale to be placed on the same chart. Generally speaking, radar charts are used to compare several key performance indicators for a player or multiple players. It may identify deficiencies in a player's game (or highlight what the player is being asked to do). As with most charts, it is all about connecting with end users and educating them on what the data does and does not say. See figure 21.1*g*.

- *Heat map:* Heat maps can be used in multiple ways; one way is to compare several key performance indicators for a team, and another may be to compare where a player spent time during the match. This example focuses on the former and on trying to show comparison between players on the team. See figure 21.1*h*.

VISUALIZATION OF UNCERTAINTY IN DATA

Sport scientists seek to communicate clear messages about insights that address their motivating questions. The ideal scenario is that the insights they communicate are useful for informing important decisions. In the elite sport context, the reality is that many decisions will have far-reaching consequences on a person's aspirations (e.g., team selection decisions), daily experiences (e.g., decisions about preparation and recovery practices), health (e.g., illness and injury management), and livelihood (e.g., recruitment, contract terms). Judgments made from data visualizations are increasingly incorporated into consequential decisions within elite sport, so accurately representing the data is critical. In doing this, sport scientists need to give thorough consideration to the various sources of uncertainty that may exist in the information being communicated, such as uncertainty arising from approximated data, estimations obtained from statistical modeling, measurement errors, and incomplete data (20).

When communicating data insights, sport scientists need to clearly communicate what the data means, and equally, what it does not mean. The principles of scientific integrity must underpin the choices they

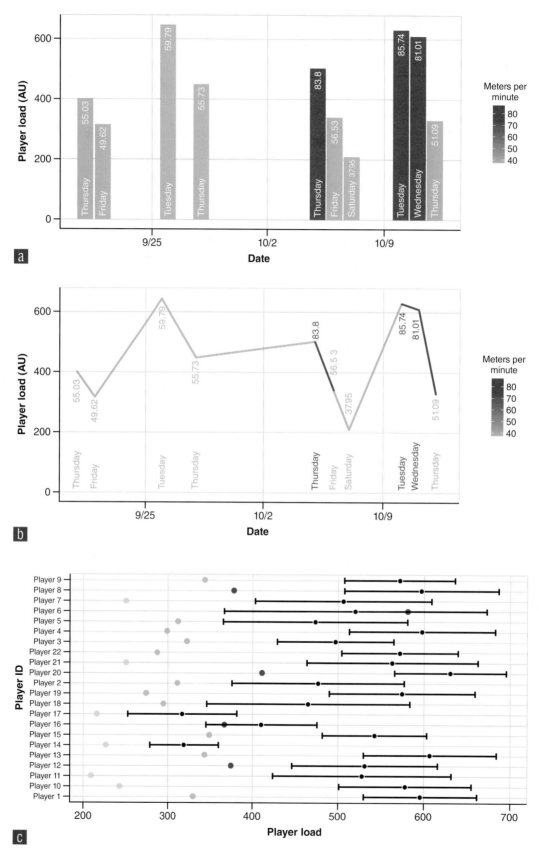

FIGURE 21.1 Common visualization types and reports in sport science: *(a)* bar plot, *(b)* line plot, *(c)* point plot,

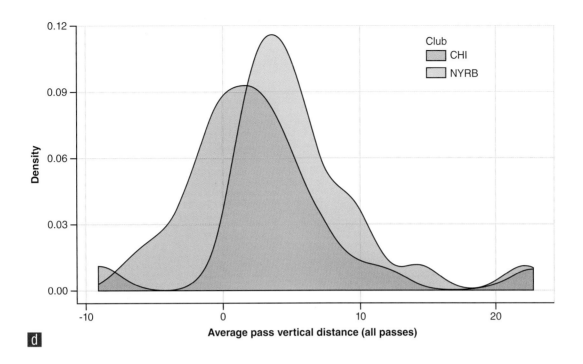

d

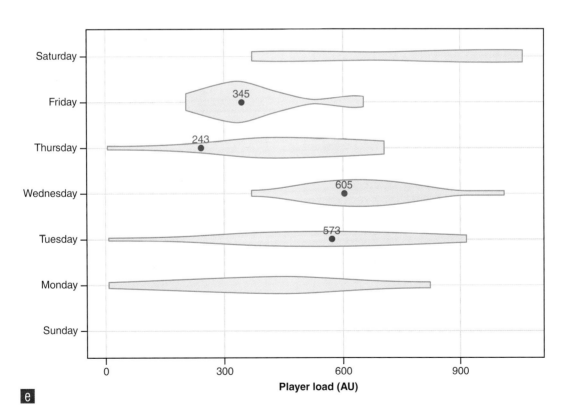

e

FIGURE 21.1   *(continued) (d)* density plot, *(e)* violin plot,

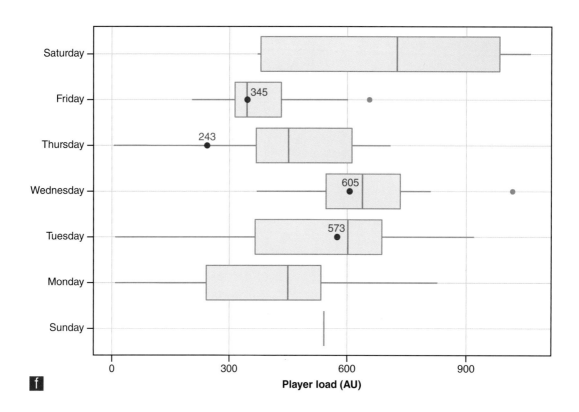

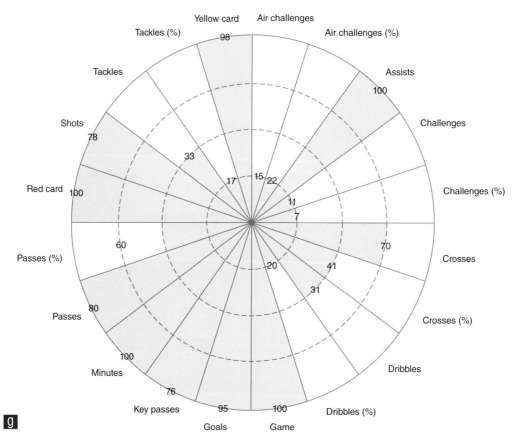

FIGURE 21.1 *(CONTINUED)* *(f)* box plot, *(g)* radar chart,

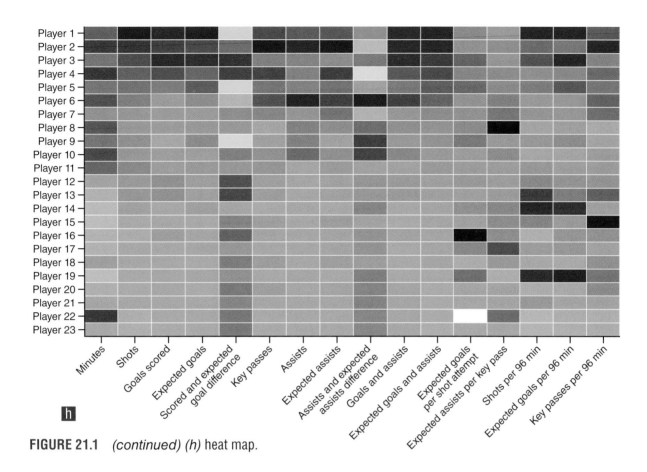

FIGURE 21.1   *(continued) (h)* heat map.

make as sport scientists, including the design choices they make when creating data displays. One principle of scientific integrity is particularly pertinent to this chapter: honesty. Ruth Bulger describes this principle as "a constellation of values including honesty, integrity, truthfulness, and objectivity in the way that scientists plan, execute, record, interpret, and publish their work" (3). To fulfill this principle, sport scientists have a responsibility to represent the data they work with as accurately as possible—this includes being honest, open, and upfront about uncertainty that exists in their measurement instruments, their methods, their analyses, their models, and their insights. An important aim is to avoid falsely conveying precision where it does not exist. By communicating insights and being honest about sources of uncertainty, sport scientists better serve those they communicate with. With a comprehensive picture of the available information, they can make data-informed decisions with levels of confidence that are appropriate for the quality of evidence available.

One of the challenges when designing data visualizations that appropriately show uncertainty is that the very process of acknowledging uncertainty requires people to grapple with complexity, which runs counter to human preferences for simplicity and ease, especially when it comes to tasks that require cognitive effort (like interpreting a data visualization!). The late Professor Hans Rosling describes it as the single perspective instinct (19):

> We find simple ideas very attractive. We enjoy that moment of insight, we enjoy feeling we really understand or know something. And it is easy to take off down a slippery slope, from one attention-grabbing simple idea to a feeling that this idea beautifully explains, or is the beautiful solution for, lots of other things. . . . It saves a lot of time to think like this. You can have opinions and answers without having to learn about a problem from scratch and you can get on with using your brain for other tasks. But it's not so useful if you like to understand the world.

How can sport scientists overcome such barriers when incorporating uncertainty into the design of data visualizations? In part, this may require repeated and ongoing discussions with other staff and decision makers to build shared understanding about why uncertainty matters: because failing to account for or recognize uncertainty when it exists can lead to misinterpretations and inaccurate conclusions (18).

The nature of the decision or problem, and the context in which the decision is being made, must also be considered when deciding how to represent uncertainty in a data visualization. For decisions that are made rapidly, visualizations of uncertainty may induce undesirable delays or feel overwhelming to the audience, so those designing the data visualizations need to consider the trade-off between precision and glanceability (11). When the decisions can be made with the luxury of time, visualizations that incorporate uncertainty may be better received by the audience, since there are more opportunities to interpret the uncertainty, seek guidance and ask questions of the sport scientist, and consider what the data means for the judgments they might make. When creating data visualizations, sport scientists can display uncertainty as a standard feature of their plots, which over time can become familiar to recipients, develop their visual reasoning skills, and reduce the cognitive burden of interpreting uncertainty in visualizations (15).

Here are some methods for visualizing uncertainty in data displays (9, 17):

- *Plotting intervals that represent areas or ranges of uncertainty:* An example is box-and-whisker plots, which display central tendency using the median and uncertainty using the interquartile range (the box) and upper and lower intervals beyond the interquartile limits (the whiskers).

- *Plotting all of the data points to show the spread or distribution of data, rather than plotting singular summary statistics on their own:* For example, instead of plotting mean values on their own, one can use density plots or histograms to show the data spread.

- *Using point opacity to indicate degree of certainty*: More certain = higher opacity; less certain = lower opacity.

- *Showing multiple looks of the same problem or motivating questions by integrating multiple sources of related information*: The aim is to convey to the audience that understanding a complex phenomenon requires consideration of multiple factors.

DATA-DRIVEN STORYTELLING

The use of storytelling to convey data insights has drawn attention for its potential "to delight and surprise and to spark creativity by making meaningful connections between data and the ideas, interests, and lives of your readers" (13). Creating and telling compelling stories with data requires some foundational knowledge of narrative structures and elements that engage audiences and convey meaning. For instance, Freytag's Triangle is one well-known structure of narrative arcs that describes five major parts comprising a story arc (8):

1. Introduction
2. Rising action
3. Climax or conflict
4. Falling action
5. Resolution

Applying this structure, Krzywinski and Cairo (13) suggest that data visualizations can exhibit a story arc by being presented in an episodic way, such that parts of the story unfold and the content and the purpose of each story part are made clear, "leaving out detail that does not advance the plot." While research on narrative visualizations is currently in its infancy, Lee and colleagues (14) have proposed the following definition of visual data stories to focus the scope of inquiry in relation to storytelling and data visualizations:

A visual data story includes a set of story pieces, that is, specific facts backed up by data.

Most of the story pieces are visualized to support one or more intended messages. The visualization includes annotations (labels, pointers, text, etc.) or narration to clearly highlight and emphasize this message, and to avoid ambiguity (especially for asynchronous storytelling).

Story pieces are presented with a meaningful order or connection between them to support the author's high-level communication goal, which can range from educating or entertaining the viewer with illustration of facts to convincing or persuading them with thought-provoking opinions.

Stories can be powerful and potentially misused, as summed up by the well-worn adage, never let truth get in the way of a good story. When stories are used to persuade, scientists risk employing cherry-picking approaches whereby, consciously or otherwise, some facts are selected for a visualization because this happens to suit a particular narrative while other pertinent facts that contradict that narrative are ignored or deemphasized. Given such risks, it is important that ethical practices be upheld when applying storytelling approaches to data visualizations (5, 14). The following are some ways sport scientists maintain integrity and honesty in their work while telling engaging and compelling stories using data visualizations:

- Avoid defining the narrative before examining and analyzing the data.
- Be wary of situations in which a confirmatory analysis may be requested to support a decision that has already been made.
- Peer review and critique (work with others to identify key messages and build the story).
- Make the underlying data and its analyses transparent, accessible, and reproducible.
- Acknowledge and outline interpretations of the data that are alternatives to the story being told, when multiple interpretations could exist.
- Explicitly identify limitations and unknowns or open questions.
- Provide opportunities for the audience to explore the data, test their own ideas, and pursue their own lines of inquiry.
- Engage in an inclusive and dynamic process in which audience insights and feedback are used and incorporated to update data visualizations over time.

CONTEXT-SPECIFIC FACTORS IN SPORT

As the saying goes, context is king. In sport, there is a lot of specific context that can be added to data. Coaches who work with a player every day will view the data within their own specific context. Similarly, performance and medical staff have unique insights that can be added to data. The goal of providing visuals, analyses, and reporting should be to engage these users and draw out their unique contextual knowledge to add to the data picture.

Timing and Formats for Delivering Data Insights

For most data types in the sporting environment, the efficiency from collection to interpretation is really important. How quickly and accurately can the data be analyzed to make informed decisions? This is an important part of the design process: understanding data pipelines and how steps in a data analysis workflow link together. These are also important to consider when identifying technologies to integrate into the environment, since getting the measured data from each system will have its own unique process that must fit into the workflow. Automating processing and reporting can increase efficiency and reduce potential user errors. Limiting any copying and pasting, manual entry, and importing or exporting of data can save the sport scientist and performance department a tremendous amount of time and increase the time available for collaborative discussions about data insights. The ultimate goals should be that as soon as the data is collected it is available to those who need it; while this is a lofty goal, thinking about the process and taking steps early to accomplish the goal can be invaluable. An often-overlooked benefit of automation is the consistency of the message and visual report. If someone is manually generating reports on a daily basis, there is a higher likelihood for variation in the message or how the report looks. Consistency of a report aids in interpretation and allows the end user to more quickly detect an abnormal pattern for the team or athlete.

Daily athlete measurements like well-being surveys, perceived exertion, or workload monitoring (e.g., distance covered, load, intensity of training) should be available before players leave for the day. This information can be useful when identifying recovery or nutrition strategies or when used by the medical staff in evaluating a player after practice. Being able to communicate this information in near real time is a strategic advantage. At worst, the data should be available before the training the next day so that it can be reviewed in full by the performance team.

Less regular (i.e., weekly, monthly) monitoring measurements (e.g., force-plate testing, isometrics, speed testing, hamstring testing) should be available immediately and within the context of that player's norms and trends over time. The purpose of performing those measurements is to evaluate how the player is responding to training and if an intervention is needed. If sport scientists cannot or do not evaluate the data immediately and communicate those results with the player and the performance team, they lose a critical opportunity to show that player the value of collecting data.

Game physical and performance metrics should be available immediately but may not need to be communicated as quickly. These measurements can be very noisy when taken on a single game sample. It is usually best to have a larger frame of reference from which to show trends or make decisions.

Using Data When Providing Feedback

Athletes in general can have a unique relationship with data. Depending on how they have been exposed to it and how it has been used by themselves on themselves, some barriers may need to be overcome. For a sport scientist, it should be a priority to make sure athletes understand why questions are asked and how their answers will be used. If athletes never get feedback or do not see the data being used, they are unlikely to trust or see value in these processes. Too often it seems that data has been used against athletes or not used at all. There should always be a plan and purpose for data collected on athletes, and there should be dedicated times to review that information with them to get their unique perspective on the data.

EXAMPLES OF DATA VISUALIZATION IN SPORT

The use of visualizations to explain and communicate information about sport performance has grown rapidly (16). Using the principles described earlier, this section examines some common examples seen in sport today.

Within-Individual Comparisons

Comparisons happen in sport. It is the job of the sport scientist to be clear when within (individual comparison) and between (comparison of at least two athletes) comparisons should take place. Reporting should be done in a way that makes it obvious what the end user should be comparing. A common technique is to use reference points to guide these comparisons.

Case 1: Self-Reported Well-Being Compared to Individual Reference Points

Well-being surveys are widely employed in many sports today, and can include asking questions about sleep, stress, mood, and rate of perceived exertion (RPE) for training (e.g., "How is your mood today?"; "How hard was training today?") and usually provide a composite score that can be tracked over time. This is used to track how athletes may be responding to training. Generally, the purpose of a well-being

survey is to understand "How are the athletes doing today?" Finding out requires the athletes to answer specific questions. Although these questions are important, they can be missing important context, that is, "Compared to what?" Any comparison requires a reference point. That is the purpose of a control group in an experiment, or baseline testing in interventions. The "compared to what" provides a framework for interpretation of the data. The comparison of that daily value to some reference point adds context to the data—so what should one compare to? The next figure shows the data from a well-being survey for a set of players. Figure 21.2a shows the raw data reporting the well-being of each player ranked from highest to lowest (comparing each player to other players). Figure 21.2b uses a scaled version of this data for all players in order to compare the players to themselves over time.

So which visualization gives better insight? Comparing players to other players or comparing players to themselves? Both of these approaches answer a question, but which answer provides information that helps make a decision? In figure 21.2 there is a dramatic difference between the raw scores and adding some context with a scaled value. This example scales the data based on the mean and standard deviation of each player to calculate a **z-score** ($z = [x - \mu] / \delta$, where x is the player's daily value and mu [μ] is the player's average value divided by the player's standard deviation [δ]).

Using this approach, all players are on the same scale, with their averages equaling zero and a positive number above the average, and a negative number below the average. Another benefit of scaled z-scores is that values correspond to the number of standard deviations and a value is above or below a player's average. For example, −0.5 would be 0.5 standard deviation below that player's normal range. This value is still within a normal range for that athlete, but a value of −1.5 or −2 is much less likely. The phrase "normal range" references the standard bell curve; in other words, this is common for this athlete. Figure 21.3 shows a standard bell curve where ±1 standard deviation about the mean represents 68.2% of the data, and if a value is below −1 standard deviation it occurs ~15.9% of the time. This type of representation can improve communication around the meaning of these numbers, such that instead of representing a value per se, they represent a concept: This response is seen less than 10% of the time, since this response has a deviation (a z-score) of −1.5. The purpose of collecting and analyzing data is to interpret and communicate results clearly, so that the end user can easily interpret the information. It is important to note, though, that this

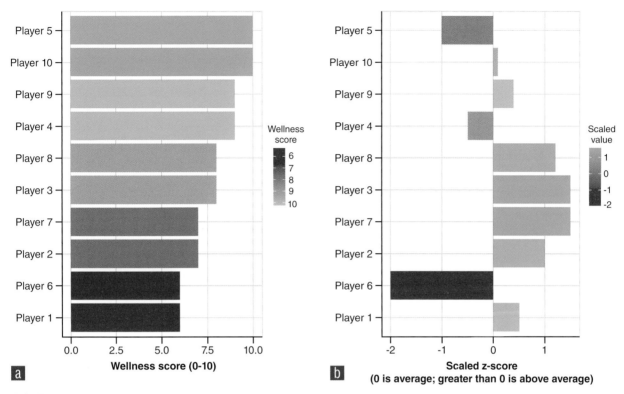

FIGURE 21.2   Presentation of well-being scores in *(a)* raw and *(b)* scaled z-score formats.

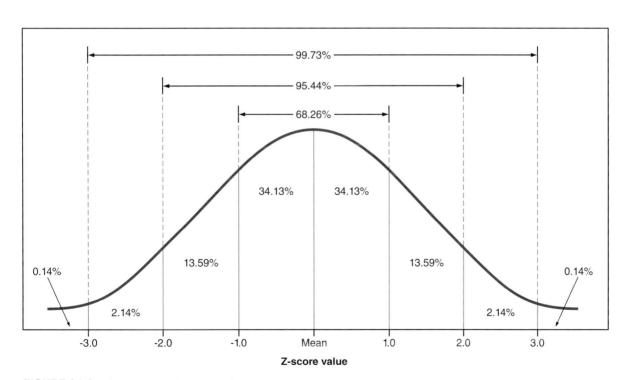

FIGURE 21.3   Standard bell curve to interpret z-scores.

transformation is valid only if the data (variable) is normally distributed (i.e., if a histogram is plotted, it should look like a bell curve). If the variable is skewed left or right (large number of observations on either side of the mean), then a z-score transformation is not an appropriate scaling method.

Scaling Data to Compare Players to Their Own Normal Ranges

Scaling data can be important when one is using subjective data, because in most cases the questions are based on a discrete scale rather than a continuous value. In the experience of the authors of this chapter, players tend to have their own scale within a scale. Some players may use only a small range of values (e.g., if the scale is from 1-5, they use only 3-5, so 3 becomes the low for them), whereas others may use the full scale (they rate their perceptions more broadly, between 0 and 5). From figure 21.2, it is clear that a player's scale tells a different story than the raw data; both parts of the figure (a and b) are ordered based on a descending total well-being score. Player 5, who has the highest raw wellness score, is actually below their own average. This suggests that this player usually answers on the upper end of the range for all questions

but deviated slightly, which is against the norm for them. Similarly, the players in the middle of the raw figure have lower scores, but they all are above their own average. This information is important because it helps to start a conversation with the athlete, and it builds trust and provides feedback on the answers given. Being able to start a conversation with questions such as "How are you doing today? You are reporting lower than normal; is anything sore or bothering you?" shows that their feelings are valued.

Recall that well-being surveys are generally composed of several questions, often with a composite score calculated. So, how can sport scientists dig a little deeper and identify what aspect of an athlete's well-being may be compromised? This then begs the question, "Are they down across all parameters, or is there a specific aspect that is below normal that can be investigated further?" Figure 21.4 is an example of how to scale responses and then visualize data to quickly communicate if athletes are below their normal range, how far below they are, and what aspects of their well-being may be compromised. Players having a score below 1 SD (yellow line) or 2.5 SD (dashed line) for a question or cumulatively for all questions could be flagged for poor well-being. This can be used to communicate how many players are responding below their normal range, adding context

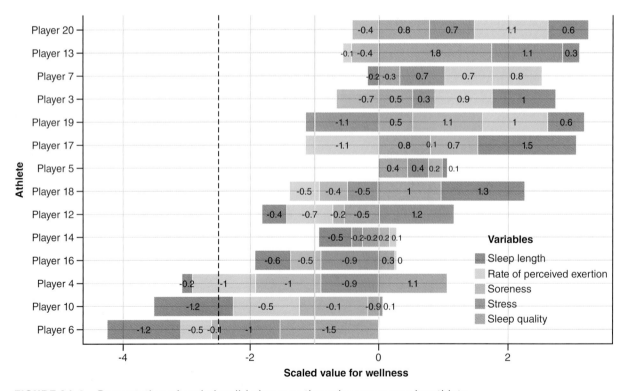

FIGURE 21.4 Presentation of scaled well-being questionnaire responses by athlete.

to the information. Since the well-being total is a composite of multiple questions, this visual also provides information about how the athletes are feeling on a more granular level. Is there a group that is not sleeping well? Or is there a group that is stressed? These subjective responses provide another layer to the sport scientist to help plan training and recovery strategies for each athlete. This information should be used to start a dialogue with the given athlete because these responses are subjective and could be more prone to biases and inaccuracies.

Changes Over Time

One of the most common findings reported by sport scientists is changes over time. This could be change as a time series (daily variations in a metric), changes in pre–post training cycle testing (e.g., 1RM, 40-m sprint time, maximum vertical jump), or how the team is improving over time for key performance metrics (e.g., time of possession, shooting percentage, defensive efficiency). These are important insights that have an impact for players, coaches, and management. Care must be taken when reporting changes over time to make sure that the information provided is clearly interpreted and unbiased. For example, time series data requires context around a player's norms. Showing a week's worth of training and games for an athlete without context does not provide the necessary information to make a decision. Is the player doing too much? Too little? The context provided should help clarify the message and leave little room for interpretation. Another important area in which clarity is needed is changes in metrics over a training cycle. Commonly this is pre–post testing. Did the athletes get stronger, faster, more powerful? These are rules to follow when reporting pre–post testing changes:

1. Show all the athletes and how they changed, not just the average for the team or position or event. Some athletes will improve; others may stay the same or get worse. This information is important as it can be used to modify training in individual and specific ways.

2. Provide some information about the size of the effect or change. Is the change meaningful or beyond the measurement error of the measurement device?

3. Use raw values when reporting change. Percent changes can be inflated when numbers are small. Focus on the actual value and units of change.

Case 2: Self-Reported Well-Being of Athletes

As discussed previously, when reporting on change over time, it is important to add context that provides a framework for how to interpret the data. The goal is that when a coach or performance staff member or even the athletes themselves see the data presented in figure 21.5, they can quickly interpret what it shows:

* How is the athlete today compared to that athlete's norms?
* How is the athlete trending over the last 7 days?
* What issues need to be addressed with the athlete and what intervention is needed?

In this case study, a combination of information types (two visuals and a list of information) is used. By combining data types, one can maximize the interpretation of the information for different end users. The ranking of the bar graph of that day's wellness reporting quickly visualizes which athletes are down, and the scaling of the data allows the user to see how far away athletes are from their normal levels. The line and point graph are then used to show the 7-day trend for the athletes, with the gray dashed line indicating the average (0 z-score) and the orange dashed line representing a z-score of −2. The purpose is to show if the athlete has dropped down for a single day or has been down for a few days (acute versus chronic low wellness). Finally, the list to the right shows which players are low for each question; the purpose is to show whether a player is down across all categories or one or two. Combining these data types in figure 21.5, the goal is that within a few seconds the user should be able to observe the critical data—in this case indicating that Player 6 is down today, that this is a big drop from where that player has been all week, and that it seems to be associated with sleep quality. Similarly, Player 16 is down today and has been down for three consecutive days. The end goal with visuals and reporting should be for the end user to draw a clear conclusion to make better decisions.

Colors are powerful within visual designs (12). The red, yellow (amber), and green traffic light has become popular in sport science, but one has to be careful about how one uses or relies on this approach. First, individuals who are colorblind will not be able to use the visual properly. While one is trying to simplify a message by using color, care must be taken not to grow too reliant on colors alone or an overuse of colors. For example, one cannot associate red with bad

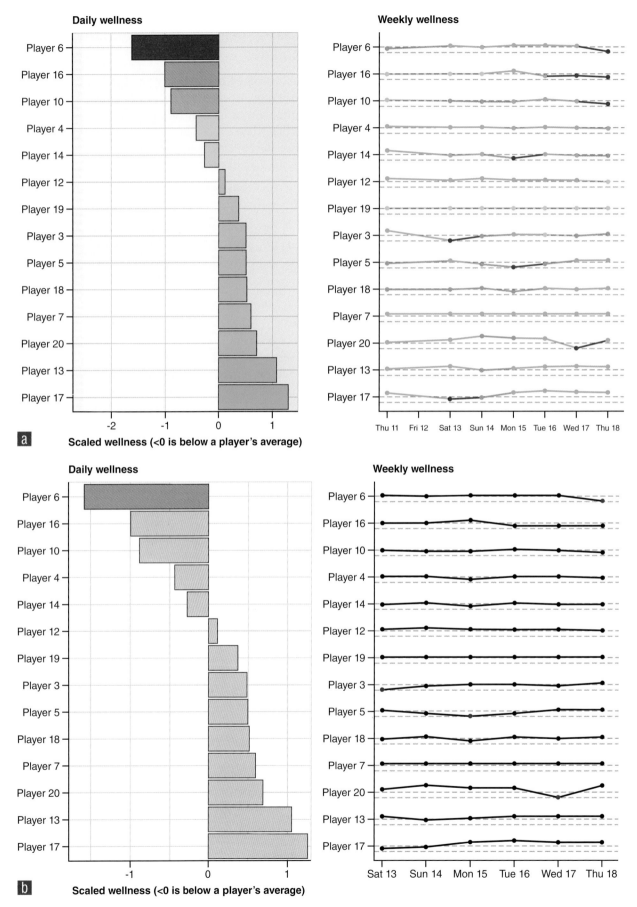

FIGURE 21.5 Presentation of daily and weekly well-being by athlete showing examples of *(a)* heavy use of color and *(b)* sparing use of color to highlight important data points.

and green with good because it is necessary to look at multiple factors with each athlete. In practice, sport scientists have to be very clear about what the colors mean and how they use them. Staff and athletes must be educated that colors are used to draw attention to information of importance, but that they must add their own context that will provide more information and help them make better decisions. How color schemes are generated can help with the interpretation. One common way people decide on color is based on a cut-point (e.g., a value less than or equal to −2 = red, greater than −2 and less than −1 = yellow, and everything else = green). Or maybe colors are assigned based on calculating the value that equals the lowest 25th percentile for training load, middle 50%, and upper 25th percentile. The purpose is to relay that red = concern, yellow = caution, and green = go or no concern. The problem, though, with cut-points is that they determine a difference between two values that can be very similar. For example, a z-score of −2 equals red, but a z-score of −1.9 would equal yellow. The cut-point determines a difference when there is not a real difference between the numbers. If the data are continuous (as with training load), using color gradients (a shifting from one color to the next) provides a better option because they better reflect the differences in the data (see figures 21.1 starting on page 318 and 21.5a). Digging into this a bit deeper, the use of color should not be overdone. Is the color adding value or used just to use color? The overuse of colors can undermine its ability to communicate a message by dulling people's eyes to what is important (7). Examine the same figure (see figure 21.5b) where the only use of color is for highlighting concern. Does the information jump out in more detail? Which is more effective? These questions underscore the importance of design and of designing with a purpose.

Case 3: Comparison of Athletes Within a Team and Over Time

The earlier examples in this chapter focused on individuals and how to represent and communicate their response to stressors, as well as how they trend over time. However, in team sports one is often interested in combining these perspectives, to understand how individuals within a team setting are responding over a period of time. When reporting and visualizing comparisons, many of the same rules discussed here pertaining to change over time still apply. Context remains critical, but more importantly, it is neces-

sary to make sure the design of the comparison is an accurate reflection of what needs to be compared.

Figure 21.6 visualizes team well-being while also adding the context of how each individual falls within the team distribution. Figure 21.6 shows the average of the scaled (z-score) well-being for the team over the last 21 days. This answers the question, "How is the team, as a whole, responding to training?" Each symbol (triangle, diamond, and inverted triangle) represents a player on the team. Showing each athlete adds context to a team average, as sometimes an average can be misleading. For example, if half the team is very low (−2 or lower) and half the team is very high (2 or higher), the team average would be around 0, but that average team value does not reflect any of the individual athlete scores. Furthermore, if the starters are the group that are very low, this is important information that needs to be clearly understood in order to make better decisions as to how to intervene.

The use of labeling for low values below a specific threshold allows the end user to identify anyone with a value less than −2.5 (i.e., outliers). This adds another layer of context to help decision makers understand the following:

- Where players are as a team
- How many players are up or high and how many are down or low
- Similarities between a group that is either very low or very high, which helps decision making for required changes or interventions

In a practical situation, if the five players who are low on the 17th (Wednesday) are starters, and there is a game on the 19th (Friday), a sport scientist may have the chance to make some adjustments and act accordingly. In the case of subjective athlete reports, design of and education on visuals should assume that important context about the athletes is going to come from the end users, and the reports should facilitate a discussion about how to proceed. There is the potential for outside stressors (e.g., academic, social) and layering the visual with team and individual information; some of these additional pieces may become evident as to where an individual or groups of individuals are relative to the rest of the team. In figure 21.6, the four players that are identified on the 17th are freshmen, and the time frame is midterms. The increased stress of academic demands may play a role in their low reporting of well-being.

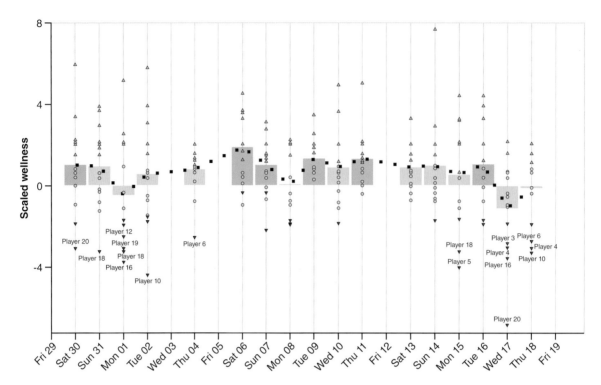

FIGURE 21.6   Team trend in well-being over 3 weeks layered with individual data for each athlete.

Integration of Multiple Information Sources

In the sport environment today, there are endless variables that one can measure and track with athletes. Identifying and grouping similar measurements together, the sport scientist can create a more detailed analysis of how the athlete is progressing and responding to training. One of the most common measurements is training load, which can be measured in numerous ways, as discussed in Chapter 2. When visualizing the training and competition load, one can think about it as volume (total amount of work done), intensity, and density (volume × intensity). Looking at load in these three ways is important because some players may respond to volume while some respond more to intensity and others respond to density. Identifying how the athletes respond to training and games will help identify the important response metrics to track.

Case 4: Training Load and Athlete Well-Being

Figure 21.7 shows examples of how to bring multiple variables together to add more context to the data using sparklines to display a lot of information for a variety of metrics in a condensed format. Sparklines can be generated with most data visualization software (e.g., Excel, Tableau, R, JavaScript); however, each may have unique ways to customize the sparklines. These examples are generated in R and can be customized to show individual norms for each person but are also interactive to show the value of each data point. Combining multiple data types can allow the end user to visually see trends at a team or individual level, incorporating multiple response variables (e.g., wellness score, cognitive load, stress, and max velocity), which allows the end user to identify if a player is more responsive to volume, intensity, or a combination of the two. In sports with congested schedules (e.g., Major League Baseball, National Basketball Associa-

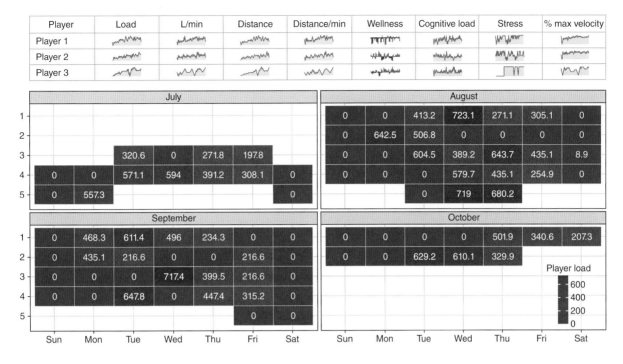

FIGURE 21.7 Integrating multiple data types and calendar view.

tion, National Hockey League), it may be more useful to use 3- to 7-day cumulative loads because there may be much less variation from day to day, but more variation with regard to acute time frames.

Adaptation of Data Visualizations for Different Audiences

One of the primary purposes of data visualization is to make it easy for the end user to see patterns or draw meaningful conclusions from the information presented. This is where design aspects of data visuals are important. Figure 21.8a through 21.8c shows three different ways to visualize the same information (4 months of loading data for the same player).

When developing data visuals, it is important to ask which format affects the audience the most. Also, what conclusions, without knowing anything else about this athlete, can be drawn from the way in which the information is presented? In figure 21.8, which view allows for a quick determination of the set of data points that belong to each week of the training calendar? For most people, it will be the calendar view. Calendars are familiar to most, so less time is spent attempting to understand what the visual is trying to represent. In figure 21.8b and 21.8c, the viewer must take time to identify the starts and ends of weeks, and days off

can result in dramatic peaks and valleys within the data. The calendar view allows for quick comparisons within and between days of the week and weeks of the month by relying on the standard presentation written text (i.e., can be read top to bottom and left to right). The audience can quickly visualize that August was a high-loading month compared to the others. This is a little more challenging in the longer time series views; it can be difficult to visualize days, weeks, and even months without studying the x-axis. This makes comparisons slightly more challenging but may be better for looking at trends and patterns for individual athletes across time.

The way in which data is presented can have a significant impact on the conclusions and interpretations that are drawn, including the layering that adds context to the visuals. In the three examples of visualization presented in figure 21.8, there are only a few layers of information. Shown are the date and the individual load that the player accumulated. The figure 21.8a (calendar) and 21.8c (dot and line) visuals use a gradient color scheme representing the player's load to add a visual layer reflecting how hard that day was for the player (the darker the red, the higher the value). As previously discussed, gradients can be useful with continuous values as they help to show subtle shifts in magnitude. In contrast, the figure 21.8b (bar plot) visual uses three distinct colors that

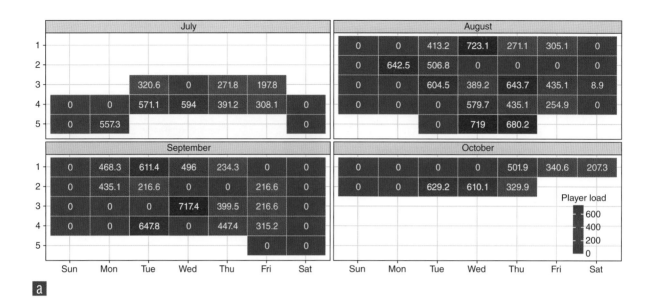

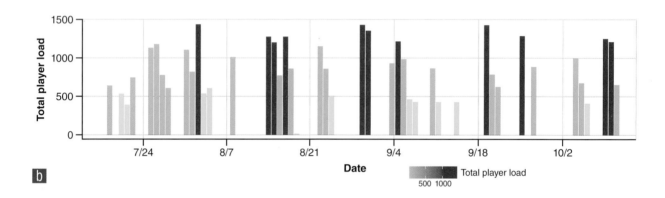

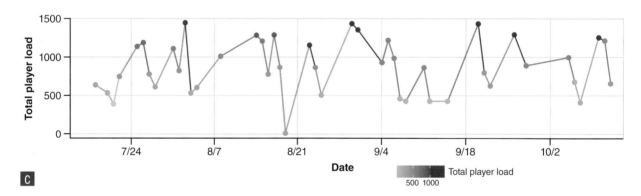

FIGURE 21.8 Data visualization design for time series data: *(a)* calendar view, *(b)* bar graph, *(c)* line graph.

represent the upper 25th percentile (red), the middle percentiles 75% to 25% (green), and the lowest 25th percentile (yellow) for that player (an example of cut-points discussed earlier). The purpose of using cut-points is to clearly identify a player's normal range of load versus high and low for that player. However, cut-points imply discrete categories and may suggest larger differences between categories than are actually apparent upon closer inspection of the underlying continuous data. Comparing the two time series plots in figure 21.8b (bar) and 21.8c (line and dot), the bar plot uses a cut-point color scheme and the line and dot plot uses a gradient color scheme. Comparing August 17th (total player load score = 1287) and 23rd (total player load score = 1159), the cut-point color scheme suggests that those two values are different, but the gradient shows how close those values really are. Use of a cut-point color scheme can communicate a difference regarding these 2 days, but the raw data difference is very small. Those 2 days placed side-by-side might cause more confusion since the end user might ask why they are different colors when the absolute difference is so small.

Communication with the end users is critical after one designs the report and visualization. Sport scientists need to be open to feedback and willing to adjust the report to meet the needs of the end user. Confusion on the part of the end user may be a design issue rather than poor understanding of the data or the concepts. Treat the end users as the experts in their field that they are and focus on inclusive design that can be interpreted accurately to allow users to add their own context. Some reports are meant to educate the end user, while others are just presenting the data in order to generate discussion. In each case, design is critical so the discussion can focus on the message and not use time explaining what the visual means. The best method comes down to the end user and the education around what these data mean and how they should be used. However, there are other ways one can use color to add context to the data. Recall that this section began with a discussion about the need to think about load, intensity, and density for the athlete. This helps to tell a more complete story within the visuals. Some ways to do that are covered next.

Data Layering to Show Load Variations

Different sections of this chapter have addressed the importance of scaling data to make comparisons both within and between athletes easier, using colors to aid the interpretation of information, and combining multiple variables to tell a complete story. The next case example looks at different ways to present time series data to end users. The goal is to present different examples of displaying information to clarify the message.

Figure 21.9 presents the same data shown in three different ways. Figure 21.9a shows raw totals and a gradient scale of the actual intensity (load per minute) to portray the volume and intensity of each day. Figure 21.9b shows the same data, but normalized to that individual using a z-score, where a positive value is above the individual's average and a negative value is below the average. In this case the color of the lines and dots is based on normalizing the load per minute (z-score), with an above-average value (positive number) more red and a below-average value (negative number) more green. The purpose of this visual is to have the user follow the trend in both volume and intensity of load over time. The design requires the end user to recognize that the line going up and a deeper red color is indicative of increasing volume and intensity. While this may be a reasonable assumption, it does require the user to consistently refer to the axis and legend. Some reference lines could easily be added to figure 21.9b at different points of the y-axis to provide a reference to 0 or whatever z-score thresholds are desired. Figure 21.9c is designed slightly differently and shows line and dot plots for normalized load, intensity, and density (where the color is the variable) and uses background coloring to help the interpretation. This visual allows the user to easily see the variation in both load and intensity (both go up, one goes up and one goes down, etc.) and the effect that can have on the density of work. Using colors in the background allows the end user to focus on the trends of the data rather than having to revert back to a legend scale. While the same information in figure 21.9c can be extrapolated from figure 21.9a and 21.9b, figure 21.9c makes the interpretation easier. It is much easier to visualize a change and variability using lines and dots as opposed to colors. The magnitude of the change is lost in a gradient scale unless there is a good reference point for what it means to shift from orange to red.

Additional layers of information can be used to add context to these figures; for example, adding the training date (or the opponent if it was a game) can allow the user to add information to this data (e.g., the player had to play extra minutes that game, or was guarding a very active player). Taking the time to think about what the visual or report is meant to

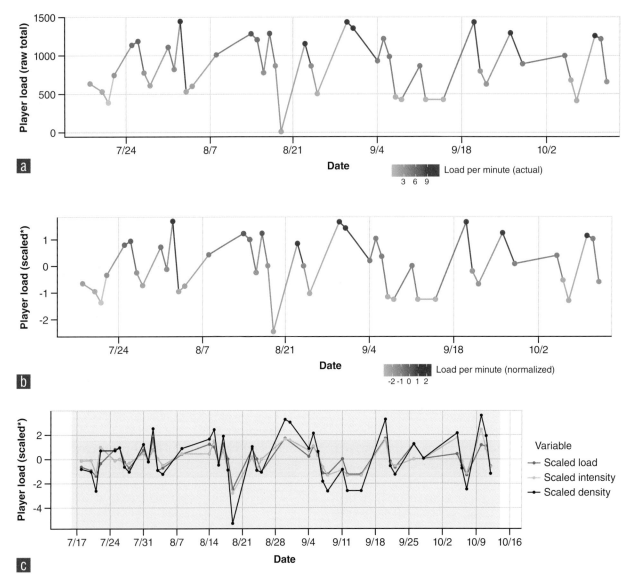

FIGURE 21.9 Data visualization design for time series data: *(a)* raw load, *(b)* normalized load, *(c)* normalized load, intensity, and density. (*Using a z-score: positive = above the player's average; negative = below the player's average)

represent and then designing the report appropriately to meet those needs can make a tremendous difference in the connection the end user makes with the report.

Visualization of Uncertainty With Sport Data

The importance of visualizing uncertainty for the sport scientist was discussed at the beginning of the chapter. The following sections present cases illustrating different ways to show uncertainty and how it can help inform a decision or create a strategic advantage.

Understanding uncertainty can have its benefits if discussed openly.

Case 5: Athlete Recruitment

With continuous measures, there are some very simple ways to show the uncertainty of a measurement or estimation. Figure 21.10 shows the relationship between age and experience (games played) in a group of athletes. The blue line and gray shaded area represent the average games played at the time of the trade at different ages and the standard error of that average. The standard error of the average is based on the standard deviation (the average deviation away from the mean) and the number of players within the sample (the larger the sample size the smaller the standard error will be, even in cases like this with a wide range of variability). This visual clearly shows that games played before being traded increases linearly with age; however, it also shows that there is a wide range for each age group. Showing the full data limits the uncertainty of the estimation by showing the wide variance that can occur. Imagine a scenario in which the front office of a professional sport team is looking for new players and is seeking to recruit younger individuals; this information could be used to target younger players with above-average experience for their age. The way this data is presented can aid in decision making and could potentially provide an advantage to the club.

Case 6: Body Composition Measurement

Another area in which uncertainty can exist is within measurements, since almost every measurement has some level of uncertainty around accuracy and reliability. It is important that when high levels of uncertainty exist, sport scientists be transparent about that uncertainty. For example, in cases in which between-individuals reliability is low (i.e., either the same measure performed by different people or the reliability of a measurement on two different people), it is necessary to either show or explain that uncertainty. One area in which this is prevalent is the measurement of body composition in athletes. Body composition is a highly variable measure, with varying amounts of uncertainty depending on the method being used. Table 21.4 presents information on the most common methods of measuring body composition: skinfold, air displacement plethysmography (ADP), bioelectrical impedance analyses (BIA), and dual x-ray absorptiometry (DXA) (2, 6). Within the table, reported data for accuracy, reliability, cost, and feasibility (time) are presented for each method. This information is important when body composition information is presented to athletes and coaches.

Figure 21.11 presents an example of the importance of showing the uncertainty of a measured value for

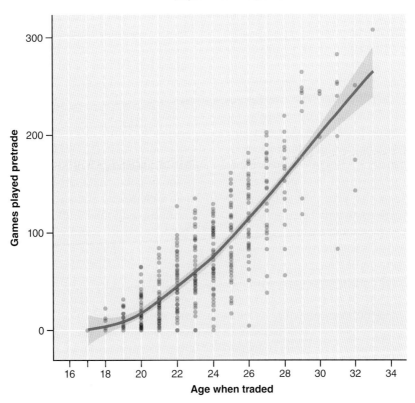

FIGURE 21.10 An example of the variation in games played by traded players with increasing age. The blue line represents the estimate of typical games played as the age of traded players increases.

TABLE 21.4 Common Methods for Measuring Body Composition

Method	Accuracy	Within-person reliability	Between-persons reliability	Cost	Time
Skinfolds	Moderate Range of difference from actual: 4%-15%	High, if method is consistently completed by the same person	Low (comparisons between people are not recommended)	Low	Short: 2 min per person (dependent on number of sites and people)
Air displacement plethysmography (ADP; e.g., BodPod)	Moderate Range of difference from actual: 4%-10%	Moderate Must be consistently calibrated	Low (comparisons between people are not recommended)	Moderate	Short: 5 min
Bioelectrical impedance analysis (BIA)	Moderate (higher for totals) Range of difference from actual: 4%-10%	High, but only for total fat mass and fat-free mass (regional measures have low within-person reliability)	Low (comparisons between people are not recommended)	Moderate	Short: 2 min
Dual-energy x-ray absorptiometry (DXA)	High Range of difference from actual: 1%-3%	High (hydration status should be normal)	High (people can be reliably compared)	High	Moderate: 3-20 min (dependent on device)

body composition measurements in two athletes (6). Body composition is measured on the same day in these athletes using various methods to better capture within-athlete and between-athletes differences for these methods. Figure 21.11a presents the measured value for each athlete for each method. Figure 21.11b shows the measured value for each method and the average error in the measurement compared to the gold standard four-compartment model. The two figures show the importance of displaying uncertainty; the default comparison made by the end user in figure 21.11a is that Athlete 2 has a higher percent body fat than Athlete 1. However, displaying uncertainty in figure 21.11b can inform the end user that the practitioner is confident that each athlete's body fat percentage is between the ranges of the error bars and that it is likely their percent body fat is similar. The reason for the large ranges is based on both the number of assumptions made using the method, and also in some cases the skill of the practitioner (e.g., skinfold). Uncertainty is very important for comparing change over time or comparing between athletes, because measured difference may not be actual differences if uncertainty is high. In figure 21.11b, if one compares Athlete 1 and Athlete 2, one assumes that Athlete 2 has a higher percent body fat than Athlete 1. While this may be true, the difference may not be quite as dramatic depending on the method used. In figure

21.11a and b, the differences between players' body composition are minimized as measures become more accurate and reliable. Problems may arise if actions are taken to lower body fat in Athlete 2, based on the comparison to Athlete 1. Using the potential error or uncertainty information from figure 21.11b, the actual values for Athlete 1 and Athlete 2 are much closer, and therefore it is more likely that they have similar percent body fat.

This type of information is also valuable in assessing change over time, because the larger the potential error in the measurement, the larger the least significant change will be. The least significant change is the absolute value above which there is certainty that a change is statistically significant (not to be confused with meaningful or clinically significant). But in lay terms, it simply means that a measure with higher error (uncertainty) will be harder to evaluate over time. If Athlete 2 is measured 2 months later at 7% (versus 9% now), is that a real change or is it just noise from a noisy measurement? Body composition is an important assessment because it can be a sensitive issue in many sports and for many individuals. There are consequences to use of the information, and it is the responsibility of the sport scientist to effectively communicate what conclusions can and cannot be drawn from the data.

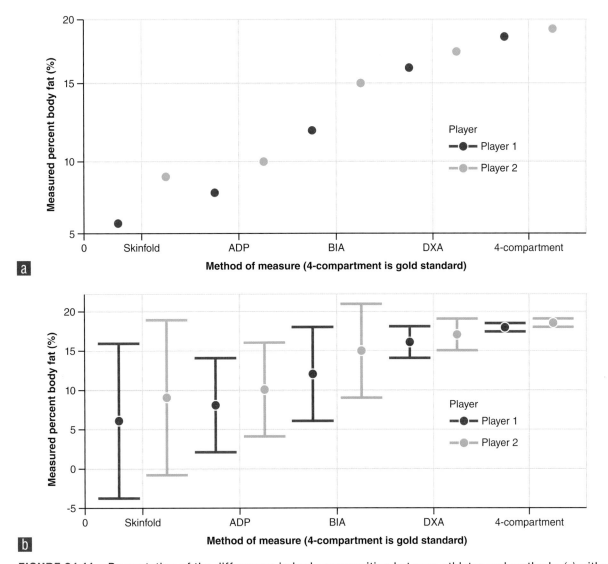

FIGURE 21.11   Presentation of the differences in body composition between athletes and methods *(a)* without error bars and *(b)* with error bars.

CONCLUSION

Communicating effectively using data visualizations requires knowing the motivating question for an analysis, understanding the audience and recognizing their capabilities, and using appropriate graphical forms that convey accurate meaning and suit the ways people perceive visual information. In elite sport contexts today, where data about preparation and performance are more available than ever before, it is critical that sport scientists have the skills to convey meaningful insights using data to inform decision making and guide practice in the daily training and competition environment. By applying universal design principles and understanding the fundamentals of human visual perception, sport scientists can create effective data visualizations that communicate accurately, clearly, and in ways that suit the needs of the audience so that they can use this information to make effective judgments and informed decisions.

RECOMMENDED READINGS

Duarte, N. *DataStory: Explain Data and Inspire Action Through Story.* Oakton, VA: Ideapress Publishing, 2019.

Few, S. *Now You See It: Simple Visualization Techniques for Quantitative Analysis.* Oakland, CA: Analytics Press, 2009.

Knaflic, CN. *storytelling with data: a data visualization guide for business professionals.* Hoboken, NJ: John Wiley & Sons, 2015.

Wilke, CO. *Fundamentals of Data Visualization: A Primer on Making Informative and Compelling Figures.* Sebastopol, CA: O'Reilly Media, 2019.

Yau, N. *Visualize This: The FlowingData Guide to Design, Visualization, and Statistics.* Indianapolis, IN: Wiley Publishing, 2011.

CHAPTER 22

Performance Interventions and Operationalizing Data

Clive Brewer, BSc (Hons), MSc

The term **high-performance sport** is often used when one is describing Olympic, collegiate, or professional athletes, whose primary objective is to achieve winning performances. Within this context, sport science is a specific discipline involving the application of scientific principles and techniques with the ultimate aim of enhancing sport performance; it may be conceptualized as distinct areas of study, such as physiology, nutrition, biomechanics, and psychology. Sport science is also often operationalized in a more interdisciplinary fashion as the science of sport (i.e., the evidential basis from which practitioners and coaches can draw to effectively enhance a component of performance that is being targeted).

In high-performance environments, sport scientists typically interact with coaching staff to provide services that affect specific aspects of performance. This may take a variety of formats related to understanding competition demands, characteristics of a specific athlete, limitations to performance, training load monitoring, or the responses to programmed training loads, among others. Sport scientists may also use scientific knowledge to inform training programming (e.g., follow researched recommendations on training methodology to program a load based on movement velocity, or use a specific work-to-rest ratio in a technical drill to target a specific bioenergetic pathway).

Whether gathering data or developing evidence-informed practice, the sport scientist is required to apply complex and sophisticated techniques in order to collect data and interpret this data to then inform training interventions and decision making. This requires the same considerations relating to data quality (i.e., validity, reliability) as would be adopted by a laboratory-based sport scientist, who is using experimental or measurement-based protocols to interpret data in order to prove or disprove an experimental hypothesis arrived at through inductive reasoning. Many of the conclusions that the research scientist may draw can form the evidential basis for interventions in the applied setting. However, there are some critical differences that need to be understood when undertaking this.

Primary is the realization that the majority of studies published in the extant literature have been undertaken with sub-elite populations. These athletes typically have very different genetic, anatomical, physiological, or biomechanical qualities from their elite counterparts, even when they are from similar sports. For example, collegiate subjects in a cycling study may have reported a $\dot{V}O_2$ max of 60 to 65 ml $\cdot$ kg^{-1} $\cdot$ min^{-1} in an endurance intervention, but how does one extrapolate the results of this to a professional road racer who may have a $\dot{V}O_2$ max of 75 to 90 ml $\cdot$ kg^{-1} $\cdot$ min^{-1}, as well as completely different cardiovascular and hematological physiology and technical (cycling) efficiencies that will cause different responses to a similar intervention? Through an understanding of how the differences in populations may affect the intervention, the experienced practitioner in these circumstances may be able to extrapolate the results of the experimental process to inform a specific intervention, but rarely will that application be direct across the contexts.

Typically, there is also a very different and highly complex motivational and psychosocial difference between elite performers and sub-elite athletes in sport that will enable performances that go beyond simple physiological explanations. Therefore, the performance of elite athletes is likely to defy the types of easy explanations sought by scientific reductionism and to remain an important puzzle for those interested in physiological integration (5).

KEY STAKEHOLDERS

For the purpose of credibility, sport science must operate in such a fashion that collected data actually affects the decision-making process within the coach–athlete program. This requires not only an understanding of the scientific process, but also an appreciation of the complex and dynamic social relationships that exist between coaches, athletes, and supporting staff.

Since about the turn of the century, there has been a significant realization that the intellectual property of sport scientists can bring great opportunity to sport performance (8), but this can happen only when the scientist proactively engages with the coaching program, and all involved are appropriately educated on the benefits provided. Sport scientists working in an applied setting within sports are in a unique and privileged position: They are able to provide quantifiable evidence that can inform and enhance player programs and empower the athlete to get better. In comparison, data that is not envisioned for use in this manner is a waste of resources and also reduces athletes' collaboration with the process; why should they engage in something that does not affect or benefit them? Such redundant practices ultimately serve to disadvantage the profession as a whole.

In practice, the success of a sport science program is built upon successful relationships with players and coaches, and these relationships are built upon mutual respect (2). This involves humility, in the sense that it is important for the sport scientist to be modest, even politely submissive (to the needs of the players and the head coach). This is often a challenging lesson to learn, especially since the academic training of many scientists is built around a process of challenging hypotheses, theories, and practices. To build trust, the scientist must instead bring value, competency, and character to the partnership.

Trust is a big component within the support team, and the sport scientist's competence at skillfully and succinctly presenting relevant data in an impactful manner to the coach is a core part of that trust. The science and data have to be valid, but more importantly, they have to be accessible to coaches, who can then own the decisions that are informed by the interpretation of data shared with them. Coaches might not need to know complex physiological theories, and they should not need to be scientists to understand what is being communicated to them, meaning that the way the information is delivered has to take into account who the receiver is and the receiver's characteristics and needs.

The lack of data application in decision making can potentially be one of the biggest failures of science within sport; scientific knowledge is recorded in scientific journals for a scientific audience, using scientific language that coaches may have difficulty engaging with. Similarly, attempts to "dumb down the science" often make the science inaccurate. However, as Einstein is often quoted as saying, "If you can't explain something simply you don't understand it well enough!" Coaches, for example, typically want to know what the sport scientist is proposing, and more importantly, why it will help them improve performance.

The ability to restructure scientific insights to build bridges with key stakeholders, and engage them with science, will be the key determinant of a sport scientist's success in the applied setting. For example, in explaining sport science to an athlete, one can use an analogy such as a car dashboard: Drivers on a journey are able to make decisions on speed, fuel efficiency, and route because of the instrumentation on the dashboard. If it were covered up, how would they know what speed they are doing (external response), or when they need to refuel (internal load)? What dashboard does an athlete have? This identifies a key function of sport science within sport performance.

PERFORMANCE AND RESEARCH DIFFERENCES

Any situation in sport, whether it be related to incidence of injury or performance enhancement, is, by its nature, **multifactorial**. Performance in sport involves solving a series of interlinking problems, defined and constrained by environmental specifics that must be solved dynamically by the athletes. The variables that are input into this process are functionally interlinking, and knowledge of how these factors interlink is imperative for the practitioner. Knowledge of this interaction of variables comes not only from researched knowledge, but from applied knowledge and experience. Indeed, athletic performance cannot be effectively explained by reductionism, which seeks to isolate rather than integrate variables. However, this does not mean that scientific principles should not be followed in the performance setting or be ignored.

A good illustration of this can be found in the researched literature around **periodization**, much of which defines periodization as a linear concept that produces significant differences in performance. This is, however, naïve in the extreme, because a **periodized plan** for a team or athlete is the logical and systematic sequencing of training factors in an integrative fashion in order to optimize specific training outcomes at predetermined time points (1). This requires a multifactorial planning paradigm that involves short-, medium-, and long-term fluctuations of training stimuli to achieve different periods of emphasis in a logical, sequential manner. This system cycles and sequences multiple training factors on a daily, weekly, monthly, and longer basis, with significant manipulation of inputs to achieve periods of different emphasis loading. Contrast this with the fact that many studies of periodization do not examine the integration of multiple training factors because a reductionist methodology requires variables to be isolated. These (usually) short-term research papers typically report training volume that consists of repetitions and intensities. This makes it difficult to interpret the training program and to determine the overall training load that the reported population (often recreational athletes) are subjected to (3).

This is important to understand, because sport scientists in the applied setting cannot simply be applying the findings from a research paper, or even a specific discipline, to their context; rather, it is important to be able to interpret data sets in the context of their application, not the body of knowledge. For example, a football player might experience greater triaxial stress in submaximal running than in sprinting due to mechanical efficiency and ground contact mechanics, whereas energetics informs us that sprinting is a more demanding activity.

SPORT SCIENCE IN THE APPLIED SETTING

In applied settings, practitioners largely operate within an interdisciplinary team or a multidisciplinary support team that has a coordinating position. This is typically the case because the role of the applied sport scientist is not to use domain-specific knowledge to advance a body of knowledge, but to solve specific sport-related problems for a team or an athlete. This requires the problem to be identified first, followed by careful consideration and integration of knowledge from a range of subdisciplines to address the problem.

It should be remembered that in most performance contexts the experiential knowledge of the coach, the athlete, and the practitioner (e.g., sport scientist, medical staff, strength and conditioning professional, nutritionist) is a great resource as a data set. Unless coaches are working with a very inexperienced team of professionals, there are few performance problems that are new or novel; most are derivatives of situations that coaches have seen before. It is important, therefore, that the sport scientist be able to use derived data to both supplement, and ultimately enhance, the coach's experiential knowledge in order to influence the program or situation and reduce the level of speculation that exists within any environment. Indeed, the objective of increased availability of data is that there should be less room for errors in execution. Data- or evidence-informed decision making is a key part of removing the guesswork from the performance process.

Using a combination of scientific knowledge represents a dichotomy in terms of the resources that are in place around the athletes. Does the team have the opportunity to employ an array of subject matter experts, or is there a generalist who can cover a breadth of knowledge, who has the capability to bring in experts for specific components of work when needed? What is clear is that regardless of whether an intervention is multi- or interdisciplinary in execution, using an appropriately coordinated multidisciplinary body of knowledge maximizes the expert resources available to solve the problem. Sharing such perspectives enables all involved in the performance process to grow their own understanding of an application and helps to ensure that no critical aspects of performance are overlooked.

By placing the athlete's needs at the center of the process, the interdisciplinary team is maximizing efficiency at the point of delivery as well. The sport scientist can then inform all involved in the player's program such that together they make that performer better. For example, in baseball, the coaches, supported by the biomechanical analytics process, may determine that in order to be better at hitting for power, a baseball player needs to adjust swing angle. The needs analysis for the player's athletic development should then focus on determining where the ranges of motion through the segments of the kinetic chain support this movement—and how to best support it—at optimal velocities, through a physio-mechanical intervention. Nutritional support can then be employed to ensure that the player's diet supports the training load and body composition to achieve this aim.

This process places the performer's needs centrally, which is crucial if the aim is to enhance the athlete's performance. It also stimulates growth in practice for all involved in the development of the plan. Coaches and practitioners begin to understand how they can best influence each other's work, and how they can learn from each other to enhance the coaching process. In this way, different knowledge perspectives and learning experiences are shared, which in turn stimulates growth in practice and begins the shaping of new ideas and opportunities. This is the cycle of the science of sport: evidence-based practice leads to practice-based evidence, which informs research and leads to evidence-based practice. This begins with collecting data that informs the assessment and subsequent plan development, examples of which are highlighted in figure 22.1.

The opportunity then for scientific process is optimized. This involves

- understanding the demands of the sport, not simply from a physical perspective but in terms of cognitive-perceptual, psychosocial, and psychomotor perspectives to inform the needs analysis;
- baseline needs analysis, which provides objective information that should be used to help the coach formulate a performance improvement plan that

is appropriately sequenced and structured, and that targets the most impactful areas to positively influence performance change;

- provision of an evidence base for specific, individualized training programs and processes to individual athletes based on their needs; and
- provision of regular monitoring and reassessment support to update and refine the plan developed for each athlete.

As figure 22.2 illustrates, the culmination of this process relates to the opportunity to educate and inform behavioral change, or program change, through application of the scientific process and operationalization of the associated data. This illustrates that there are numerous opportunities to affect a team, individual, or program throughout the training or performance process, and that these opportunities can be led either by one person or more typically based on a range of expert inputs. Indeed, the examples that can be incorporated into the evidence-based practice arrow (the green arrow in figure 22.2), or replacement of the training process with a learning or performance process, significantly increases the number of examples of building blocks that can be incorporated.

Bioenergetics

Nutritional status
Hydration status
Environmental sweat response
Macronutrient status
Metabolics
Neuroendocrine status

Information processing

Dynamic visual acuity
Visual-spatial processing
Simple and choice
  reaction times

Adaptive skill potential

Learning efficiency
Decision-making
Conscientiousness

Performance under pressure

Competitiveness
Grit
Optimism
Composure
Focus

Load management

Volume of high-intensity
movements:
  • Accelerations
  • Decelerations
Total volume of work:
  • Defense
  • Offense
  • Practice
  • Off-field training
Acute load versus conditioned
(chronic) load:
  • Volume
  • Intensity
  • Density

Preparedness

Sleep quality
Sleep quantity
Cumulative fatigue
Cumulative stress
Neuromuscular status
Motivation

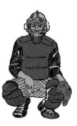

Athleticism

Range of movement
Postural strength and endurance
Speed:
  • Linear (time to 1st)
  • Agility
  • Throw to 2nd
Strength and explosive power
Repeated high-intensity endurance

Functional risk management

Current medical data
Injury history
Body composition
Training status (readiness and
  load management factors)

FIGURE 22.1   Sample sport science data points that can inform a catcher's personal development program in professional baseball.

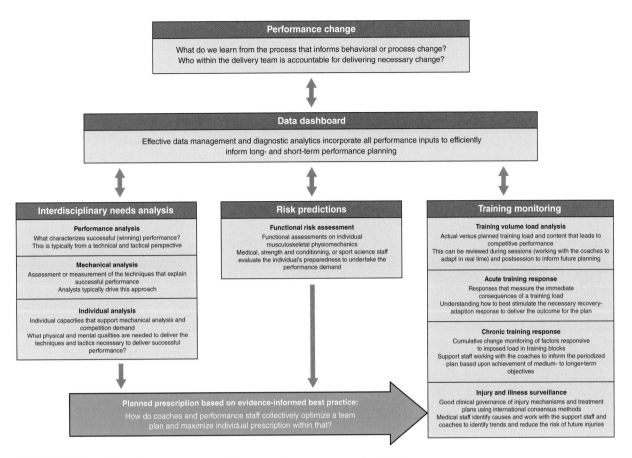

FIGURE 22.2   Data-driven processes inform performance development.

Figure 22.2 also introduces the art of the science. For example, note that several of the blocks incorporate the concept of risk in performance terms. This is a multifactorial concept based upon a combination of probabilities, whose dimensions are conceptualized in different fields of science. For example, in injury one might refer to epidemiology, kinesiology, and physiomechanics related to movement. The choice may also depend upon exposure; an athlete who is required to perform in every match has an element of risk different from someone who has a backup role. So it is a concept, rather than an absolute science, that is predictive or correlational. Understanding concept analysis is critical for developing an empirical knowledge base in applied sport practice, which will be illustrated in the remainder of this chapter.

DATA, CRITICAL THINKING, AND DECISION MAKING

As previously identified, the role of the sport scientist is to affect the performance process of the athlete or team. This can be achieved in several ways that integrate evidence from a range of sources, as well as experiential interpretation from a range of perspectives. The following examples explore how this might take place within applied sport. The information they convey is not exhaustive, but they illustrate how scientific knowledge can be used to create data sets that provide evidence to better guide decision making and the operationalization of performance interventions within the environmental constraints. The potential impacts for such interventions can be broadly described via these themes:

- Enhancing performance
- Optimizing health
- Solving problems
- Determining the evolution of technical components of performance

In any training process, the coach is required to create a periodized plan that will ultimately present the athlete with the best chance of success in a target competition. This involves optimizing the performance potential at a predetermined time point, and in many team sports this performance capacity must be maintained throughout the duration of a season. This peaking requires the structuring of precise training interventions to target specific outcomes, as well as to ensure that they are sequenced in such a way that prerequisite capacities are put in place, emphasizing certain training characteristics at specific times (without being an exclusive focus). The plans should also manage the training stressors so as to reduce the potential for overtraining yet promote the long-term development of the athlete. Regardless of the performer's level, the performer should be attempting to get better.

A regular season in Major League Soccer (MLS) is 34 weeks long, with successful teams qualifying for playoffs after the season. During the season, games are played every 3 to 8 days, with the training program in between games adapted by the club to ensure recovery from the previous game, technical and tactical preparation for the forthcoming game, and maximization of physical and psychological capacities coming into the game. This requires not simply an understanding of the stressors that influence the fitness (or fatigue) of the squad, but also an ability to quantify these at an individual level in order to best understand, and therefore manage, them within each player. The stressors are not necessarily negative, however; a review of any basic training process will identify that a stressor must be applied in order to elicit a programmed adaptive response (7).

A number of staff must come together with the common purpose of directing the daily training process. Principal among these is the head coach, who is ultimately accountable for the team's performance and the environmental constraints under which they practice and compete. Coaches have a number of assistants who help with guiding the technical and tactical preparation of the team. Working in collaboration with the coaching team is the performance team (which has different names across different organizations); the role of the members is to guide the physical and mental components of team preparation. Typically, the performance team consists of medical staff, strength and conditioning professionals, data analysts, nutritionists, mental performance coaches, and mental health experts. There may also be a sport science function, or the head of the program (e.g., a performance director) may be the sport science expert, depending on the structure at the club.

Figure 22.3 presents a typical example of how the underlying training processes can be divided into on-field and off-field for the individual soccer player within a team setting. On-field stressors can be quantified through athlete tracking systems such as Global Positioning System (GPS) technology. These typically allow the quantification of daily training volumes through external variables such as distances covered, intensity (speeds achieved), and meters per minute. They also use accelerometry to record internal variables, such a triaxial stress in the posture in response to the external loads.

In order to determine players' readiness to train, daily monitoring processes are also typically used to quantify their status. These processes vary with each team, and how they are constructed is determined by a range of factors such as available expertise, available budget, and the culture of the club. Typically, there is some form of neuromuscular assessment and a form of player self-report, but this can be as extensive as the resources available and the time to collect and analyze the data. As an example, figure 22.4 shows an example of interdisciplinary monitoring of daily fluctuations in peak power output.

In this scenario, the sport scientist must answer these questions: What level of fluctuation is significant enough to warrant an intervention? What type of intervention is required? These questions are not insignificant to consider on a daily basis for the sport scientist, whose primary aim is to maximize the training potential for the player (i.e., sport scientists should be doing everything they can to keep players on the field). This means being curious about why there is a variance in the score, as well as what the level of variance might be. Beyond understanding that there might be diurnal and environmental variation in power outputs, there is little published literature to suggest what might constitute a significant drop in peak power output. Suggestions might therefore be to identify an absolute value (e.g., 5%-10%) or a relative value (e.g., more than 1 standard deviation from the athlete's normal) that might trigger an alert for further investigation.

It is also important to understand that variance does not usually require the athlete to reduce the training load, although this may happen on occasion. This variance may be an opportunity for the athlete to use the results to direct an intervention that will enhance preparation for the day. For example, in baseball, one of the tests that can be run daily with pitchers is a dynamic shoulder motor control test. Once assessments have been done for a certain period of time to establish a baseline, all the athletes can identify what the ideal range in this test is for them. This means that

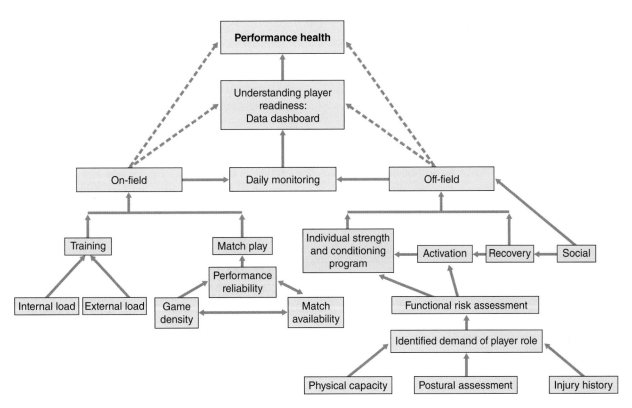

FIGURE 22.3 Understanding the role that sport science plays in the management of player performance health in a Major League Soccer (MLS) team.

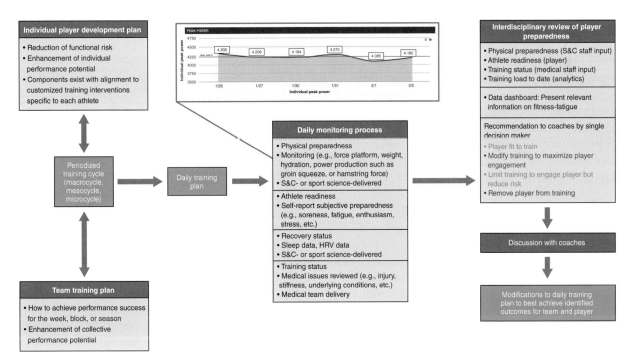

FIGURE 22.4 An example of an interdisciplinary process for reviewing training plans based upon daily screening processes.

if they had greater motion than is ideal, they could undertake motor control and stabilization work in the weight room, such as Indian club routines or loaded arm-bar work. However, if the active range of triaxial motion achievable is reduced, they may instead seek soft tissue work, either self-directed or on the treatment table with a therapist.

Similarly, linking data sets is an important process in order to gain full insight into an athlete's status. For example, if reduced power output occurs on a day following poor sleep, this may be a reason for the decline in performance. However, unless the athlete has time to power nap and wake up before training, it is difficult to overcome this circumstance. Instead, the information may guide some activation work or neural excitation practices that will help the athlete prepare, as well as guiding appropriate recovery interventions that will aid sleep following training that day.

It is important that in each situation, the decision to intervene rests with one person on the staff. For example, self-report surveys are excellent in terms of providing a basis for a discussion with athletes and just checking in with them. If athletes self-report high stress or high fatigue, it is often a good idea to follow up, asking them how they are doing, checking whether everything is good, and so on. After all, stressors are additive, and if there are things going on away from training that influence performance, discussing them and showing that you care can help significantly. But if five staff members ask the same question in succession, this becomes stressful for the performer and hinders the relationship and the management process. Similarly, it would not be appropriate to present three different versions of an athlete's readiness, based upon different individual interpretations of the data, to the coach. Thus, it is important that the sport scientist review the data in its entirely and then make an appropriate recommendation.

An important consideration is that the closer a training stimulus is to maximal neuromuscular demand, the more conservative decision making should likely become in an effort to reduce injury, risk of underperformance, or both. For example, sprinters doing maximal sprint work or very high-intensity plyometrics might have their training adapted (i.e., reduced) consequent to a very small (5%) variance in force production on a groin squeeze test. In comparison, soccer players participating in a high-intensity practice session that consists of low yet maximal sprint volume can potentially have training adaptations implemented following a larger (10%) change in a groin squeeze diagnostic because maximal neu-

romuscular strain was likely lower. Note that this is not a perfect science; instead, it requires data to be collected over long periods of time before it is used to guide interventions in an impactful way. Some of the worst decisions are ultimately made by practitioners analyzing data before there is enough data to really base a decision upon. Also required is an understanding of what is normal for the population and normal for the individual player. Many have learned from experience that the worst decisions are made based on monitoring data before there is enough to truly understand what influences the trend.

CASE STUDY: THE ROLE OF SPORT SCIENCE IN THE PERFORMANCE DEVELOPMENT OF MAJOR LEAGUE PITCHERS

At every level of sport, the aim of practitioners is to make the player better, whether the player is a young athlete or an All-Star. A major league pitcher in baseball is a highly skilled and physical athlete who requires dexterity, power, and durability to achieve success at the highest level. A sport science program can provide data-informed decisions that can guide both the physical and technical development of a player and how the coaches manage the player. This is based upon the premise that certain movement qualities underpin not simply successful execution of a skill, but also the ability to repeat the execution of a skill without injury. These movement patterns must be maintained despite multiple repetitions of actions with high neuromuscular demands that could, without appropriate management, impair the movement.

To be a successful starting pitcher in Major League Baseball (MLB), a player should have the durability to be able to pitch every 5 days (i.e., the approximate starting rotation in the regular season) and throw five to eight innings per start (for an average total of 80-120 pitches). The velocity of each pitch will be between 90 (145 kph) and 105 mph (169 kph) depending on the pitcher, and each type of pitch will have a different neuromuscular demand. For example, fastballs are maximal-effort deliveries but place less mechanical stress on the pitcher's shoulder and elbow than a curve ball.

The player development process is complex and necessitates the identification of a plan that determines how a player can meet the required performance demands from a physical, mental, technical, and tactical perspective. As identified previously, there is a strong interrelationship between skill execution and the player's movement (physical) ability to execute that skill. The key requirement for a sport scientist in this field is to work with the skill-specific coach (who may have little or no background in functional anatomy) in order to inform the development process from a physio-mechanical (in this example) perspective. As figure 22.5 illustrates, the motor requirements for a pitch delivery are known (with much individual variation accepted). However, the ability to assess the athlete's capacity to match these requirements and inform an ongoing training and playing process that delivers and supports sustained performance improvement is crucial.

Data can be used to inform the coaching process around players' ability to enhance their motor control, generate and accept force, and give context to efficient technique in delivery. In providing this information sport scientists can also enhance durability by increasing the resistance to fatigue and creating a more robust movement system. The important context for this data is that it be interpretable to the respective target professionals who will translate the identified requirements into action plans.

This can be explained through the process detailed in figure 22.5. Kinematic analysis of the pitching delivery indicates that a comprehensive physical assessment process is necessary to inform the training plan. Joint assessments cannot be limited to range of motion alone (for example), since while the shoulder may need to rotate through more than 165° of motion externally and internally, this is predicated on high internal torque and dependent upon trunk angular velocity for 60% of the variance (6). Through quantification of the underpinning physio-mechanical characteristics a player has, the sport scientist, in conjunction with medical and conditioning specialists, can use a gap analysis that compares current and required physical characteristics.

In determining this, in the context of expert knowledge about the player's potential to achieve, the support team can provide a plan that enables the player to address areas such as factors that may exacerbate injury risk or reduce performance potential. The basis of such programs is typically to treat pain, correct dysfunction, train deficiency, and load competent patterns. Each stage of this process yields data that can then be tracked to monitor progress over time.

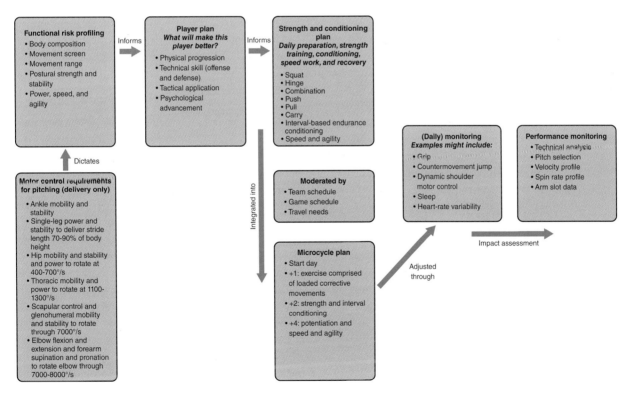

FIGURE 22.5 Sport science application in the player-performance development process for baseball pitchers in a Major League Baseball (MLB) organization.

The Importance of Evidencing a Differential Diagnosis

With appropriate interpretation, data should be extremely influential in a differential diagnostic process for a player development plan. Suppose, for example, that the coaches identify that a player needs to do more agility work because that player is always slow off the mound in fielding a ball. However, the reactive agility testing data demonstrates that the player has really good movement times for the position, and the video shows good movement skills. This, then, helps to provide evidence for the discussion that perhaps contextual application of these skills is what is needed in practice, and that the apparent slowness is not actually physical, but more related to reading and reacting to the game situation.

Similarly, when a pitching coach suggests that a player does not use the lower body enough in the delivery (forward momentum and hip rotation is enabled with leg drive), it is useful to be able to look at vertical jump data and compare hands-on-hips jumping performance with a countermovement jump: The hands-on-hips jump is indicative of lower-body power, so a low number here may illustrate that the player needs more focus to develop this as a strength-power movement quality, and the program can be tailored accordingly. The total-body jump should be significantly higher (deterministic modeling of the countermovement jump suggests that this might be as high as 40% in good jumping athletes [4]). If this significant difference is not seen between the two styles of jump, it may indicate that the player lacks the coordinative ability to synchronize ground-based movements through the kinetic chain. This may require the addition of increased medicine ball throws and plyometric drills that require the lower limb to generate forces and transfer these to high impulse to the ball. These may be the focus of the program or be needed to build on top of a strength generation focus. Conversely, the player may have really high power-producing capacity and jumping skill execution but need specific pitching drills to learn to apply impulse to the baseball in the specific drill context.

Audience-Specific Data Analytics and Communication

Figure 22.5 presents an overview of an involved and continuous process, and it is outside the scope of this chapter to explore each stage in detail. However, specific examples of interventional opportunities merit further exploration to illustrate the impact that the scientific process can have upon a player's program. It is also important to consider who the data is affecting and the respective time frames that need to occur for professionals to undertake their roles. An earlier section of this chapter provided an example of instantaneous feedback required to guide intervention following a daily shoulder motor control screening.

Evidence-guided decisions are also important for the coach, who will need data to inform daily and weekly decision-making processes that relate to adjustments to the player's program, and ultimately selection. As figure 22.6 illustrates, tools should be produced that enable the coach to manipulate program or environmental variables based upon the information available. Specific monitoring examples highlighted earlier in the chapter illustrate this principle well.

Recording and analyzing such data sets enables the establishment of trends that can be traced at a system level through reports and surveillance techniques. These enable professionals whose role is more about program guidance or roster management (rather than direct player program delivery) to undertake reviews and inform their decision making for more longitudinal impact. This may inform discussions between experts, strategic program decisions, or educational processes for staff that will address the gap analysis between what the system needs and what the system can deliver. What is crucial is that although the required techniques are different at each delivery level, the time frames for making and acting upon decisions are different, and the data reporting may be different, the actual raw data sets that inform each of these processes are typically the same. It is the presentation and analysis of the data that are typically adapted to enable decisions to be made at an individual or program level.

It is also important to respect the fact that data collected with the intent of benefitting a player's performance health can be taken out of context if the correct management process is not used. For example, the practitioner taking the shoulder measurement needs to know the specific data point at which to make a decision, the coach needs to know that the player is good to go as planned or if today's workload needs to be modified, and the front office needs to know if the player is on track with meeting the target objectives within the defined player development plan. Ultimately, players who cannot maintain their performance trajectory (or those who exceed it) will be determining roster moves.

Sport scientists should consider that modern-day athlete development requires a multifaceted and

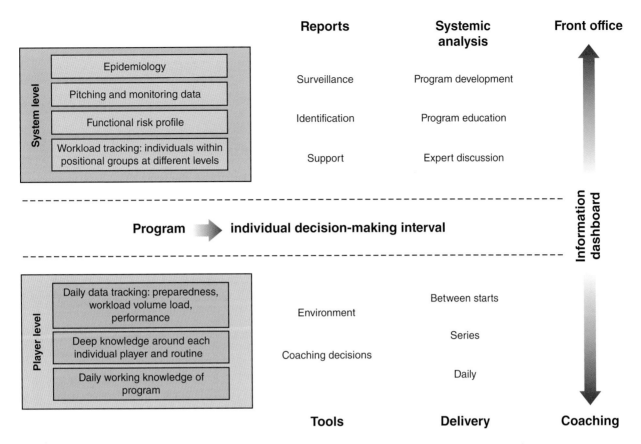

FIGURE 22.6 The information management process is dictated by the decision interval within a system.

modular approach with all practitioners working in synergy toward a commonly identified, monitored, and quantifiable goal that has the athlete as the central focus of the delivery process. It is necessary to be able to evidence the systematic process of athletic training and management so that it is possible to interrogate, explain, and replicate or eradicate emergent patterns (e.g., injury trend, peak performance). This informs the decision-making process for training programming, scheduling recovery, and optimizing performance. It also enhances the human interaction that is central to performance sport, and the athletes' trust that the data is being collected, interpreted, and used in the interest of their further development is central to this process.

Problem-Solving the Travel Schedule

MLB requires the players to play 162 games in 183 days. This means that team travel is an occupational necessity, and the resulting jet lag can be a problem. Laboratory studies and the examination of athletic performances have demonstrated that circadian rhythm aligns physiology, performance, and behavior to 24-hour environmental cycles, so travel between time zones can have an impact upon pitchers' routines. Similarly, sleep disruption can have a major impact upon a player's preparedness. This originates not just from traveling after games to the next city, but also from playing games late at night, when levels of adrenaline and caffeine are high, and sufficient relaxation to achieve sleep is tough to achieve. The effects of both acute sleep loss and chronic sleep deprivation are well documented within the extant literature; therefore monitoring sleep is important to inform decisions on the players' routine. While conventional wisdom is that consistency in sleep schedule is key, and that yo-yo schedules with more effort on one night and less on another should be avoided, this is not practical in the world of travel baseball.

However, using the sleep literature to appropriately plan for sleep and detailing for the team's and players' routines as the squad travels between games is important. This may typically involve the integration of a sleep scientist to support the team, who can interpret the players' actigraphy data to inform decisions about routines. Understanding the role that naps play for the athlete is also important. Indeed, they may be used to make up acute sleep debt, but more appropriately they can be used as a temporary boost for alertness and performance. Planning these with a limit of 20 to 30 minutes is important. This keeps the athlete from going into a deep sleep and then waking, causing the player to feel sleep inertia (sluggishness and grogginess). Table 22.1 demonstrates how sleep data, in conjunction with expert knowledge, can be used to plan a travel schedule for a player on a major league schedule.

PERFORMANCE INVESTIGATION

The role of the sport scientist is to inform evidence-based discussion. Indeed, key decisions are made as a result of expert discussion around data, not the data itself. Therefore, analysis of data trends can bring to life important issues that might otherwise go undetected in a player's performance. This is demonstrated in figure 22.7, which uses TrackMan, a popular technological tool in baseball, to record release-side data in a major league pitcher.

It is also important to understand that singular data sets do not typically present the full picture, but when a scientist is curious about a data trend and can look at this in relation to other data sets (for example, velocity data, or even monitoring data trends), then questions can be posed that others can follow up on.

Figure 22.7a shows an ongoing trend for the pitcher to alter the arm slot as the start progresses. This in itself may not be alarming for the coach, but when combined with other data sets (such as shoulder motor control and grip strength), this data can initiate a discussion between the player, the coach, and the medical staff. In this example it was discovered that the player had some unreported residual shoulder tightness that was limiting his action. With treatment during the next 4 days, this was resolved, his performance data was enhanced, and his monitoring data improved. The key outcome here is that discussion around the data resulted in both a successful intervention and the athlete's not missing any performance time. This educated the athlete about the importance of trusting the medical staff with consistent communication about how his body felt at all times.

Successful outcomes do not always have to be about the medical or even the physical state of a player. The sport scientist is typically required to be curious and ask "Why" questions, which can be particularly influential in directing discussions among coaches and other interdisciplinary team members. For example, in figure 22.7b, the data demonstrates that the player has a fairly obvious change in arm-slot position. If the scientist raises questions with the coach about why this might be, it can direct the coach's attention to particular aspects of the delivery that may be desirable to attend to. In this specific example, the player has switched sides of the rubber, which is a move that is not always obvious during the game. The performance data can then be reviewed in light of this (i.e., was it a successful decision for enhancing performance?) and appropriate technical adjustments to the player's subsequent plan can be made.

CONCLUSION

The performance environment comprises a wide range of experts with specific experiential knowledge sets. It should always be remembered that this experiential

TABLE 22.1 Planning a Travel Schedule Between Major League Games Requires the Appliance of Sleep Data and Expert Knowledge to Optimize Players' Readiness to Perform

Game	Postgame flight time	Nap strategy	Postgame target bedtime	Target wake-up time the next day
7:07 p.m. (Pacific Time)	4 h	1.5-h nap on the plane after the game	6:00 a.m. (Central Time)	12:00 p.m.
7:15 p.m. (Central Time)		30-min nap (before the game at about 4:00 pm)	12:00 a.m. (Central Time)	10:00 a.m.
7:15 p.m. (Central Time)			12:00 a.m. (Central Time)	8:00 a.m.
12:45 p.m. (Central Time)	2 h		Home at 12:00 a.m. (Eastern Time)	10:00 a.m. or later

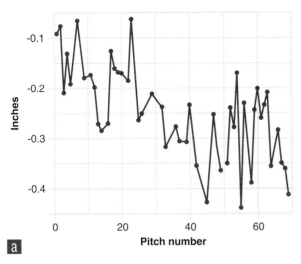 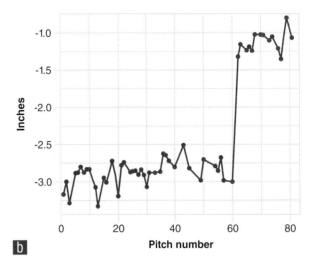

FIGURE 22.7   Curiosity about delivery data can inform interdisciplinary discussions between support staff and coaches: *(a)* release-side data from a pitcher with shoulder tightness during a game and *(b)* a pitcher who has moved to the other side of the rubber for technical reasons.

knowledge is the biggest data set that a team possesses. The role of derived data is to inform specific decisions that can remove speculation from the process and also enhance the practitioner's experiential data set (i.e., learning). Expert interpretation of the data is essential before it is presented for discussions so that the questions posed are either "Why is this happening?" or are followed by "What will we do about it?" The application of differential diagnostic processes to understand the impact of specific interventions upon outcomes for the athletes is crucial in this process.

This enables sport scientists to make decisions around what is working or what requires changing. The sport scientist therefore must be skilled in identification of what data needs to be monitored, how to best collect it, and crucially how this can be communicated to an expert audience so that discussions and decisions can be made in the best interests of the players' development. Curiosity and communication are essential qualities that the applied practitioner must possess to be successful in this environment.

RECOMMENDED READINGS

Bourdon, PC, Cardinale, M, Murray, A, Gastin, P, Kellmann, M, Varley, MC, Gabbett, TJ, Coutts, AJ, Burgess, DJ, Gregson, W, and Cable, NT. Monitoring athlete training loads: consensus statement. *Int J Sports Physiol Perform* 12:S2161-S2170, 2017.

Collins, D, Cruickshank, A, and Jordet, G, eds. *Routledge Handbook of Elite Sport Performance.* Milton Park, Abington, UK: Routledge, 2019.

McGuigan, M. *Monitoring Training and Performance in Athletes.* Champaign, IL: Human Kinetics, 2017.

Thornton, HR, Delaney, JA, Duthie, GM, and Dascombe, BJ. Developing athlete monitoring systems in team sports: data analysis and visualization. *Int J Sports Physiol Perform* 14:698-705, 2019.

Wexler, S, Shaffer, J, and Cotgreave, A. *The Big Book of Dashboards: Visualizing Your Data Using Real-World Business Scenarios.* Hoboken, NJ: John Wiley & Sons, 2017.

PART VI

Special Topics

CHAPTER 23

Recovery and Sleep

Jessica M. Stephens, PhD

Shona L. Halson, PhD

Recovery from the stressors of training or competition (or both) is complex and varied depending on the demands placed on the athlete. The area of athlete recovery has grown considerably, and the incorporation of recovery strategies into high-performance programs has become routine. Alongside the increase in the practical usage of recovery strategies has come an increase in research examining these strategies. Although there is still more work to be done to fully examine the mechanisms and the efficacy of many recovery strategies, currently sufficient evidence is available regarding many interventions to enable practitioners to make informed decisions for incorporating recovery into a high-performance program.

RECOVERY STRATEGIES

While research on the effects of recovery on performance continues to advance, not all of this research has concurrently investigated the underlying mechanisms of the various recovery strategies. Therefore, many of the exact mechanisms of recovery are unclear. Research in this area typically uses varying measures of performance (specific to the type of exercise performed and fatigue induced), markers of muscle damage and inflammation (e.g., creatine kinase, myoglobin), changes in blood flow, and perceptual measures of recovery, fatigue, and soreness. In general, the aim of recovery is to decrease the time taken to return the body to homeostasis, from both a physiological and a psychological perspective. Therefore, the majority of recovery strategies target the metabolic and mechanical or cognitive alterations (or both) that result from exercise. Common recovery strategies typically target muscle or body temperature, muscle soreness and inflammation, blood flow, and mental fatigue.

The recovery pyramid presented in figure 23.1 outlines the main recovery strategies currently being used in high-performance sport. The **recovery pyramid** is built on the foundation of sleep, followed by nutrition and hydration. These three areas have the potential for the greatest impact on athletic performance. This foundation can then be built upon by incorporating other strategies such as hydrotherapy, compression, and massage, which have been the focus of less research attention. The top of the pyramid includes strategies based on minimal or no evidence and may be considered fads that are momentarily popular.

This pyramid can be used to provide advice and education to athletes regarding prioritization of recovery strategies. For example, the base is the most important aspect to focus on and can have the highest influence on recovery and performance. The middle section of the pyramid may also be effective and can be appropriate when used in a comprehensive recovery plan. However, these strategies should be incorporated only once the foundation of the pyramid has been addressed. The top of the pyramid includes emerging strategies that may have little or no evidence and, therefore, their effectiveness is unknown or questionable. These strategies should either be avoided or used with the knowledge that they may be ineffective. Importantly, these recovery strategies may be undertaken in place of more effective techniques, thereby decreasing the effectiveness of the overall recovery plan.

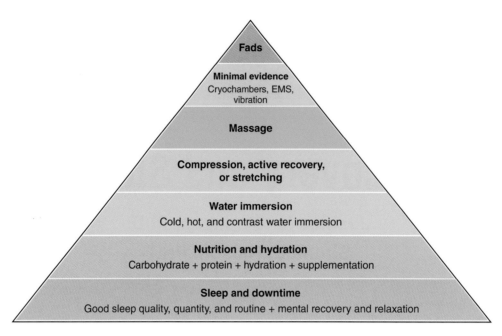

FIGURE 23.1 The recovery pyramid.

Sleep

Sleep is considered the foundation of the recovery pyramid due to its importance for athlete performance and well-being. Sleep deprivation has been shown to have negative effects on performance, mood state, metabolism, and immune and cognitive function (15). Research in elite athletes suggests that their sleep quality, quantity, or both are often less than optimal (25, 26) and that improvement in sleep is warranted in many athletes. Training and competition times (36, 37) and travel, as well as stress and anxiety (20), may contribute to poor sleep in athletes. However, appropriate education and behavior change strategies are often needed to minimize the influence of social media or video games on sleep. Smartphones and video games emit blue wavelength light (which can decrease melatonin release) and may also be a source of stress, worry, or competition at a time when light and stimulation should be avoided before sleep (28a).

The intensity of training may also influence sleep; while sleep would be expected to improve during intensified training (due to an increased need), evidence suggests that this does not occur (21, 24). Other factors such as caffeine consumption, muscle soreness, injury, jet lag, and travel (i.e., sleeping in foreign environments) are anecdotally reported to have a negative effect on an athlete's sleep if not managed appropriately. Only a small number of studies have investigated the effects of sleep extension in athletes; however, based on the available information it is suggested that a minimum of one week of increased sleep duration results in improvements in a range of performance metrics in athletes (6a).

Figure 23.2 describes the objectives and presents some recommendations for obtaining quality sleep in athletes (11).

Nutrition

Chapter 24 covers fueling and nutrition in depth; however, it is important to acknowledge here that nutrition is also a key component of athletic recovery. For greater insight into the role of fueling and nutrition in athlete recovery, readers are directed to the information in chapter 24.

Water Immersion

The use of water immersion or hydrotherapy has been a highly popular area of recovery for many years. A number of water immersion options are used to aid performance recovery. Most commonly athletes will perform cold-water immersion, contrast-water therapy, or hot-water immersion (38, 44). These water immersion strategies have been reasonably well examined in research to date, and the choice of which

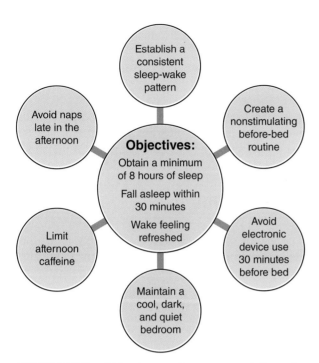

FIGURE 23.2 Objectives and recommendations for obtaining quality sleep in athletes.

Adapted by permission from Caia, Kelly, and Halson (2017).

strategy to implement should be based on what the athletes are trying to recover from and for.

Cold Water Immersion

Cold-water immersion (CWI) typically involves either full-body (excluding head) or limb-only immersion in water temperatures ranging between 40 °F (5 °C) and 68 °F (20 °C) for up to 20 minutes. This may be performed either continuously or intermittently (44). The main aim of CWI is to reduce body tissue temperatures and blood flow, which then leads to reductions in swelling, inflammation, cardiovascular strain, and pain (39). It is these physiological changes that lead to enhanced recovery by reducing hyperthermia-mediated fatigue, reducing the previously mentioned swelling and inflammation associated with delayed-onset muscle soreness (DOMS) and improving autonomic nervous system function (18).

At present there is no gold standard or optimal combination of water temperature, depth, duration, and mode of immersion (39) for CWI. The choice of protocol for CWI should vary depending on the athlete and what the athlete is recovering from. It has been observed that temperatures between 52 °F (11 °C) and 59 °F (15 °C) for durations of 11 to 15 minutes are optimal for the reduction of muscle soreness (27). However, regarding the use of CWI for the reduction of thermal strain or improving autonomic system function, there is less scientific evidence to suggest an optimal protocol.

Another factor to consider when determining the CWI protocol to use is the physical characteristics of the athletes, since it has been shown that body composition, sex, age, and ethnicity all affect the physiological responses to CWI (38). Less intense protocols (e.g., warmer water temperatures or shorter durations) are recommended for athletes with low body fat and low muscle mass. Female, youth, and masters athletes are also likely to require less intense protocols compared to the average adult male athlete (38).

Practically, CWI is best used in hot environments to aid the recovery from thermoregulatory fatigue, and it may also provide a precooling advantage if subsequent performance is required on the same day. Cold-water immersion is also effective for managing muscle soreness and damage, as is evident from studies examining circulating creatine kinase, which is often used as an indirect marker of muscle damage (1a). Research has shown that CWI significantly enhanced the recovery of squat jump and isometric force and significantly reduced creatine kinase concentration compared to a passive control condition 48 hours after muscle-damaging exercise (40a). Additionally, it has been found that CWI improved the recovery of sprint speed and attenuated the efflux of creatine kinase compared to a control condition during a simulated team sport tournament (26a). Therefore the regular use of CWI in-season or during tournaments is recommended to aid recovery of DOMS and general soreness.

Hot Water Immersion

Hot-water immersion (HWI) typically involves either full-body (excluding head) or limb-only immersion in water temperatures above 96 °F (36 °C). Hot-water immersion is usually performed in one continuous immersion and often involves the use of underwater jets to massage the muscles (44). When used for recovery purposes, the main aim of HWI is relaxation and easing of muscle tension. Physiologically, HWI leads to increases in body temperatures and blood flow (40). Through this increase in blood flow, HWI is thought to improve the removal of metabolic waste and increase nutrient delivery to and from the cells (45). These physiological responses are believed to aid healing and the recovery of neuromuscular performance (40, 45); however, this is theoretical at present, and future research is required to prove this theory.

There remains minimal research supporting the use of HWI for performance recovery; therefore it is difficult recommend optimal protocols. Similar to findings for CWI, the maximum duration suggested from research is approximately 20 minutes. Despite the lack of scientific evidence to support the benefits of HWI, anecdotally it remains a popular recovery method. Athletes often prefer the use of HWI over CWI because they find it more comfortable and relaxing. Practically, HWI can be used to aid psychological recovery since it provides relaxation benefits. It may also be useful on rest days and before massage to relax tight muscles. However, HWI should be applied with caution when soft tissue injuries are suspected because the increased blood flow may theoretically exacerbate swelling, bruising, and inflammation. Likewise, HWI is not recommended when athletes are in a hyperthymic state postexercise since the warm water will likely maintain elevated body temperatures, prolonging thermoregulatory stress.

Contrast Water Therapy

Contrast-water therapy (CWT) involves the athlete alternating between CWI and HWI; typically athletes will transfer between hot and cold pools three to seven times and spend 1 or 2 minutes in each (44). The aim of using CWT recovery is to enhance blood flow and the clearance of metabolic waste products. This is achieved by alternating between the CWI, which has a vasoconstrictive effect, and HWI, which has a vasodilating effect; this is then thought to cause a pumping action to occur to enhance blood flow and waste clearance (40, 42). Contrast-water therapy has been shown to enhance the recovery of fatigue and muscle damage through changes in body temperature, reductions in muscle spasm and inflammation, and improved range of motion (40).

Protocol selection for CWT still remains largely anecdotal because minimal research has been conducted to determine what is optimal. Although it has been shown that there is no dose–response relationship for the overall duration of CWT and the recovery of running and cycling performance (42, 43), it is still unknown how many rotations and the duration per rotation are optimal. However, research has shown that a 1:1 ratio of hot to cold can have positive performance effects (14), with 6 minutes of CWT at a 1:1 ratio

improving cycling time trial and sprint performance compared to control by 1.5% and 3%, respectively (42).

Practically, CWT is used more in scenarios in which athletes are fatigued and tired rather than recovering from DOMS or exercise-induced hyperthermia. Contrast-water therapy is also suggested to be an effective recovery strategy for non-weight-bearing sports such as swimming and cycling in which the main recovery priority is the clearance of metabolic waste (14).

Compression

The use of compression to aid recovery is another recovery modality that is growing in popularity. Compression is applied to the limbs of the athlete by way of compression garments (e.g., tights or socks) or pneumatic compression boots and sleeves. There is a growing body of evidence to support the use of compression to aid recovery; however, this is an early area of research particularly with regard to the pneumatic compression.

Compression Garments

Compression garments such as tights, socks, long-sleeved shirts, and arm or leg sleeves have become a common recovery method for athletes to enhance circulation following exercise (8). Compression garments originated in the medical industry and are used for their ability to enhance circulation, lymphatic flow, and venous return (8). These physiological changes are believed to make compression garments effective for recovery by reducing swelling, inflammation, and edema (8, 10). Research has shown compression garments to be effective at enhancing the recovery of strength, power, and cycling performance (10). Compression garments have been shown to increase sprint cycling performance, with the work per sprint increased by 4.3% compared to control (7). For further information about the various performance impacts of compression garments, refer to the meta-analyses by Hill and colleagues (17) and Brown and colleagues (10).

Although previous research has shown compression garments to enhance recovery (8, 10, 17), the optimal combination of when to wear them, how long to wear them, and which type of garment (e.g., tights versus socks) remains unclear. Compression garments have been found to be effective for enhancing recovery when worn for as little as 20 minutes between exercise bouts (1); however, it has been suggested that the longer the athlete is able to wear the garments the greater the benefits will be (40).

Compression garments have also been shown to be beneficial for recovery following long-haul air travel. Wearing compression socks during travel has shown improvements in athletes' subjective ratings of fatigue and muscle soreness, in addition to reductions in lower limb swelling (7). Wearing compression during long flights has also shown benefits on the recovery of countermovement jump performance and a reduction in creatine kinase compared to the control group (7, 23); therefore it is recommended that athletes wear compression during travel especially when they will be required to perform in competition or training soon after arrival.

Pneumatic Compression

Pneumatic compression typically involves the application of compression boots or sleeves to the legs or arms. These sleeves are inflated to apply external compression to the limbs, and the amount of compression applied by pneumatic devices is much greater than that of compression garments (boots apply up to 110 mmHg whereas compression garments apply up to 30 mmHg) (9, 47). Most commercially available devices offer compression that is applied sequentially starting at the foot and moving up the leg in segments, with the previous segment staying inflated until the full leg is released. However, there are also options for peristatic compression and segment-by-segment compress and release cycles. Much like compression garments, pneumatic compression is thought to improve circulation and venous return to enhance the removal of metabolic waste products (29).

Pneumatic compression is an emerging technology, and as such, minimal research has been conducted to examine the efficacy or optimal protocols for use. Anecdotally, pneumatic compression is popular among athletes and has been shown to be effective for improving subjective ratings of muscle fatigue, pain, and soreness (16). However, pneumatic compression is yet to show strong benefits for the recovery of performance (16, 29, 47). Future research is required to fully determine the impact of pneumatic compression on performance and the optimal protocols for its use.

Active Recovery

An active recovery, or cool-down, performed immediately following exercise is one of the most well-known recovery strategies (41). **Active recovery**

is typically performed at the end of a training session or competition for a duration of 5 to 15 minutes and involves low- to moderate-intensity aerobic exercises (41). The aim of active recovery is to maintain an elevated blood flow, which is thought to enhance the removal of waste products such as blood lactate (41). Research to date has shown mixed results, with some studies supporting and others showing no benefits from the use of active recovery (40). It has been shown that active recovery is largely ineffective at enhancing performance recovery and unlikely to prevent injuries when subsequent performance is required more than 4 hours later (41). However, it has also been shown that when repeat performances are required in a short period of time (<30 min), active recovery is effective and should be incorporated (19). Although it appears that active recovery is useful for short recovery periods but not longer time frames, there remains a lack of consensus on the benefits of active recovery, and further research is required.

In summary, active recovery is a widely used and routine or ritualistic practice performed by athletes, so despite the mixed results in the research, a strong negative impact on performance recovery has not been observed. Therefore, it is recommended that athletes still perform an active recovery if they feel it is beneficial.

Stretching

Stretching is another recovery method that is widely used but is not supported by strong scientific evidence to suggest a positive effect on performance recovery (3). When used for recovery purposes, the aim of stretching is to reduce muscle soreness and stiffness as well as relaxing the muscle and improving range of motion (35). Stretching has been suggested to aid recovery of muscle soreness by dispersing the accumulated edema in damaged muscle tissue; however, this has yet to be demonstrated in research (3).

When stretching is used for recovery it is often done in conjunction with an active recovery or cool-down, and it is generally recommended that static stretches be performed for the major muscle groups used during exercise and held for 15 to 30 seconds (33). It is also advised that stretching should not cause discomfort or pain.

Massage

Massage is one of the most frequently used recovery strategies (31) and is typically performed by a trained therapist; however, athletes can also learn self-massage techniques and use devices such as foam rollers for myofascial release and trigger points. Massage is thought to increase blood flow, decrease muscle tension, decrease muscle excitability, and improve overall perceptions of well-being (19). Moreover, massage has been found to have the best effect on acute recovery (10-20 min), especially when shorter in duration (1-12 min); however the benefits of massage on performance recovery remain small and unclear (31).

The use of foam roller self-massage has yielded stronger evidence of benefit in research to date, with studies showing that foam rolling attenuates decreases in sprint and strength performance, decreases perception of pain, decreases DOMS, and increases range of motion (5, 46). Athletes can also use devices such as a massage ball, massage roller sticks, or percussion massage devices to perform self-massage. It is important that athletes be well educated on how to use self-massage because they can increase soreness, swelling, and bruising by using these techniques incorrectly. It is recommended that athletes consult with a trained therapist to learn how to safely use self-massage techniques that will be of specific benefit in relation to their needs.

Recovery Technologies

Recovery technologies are constantly advancing, and new options often claim to have superior effects on athlete recovery. Some of the technologies mentioned later have been available for many years, but there remains minimal scientific evidence to support their use. The technologies in this section should be approached with more caution since support for their effectiveness is minimal, and their benefits to recovery are likely to be smaller than the those of the previously mentioned strategies.

Cryotherapy and Cryosaunas

There are typically two forms of whole- or partial-body cryotherapy: cryochambers and cryosaunas. **Cryochambers** are single- or multiple-person chambers where the athlete, including the athlete's head, is completely exposed to the very low temperatures. In **cryosaunas** (also sometimes referred to as cryocabins), the athlete's head is not exposed because the liquid nitrogen used for cooling is not breathable.

Cryotherapy involves exposing the athlete to extremely cold air, usually below −166 °F (−110 °C)

for 2 to 5 minutes (6). Much like CWI, cryotherapy is believed to enhance recovery through reductions in tissue temperatures and blood flow, which decreases swelling and inflammation and provides an analgesic effect (2). Research to date has shown cryotherapy to have no negative effects on recovery, but it also has not yielded clear and consistent benefits to recovery (12). Therefore, it would be recommended that given the cost and practical difficulties associated with accessing cryotherapy, athletes instead choose CWI as a more practical way of using cold-temperature exposure to aid recovery (6). Still, if access to cryotherapy is available, this option may be a means of reducing monotony with respect to cold exposure.

Particular care must be taken with regard to safety in the chambers and ensuring adherence to the appropriate exposure time. Overexposure to cryotherapy may lead to hypothermia, cold burn (skin damage), hypertension, discomfort, reduction in nerve conduction, and reduced peripheral blood flow in fingers and toes. These are some important safety considerations for cryotherapy use:

- Athletes should be supervised at all times when in either cryochambers or cryosaunas; for multiple-person cryotherapy chambers, supervising personnel should remain outside the chamber.
- The cold-sensitive parts of the body (hands, feet, and mouth) should be protected against cold exposure.
- Skin surface should be completely dried to remove all sweat and moisture.
- Athletes should not breathe the liquid nitrogen when using cryosaunas (this may occur if they faint or bend down and are exposed to the cold vapors inside the sauna).

Muscle Stimulation

Electrical muscle stimulation (EMS) devices are another emerging recovery strategy. **Electrical muscle stimulation** involves placing electrodes over fatigued muscles, which then deliver transcutaneous stimulation to the muscle. Electrical muscle stimulation is thought to increase blood flow and venous return, therefore enhancing recovery by accelerating the removal of metabolites (4, 30). As with whole-body cryotherapy, research examining EMS has not identified negative effects on recovery (13), but also has not demonstrated conclusive benefits to performance recovery (30). Electrical muscle stimulation was, however, shown to have positive perceptual benefits when athletes were asked to rate their perceived muscle soreness, energy, and mood (4, 13) and therefore may be a beneficial recovery strategy. Further research is required to enable recommendations on use and on protocols to be provided. Some devices have modes for training recovery, competition recovery, and reducing muscle soreness. Because research is limited in this area, it is recommended that athletes follow the device protocols and recommendations or their own individual preferences.

Percussion and Vibration Massage Devices

Whole-body vibration and **percussion devices** such as foam rollers, massage balls, and massage guns, which deliver vibration or percussion treatments to the muscle, are becoming popular. These devices are believed to promote circulation, decrease muscle stiffness and tension, and increase range of motion (22, 32). Percussion and vibration massage devices do show promise for enhancing recovery; but as with many of the emerging technologies, the evidence so far suggests only positive perceptual benefits, and more research is needed to examine the physiological and performance effects (22). Similar to the situation with EMS devices, recommendations for use are not standardized and are generally based on athlete preference or manufacturer's guidelines if available (or both).

Mental Recovery

Increasing evidence suggests that cognitive fatigue can impair physical, technical, tactical, and psychological components of sporting performance. As a consequence, methods to enhance recovery from the cognitive load experienced by athletes are emerging. Methods include relaxation strategies, mindfulness, meditation, biofeedback, neurofeedback, and various forms of technology that targets brain activity. There is a distinct lack of research in this area; however, it is anticipated that reducing mental fatigue will become increasingly important for today's athlete (34a).

Recovery Fads

Due to the popularity of recovery, many companies view recovery strategies as an opportunity for significant financial gains. This is highlighted by the fact that the majority of new technologies go to market with an absence of independent scientific research. When examining recovery strategies that involve

new or emerging technologies it is important for the sport scientist to ask the manufacturers questions about suggested mechanisms of action and available research. However, since research often significantly lags behind practice, practitioners should have a basic understanding of the mechanisms of physiological and psychological recovery to be able to make appropriate judgments on the use of new equipment and technology. It is also acknowledged that the belief effect can have a powerful and important influence on recovery, and therefore this should not be discounted when a lack of scientific evidence exists. However, it is important that athletes not engage primarily in technologies that may be popular and lack scientific rationale at the expense of strategies that have strong scientific as well as anecdotal evidence.

RECOVERY AND ADAPTATION

Traditionally, recovery has always been considered an integral part of adaptation to training, whereby recovery is required following the training stimulus to ensure that an athlete does not become excessively fatigued and adapts to the training program. However, there is currently some debate regarding the role of recovery in potentially decreasing adaptation by blunting the inflammatory and signaling response necessary to promote certain adaptations (34). At present the focus of this debate is centered on CWI, with a lack of consensus in the research findings. A conservative approach to this issue would be the removal of recovery after resistance training sessions since this aspect of the training program has been shown most to be negatively influenced with respect to adaptation. However, it must be noted that there is no research on elite athletes to date.

A more suitable approach may be to periodize the use of recovery for the elite athlete. In the same ways training and nutrition are periodized, consideration should be given to periods in the training program when recovery may be minimized (e.g., in cardiovascular endurance training phases) and when it may be emphasized (e.g., during a competition phase). Given this information, the most important aspect to consider is whether the athlete's goals are short or long term. Is the current aim to enhance adaptation to training or minimize fatigue for quality training sessions, competition, or performance enhancement? For a comprehensive review on periodizing recovery in individual and team sports, refer to the review by Mujika and colleagues (28).

RECOVERY PROGRAM DESIGN

For the design of a recovery program, no gold standard or best practice protocol can be recommended. Recovery is a unique challenge that will vary from athlete to athlete and sport to sport. To determine which strategy or strategies to implement it is recommended that sport scientists start by asking themselves the following questions:

1. What is the main stress that the athlete is trying to recover from (e.g., thermal strain, muscle damage, metabolite accumulation, energy system depletion, mental fatigue)?

2. What is the time frame for recovery? When does the athlete need to train or compete again? Is high quality required in the next session?

3. Are there any environmental factors that could affect the athlete's recovery (e.g., heat, altitude, cold)?

4. Is the athlete excessively fatigued (e.g., is the risk of negative consequences from fatigue greater than the risk of potentially affecting adaptation)?

5. Is the athlete in a competition or a preparation phase (e.g., what is the current priority of the athlete's long-term plan)?

6. What facilities will the athlete have access to?

Once the aim of and challenges to recovery have been identified, a program can be developed. It is important for athletes to trial different recovery strategies in the training environment, before implementing them in competition, to know how they individually respond and feel after using different strategies. Although it is important that the sport scientist understand the aims of recovery in athletes' specific individual circumstances, some generalized recommendations can be made for different situations. The scenarios presented next may be used by practitioners as a starting point for planning recovery but should be individualized to their own specific contexts.

Scenario 1: Team Sport, In-Season, Participating in One Game per Week

- *Postgame recovery timeline:* The timeline in figure 23.3 represents the postgame recovery steps that should be taken.

- *Game day plus one:* If the athlete is still feeling excessively fatigued or sore the day after the game,

further recovery strategies could be incorporated. Massage, compression boots, or water immersion strategies may be effective here.

Scenario 2: Tournament (Team or Individual Sport), Multiple Games or Events per Day or Over Multiple Days

If there are 60 minutes or less between games or events, the athlete could follow these strategies:

1. Active recovery
2. Stretching
3. Nutrition and hydration
4. Massage or compression

Generally, when the turn-around between games or events is short, water immersion strategies are not recommended for a number of reasons. Firstly, the practicalities of the athlete needing to get changed and dry may be infeasible if time is short. Secondly, CWI may cool the muscles and have a negative impact on performance (38). However, CWI may be considered between non-sprint events with a short turn-around if the environment is hot because it is likely to have a positive precooling benefit in relation to subsequent performance. If there are subsequent days of competition, the athlete could follow the process suggested in scenario 1, upon completion of each day.

When designing recovery programs, one of the most important considerations for sport scientists is the practicalities of implementation. For example, during travel, access to plunge pools or spas can be difficult; often portable pools or plastic tubs are used in change rooms. The practicalities of getting a large team through CWI with only a small pool that fits one or two people can be time-consuming. In this scenario, the athletes who have had more game time could be prioritized for water immersion, while those who have not played as long could use a different recovery strategy such as pneumatic compression. Additionally, athletes could use a shower for cold or contrast benefits. Although showers do not provide the hydrostatic pressure benefits of water immersion, they still provide thermal changes and may have some positive benefits when immersion is not possible.

CONCLUSION

Recovery is multifaceted, and both the choice of recovery strategy and the ways in which recovery

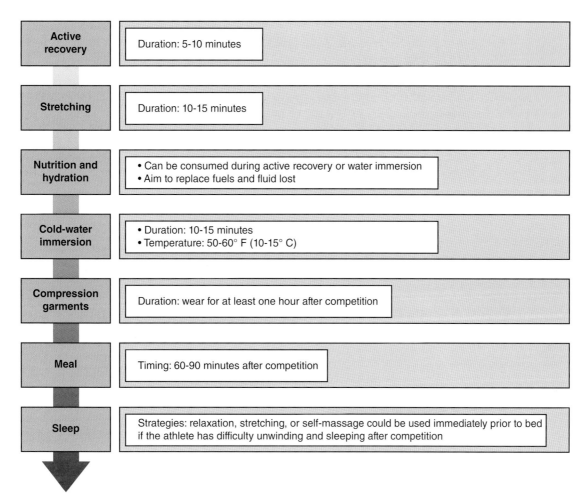

FIGURE 23.3 Postgame recovery timeline.

strategies are combined in athletes involve many considerations. Initial considerations should have to do with the effectiveness of the available recovery strategies and prioritizing simple strategies that provide the foundation to recovery, such as sleep and nutrition. Further, the dose of recovery should be considered within the context of the training program and periodized to maximize performance and adaptation.

RECOMMENDED READINGS

Brown, F, Gissane, C, Howatson, G, van Someren, K, Pedlar, C, and Hill, J. Compression garments and recovery from exercise: a meta-analysis. *Sports Med* 47:2245-2267, 2017.

Caia, J, Kelly, VG, and Halson, SL. The role of sleep in maximising performance in elite athletes. In *Sport, Recovery and Performance*. Kellman, M and Beckman, J, eds. Abington, UK: Routledge, 151-167, 2017.

Halson, SL. Sleep in elite athletes and nutritional interventions to enhance sleep. *Sports Med* 44(suppl 1):S13-S23, 2014.

Hill, J, Howatson, G, Van Someren, K, Leeder, J, and Pedlar, C. Compression garments and recovery from exercise-induced muscle damage: a meta-analysis. *Br J Sports Med* 48:1340-1346, 2014.

Ihsan, M, Watson, G, and Abbiss, CR. What are the physiological mechanisms for post-exercise cold water immersion in the recovery from prolonged endurance and intermittent exercise? *Sports Med* 46:1095-1109, 2016.

Mujika, I, Halson, S, Burke, LM, Balagué, G, and Farrow, D. An integrated, multifactorial approach to periodization for optimal performance in individual and team sports. *Int J Sports Physiol Perform* 13:538-561, 2018.

Stephens, JM, Halson, S, Miller, J, Slater, GJ, and Askew, CD. Cold-water immersion for athletic recovery: one size does not fit all. *Int J Sports Physiol Perform* 12:2-9, 2017.

Fueling and Nutrition

Louise M. Burke, PhD

Eric S. Rawson, PhD

An athlete's diet plays a number of key roles in the achievement of a lengthy and successful sporting career. In the training phase, eating plans must provide the fuel to train hard, as well as the nutrients needed to adapt optimally and recover well. Energy, macronutrients, and **micronutrients** (food chemicals) are also part of staying healthy and injury-free. Achieving and maintaining an optimal body composition without undue food stress or restrictiveness involves judicious manipulation of energy and protein intake. In the competition phase, an athlete needs to recognize physiological factors that cause fatigue or suboptimal performance, and where possible, use nutritional strategies before, during, or between events to reduce or delay the onset of these issues. Finally, although a "food first" policy provides the best approach to sports nutrition, there are occasions when sports foods or supplements might be a practical way to address nutrient needs or to provide a direct performance boost.

With the variety of training strategies and event characteristics that make up the world of sport, it is not surprising that the specific needs of each athlete are unique and constantly changing. Indeed, sports dietitians promote the importance of personalization, periodization, and practicality in the development of each athlete's dietary plan. It is beyond the scope of this chapter to provide a detailed account of every goal or strategy within the sports nutrition toolbox or to explain the complexities of the skills used by sports dietitians and nutrition experts in assessment, counseling, and monitoring with regard to an athlete's diet. Nevertheless, an appreciation of the key principles of sports nutrition can assist sport scientists and other members of the performance staff to provide an environment and culture that reinforces sound knowledge

and practice, as well as to identify opportunities to address problems or opportunities at an early stage. The aim of this chapter is to provide practical insights that highlight the role of performance nutrition.

ENERGY AND BODY COMPOSITION MANAGEMENT

Energy intake (EI) is the starting point for assessing and educating an athlete about sports nutrition. EI determines athletes' capacity to consume the macronutrients, micronutrients, and other forms of nutritional support that fuel and optimize their training and health needs. It also underpins athletes' capacity to alter their body composition, for example, to gain muscle mass or reduce body fat content. Determining the proper amount of daily kilocalories (i.e., EI) needed to support athletic performance and optimize body composition is critical. The **estimated energy requirement** (EER) is the sum of total daily energy expenditure, which includes resting metabolic rate, the thermic effect of feeding, and the energy expenditure related to physical activities. The EER can be estimated using equations that include variables such as age, weight, height, and physical activity. Accurate measures of age, weight, and height are easily obtained, but estimates of physical activity are more complex. For example, using the Institute of Medicine equation (43a), a 22-year-old male, who weighs 176.4 pounds (80 kg), is 5.6 feet (1.7 m) tall, and reports a physical activity level (PAL) of very active (PA coefficient = 1.48), has an EER of 3,694 kcal/day. For the same individual, a reported PAL of active (PA coefficient = 1.25) reduces the EER to 3,190 kcal/day.

Thus, these estimates should be used cautiously, with use overseen by a qualified professional and the resulting estimates paired with body composition goals and tracking. The following are equations used for the calculation of EER in males and females (note that age is in years; weight is in kilograms; height is in meters; the physical activity coefficient is based on the PAL as outlined in table 24.1).

Estimated energy requirement for males >19 years:

$$662 - (9.53 \times \text{age}) + \{\text{physical activity coefficient} \times [(15.91 \times \text{weight}) + (539.6 \times \text{height})]\}$$

Estimated energy requirement for females >19 years:

$$354 - (6.91 \times \text{age}) + \{\text{physical activity coefficient} \times [(9.36 \times \text{weight}) + (726 \times \text{height})]\}$$

Other methods are available to estimate energy requirements (see https://globalrph.com/medcalcs/estimated-energy-requirement-eer-equation/), but these too are estimates and so require proper supervision. In some instances, resting metabolic rate might be more precisely measured using indirect calorimetry. However, the other components of energy expenditure, thermic effect of feeding and physical activity energy expenditure, will still be estimates. The dietary apps that combine EI and physical activity energy expenditure are popular, but they cannot replace consultations with, and tracking by, a sports dietitian or sport scientist.

Traditionally, energy transactions in the body have been viewed in terms of energy balance, where EI in excess of expenditure leads to a gain in body energy stores (fat mass, and perhaps muscle mass) while an energy deficit, created by greater expenditure than intake of energy, leads to a loss of body energy stores (loss of fat and muscle mass). Before discussing the deliberate adjustment of energy metrics to promote a change in body composition, it is important to address the concept of **energy availability** (EA). This term was first popularized by Anne Loucks (35) to describe the difference in EI and exercise energy expenditure

in relation to **fat-free mass** (FFM). A numerical value can be derived from this concept:

$$\text{EA} = (\text{EI} - \text{energy cost of exercise [kcal]}) / \text{FFM (kg)}$$

Optimal EA when an athlete is in energy balance and achieving the energy needed to support all body functions is suggested to be ≥40 to 45 kcal/kg FFM per day (41). Problems arise when energy deficits are created, either deliberately or accidentally (as will be discussed later). While this can temporarily lead to a loss of body energy stores (i.e., weight loss), the body usually adjusts to this (as a survival mechanism) to conserve energy expenditure. This adaptation produces two practical outcomes: (a) The body now has a new and lower point at which energy balance is achieved (thus making it more difficult to achieve an energy deficit to produce fat or weight loss), and (b) the body spends less energy on processes that are not essential for survival (e.g., reproductive system, bone health, protein synthesis) (41). Suboptimal support for such activities can interfere with optimal health, training adaptation, and sport performance. Energy availability represents a new way to assess an athlete's energy considerations and capacity to meet sports nutrition goals. It can be difficult to conceptualize; and in real life, it is almost impossible to measure with accuracy and validity (i.e., to capture an account that represents habitual behavior) (9). However, it helps to clarify the high risk of injury, illness, and poor performance in groups of athletes who under-eat or over-exercise and thus risk low EA (often defined as <30 kcal/kg FFM; [41]). This also means that judgments cannot be made about the suitability of an athletes EA based on whether the athlete is weight stable or has high or low body fat levels. As explained by Melin and colleagues (41), two athletes can have similar body composition, energy intakes, and be weight stable, yet one may have a healthy EA while the other has a low EA (LEA) due to remarkable differences in energy expenditure. An assessment of

TABLE 24.1 Physical Activity Level Values and Activity Coefficients

Physical activity level (PAL)*	Examples	Physical activity coefficient (males/females)
Sedentary (≥1.0 to <1.4)	Common activities of daily living (ADLs)	1.00/1.00
Low active (≥1.4 to <1.6)	ADLs *and* 30-60 min of daily moderate activity	1.11/1.12
Active (≥1.6 to <1.9)	ADLs *and* ≥1 h of daily moderate activity	1.25/1.27
Very active (≥1.9 to <2.5)	ADLs *and* ≥1 h min of daily moderate activity and 1 more h of vigorous activity or 2 h of moderate activity	1.48/1.45

* PAL = ratio of total energy expenditure to basal daily energy expenditure ("1.0" means total energy expenditure equals basal daily energy expenditure).

EI and expenditure must allow for the concept of EA to support optimal function. This should be undertaken by an expert (e.g., sports dietitian) and may require tests of health and metabolic function to confirm a suspicion that LEA has occurred.

For athletes attempting to reduce body fat, modest reductions in EI (e.g., about 300 kcal/day) are recommended; while for weight gain, modest increases (about 500 kcal/day) are recommended. Such targets allow for optimal changes in body composition without the consequences of large changes in EA. These figures are estimates and must align with the goals of an individual athlete and the timetable for achieving the desired body composition. There is not an ideal macronutrient distribution for fat loss, maintenance of muscle mass, or muscle gain (carbohydrate recommendations are discussed later in the chapter). Beyond health, and provision of adequate amounts of energy, macro-, and micronutrients, the most important feature of the diet is **sustainability** (i.e., it can be maintained). Protein plays a critical role in achieving desired body composition in athletes, since it augments strength gain and the hypertrophic response to resistance training, aids in muscle maintenance during energy restriction and weight loss, and enhances satiety. The recommended protein intake for sedentary individuals ($0.8 \text{ g} \cdot \text{kg}^{-1} \cdot \text{day}^{-1}$) is too low for athletes. Witard and colleagues (61) recommend 1.3 to 1.7 g protein per kg body mass per day for athletes attempting to maintain or gain weight. Higher protein intakes, up to 2.4 g/kg, are recommended for athletes attempting to lose weight while maintaining or gaining muscle mass. Finally, it should be noted that weight or fat loss is an activity undertaken (or desired) by most people at some stage of their lives, and it may seem a simple task. However, as shown by the common lack of success in the wider community, it is a challenging activity that should be undertaken with professional support to ensure that realistic targets and sustained success are achieved, within the athlete's larger sports nutrition goals.

FUELING FOR TRAINING AND COMPETITION

In most sports, success is achieved by the athlete who can produce the most chemical energy over the duration of the event, translating this into power, speed, force, or strength, often with an overlay of skill or concentration. Four energy-producing pathways contribute to the muscle's ability to regenerate adenosine triphosphate (ATP), the fuel currency of the cell. The phosphagen system and anaerobic glycolysis yield rapid but short-lived ATP production in the absence of oxygen, while oxidative pathways in the mitochondria generate ATP from carbohydrate (muscle glycogen, blood glucose) and fat (muscle triglycerides and blood-free fatty acids derived from adipose tissue) at a lower rate but for a longer duration. All systems contribute to energy production, but their relative contribution is determined by a range of factors including the availability of substrate and oxygen supply, the rate of energy demand (e.g., intensity of exercise), the athlete's training status, and the presence of by-products from reactions (e.g., excess H^+ ions or reactive oxygen species) that interfere with homeostasis. For greater insight on the energetic characteristics of a range of sports, the reader is referred to the textbook by Maughan and Gleeson (39).

A key issue for athletes is to understand the factors that limit a steady supply of fuel for their event and to undertake specific training and nutritional strategies that can overcome some of these issues. For example, fatigue during repeated bouts of high-intensity exercise is often associated with the failure to regenerate muscle phosphocreatine (PCr) during the recovery between sprints or efforts. Creatine supplementation can support the function of this phosphagen pathway by increasing muscle concentrations of creatine and PCr (30). Buffering supplements (bicarbonate and β-alanine) can be used to extend the capacity of the anaerobic glycolytic system by neutralizing the disturbance to acid–base balance that occurs with excess production of H^+ ions (12, 53).

For aerobic endurance sports, where oxidative fuels provide the bulk of the energy supply, there are two (apparently competing) issues: how to extend the finite carbohydrate stores in the body and how to make better use of the relatively unlimited fat stores in even the leanest athlete. The process of aerobic endurance training enhances both goals, increasing the muscles' glycogen and intramuscular triglyceride stores and increasing the capacity of both metabolic pathways via adaptations in regulatory enzymes and transporter proteins (48). For most of the time in the evolution of sports nutrition since about the 1960s, the spotlight has focused on carbohydrate-based strategies that attempt to increase body carbohydrate stores to meet the needs of the training session or event. Such strategies, known as achieving **high carbohydrate availability**, include consuming carbohydrate-rich meals in the hours and days before the session to maximize muscle glycogen content or consuming carbohydrate during sessions of longer duration (8). There is clear evidence that these approaches enhance aerobic endurance performance when sustaining high rates of carbohydrate oxidation in the muscle throughout exercise (22, 49) and that they have central nervous system effects that include improved pacing and perception of effort (10). Guidelines for strategies that achieve these goals are provided in table 24.2 (52). It should be noted that athletes are encouraged to consume carbohydrate according to the fuel costs and goals of each exercise or training session, rather than eating a high-carbohydrate diet per se. Indeed, it is recognized that such needs and goals vary between athletes, but also from day to day for the same athlete. This concept of a periodized and personalized approach to carbohydrate intake in the athlete's diet is often misunderstood and misrepresented (8).

TABLE 24.2   Guidelines for Carbohydrate Intake in Training and Before and During Exercise When High Carbohydrate Availability is Desired

DAILY NEEDS FOR FUELING AND RECOVERY*		
Situation	**Description**	**Carbohydrate targets**
Light training load	Low-intensity or skill-based activities	$3\text{-}5\ g \cdot kg^{-1} \cdot day^{-1}$
Moderate training load	Moderate exercise program (e.g., ~1 h/day)	$5\text{-}7\ g \cdot kg^{-1} \cdot day^{-1}$
High training load	Aerobic endurance program (e.g., 1-3 h/day moderate- to high-intensity exercise)	$6\text{-}10\ g \cdot kg^{-1} \cdot day^{-1}$
Very high training load	Extreme commitment (e.g., >4-5 h/day moderate- to high-intensity exercise)	$8\text{-}12\ g \cdot kg^{-1} \cdot day^{-1}$
ACUTE FUELING STRATEGIES**		
General fueling up	Preparation for events <90 min exercise	24 h @ 7-12 g/kg as for daily fuel needs
Carbohydrate loading	Preparation for events >90 min of sustained or intermittent exercise	36-48 h @ 10-12 g/kg body mass per day
Pre-event fueling	Before exercise >60 min	1-4 g/kg consumed 1-4 h before exercise Timing, amount, and type of carbohydrate foods and drinks chosen to suit the practical needs of the event and individual preferences and experiences
During brief exercise	<45 min	Not needed
During sustained high-intensity exercise	45-75 min	Frequent 5- to 10-s contact of the mouth and oral cavity with carbohydrate to promote central nervous system benefits
During aerobic endurance exercise including stop-and-start sports	1-2.5 h	30-60 g/h to provide a source of muscle fuel to supplement endogenous stores
During ultraendurance exercise	>2.5-3 h	Up to 90 g/h to support greater reliance on exogenous carbohydrate stores Products providing multiple transportable carbohydrates (glucose/fructose mixtures) to achieve high rates of oxidation of carbohydrate consumed during exercise

Adapted from D.T. Thomas, K.A. Erdman and L.M. Burke (2016, pg. 543-568)

*These targets, especially when consumed acutely around a specific session, are intended to provide high carbohydrate availability when it is important to exercise with high quality or at high intensity or both. These theoretical recommendations should be fine-tuned with individual consideration of total energy needs, specific training needs, and feedback from training performance.

**These promote high carbohydrate availability for optimal performance in competition or key training sessions.

Periodically, interest has switched toward strategies that reduce the muscle's reliance on finite substrates while exploiting its relatively unlimited stores of fat (6). This includes short or chronic adherence to a low-carbohydrate, high-fat diet (LCHF), a popular concept at the time of preparing this chapter. Although this approach has been shown to dramatically increase the muscle's capacity to use fat as an exercise fuel even in well-trained athletes (56), and it is supported by testimonials of successful (or least not impaired) performance on social media, there are some caveats to this approach. Several studies of athletes who have adapted to a LCHF diet, including a ketogenic version in which daily restrictions of carbohydrate <50 grams per day caused chronic ketosis (high circulating levels of ketones), show that although exercise performance at low to moderate intensity levels was maintained on LCHF, there is an impairment of performance at higher intensities of exercise (11, 45). The reason may be that fat oxidation requires greater (~5%) amounts of oxygen to produce an amount of ATP similar to that produced by the carbohydrate oxidation pathways, and, at higher intensities of exercise, oxygen delivery to the muscle rather than substrate availability becomes limiting (11). Furthermore, attempts to increase carbohydrate availability around a single performance, to get the best of both worlds, might have some value (59), but are inferior to performance supported only by high carbohydrate availability (21). It appears that fat adaptation has separate effects that downregulate the use of carbohydrate as a muscle fuel even when it is available (50). Therefore, while LCHF diets may have some role in athletic performance, this might be restricted to ultraendurance sports in which exercise intensities throughout the event are modest. It is noted, of course, that even in events greater than 3 hours in duration, success requires shorter bursts of higher-intensity work in the form of tactical changes in pace, uphill efforts, and sprints to the finishing line. Indeed, a case history of elite cyclists in grand tours (3 weeks of cycling with daily stages of 5-8 hours with mean power outputs suggesting modest exercise intensities) shows that these athletes concentrate on matching carbohydrate availability to the needs of each stage, including tactics to achieve extremely high rates of carbohydrate intake to match the fuel costs of hilly and tactical riding (60).

With specific regard to carbohydrate intake during exercise, table 24.2 shows a sliding scale of recommended intakes according to the duration and intensity of the session. The benefits of these practices range from central nervous system responses, to the inter-action between carbohydrate intake and receptors in the oral cavity in shorter events (14), to the provision of a substantial amount of the muscle's fuel requirements in ultraendurance events where exogenous sources are needed to replace the muscle's dwindling glycogen stores (17). To achieve the practicalities of intake during competition, athletes must make use of the unique opportunities to consume foods and drinks within the rules and logistics of their sport. When aggressive intakes are desired, athletes should also choose items that combine carbohydrates with different intestinal absorption characteristics to maximize the total uptake into the bloodstream (25). Practicing the use of these products during training (**gut training**) will adapt the gastrointestinal tract to better tolerate and absorb intake during exercise, potentially leading to better fueling and an enhancement of competition performance (16).

HYDRATION

A decrease in body water, or **dehydration**, resulting in a hypohydrated state, impairs performance in most sports (13, 15, 46). A small decrease in body mass due to water loss, with 2% often used as the cut-point, can reduce aerobic endurance and intermittent exercise performance (15). Further, Savoie and colleagues (46) reported that dehydration reduces maximal strength and power production 5.5% and 3.5%, respectively. Although it is unlikely that an athlete will become dehydrated during a sprint or power-type activity (e.g., throwing, sprinting, weightlifting), performance in these sports would be impaired if athletes were already dehydrated when they began their competition. Additionally, dehydration can potentially reduce performance during both sport practice and strength and conditioning sessions, thereby decreasing training effectiveness and, subsequently, suboptimal training adaptations. Even athletes competing in cold environments, such as in ice hockey, with ample fluid availability, can become dehydrated. As an example, Logan-Sprenger and colleagues (34) reported that about 22 minutes of ice hockey in euhydrated players resulted in sweat loss (3.2 L) greater than fluid intake (2.1 L), weight loss (up to 4.3% body mass), and a significant sodium deficit. Finally, a 2% decrease in body mass from dehydration negatively affects mood, including perceived fatigue (15) and cognitive performance (62). Thus, dehydration can impair performance through multiple mechanisms and across many sports, making proper assessment and maintenance of hydration critical.

Prevention and Assessment

Casa and colleagues (4, 13) describe practical solutions to reduce risk of dehydration in athletes, including these:

- Using first morning (body) weight, urine (color), and thirst (sensation) (**WUT**) to guide fluid and electrolyte consumption
- Incorporating electrolytes, including sodium and potassium, along with rehydration at mealtime
- Personalizing fluid needs by estimating sweat loss from changes in body weight
- Incorporating competition drinking strategy into training
- Training during the coolest times of day, in air-conditioned facilities rather than in extreme heat, and using active cooling techniques (e.g., cold towels) (For more detailed information, see chapter 25.)

According to Belval and colleagues (4), there is no single best method to assess hydration in all situations. In research and clinical settings, plasma osmolality and volume, urine volume, osmolality, and specific gravity are useful, but these are often impractical in field settings. In the field, because acute changes in body mass are primarily driven by changes in body water, assessments of body mass can be very informative. Techniques can be combined (e.g., body mass and urine color) to monitor hydration and identify dehydration. A best practice would be to review the characteristics of a given sport that increase risk of dehydration, such as fluid availability, environment, and exercise intensity. For a more detailed analysis, the interested reader should consult reviews by Belval and colleagues and Casa and colleagues (4, 13).

Fluid Intake Recommendations Before and During Practice and Competition

Evidence-based recommendations to prevent dehydration and encourage rehydration exist in the following three domains:

- *Before competition and practice:* The goal is to start euhydrated and with normal plasma electrolyte levels. This includes reversing fluid deficits that might have occurred from previous exercise sessions, weight-making strategies, or exposure to hot weather. Athletes are often advised to consume a drink (e.g., 5-7 ml/kg) in the hours before exercise to restore fluid levels while leaving sufficient time for excess to be urinated.
- *During competition and practice:* The typical goal is to prevent excessive dehydration (>2% body mass loss from water), and the practicality of achieving this depends on the likely rates of sweat loss (due to factors such as the intensity of exercise and environmental conditions), as well as the opportunities to drink during the session or event (availability of fluids, breaks in play or exercise, willingness to slow down to grab and consume a drink during continuous exercise, etc.). Because of the many permutations of these factors, actual fluid losses by athletes in real-life conditions can vary from large deficits to occasional but worrying levels of excessive fluid intake. The latter, which are associated with an increase in body weight over the exercise session, can lead to the rare but potentially fatal condition of hyponatremia (23).
- *After competition and practice:* The goal is to replace fluids and electrolytes. For athletes who need rapid replacement due to a subsequent athletic event, drinking 1.5 L fluid for every kilogram body mass lost is recommended. Secondary goals when rapid replacement is needed are to consume 1.0 to 1.5 g carbohydrate/kg/h for 3 to 4 hours (for more details see table 24.3) and adequate sodium. For more leisurely replacement, athletes should follow healthy eating and drinking practices, and add salt when sodium losses are high.

Presenting advice to athletes about fluid intake during exercise has become a contentious issue, due to disagreement around the point at which dehydration impairs performance (and therefore warrants addressing), as well as the danger that the information might be incorrect or misinterpreted, leading to excessive consumption (20, 26, 27). A simple summary might be as follows:

- Drink 0.4 to 0.8 L/h ad libitum (as much or as often as necessary or desired) or as time, comfort, or opportunity permits to reduce thirst and a level of fluid deficit that appears to interfere with optimal performance.
- Drink water unless there is benefit from replacing carbohydrates during exercise to supply muscle fuel (events of >60-75 min) or to provide a boost to the central nervous system. Targets for such activities are provided in table 24.2 but should be manipulated based on specific need and experience.

A thorough understanding of the evidence-based fluid intake guidelines from professional societies is essential for athletes and all members of the team involved with athlete care (3, 40, 52).

RECOVERY AND ADAPTATION

Postexercise recovery is a hot topic in sports nutrition, with interest in the quantity and the timing of intake of nutrients to optimize recovery issues such as refueling, rehydration, and protein synthesis for repair and adaptation. Recovery processes that help to minimize the risk of illness and injury are also important and are covered separately. In some cases, there is little effective recovery until nutrients are supplied, while in others, the stimulus for recovery is strongest in the period immediately after exercise. Recovery between exercise sessions may have two separate goals:

1. Restoration of body losses or changes caused by the first session to restore performance levels for the next

2. Maximizing the adaptive responses to the stress provided by the session to gradually make the body better at the features of exercise that are important for performance

Lack of appropriate nutritional support can interfere with the achievement of one or both of these goals. However, a side effect of the interest in recovery eating is an industry that appears to promote an aggressive and one-size-fits-all approach to postexercise nutrition, when in fact, the optimal approach is individual to each session and each athlete. Each athlete should use a cost–benefit analysis of the various approaches to recovery following different types of exercise and then periodize different recovery strategies into training or competition programs. An understanding of the needs of each training session or event and the overall goals of the program will help the athlete to distinguish between scenarios in which a proactive approach to recovery eating is warranted and the situations in which it may actually be beneficial to withhold nutritional support (see table 24.3).

A particular case in which the withholding of nutritional support is justified involves the evolving area of "train low" with respect to carbohydrate availability. Over the past decade it has been recognized that undertaking exercise with low carbohydrate availability (in particular low muscle glycogen, and to a lesser extent, lower blood glucose) may amplify the training stimulus and increase the expression of enzymes that promote fat metabolism as well

as increase mitochondrial mass and function (24). Although there are various strategies to achieve a train low scenario (8), a clever protocol involves the sequencing of a key or quality training session undertaken with high carbohydrate availability, followed by the restriction of carbohydrate intake in the hours after the session to delay the restoration of muscle glycogen (7). This allows the first session to be undertaken without sacrificing performance; it prolongs the period of enhanced adaptation and cellular adaptation that accompanies aerobic endurance exercise (i.e., "recover low"), and then creates the opportunity for the next exercise session to be undertaken with low glycogen stores. The integration of such strategies into an athlete's larger training program has been shown to create superior performance outcomes in sub-elite athletes (37), although not with elite competitors (11). Further work on such periodization of carbohydrate availability around training sessions is warranted and has been formally recognized in sports nutrition guidelines (8, 52).

NUTRITION FOR HEALTH AND INJURY PREVENTION

Staying healthy and injury-free is a key ingredient in a sporting career, since it supports consistent training and ensures that athletes can be at their peak for important competitions. However, the intensive exercise programs undertaken by many athletes straddle the fine line between providing the maximum stimulus for performance improvements and increasing the risk of illness and injury. Although evidence is not sufficient to set recommendations for nutritional practices that will guarantee minimum downtime or loss of training quality, some issues for the opposite outcome can be identified. These can be divided into risks of infectious illnesses, nutrient deficiencies, and injury.

There is a general belief that athletes are at increased risk of succumbing to infectious illnesses, particularly upper respiratory tract infections, during periods of high-volume training or after strenuous competitive events (57). Indeed, markers of acquired immune function are suppressed during the acute response to a bout of exercise, and it is intuitive that an exacerbation of the duration or severity of such effects beyond the level tolerated by the body could lead to compromised resistance to common infections (57). Nutritional factors that may exacerbate this risk include inadequate fueling (low carbohydrate availability) around exercise sessions and poor EA.

TABLE 24.3   Guidelines for Recovery: Refueling, Rehydration, and Adaptation

	Refueling	Rehydration	Repair and adaptation
Strategies to maximize goal	• Start carbohydrate intake soon after the session finishes; aim for a meal or snack providing ~1 g/kg body mass of carbohydrate • Continue with more snacks, drinks, or meals to achieve a carbohydrate target of 1-1.5 g · kg^{-1} · h^{-1} for the first 3-4 hours of recovery, then resume an eating pattern that meets overall fuel and energy goals; total carbohydrate requirements can range from 3-12 g/kg body mass per day • Choose carbohydrate forms consistent with other goals (e.g., energy needs, benefits of ingesting fluids and protein at the same time) • Choose carbohydrate-rich foods according to appetite and practicality	• Have a supply of fluids on hand that are palatable, suited to the conditions, and suited to other recovery nutrition needs of the athlete • When the fluid deficit is moderate to large (e.g., >2 L) and the rehydration period is <6-8 hours, have a planned fluid intake based on the deficit that needs to be replaced • Note that an approximation of the net fluid deficit is provided by the body mass change over the exercise session (~1 kg = 1 L); it may require the intake of a volume of fluid that is ~125% of the estimated deficit to allow for ongoing fluid losses (urine and sweat losses) • Start to consume fluids soon after the session finishes and aim to consume the target volume over the next 2-4 hours • Replace sweat electrolyte losses at the same time as consuming fluids, since this will maintain thirst and maximize fluid retention via smaller urine losses; choose fluids with added electrolytes (principally sodium) or consume salt-rich foods at the same time • Avoid excessive intake of alcohol since this is counterproductive to recovery goals, and the diuretic effect of alcohol is likely to reduce the effectiveness of rehydration	• Consume a high-quality protein-rich food providing ~20-25 g protein soon after the exercise session has finished; these targets might need to be expanded (e.g., 15-40 g) to account for the extreme range in athlete body size and muscle mass • Plan a pattern of snacks and meals to suit energy needs and other nutritional goals and lifestyle needs • Incorporate protein into meals and snacks every 3-5 hours • Include a protein-rich snack or meal before bed to allow protein synthesis to remain optimized overnight • Together, these patterns should lead to an intake of ~1.4-1.7 g/kg body mass per day (or for weight loss, up to 2.4 g · kg^{-1} · day^{-1})
Benefits	Maximizes muscle fuel for next demanding workout or event	Quickly restores hydration status for next demanding workout or event	Maximizes muscle protein synthesis after exercise to promote adaptations to the training stimulus; note that the elevated response lasts at least 24 hours
When should it be undertaken?	• After races or fuel-depleting training sessions when the athlete is backing up for the next session in 8 hours or less • When total fuel needs are high—high-volume training, demanding competition schedule (e.g., cycling tour, tennis tournament)	Following sessions that cause large sweat losses when the athlete is backing up for another session in 8 hours or less and will be exercising in hot conditions	• After competitive events or key training sessions (resistance sessions, high-intensity sessions) in which there is a major exercise stimulus or the occurrence of muscle damage • When gains in muscle mass and size are a priority

	Refueling	**Rehydration**	**Repair and adaptation**
Downsides	• May encourage intake of more kilojoules than needed (leading to weight gain) or a pattern of eating that is more risky for dental health • May encourage the intake of nutrient-poor foods since these are more accessible or easy to eat immediately after exercise • May reduce the period of enhanced adaptation after exercise	• May encourage the athlete to consume more kilojoules than needed (leading to weight gain) if the energy content of fluids is not accounted for • May cause gastrointestinal discomfort or the need for urination if large volumes of fluid are consumed quickly	• May encourage the athlete to think that expensive protein supplements are necessary • May require a reorganization of eating practices since most Western diets tend to be heavily loaded with protein at the evening meal rather than equally spread over the day
When is it expendable?	• When sessions are light or low in intensity and muscle glycogen is not likely to become depleted or limit performance • When the available recovery eating choices are low in nutritional value, and it makes more sense to wait a little until the athlete can have a more nutritious meal or snack • When the athlete has periodized some "train low" sessions into the training program, which may require a delay in refueling in the attempt to prolong the adaptation to the session just done, or commence the next session with depleted glycogen stores	• Just before bed, otherwise the athlete risks the interruption to sleep due to overnight toilet visits; it may be preferable to drink little before bed, then rehydrate in the morning • When fluid losses are mild and further sessions are undertaken in cool conditions	• When sessions are light or low in intensity and unlikely to promote great adaptation, and it does not suit the athlete's practical opportunities or energy restraints to include another food opportunity • If maximized protein-based recovery is desired but restricted energy requirements do not allow extra intake of food in the day, the athlete should consider changing the timing of training so that an existing meal can be consumed just after the workout to promote the enhanced protein synthetic response

Adapted from Thomas, Erdman, and Burke (2016).

Athletes are advised to follow nutritional practices that avoid such deficiencies, particularly in scenarios in which there are other immune system challenges. This includes individuals with history of recurring illnesses, periods of travel and communal living in which athletes encounter an increased risk of exposure to pathogens, and the periods around important events or intensified or specialized training (e.g., altitude training) in which the outcomes of immunodepression create greater penalties if illness were to occur. Meanwhile, nutritional supplements have been promoted as offering immune protection. However, there is limited evidence of benefits from supplementation with vitamin C and herbal products such as echinacea and glutamine, and mixed support for the use of colostrum and probiotics (58).

Athletes who consume moderate to high energy intakes from a varied diet based on nutrient-dense foods typically report intakes of vitamins and minerals well in excess of recommended dietary intake and are likely to meet any increases in micronutrient demand caused by training. This explains why routine supplementation with vitamins is not justified based on the absence of evidence of enhanced performance following vitamin supplementation except when it was used to correct a preexisting deficiency. Energy restriction, fad diets, and disordered eating are typical causes of inadequate micronutrient intakes of some athletes. Food range may also be restricted by poor practical nutrition skills, inadequate finances, and an overcommitted lifestyle that limits access to food and causes erratic meal schedules. Athletes require education about the quality and quantity of food intake, but a low-dose, broad-range multivitamin or mineral supplement may be useful when an athlete is unwilling or unable to make dietary changes, or when traveling to places with uncertain food supplies or eating schedules.

There are a few micronutrients at greater risk of inadequate intake in the diets of athletes. Inadequate **iron status** can reduce exercise performance via suboptimal levels of hemoglobin, and perhaps muscle-related iron functions. However, it may be difficult to distinguish true iron deficiency from alterations in iron status measures caused by exercise itself (e.g., changes in plasma volume, acute-phase responses to training). Reduction of blood hemoglobin concentrations due to plasma expansion, sometimes termed sports anemia, does not impair exercise performance. Nevertheless, some athletes are at true risk of an iron drain due to increased iron requirements to cover growth or increased gastrointestinal or hemolytic iron losses (47). Changes in plasma levels of the iron-regulating hormone hepcidin in response to strenuous exercise, especially with low carbohydrate availability, may reduce gut iron absorption and recycling of iron released through hemolysis; however, the chronic effect on iron status is still unclear (47). Meanwhile, the most common risk factor among athletes, as in all young people, is a low-energy diet or low intake of available iron. Female athletes who restrict dietary EI or variety, vegetarians, and athletes eating high-carbohydrate, low-meat diets are most at risk (18). Evaluation and management of iron status may need assessment by a sports medicine expert. Low iron status (serum ferritin levels lower than ~30 ng/ml) should be considered for further assessment and treatment. Although the effect of low iron status without anemia on performance is unclear, many athletes with low iron stores, or a sudden drop in iron status, complain of fatigue and inability to recover after heavy training or a failure to respond to altitude training. Many of these respond to strategies that improve iron status or prevent a further decrease in iron stores. In any case, routine screening of athletes or scenarios of high risk of inadequate iron stores can provide early intervention to prevent the outcomes of iron deficiency (47).

Although prevention and treatment of iron deficiency may include iron supplementation (47), long-term management should be based on dietary counseling to increase intake of bioavailable iron (increasing intake of heme iron sources and complementary intake of vitamin C or meat foods with non-heme iron foods). Evolving knowledge about hepcidin may lead to more definite recommendations around the timing of iron intake after exercise sessions to reduce its effect on iron absorption. These strategies can be integrated with the athlete's other exercise and nutrition goals.

Vitamin D deficiency or insufficiency is now recognized as a potential problem in some sections of the general population, with the major risk factor being not appropriate exposure to sunlight. Athletes at risk include those undertaking indoor training (e.g., gymnasts, swimmers); those residing at latitudes greater than 35°; athletes who train in the early morning or late evening, thus avoiding sunlight exposure; and those wearing protective clothing or sunscreen and consuming a diet low in vitamin D (31). Athletes with these characteristics should seek professional advice and have their vitamin D status monitored. Prevention or treatment of vitamin D insufficiency may require supplementation, although there is some debate over the levels that could be considered suboptimal and how these should be addressed (44).

Injuries generally occur via two mechanisms: acute problems that often follow a collision or impact, or chronic problems that result from inadequate resilience to continual high levels of exercise (e.g., stress fracture). Nutritional factors may be indirectly involved with some aspects of acute injury if inadequate nutrition contributes to the fatigue that tends to lead to poor concentration and technique or an increased risk of accidents. Meanwhile, they are more often involved in the development of chronic injuries such as stress fractures and the low bone density with which they are commonly associated (5). Although this seems contradictory in the face of the general bone protection afforded by exercise, many athletes suffer from either direct loss of bone density, or failure to optimize the gaining of peak bone mass that should occur during the 10 to 15 years after the onset of puberty (28). Poor bone health is considered a hallmark feature of low EA as recognized in the **female athlete triad** (43) and **relative energy deficiency in sport (RED-S)** syndromes (42). However, although poor bone health was first identified as a common problem among groups of female athletes (1), the link between menstrual issues, bone problems, and low EA is not universally expressed (33), and symptoms are also seen in male athletes (51).

As briefly outlined earlier in this chapter, **low energy availability** (LEA) represents a mismatch between an athlete's EI and that athlete's daily energy commitment to exercise. LEA can be caused by restrictions in EI, a high training or competition workload, or a combination of both. Although LEA was first considered to be a proxy for an eating disorder, further investigation of the female athlete triad (LEA, menstrual dysfunction, and poor bone health) revealed that this energy mismatch could also occur as an inadvertent outcome of poor food knowledge or availability or a misunderstood attempt to manipulate body composition (36). Irrespective of the cause of LEA, it appears to interact with other personal, life-style, and exercise-related factors to create a range of health and performance outcomes. Simply put, in the face of chronic LEA, an individual's body adapts by reducing its metabolic expenditure (i.e., resting metabolic rate) on processes that it might consider to be nonessential. A range of hormonal, metabolic, functional, and psychological adjustments has been described, including effects on performance (55), which have become known collectively as RED-S (42). There is still debate over the range of these outcomes and whether they affect male athletes in the same way (31). Further research is needed to explain all the direct and indirect associations between LEA and impaired body health and function. In the meantime, athletes are advised to seek expert opinion on maintaining healthy EA or moderating and periodizing phases of reduced EA (or both) (e.g., required or desired weight loss programs, periods of intensified training) within their overall nutrition plans (42). Treatment of diag-nosed cases of RED-S should be undertaken with the inclusion of expert medical, psychological, and nutritional support.

In addition to an environment of adequate avail-ability of energy, healthy bones require adequate bone-building nutrients, and potentially, carbohydrate. Adequate **calcium** intake is essential, with suggestions that calcium recommendations be increased to 1,300 to 1,500 mg/day in female athletes with impaired menstrual function, as is the case for postmenopausal women (28). Where adequate calcium intake cannot be met through dietary means, usually through use of low-fat dairy foods or calcium-enriched soy alterna-tives, a calcium supplement may be considered.

SUPPLEMENTS AND SPORTS FOODS

Sports products represent a lucrative portion of the worldwide explosion in the manufacture and mar-keting of supplements following the 1994 Dietary Supplement Health and Education Act. According to one report, sports supplements generated global revenue of US$9 billion in 2017, with a doubling of this value forecast by 2025 (37). Surveys confirm the high prevalence of sports foods or supplement use among athletes, including greater use at higher levels of competition (38). Despite earlier reluctance, many expert groups, including the International Olympic Committee (38), now pragmatically accept the use of supplements that pass a risk-benefit analysis of being

safe, effective, legal, and appropriate to an athlete's age and maturation in the sport. Supplements used by athletes fall into different categories:

- Medical supplements for treatment or prevention of nutrient deficiencies
- Sports foods providing energy and nutrients when it is impractical to consume everyday foods (e.g., sports drinks, protein supplements)
- Performance supplements that directly enhance exercise capacity or provide indirect benefits via recovery, body composition management, and other goals

The justified uses of medical supplements have already been discussed, and the valuable uses of sport foods are summarized in figure 24.1. However, despite limited evidence to support enthusiastic claims, performance supplements are the ones that receive most attention from athletes and coaches. The exceptions, which have efficacy as to their beneficial effect on sports performance, include caffeine, creatine monohydrate, bicarbonate, beta-alanine, and beetroot juice or nitrate.

Any benefits associated with supplement use must be balanced against the financial costs, the opportu-nity for adverse outcomes arising from poor protocols of use (e.g., excessive doses, interactions with other supplements), and the risks inherent in using products that are manufactured and regulated less stringently than foods or pharmaceutical goods. Apart from the health concerns, there is a small but real risk that supplements will contain substances that are prohibited by anti-doping codes such as the World Anti-Doping Agency (WADA) code (19). The use of confusing and variable chemical names on product labels may cause an athlete to fail to recognize a banned ingredient. In addition, supplements have been found to contain a variety of prohibited substances as contaminants or undeclared ingredients: These include stimulants, ana-bolic agents, selective androgen receptor modulators, diuretics, anorectics, and β2 agonists. Unfortunately, strict liability codes mean that an athlete who returns a positive urine test will record an adverse doping rule violation and receive sanctions such as being fined or banned from sport (or both) for a lengthy period, even if the substance was ingested unintentionally or in minute doses. Supplement contamination deservedly receives a large amount of attention in education around supple-ment use (54) and should remain a major issue in the athlete's process of decision making around supplement use (see figure 24.2). Third-party auditing of products can help elite athletes make informed choices about

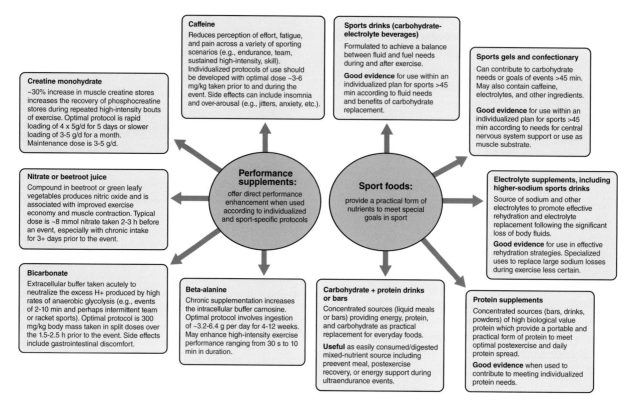

Creatine monohydrate
~30% increase in muscle creatine stores increases the recovery of phosphocreatine stores during repeated high-intensity bouts of exercise. Optimal protocol is rapid loading of 4 x 5g/d for 5 days or slower loading of 3-5 g/d for a month. Maintenance dose is 3-5 g/d.

Nitrate or beetroot juice
Compound in beetroot or green leafy vegetables produces nitric oxide and is associated with improved exercise economy and muscle contraction. Typical dose is ~8 mmol nitrate taken 2-3 h before an event, especially with chronic intake for 3+ days prior to the event.

Bicarbonate
Extracellular buffer taken acutely to neutralize the excess H+ produced by high rates of anaerobic glycolysis (e.g., events of 2-10 min and perhaps intermittent team or racket sports). Optimal protocol is 300 mg/kg body mass taken in split doses over the 1.5-2.5 h prior to the event. Side effects include gastrointestinal discomfort.

Caffeine
Reduces perception of effort, fatigue, and pain across a variety of sporting scenarios (e.g., endurance, team, sustained high-intensity, skill). Individualized protocols of use should be developed with optimal dose ~3-6 mg/kg taken prior to and during the event. Side effects can include insomnia and over-arousal (e.g., jitters, anxiety, etc.).

Beta-alanine
Chronic supplementation increases the intracellular buffer carnosine. Optimal protocol involves ingestion of ~3.2-6.4 g per day for 4-12 weeks. May enhance high-intensity exercise performance ranging from 30 s to 10 min in duration.

Performance supplements: offer direct performance enhancement when used according to individualized and sport-specific protocols

Sport foods: provide a practical form of nutrients to meet special goals in sport

Sports drinks (carbohydrate-electrolyte beverages)
Formulated to achieve a balance between fluid and fuel needs during and after exercise.
Good evidence for use within an individualized plan for sports >45 min according to fluid needs and benefits of carbohydrate replacement.

Carbohydrate + protein drinks or bars
Concentrated sources (liquid meals or bars) providing energy, protein, and carbohydrate as practical replacement for everyday foods.
Useful as easily consumed/digested mixed-nutrient source including preevent meal, postexercise recovery, or energy support during ultraendurance events.

Sports gels and confectionary
Can contribute to carbohydrate needs or goals of events >45 min. May also contain caffeine, electrolytes, and other ingredients.
Good evidence for use within an individualized plan for sports >45 min according to needs for central nervous system support or use as muscle substrate.

Electrolyte supplements, including higher-sodium sports drinks
Source of sodium and other electrolytes to promote effective rehydration and electrolyte replacement following the significant loss of body fluids.
Good evidence for use in effective rehydration strategies. Specialized uses to replace large sodium losses during exercise less certain.

Protein supplements
Concentrated sources (bars, drinks, powders) of high biological value protein which provide a portable and practical form of protein to meet optimal postexercise and daily protein spread.
Good evidence when used to contribute to meeting individualized protein needs.

FIGURE 24.1 Evidence-based performance supplements and sport foods.

supplement use but cannot provide an absolute guarantee of product safety (38).

NUTRITIONAL ASSESSMENT AND REFERRAL FOR EXPERT ADVICE

The professionals who often have the most contact with athletes, such as coaches, strength and conditioning coaches, and athletic trainers, may not always be the best choice to manage the common nutrition problems and concerns that arise. For example, body composition assessment might fall under the direction of athletic trainers or assistant coaches, but interpreting body composition data for a given athlete or providing meal plans for an athlete attempting to alter body composition is likely outside their scope of practice. The list of nutrition-related issues that athletes experience is seemingly endless, but can include poor hydration practices, low EI, poor micronutrient intake, improper macronutrient distribution, inappropriate or improperly managed body composition goals, fatigue, poor sleep quality or quantity, disordered eating, and more. This highlights the need for a well-defined, well-informed team that includes a sport scientist. In fact, sport scientists often have a breadth of training that allows them to bridge the gaps between team members whose

education and professional scope of practice include minimal nutrition expertise.

In some cases, effective monitoring and athlete education can come from a professional who has some training in nutrition. For example, hydration assessment and fluid provision are often under the direction of athletic training. It is common for athletic trainers to use techniques such as specific gravity or pre- and posttraining weight checks to track hydration status. Indeed, athletes can be involved in their own self-assessment via tracking of body weight, urine volume and color, and thirst (4, 13). However, athletes can have marked differences in fluid intake and sweat rate or content between individuals, sports, fitness levels, and environments. Athletes identified as having poor hydration status would be best served by referral to a dietitian or nutritionist to develop a proper plan. Further, not all techniques have the same accuracy and value. As an example, Adams and colleagues (2) compared urine reagent strips to refractometry and concluded that the urine strips were not valid in assessing hypohydration. Recovery after injury provides another scenario in which an athlete might benefit from specialist advice. Changes in EI and macronutrient distribution should be handled by a sports dietitian or nutritionist, while education about dietary supplements purported to aid in recovery from injury could be conducted by sport scientists, athletic trainers, or strength and conditioning

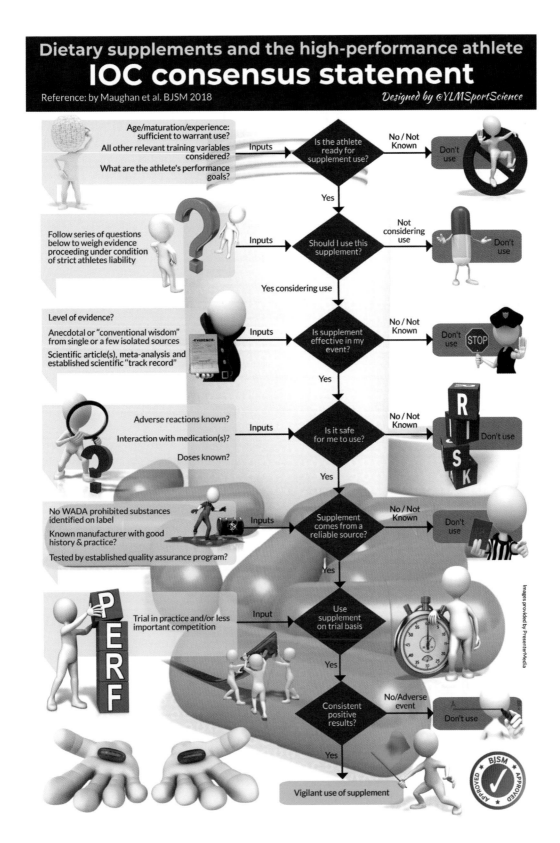

FIGURE 24.2   Decision making around supplement use.

Reprinted from R.J. Maughan, L.M. Burke, J. Dvorak, D.E. Larson-Meyer, P. Peeling, R.M. Phillips, E.S. Rawson et al. (2018, pg. 439-455).

coaches who have received guidance from the nutritional support team.

Knowing when to refer to an expert, such as a sports dietitian or nutritionist or physician, is critical, and sport scientists often have sufficient nutrition education to know when to educate and when to refer. Ideally, a properly credentialed sports dietitian or nutritionist should perform nutrition assessment of athletes. Indiscriminate use of nutritional assessment tools such as diet records or recalls and food frequency questionnaires is ill advised. The utility and limitations of such techniques are well described (32), and use should be limited to properly credentialed sports nutrition professionals. Estimating dietary intake includes many confounding influences, requiring many more assessments than possible in most cases. For example, Larson-Meyer and colleagues (32) described the number of days of diet records required to estimate a true average intake for a given individual as 27 to 35 days for energy, 37 to 41 days for carbohydrate, and 390 to 474 days for vitamin A. The development of a framework that includes things like day-to-day nutrition responsibilities and education, based on professional scope of practice, should be established before athletes arrive for their competitive season. Signs and symptoms of more serious issues and when to refer to another professional should also be established preseason. Proper management of athlete nutrition has become more difficult with the widespread use of smartphones and diet apps, whereby athletes and even entire teams track nutritional intake without ever meeting with a qualified professional.

While this is unacceptable, in reality, in some levels of sport, both nutrition and strength and conditioning are the responsibility of the head coach or assistant coaches or both. Ultimately, in the absence of qualified professionals, and in the case of people advising athletes outside of their scope of practice, sport teams expose themselves to both ethical and legal issues. For example, an athlete who reports unusual symptoms of fatigue may have an underlying nutrient deficiency or perhaps an eating disorder. If the symptoms are noted but left unchecked, or improper advice is provided, the underlying cause could be ignored and the condition will worsen. Using dietary supplements as another example, athletes who are subject to drug testing must be educated on the potential of supplement contamination with banned substances or impurities, as well as supplement, food, medication, and condition interactions.

CONCLUSION

Although nutrition cannot turn an ordinary athlete into an Olympic champion, support of training and competition needs is important in allowing all athletes to reach their potential, including optimal performance outcomes and longevity in their sport. A range of personalized and targeted nutritional strategies can help to keep athletes healthy and injury-free, in ideal physical shape, able to adapt to training, and ready to compete at their best. Sport scientists, athletic trainers, and coaches play an important role in the identification (and referral) of athletes with nutrition problems, in providing or supporting education about nutrition practices, and in the management of an environment that allows nutrition goals to be met. Collaboration with a sports dietitian or nutrition expert provides a partnership that allows expertise to be personalized and implemented in sport.

RECOMMENDED READINGS

Burke, LM, Castell, LM, Casa, DJ, Close, GL, Costa, RJS, Desbrow, B, Halson, SL, Lis, DM, Melin, AK, Peeling, P, Saunders, PU, Slater, GJ, Sygo, J, Witard, OC, Bermon, S, and Stellingwerff, T. International Association of Athletics Federations consensus statement 2019: nutrition for athletics. *Int J Sport Nutr Exerc Metab* 29:73-84, 2019.

Burke LM, and Hawley, JA. Swifter, higher, stronger: what's on the menu? *Science* 362:781-787, 2018.

Larson-Meyer, DE, Woolf, K, and Burke, L. Assessment of nutrient status in athletes and the need for Supplementation. *Int J Sport Nutr Exerc Metab* 28:139-158, 2018.

Maughan, RJ, Burke, LM, Dvorak, J, Larson-Meyer, DE, Peeling, P, Phillips, SM, Rawson, ES, Walsh, NP, Garthe, I, Geyer, H, Meeusen, R, van Loon, L, Shirreffs, SM, Spreit, LL, Stuart, M, Vernec, A, Currell, K, Ali, VM, Budgett, RGM, Ljungqvist, A, Mountjoy, M, Pitsiladis, Y, Soligard, T, Erdener, U, and Engebretsen, L. IOC consensus statement: dietary supplements and the high-performance athlete. *Br J Sports Med* 52:439-455, 2018.

Rawson, ES, Miles, MP, and Larson-Meyer, DE. Dietary supplements for health, adaptation, and recovery in athletes. *Int J Sport Nutr Exerc Metab* 28:188-199, 2018.

CHAPTER 25

Environmental Stress

Yasuki Sekiguchi, PhD

Courteney L. Benjamin, PhD

Douglas J. Casa, PhD

Sport scientists are given the task of preparing athletes, both mentally and physically, to compete in a wide range of environmental conditions. Various environmental conditions, such as heat and altitude, can have a significant impact on an athlete's performance and safety (36, 61). Major sporting events, such as FIFA World Cup Soccer and the Olympics, are often held in locations where heat or altitude or both come into play. Predetermined, uniquely designed programs for each environmental condition can induce positive adaptations and ensure peak physical condition for the individual- and team-sport athlete. Therefore, it is critical for sport scientists to have an understanding of the physiological responses to competing in these environments and practical methods to ensure elite performance and safety.

PERFORMANCE AND SAFETY IN THE HEAT

Reaching peak performance in the heat creates unique challenges for athletes, coaches, and sport scientists. An understanding of the physiology of exercise in the heat and the implementation of various strategies to overcome these challenges can be the deciding factor in an athlete dropping out or thriving in a competition.

Physiology of Exercise in the Heat

Shortly after the initiation of exercise, internal body temperature increases from metabolic heat production (11). During physical activity in extreme heat or with heavy personal protective equipment, the body cannot thermoregulate efficiently, which leads to an elevation in internal body temperature and is known as **uncompensable heat stress** (11). To dissipate heat, blood vessels vasodilate, skin blood flow increases, and the sweating response is initiated (5). Most heat dissipation is achieved via evaporation of sweat from the skin; however, this mechanism is hampered in extreme humidity (5). Heat can also be gained or lost, depending on environmental conditions, through radiation, convection, and conduction (28). Figure 25.1 demonstrates the mechanisms involved in the heat balance equation.

Heat Illness

While sport scientists are not necessarily licensed medical professionals (i.e., athletic trainers, physical therapists, or physicians), it is important for all individuals on the performance staff to be aware of signs and symptoms of exercise-induced illnesses and the appropriate life-saving treatment. Exertional heat illnesses, including heat exhaustion, heat syncope, and heat cramps, are a prevalent and recurring issue across all levels of sport (18). **Heat exhaustion** refers to collapse resulting from physiological exhaustion (11). **Heat syncope** is fainting due to hypotension resulting from lack of heat acclimatization or acclimation, upright posture, and gravitational pooling of blood in the leg when not enough blood is returned to central circulation (5). **Heat cramps** are painful spasms of skeletal muscle that are often observed following prolonged, strenuous exercise in

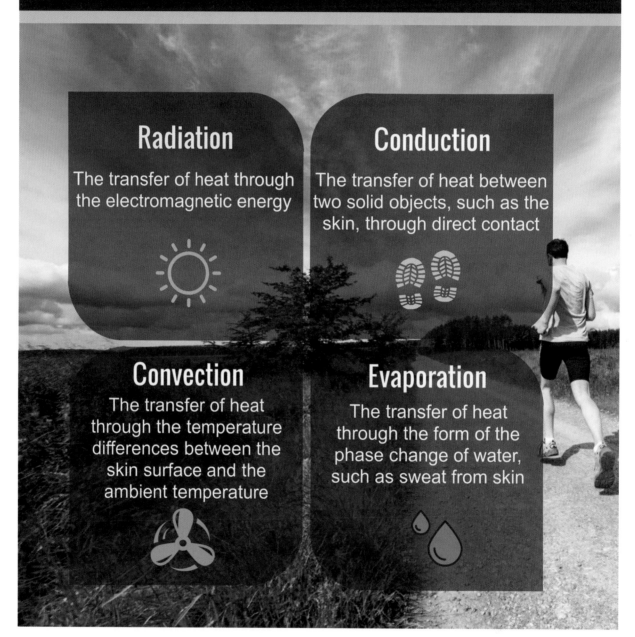

FIGURE 25.1   Radiation, conduction, convection, and evaporation in terms of human heat exchange.

the heat (11). **Exertional heatstroke** is among the top three leading causes of death in sport, despite the 100% survival rate with gold standard medical treatment (rapid recognition using valid internal body temperature and on-site cold-water immersion [CWI]) (18). Factors associated with exertional heat illness include fatigue, electrolyte losses, cardiovascular inefficiency, and hypohydration (18).

Performance in the Heat

Training and competing in the heat have negative implications for performance and safety, including a higher internal body temperature, increased heart rate, changes in perceptual measures, and slower time trials (62). Sport scientists can use several strategies to maximize athlete performance and safety in the heat.

Heat Acclimatization and Acclimation Strategies

One of the most simple and effective strategies to reach peak performance during exercise in the heat is **heat acclimatization** (natural, outside environment) or **heat acclimation** (artificial environment) (3). For the purposes of this chapter, HA refers to heat acclimatization or heat acclimation, depending on the environment. Heat acclimatization or heat acclimation is the process of gradually and systematically increasing physiological stress by training in the heat (9). Sport scientists can implement HA to maximize athletes' performance and safety.

HA Impacts on Performance in Heat and Cold

HA or acclimation not only is useful for competing in hot environments, but data demonstrates that this strategy can also be used to improve performance in cooler conditions (50). The appropriate use of HA policies reduced heat illness by as much as 55% at the U.S. high school level (48). In the team-sport setting, promising data demonstrated a 33% improvement in intermittent exercise in a group of female team-sport athletes following just four short HA sessions (77). With knowledge of the physiological and perceptual adaptions that occur from HA and strategies for inducing these improvements, sport scientists can effectively design a plan to optimize performance for both individual and team sports in hot and cool environmental conditions.

Adaptations to HA Induction, Decay, and Maintenance

Several positive physiological and perceptual changes known to improve exercise performance occur throughout HA (see figure 25.2). Plasma volume expansion, one factor that leads to lower heart rate and rating of perceived exertion, can be seen in as little as 3 days of HA (63). Other factors associated with a lower heart rate and improved perceptual measures include lower skin temperature and internal body temperature (62). The majority (~95%) of the internal body and skin temperature adaptations occur in 5 to 8 days of HA (62). Sweat responses, including an increase in sweat rate and a decrease in sweat electrolyte concentration, occurs within 5 to 14 days (78). While fewer studies have investigated this topic, there appears to be a reduction in lactate accumulation following HA, most likely due to an increased ability to clear lactate (73, 81).

The adaptations that occur with HA occur extremely fast; however, these will be lost relatively quickly without continued heat exposures and are typically referred to as **HA decay**. Following HA, heart rate and internal body temperature typically diminish at a rate of 2.5% decay per day without heat exposure (31). The ability to maintain a lower internal body temperature also decays without continued heat exposure; however, several factors (discussed later in this section) contribute to the rate at which this occurs. Few studies have examined the decay in sweat rate and other physiological variables following HA; therefore, the rate of decay is unknown. Even though there are known improvements in performance and safety with HA, one study has investigated strategies to maintain these benefits for an extended duration following HA induction (65). This strategy involved an exercising heat exposure once every 5 days and yielded positive physiological benefits compared to a control group (65). The benefits of this strategy are critical for athletes and sport scientists aiming to periodize performance optimization for specific competitions without interfering with sport-specific training.

Strategies for Optimal HA

The drastic improvements in physiological and perceptual responses, as well as exercise capacity and performance, following HA demonstrate the value of sport scientists developing programs using

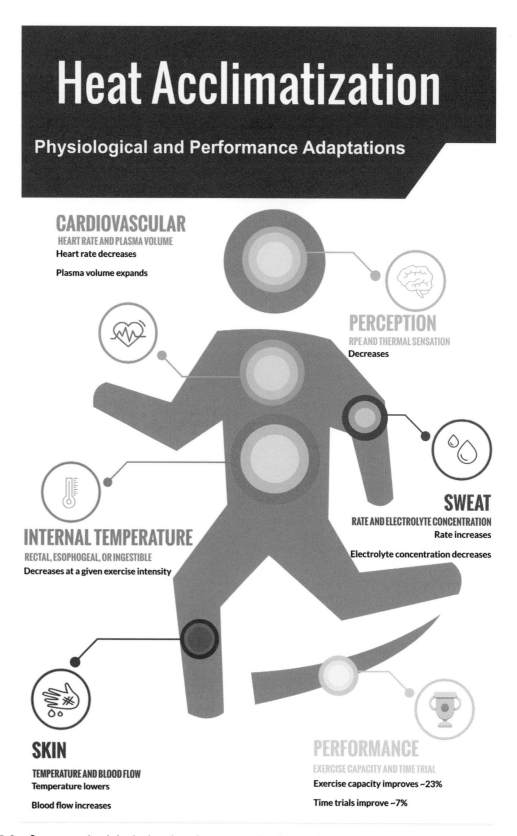

FIGURE 25.2 Common physiological and performance adaptions following a heat acclimatization program.

this strategy. Much as with the periodization of resistance training, conditioning sessions, or team practice, developing an effective HA strategy entails programming activities based on several internal responses and external variables that can be manipulated to achieve the desired predetermined goal (see figure 25.3). A sport scientist's role in managing the training stress balance of the athletes while using this strategy is critical to their success. If a HA protocol is implemented, the volume, intensity, and duration of the usual training should be modified to ensure that overtraining does not occur.

Internal Factors to Consider for the Development and Implementation of a HA Plan

Two primary individual athlete characteristics that can influence the effectiveness of a HA plan are aerobic fitness before the start of HA and the resting and exercising internal body temperature responses of that athlete. Athletes who are aerobically trained appear to exhibit physiological and perceptual adaptations induced by training alone that mirror partial HA responses (61). While reaching peak fitness is clearly essential in any sport, the role of aerobic fitness in heat tolerance should not be underestimated. Even athletes who are not considered aerobic (e.g., offensive linemen) may benefit from additional programmed aerobic training to improve their tolerance to exercise in the heat (61). Training programs for most field sports include some form of aerobic training; therefore, many elite athletes already demonstrate positive adaptations that improve exercising heat tolerance. Despite this fact, one of the most fascinating results of HA induction is the improvement observed in maximal oxygen consumption ($\dot{V}O_2$max), with reported improvements as much as 9.6% (45).

An increase in internal body temperature during exercise (accurately measured only through rectal, esophageal, or ingestible thermistors) is essential to drive the adaptations seen from HA (25, 78). To ensure full HA adaptations, including improvements in the sweat response, which is typically the last adaptation to occur, previous research has pointed to an **isothermal** method of HA induction, in which exercise intensity is adjusted to maintain a predetermined internal body temperature (typically 38.5° [101.3°F]) (39). This critical temperature threshold has been questioned as to whether it is the best method of HA, and some have postulated that even higher internal body temperatures may elicit adaptations of larger magnitude; however, future research is required (78). Two other methods that have produced promising results include **controlled work rate** and **clamped heart rate** (31). The controlled work-rate method involves setting a predetermined exercise intensity (for example, speed 12 km/h) and continuing this intensity throughout HA induction (78). One limitation of this method is that the relative intensity, and consequently, the amount of time spent at an elevated internal body temperature, typically decrease each day throughout HA induction due to the positive adaptations that occur. The clamped heart rate method involves setting a predetermined heart rate response (e.g., 150-155 beats per minute) for the entire length of HA induction. This method foregoes the limitation of stagnant physiological stress as seen in the controlled work-rate method; however, protocol development is crucial to ensure that the desired internal body temperature is achieved. One additional consideration for designing a HA program is that resting internal body temperature typically decreases over the course of HA, making the desired high internal body temperature increasingly more difficult to achieve.

External Factors to Consider for the Development and Implementation of a HA Plan

There are several components of a HA plan that are important for a sport scientist to consider during a programming phase. These include the following:

- Environmental conditions
- Length of induction
- Duration of sessions
- Frequency of sessions
- Exercise intensity
- Balance between HA and sport-specific training
- Alternative strategies

The majority of these, with the exception of environmental conditions in a natural environment, can be manipulated to ensure the appropriate training stress and adaptations. Understanding how to assess, manipulate, and alter these variables for specific training goals is imperative for sport scientists (64).

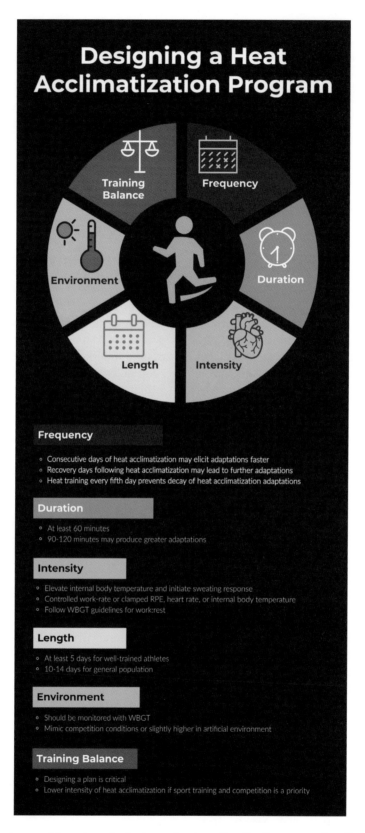

FIGURE 25.3 Factors to consider when designing a heat acclimatization or acclimation program to optimize performance and safety.

Environmental conditions are controlled only with access to an environmentally controlled room and therefore may not be practical for some programs. In cases in which an environmental laboratory or room is available, the predicted competition environment conditions, or slightly higher temperature or humidity or both, could be used for HA. In both artificial and natural environments, the use of a **wet-bulb globe temperature** (WBGT) monitor is the gold standard method for assessing the conditions. WBGT is the way to assess environmental heat stress because it measures ambient temperature, solar radiation, relative humidity, and wind, which are all known to influence physiological variables in the heat (24). A WBGT device is small, handheld, and portable. Guidelines for the use of a WBGT device should be based on each instrument's manual. Several military, occupational, and sport organizations have safety guidelines related to WBGT to guide practitioners in designing work-to-rest ratios (49).

Length of induction refers to the total number of days specifically designated for HA training. In the general population, it seems that the full benefits of HA are present in 10 to 14 days of training in the heat (9). Due to the interaction of HA and physical fitness discussed previously, it appears that elite athletes may obtain HA benefits from relatively short induction programs (5 days) (37, 38). However, there are a wide variety of individual responses and starting fitness levels, leaving sport scientists the discretion to take into account individual responses to determine the appropriate induction length (64).

The duration of HA sessions typically ranges from 60 to 120 minutes; the longer exercise duration seems to be favorable as well, since it gives the body a longer time to elicit the desired internal body temperature and the sweating responses needed to induce adaptations (72). While longer duration seems to be best to elicit HA, these session durations are not always practical to implement in other sport-specific training. While duration is an important component to consider for effective HA, there are other strategies that can be used to fit this strategy into a training plan as discussed later in this section.

The **frequency of HA sessions** refers to the number of days between sessions, with some programs completing sessions consecutively or with days of rest scheduled in between (64). If the HA is occurring, for example, during preseason periods of training, these sessions will be implemented consecutively. While this may be applicable to skill-based training, research

provides evidence that two sessions per day may not lead to faster HA adaptations than one session per day (80). Therefore, although consecutive HA may lead to faster complete adaptations, there is evidence to suggest that recovery following HA is crucial in order to attain the complete benefits (30). Hence, programming recovery days following an intense HA training regimen would be ideal for obtaining performance benefits. If a HA maintenance program is implemented, promising data suggests that heat exposure every 5 days can be used to prevent the decay of these positive adaptations (65).

There are a few factors to consider when determining the exercise intensity of a HA program, since the majority of the drive for adaptations is an increase in internal body temperature and the initiation of the sweating response. If HA is occurring naturally during sport-specific training, such as team practices, monitoring heart rate and using the appropriate work-to-rest ratios based on the WBGT may serve to determine exercise intensity. If an artificial laboratory is used, exercise intensity can be based on the internal body temperature, a percentage of the athlete's fitness level (e.g., a percentage of $\dot{V}O_2max$), clamped rating of perceived exertion, or clamped heart rate (62). The key to any of these methods is ensuring that the internal body temperature and sweating response is high enough to induce adaptions, while keeping the athlete safe.

Whereas it is ideal to control all of these factors during a HA program, logistical concerns sometimes arise when designing the plan, such as time commitment, financial resources for appropriate technology (i.e., internal body temperature monitoring), or training phase. Several programming frameworks have been proposed to overcome some of the barriers of HA and training (64). One component is the implementation of a HA maintenance plan. Another example of a strategy that can be used to overcome these barriers is alternative strategies to drive HA. One strategy that has been suggested is sauna bathing or hot-water immersion following a bout of exercise to maintain an elevated internal body temperature; however, future research is needed to determine the effectiveness of this latest strategy (26).

Hydration Strategies

Maintaining appropriate hydration status is important for athletes to optimize exercise performance (71).

Thus, it is critical that sport scientists understand the effects of hydration status on exercise performance, the method of hydration assessment, and hydration strategies.

Hydration Impacts on Performance

It has been shown that greater than 2% body mass loss decreases aerobic exercise performance, while some research has indicated that mild dehydration (about 1.5% body mass loss) can also impair aerobic performance (16, 71). It has been also reported that 3% to 4% body mass loss leads to reduced muscular strength and power (42). Dehydration is also associated with poor performance in sport-specific cognitive, motor, and skill execution (13). In addition to decreases in exercise performance, dehydration is a risk factor for heat illness, including heat exhaustion, exercise-associated muscle cramps, and exertional heatstroke (11). Even though it is well established that dehydration negatively affects exercise performance and safety, significant dehydration has been reported in both the team- and individual-sport settings (28, 59). Additionally, athletes are often dehydrated even before the start of exercise and do not consume appropriate amounts of fluid to optimize body fluid balance (2, 12). Thus, it is important for sport scientists to understand the methods used to assess hydration status and develop the skills to make a plan to maintain optimal hydration.

Hydration Assessment

Assessing athletes' hydration status is the first step to optimize body fluid balance in athletes, and understanding the valid and reliable methods to assess this is critical. There is no gold standard for assessing hydration status. Measurements to assess hydration in laboratory settings include plasma osmolality, urine osmolality, and 24-hour urine collection (6, 71). While these methods are commonly used in research, they are often difficult to use in a field setting. Valid field methods are also discussed here.

Body Mass Loss Tracking changes in body mass is an easy method to assess acute changes in hydration status (43). Based on two measurements of body mass, such as before and following exercise, **percent body mass loss** can be calculated by the following equation:

(Pre-exercise body mass − Postexercise body mass) / (Pre-exercise body mass) × 100

The goal of a sport scientist should be to prevent athletes from losing 2% of their body mass. While percent body mass loss is often used to track acute changes in hydration status, it can be used to monitor daily fluid balance, when appropriate baseline body mass has been established, by assessing first morning body mass for 3 consecutive days (7). Additionally, when 100% of sweat losses from the previous day of exercise have been replaced, the fluctuation of body mass is likely less than 1% (27). Thus, this method can also be used to check whether athletes have successfully recovered from a previous session.

Urine Color and Urine Specific Gravity Urine indices, such as urine color (7, 10, 44, 54) and urine specific gravity, are also easy for sport scientists to use. A urine color chart (see figure 25.4; this chart is not validated so it is for example purposes only) can be used as a marker of current hydration status. Urine color 4 or greater indicates dehydration. Urine color 5 or greater may indicate >2% body mass loss. Maintaining pale yellow or straw-colored urine corresponds to appropriate hydration (7, 44, 54).

Urine specific gravity (USG) refers to the density of a sample compared to pure water (6) and is another way to assess hydration status, performed using a refractometer that sport scientists can use. A USG ≥1.020 indicates dehydration (71). These urine measurements are accurate assessments of hydration status; however, values may be altered by rapid rehydration without altering the actual level of hydration (35, 43). Drinking rapidly can result in lower antidiuretic hormone (AVP), and this leads to diluted urine, which does not truly represent hydration status (43). Therefore, assessing urine color and USG based on the first morning urine sample provides the most accurate results (43). Interestingly, urine indices collected from an afternoon spot sample measurement give as accurate results as a 24-hour urine collection, which, as already mentioned, is the appropriate method to track the regular hydration status (21). Hence, to assess an athlete's habitual hydration status, an afternoon spot sample is also an accurate and practical method. These values may be affected by exercise or large amounts of fluid intake (or both) during the day; thus this method should be used only when athlete's do not participate in physical activity during the day.

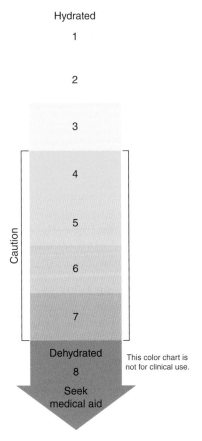

Urine Color Chart

Hydrated
1
2
3
4
5
6
7

Caution

Dehydrated
8
Seek
medical aid

This color chart is
not for clinical use.

FIGURE 25.4 Urine color chart.

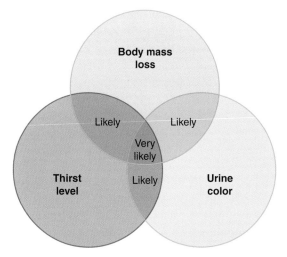

The criterion of dehydration
• Body mass loss > 1%   • Urine color > 5   • Feeling of thirst

FIGURE 25.5 A Venn diagram shows body mass loss, urine color, and thirst level.

Adapted by permission from S.N. Cheuvront and R.W. Kenefick (2016, pg. 1).

A Venn Diagram With Body Mass Loss, Urine Color, and Thirst Level   In addition to these measurements, a Venn diagram as suggested by Cheuvront and colleagues (29) is widely used in field settings to show hydration status (see figure 25.5; 29). The **Venn diagram** shows assessments of body mass loss, urine color, and thirst level. When all three markers indicate dehydration levels, an athlete is very likely to be dehydrated, and when two markers indicate dehydration levels, an athlete is likely dehydrated (29). The criteria for dehydration levels used in this diagram are body mass loss >1%, urine color >5, and feelings of thirst (29). Sport scientists can use Venn diagrams in field settings to evaluate hydration status. The Venn diagram is best used daily, in the morning, when the athlete first wakes up.

Sweat Rate Assessment

Assessment of sweat rate is critical to make a fluid intake plan. **Sweat rate** (L/h) is calculated by the following equation:

[Pre-exercise body mass (kg) − Postexercise body mass (kg) + Fluid intake (L) − Urine (L)] × 60 / Exercise duration (min)

Several factors affect sweat rate, including body mass, HA state, exercise efficiency, and environmental conditions (71). There is considerable variability in sweat rate between athletes, even in those who compete in the same sport (71). Thus, it is important for sport scientists to calculate individual sweat rates. Sweat rate can be used to create a planned drinking strategy, which is explained later in this section, to minimize fluid loss by estimating sweat loss based on the length of an exercise.

Sweat Electrolyte Assessment

In addition to hydration assessment, measurements of electrolytes are also important for performance and safety considerations. When an athlete exercises in the heat or performs multiple sessions, sweat electrolyte losses can exceed dietary intake (8). Among electrolytes, sodium is considered the most important

(75). Sodium promotes water absorption and stimulates glucose absorption (75). Additionally, sodium is associated with the etiology of exertional heat exhaustion, exertional heat cramps, and exertional hyponatremia (5). The gold standard to measure sweat electrolyte concentrations is the **whole-body wash-down method** (8). The procedure is presented next.

The clothes and towels that are used for the test are washed without soap or detergent to remove electrolyte content from the fiber of the clothing before starting the test. The clothes are then dried without fabric softeners or any other fabric care products. Just before entering the environmental chamber for testing, athletes are instructed to shower without the use of soap or any other product to remove all electrolyte content from the surface of the skin. The athlete then dries off with the washed towel and dresses in the washed clothes. Athletes then undergo the exercise test and are instructed to continuously capture sweat throughout the duration of the test by using towels. Upon cessation of exercise, athletes are rinsed with approximately 2 gallons (7.5 L) of distilled water. Athletes change into different clothes and add their clothes to the wash-down tub. The clothes are then thoroughly mixed in the tub and samples are collected from the tub for analysis with the use of an electrolyte analyzer.

While the whole-body wash-down method is the gold standard to assess sweat electrolytes, it might be unrealistic to use this method in an applied setting. Some research has pointed to the use of a regional sweat patch. Sweat patches are attached to different regions of the body, including forearm, back, chest, forehead, and thigh (14). These patches collect local sweat, which is then assessed with an electrolyte analyzer to measure electrolyte concentrations. However, the values from these patches are not as accurate as with the whole-body wash-down technique (15). Indeed, sweat patches generally overestimate sodium and potassium concentrations (14). If the sweat patch method is employed, a regression equation may be used to get better predictive values of sweat electrolyte concentration (15). The best regions in which to predict electrolytes measured by whole-body wash-down are the thigh for sodium and the chest for potassium (14).

Hydration Strategies

After analyzing hydration status, it is important to implement strategies to optimize hydration status. In general, there are two methods that are highly debated in the discussion of hydration strategies, which include planned drinking and drinking to thirst.

Planned Drinking and Drinking to Thirst   In terms of drinking to thirst, previous research has discussed the limitations of using thirst level in isolation, because this measurement might not be appropriate to assess hydration status when athletes perform exercise for longer than 1 hour to 90 minutes at high intensities in hot conditions (43, 47). One of the reasons for this is that thirst is initially perceived when 1% or 2% body mass loss occurs (7). Additionally, when athletes consume fluid based on thirst, they tend to replace about 60% of fluid losses, which is characterized as voluntary dehydration (43, 52). In these situations, a drinking plan should be created before exercise based on sweat rate to achieve 2% or less body mass loss throughout exercise without total-body fluid gains (46, 52). However, drinking to thirst could be used when exercise lasts less than 1 hour to 90 minutes, during exercise in cooler conditions and at lower exercise intensities (47).

Pre-Exercise, During Exercise, and Postexercise Hydration Strategies   Establishing and using a hydration plan for before, during, and following exercise will help ensure optimal hydration (see figure 25.6). The goal for any athlete is to begin exercise well hydrated and with the appropriate electrolyte balance (71). The American College of Sports Medicine consensus position recommends the consumption of 5 to 7 ml fluid/kg body mass at least 4 hours before exercise (71). If an athlete does not produce urine, or the urine is dark, the athlete needs to consume another 3 to 5 ml fluid/kg body mass about 2 hours before exercise (71). However, the amount of sodium consumed should be determined by the results of the whole-body wash-down test. Enhancing fluid palatability promotes rehydration, and several factors influence this, including fluid temperature, sodium content, and flavoring (71). The preferred fluid temperature is between 15 °C and 21 °C (59-70°F), which increases palatability and fluid intake (71).

The goal of hydration strategies during exercise is to prevent excessive dehydration (>2% body mass loss) and electrolyte losses (71). Planned drinking strategies can be created based on sweat rate and electrolyte balance tested beforehand (71). Carbohydrate consumption can be beneficial during high-intensity exercise that lasts ~1 hour or during low-intensity exercise of longer duration (71). Carbohydrate consumption of 30 to 60 g/h has been recommended to maintain blood glucose levels and sustain exercise performance (71). However, the concentration should not exceed 8%, at which point gastric emptying starts slowing (71). The goal of hydration strategies following exercise are to

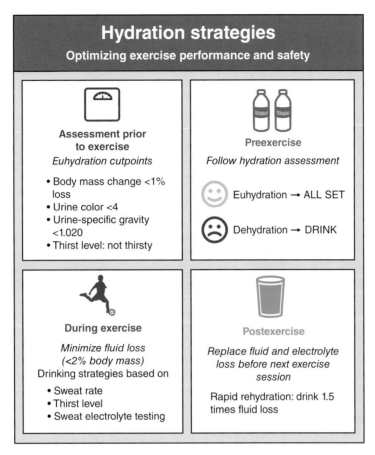

FIGURE 25.6 Methods for assessing hydration status before exercise, minimizing fluid loss during exercise, and rehydrating after exercise.

replace any fluid and electrolyte loss from exercise (71). When athletes have another exercise within about 12 hours and need rapid rehydration, they should consume 1.5 times the body mass loss (71, 76).

Cooling Strategies

A rise in internal body temperature can have a negative impact on performance and safety. Cooling strategies to mitigate this rise may be of interest to sport scientists (33, 56). A rise in internal body temperature alone could lead to decrements in metabolic and neuromuscular performance, even in the presence of **euhydration** (adequate hydration) (60).

Cooling Impacts on Performance

Several cooling strategies and the timing of these interventions have been investigated as a method to optimize performance, and it appears that a **mixed-method approach**, which refers to the use of multiple cooling modalities, is the optimal approach (20). While

the effectiveness of using cooling strategies is clear, there are practical considerations for sport scientists to keep in mind to determine the most appropriate modality (66).

Cooling: Timing and Modality Selection

When selecting a cooling modality, one must first determine the timing and feasibility of implementing this strategy during a training session or competition. The timing of cooling interventions is typically categorized into three possibilities: precooling, percooling (i.e., during exercises or competition or both), and postcooling (20). The use of precooling and percooling is typically considered when the goal is to mitigate a rise in internal body temperature for performance and safety optimization. Postcooling is used for recovery purposes to prepare athletes for future training and competition.

Since **precooling** will occur before a competition or training session, planning an appropriate warm-up is also warranted to ensure that athletes are at their best before the start of competition. Well-established evidence shows that a warm-up before competition is important for improved physical and psychological performance (67). However, if the warm-up is not altered appropriately based on environmental conditions, the athlete is at risk for heating up, which can have negative performance implications (67). Still, the use of cooling modalities before competition may allow athletes to warm up according to their physical and psychological needs without causing a rise in internal body temperature. In addition, cooling modalities are more effective than HA, fluid ingestion, or aerobic fitness in lowering internal body temperature at the onset of exercise (3).

Based on a review, ice slurry ingestion and CWI appear to be the most effective for reducing internal body temperature before exercise (20). The current research related to ice slurry ingestion suggests the consumption of ~1 L of crushed ice that is ≤4°C (≤39°F) before the start of exercise (66). Whole-body CWI at 22 °C to 30 °C (72-86°F) for 30 minutes appears to be the most common; however, partial CWI (legs only) at 10 °C to 18 °C (50-64°F) has also been used. One concern with the latter method is the need to rewarm the muscles due to the lack of nerve conduction and muscle contraction velocities that result from this water temperature, thereby creating a temporary reduction in power output (32). Other methods of precooling, including the use of fans, cooling or ice vests, or cooling packs may also be beneficial to use for precooling (1).

Percooling refers to cooling during an event or competition to attenuate the rise in internal body temperature during exercise and may be of interest since the benefit of precooling diminishes after 20 to 25 minutes of physical activity (19). Due to the need for feasible products to provide cooling during exercise, several options have been made available for use during such activities. Ice slurry ingestion, ice or cooling vests, wind or water dousing, cooling packs, and menthol cooling have all been investigated as potentially effective cooling modalities (20, 51, 53, 66) (see figure 25.7).

Postcooling is a term used to describe any cooling modality following a bout of exercise and is typically used to heighten recovery. The most common methods of postcooling are CWI and cryotherapy, although cold-air exposure and cooling packs have been used (20, 66). Cold-water immersion appears to decrease delayed-onset muscle soreness and perceived fatigue; however, this postcooling modality does not seem to affect any objective measures of recovery (20, 34). Cryotherapy is becoming an increasingly popular

modality and seems to be beneficial with regard to both subjective and objective markers of recovery, including reduced delayed-onset muscle soreness, increased muscular strength, and improvements in inflammatory blood biomarkers (20). In addition to physical recovery, markers of central nervous system function (heart rate variability) may also be improved following water immersion (thermoneutral and CWI); however, future research on this is needed (4).

Overall, a mixed-method approach for precooling and percooling should be considered for optimal results (66). While cooling strategies can be useful for both performance and recovery, a cost–benefit analysis is needed in order for each organization to determine the balance between practicality and usefulness of specific modalities and the best method for implementation. See table 25.1 for information that can be used for the development of an optimal cooling plan (20, 51, 53, 66).

PROGRAMING AT ALTITUDE

Altitude training is popular especially among aerobic endurance athletes. It is critical for sport scientists to understand the significance and practical implications of altitude training.

The Importance of Altitude Training

Aerobic performance is generally impaired above 1,000 meters, and aerobic capacity is reduced 7% to 8% for every 100 meters above 1,500 meters from sea level (40, 58). Short-duration anaerobic exercise may not be influenced by altitude; however, repeated intermittent exercise performance is decreased compared to this exercise at sea level (40). Team sport performance is also affected by altitude (58). For example, total distance covered in the FIFA World Cup was reduced at altitude compared to sea level (58). However, exposures to hypoxic conditions have been shown to improve exercise performance at normal conditions (23). Therefore, understanding altitude training is important for sport scientists when athletes perform exercise at altitude as well as at sea level (36).

Adaptations to Altitude

Increased hypoxic stress at altitude promotes key physiological adaptations (36). Decreased **partial pressure of oxygen** (PaO_2) at altitude reduces

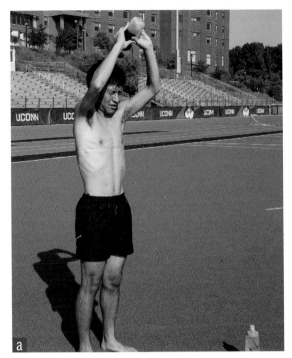
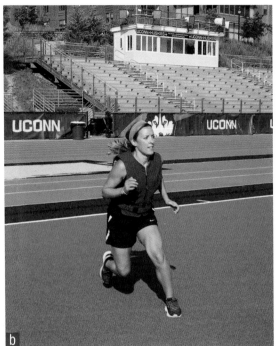
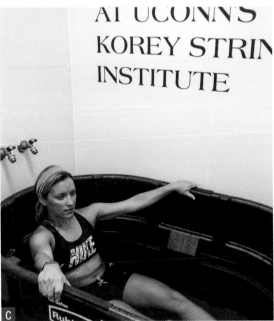
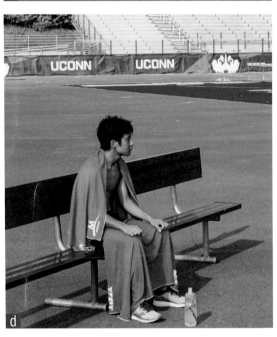

FIGURE 25.7   The use of cooling strategies includes *(a)* ice-water dousing, *(b)* cooling vest, *(c)* cold-water immersion, and *(d)* ice towels.

hemoglobin-oxygen saturation and decreases total oxygen content of the blood (36). Adaptations, including ventilatory, cardiovascular, hematological, and skeletal muscle, following altitude training are due to the compensation for this hypoxic stress (36). Hypoxic stress elevates respiratory rate in

the early stages of altitude exposures (36, 68, 74). Hyperventilation caused by altitude exposure increases PaO_2, and this increases oxygen loading in the lungs (36). These ventilatory adaptations might have advantages with respect to exercise when athletes return to sea level. The hematological improvements

TABLE 25.1 Considerations for Selecting a Cooling Modality for Optimizing Performance in the Heat

Cooling modality	Preferred use	Cooling rate	Advantage	Disadvantage	Estimated cost
Cooling garment	• Temperature: 0-20 °C (32-68 °F) • Precooling or percooling	• Ice towels: 0.11 °C (0.198 °F) /min • Major artery ice pack: 0.028 °C (0.05 °F) /min • Cooling blanket: 0.01 °C (0.018 °F)/min	• Possible to use during exercise • Available to full team at once • Easy to prepare • Practical for sport settings	• Not long-lasting effects • Must recool the product often	$100-$400 per garment
Ice slurry ingestion	• Temperature: ≤4°C (≤39°F) • Volume: ~1 L • Precooling or percooling	Not applicable	Multipurpose modality—cooling and hydrating	• Relies on location of machine • Electricity needed	~$1,000 dependent on machine brand
Dousing	• Temperature: 15 °C (59 °F) • Precooling or percooling	Mixed-method dousing with fan: 0.15 °C (0.27 °F)	• Possible to use during exercise • Available to full team at once • Easy to prepare • Practical for sport settings	Hard to cover large surface area comfortably	$0
Fan	• High speeds • Precooling or percooling		• Easy to prepare • Easy to implement	• Can use only during breaks from exercise • Electricity needed	$100-$400 per unit
Cold-water immersion	• Temperature: 2-25 °C (35.6-77 °F) • Time: 10-30 min • Cover as much body surface area as possible • Precooling or postcooling	• 2 °C (35.6 °F) CWI: 0.35 °C/min • 8 °C (46.4 °F) and 20 °C (68 °F) CWI: 0.19 °C/min	High cooling rate	Preparation required	$90 per tub
Cryotherapy	• Temperatures lower than –100 °C (–148 °F) • Time: 2-4 min • Postcooling	Not applicable	Appears to improve recovery	Not practical for sport settings	$60-$100 per session

that result from altitude training is an important adaptation (36).

Erythropoietin (EPO) is primarily produced in the kidneys and improves oxygen-carrying capacity in the blood (70). In general, EPO concentration peaks from day 1 to day 5 following hypoxic exposures (36). The adaptations that occur in skeletal muscle following hypoxic exposure include improvements of muscle metabolism economy and buffering capacity (36). Hypoxic exposures promote the ability to uptake glucose during exercise (82), the formation of capillaries, and increases in blood flow to exercising tissues (22, 57). Additionally, mitochondria density and oxidative enzyme concentration increase, which contributes to improvement of muscle oxidative capacity (36, 41).

Strategies to Optimize Performance at Altitude

The effects of each altitude training method tend to be controversial. There are typically three models, which include live high, train high; live high, train low; and intermittent hypoxic training (36). The **live high, train high model** refers to living and training at moderate altitude (1,800-2,500 m) for 2 to 3 weeks (36). This training can increase aerobic endurance performance for 6 to 8 weeks. However, it might be challenging to maintain the same intensity for long exposures of time, and it might be recommended exercising at sea level to avoid overtraining and immune suppression (36, 69). The **live high, train low model** was introduced to overcome the limitations of the live high, train high model. This method involves athletes living at 2,000 to 2,500 meters for ~4 weeks (36). This method has been shown to increase aerobic endurance performance; however, it requires significant travel between training sessions, and alternative strategies (i.e., the use of hypoxic tents) have been suggested (36, 79). **Intermittent hypoxic training** consists of athletes using a short interval of hypoxic stress via inspiration of hypoxic gas during training while they are living in **normoxic** conditions, which have a normal oxygen concentration (36). Aerobic endurance performance might be improved due to muscle adaptations whereas hematological adaptations might not be observed (36, 55). In addition to these three methods, previous research investigated the combination of heat and hypoxic exposures during sleep and training to promote adaptations in hemoglobin and plasma volume compared to a nonhypoxic exposure group in team-sport athletes (23). Further studies are required to conclude on the effect of the combination of heat and hypoxic exposures, which manipulates the amount of oxygen level as well as hyperbaric interventions or exposures, which manipulates atmospheric pressure.

CONCLUSION

Training and competing in extreme environmental conditions introduce several obstacles to reaching peak safety and performance during physical activity; however, there are several strategies and guidelines that sport scientists can use to overcome these obstacles (5, 36, 62). Developing a HA plan, hydration strategies, and determining optimal cooling methods are tools that sport scientists can implement with the athletes who compete in extreme conditions (i.e., heat). Sport scientists can also use altitude strategies, including the live high, train high strategy, the live high, train low strategy, or intermittent hypoxic training to ensure peak performance while guaranteeing safety both in hypoxic situations and at sea level. In addition to helping athletes reach peak performance and stay safe in these extreme environments, these strategies may also improve performance in less extreme or cooler circumstances. With appropriate knowledge and application, sport scientists can apply these strategies to elevate athletes to new levels of accomplishment and ensure their well-being throughout competitive sports.

RECOMMENDED READINGS

Armstrong, LE. *Performing in Extreme Environments.* Champaign, IL: Human Kinetics, 1999.

Casa, DJ. *Sport and Physical Activity in the Heat: Maximizing Performance and Safety.* Cham, Switzerland: Springer, 2018.

Casa, DJ, and Stearns, RL. *Preventing Sudden Death in Sport and Physical Activity.* Burlington, MA: Jones & Bartlett Learning, 2017.

Cheuvront, SN, and Sawka, MN. Hydration assessment of athletes. Gatorade Sports Science Institute 18, 2005.

Periard, JD, and Racinais, S, eds. *Heat Stress in Sport and Exercise.* Springer International Publishing, 2019.

CHAPTER 26

Psychobiology: Flow State as a Countermeasure to Mental Fatigue

Chris P. Bertram, PhD

Mental fatigue is a psychobiological state that can manifest as feelings of lethargy, disinterest, or decreased motivation and often results in a general reduction in cognitive or motor proficiency or both. Conversely, the psychobiological state of **flow** is described as a state of mind in which a person is completely and effortlessly immersed in an activity; flow is considered a hallmark of peak performance. Synonyms for flow, such as "the zone" or "runner's high," are used colloquially to describe episodes of peak performance or deeply enjoyable experience. Historically, however, these states were seen to be elusive and fleeting in nature (87, 88). Advances in imaging technology and neuroscience have allowed for a much broader understanding of the neurological, psychological, and phenomenological nature of flow states. Likewise, similar approaches have strengthened the understanding of mental fatigue and its deleterious impact on physical, as well as cognitive, performance in sport. As a result of insights into the opposing forces of mental fatigue and flow state, scientists and practitioners are now beginning to explore ways of eliciting flow states on demand in order to expedite learning and optimize performance. This chapter overviews the relevant background and neurological processes underlying flow states. Furthermore, the chapter addresses the topic of mental fatigue for an in-depth examination of the phenomenon and its broader impact on sport performance. The chapter concludes by presenting several evidence-based suggestions for how sport scientists can create the preconditions for flow, leverage them to counteract mental fatigue, stimulate higher rates of learning, and drive more optimized levels of performance.

FLOW STATE AND ITS IMPACT ON PERFORMANCE

While the neuroscience of flow is a relatively new concept in human athletic performance, the concept itself has been talked about in one way or another for longer than most people realize. After witnessing celebrations at a Roman carnival in 1789, the German writer Johann Wolfgang von Goethe used the term **rausche** to describe "an acceleration of movement leading to flowing joy." The philosopher Nietzsche frequently referred to *rausche* as that which is inspired by great works of art or aesthetic beauty, famously noting in his 1901 work *The Will to Power* (79):

> Art reminds us of states of animal vigor; it is on the one hand an excess and overflow of blooming physicality into the world of images and desires; on the other, an excitation of the animal function through the images and desires of intensified life - an enhancement of the feeling of life, a stimulant to it.

More modern examinations of flow began in the 1940s and 1950s with the work of American humanist psychologist Abraham Maslow. Known best for his development of the now-famous hierarchy of needs, Maslow dedicated his career to a deeper understanding of the quest for ultimate happiness, or what he termed **self-actualization** at the pinnacle of the pyramid of human existence. Maslow seemed intuitively aware of the reality of **flow states** many years before the term had been coined. Instead, however, Maslow (73) talked of peak experiences as those "rare, exciting, oceanic, deeply moving, exhilarating, elevating experiences that generate an advanced form of perceiving reality and are even mystic and magical in their effect upon the experimenter."

Building on Maslow's work, psychologist Mihály Csíkszentmihályi reconceptualized the notion of peak performance, and in 1975 coined the term "flow" as a descriptor for the nonordinary state of consciousness that drives peak experiences (18). Csíkszentmihályi's notion of flow stemmed from studies conducted around the globe looking at the nature of happiness, and he eventually identified nine key characteristics of the flow experience (18):

1. *Goals are clearly defined:* There is a distinct feeling of certainty about what needs to be done. There are no contradictory or ambiguous signals interfering with the idea of what actions need to be taken next. Clear goals reinforce a sense of purpose and evoke action.

2. *Unambiguous feedback is available:* Immediate and clear feedback is received (from internal or external sources or both), providing reassurance that things are going according to plan. This feedback also helps provide guidance when actions need to be altered to meet changing and often unpredictable task demands.

3. *An appropriate ratio of skill level and challenge is present:* There is a feeling of balance between the demands of the task and one's ability. When the challenge is too high, the experience can be met with frustration or anxiety. If the challenge is too low, there can be boredom or disengagement. In flow, there is a perceived match between challenge and skill (or perhaps a slightly higher level of challenge relative to skill) that drives engagement in the task while maintaining a state of calm.

4. *Action and awareness merge:* A deep level of involvement is experienced whereby actions or activities feel spontaneous and automatic. Often thoughts can be preoccupied with events that have happened in the past, or worries about things yet to come; however, in flow, thoughts and actions merge seamlessly and skilled movement seems to happen automatically.

5. *Concentration on the task is high:* Irrelevant information is filtered from consciousness and there is a heightened alertness and focus on a profound singleness of purpose. Furthermore, this intense concentration is perceived to be effortless despite the high risk or demands that may be present.

6. *One has a sense of control:* In a state of flow, there is a deep sense of autonomy and command of one's self and the environment. There is an abiding confidence that goals will be achieved, as well as a strong sense of personal agency over one's ability to meet or surpass those goals.

7. *The ego vanishes:* Flow decreases immediate concerns with oneself during engagement in the activity. While at the extremes this can lead to increased risk-taking behaviors, more commonly this loss of self is met with a feeling of liberation from ordinary self-consciousness along with increased freedom of expression, confidence, and creativity.

8. *Time becomes distorted:* In flow, time is experienced differently than normal. In some instances, it can feel slowed down to almost a freeze-frame effect. More commonly, time can seem to pass by at a greatly accelerated rate, with hours seeming like minutes.

9. *The experience is autotelic:* Flow is intrinsically rewarding and enjoyed for its own sake. The action or activity itself is reason enough to continue without a need for any kind of extrinsic reward or future benefit.

Subsequent research has supported the notion of these nine flow dimensions (21, 50, 72), while additional studies have provided evidence for the ability of the model to predict these characteristics in numerous areas of sport (48, 51, 102), musical performance (108), and video game play (52).

Establishing the nine primary characteristics was central to the development and validation of the Flow State Scale (50) and later the Flow State Scale-2 (49). Formulating these instruments was critical because it allowed researchers to quantify a flow state for the first time, and it created the opportunity to use flow as a variable in a host of experimental settings (44, 54).

The Anatomy of Flow

With upward of 100 billion individual nerve cells capable of forming approximately 100 trillion separate connections, the complexity of the human brain is extraordinary. The extent of this complexity has led to some interesting (and often misguided) theories about the nature of human performance and the role of the brain in that process. For example, there is a persistent saying that people use only 10% of the brain at any given time, and that as skills evolve, more of the brain comes online, thus leading to better levels of performance. As it turns out, in many ways, the exact opposite is true. The reality is that when our brains are in a flow state, certain parts of the brain actually deactivate. Dietrich (24, 25) first described this selective deactivation and termed it **transient hypofrontality**. Dietrich's suggestion was that many altered states of consciousness (of which flow is one) could be explained by the temporary deactivation of certain areas of the prefrontal cortex (PFC). The PFC is generally regarded as the site of executive function in the brain, and is thought to oversee many basic cognitive processes such as attentional control, inhibition, and working memory, along with higher-order functions such as reasoning and critical problem solving (see Baggetta and Alexander [2] for a review). Empirical evidence also suggests that the frontal cortex plays a significant role in the perception and calculation of time (38) and the perceptions of self and ego (29), as well as self-criticism and self-defeating thoughts (66). Importantly, many of these findings (i.e., a distorted sense of time, decreased self-consciousness, increased positive self-concept) relate to the typical phenomenological experiences that athletes report during flow states (44, 50, 51, 74).

Support for the transient hypofrontality hypothesis has come, in part, from functional magnetic resonance imaging (fMRI) studies looking at brain activation patterns during heightened states of creativity. Limb and Braun (62) conducted a study in which the brain activity of jazz musicians was observed while they were playing either an overlearned (i.e., memorized) piece of music or a spontaneously improvised piece of music. The results showed marked differences in activation-deactivation patterns across the two conditions. Specifically, it was demonstrated that improvisation led to extensive deactivation across parts of the PFC (specifically in the dorsolateral prefrontal cortex or DLPFC), along with corresponding deactivations in brain areas (amygdala and hippocampus) associated with increased mood and pleasure. A similar study conducted by Liu and colleagues (64) looked at the brain activity of professional freestyle rap artists while they performed either memorized lyrics or spontaneously improvised lyrics. Results from the fMRI scan indicated that brain areas associated with close self-monitoring and editing (i.e., the DLPFC) were deactivated when rappers were "freestyling" compared to when they simply recited memorized lyrics. These authors also reported accompanying increased activity of the premotor and cingulate cortex (in the anterior cingulate cortex) in the improvisation condition. Taken together, the results suggest that transient hypofrontality causes downregulation of the DLPFC, which in turn decreases hyper-analytical thinking while simultaneously creating an opportunity for the brain to conjure the type of remote associations that appear in moments of heightened creativity and the state of flow (74).

The Flow of Brainwaves

One of the more reliable ways that brain activity can be quantified is through measurement of its electrical output (see chapter 15). Along with an assortment of chemical neurotransmitters, the propagation of brain waves, especially the neocortex, is thought to represent one of the key forms of communication between various regions and networks of the brain (114). To varying degrees, the brain is active 24 hours a day, and the electricity it produces is sent out in waves of fluctuating amplitude and frequency. The number of waves measured per second is termed **hertz** (Hz), and these frequencies are known to correlate well to the both the emotional and the cognitive state of the brain (13, 77). For example, as you are sitting and reading this chapter, there is a good chance your brain is emitting relatively fast-moving waves that are measurable at a frequency between 13 and 30 Hz (also called **beta waves**). Fear and anxiety are likewise highly engaging brain states (sometimes negatively so) and also exist at the higher end of the beta spectrum (55). On the other hand, feelings of relaxation tend to produce slower, longer waves (and hence fewer of them each second). These waves, between 8 and 12.9 Hz, are called **alpha waves**. Alpha waves tend to appear when the mind is in a state of wakeful relaxation or even daydreaming. Alpha waves are also associated with increased creativity and the ability to move from thought to thought with very little in the way of internal judgment or resistance (69). An even slower wave called **theta** appears when the brain's output moves into the range of 4 to 7.9 Hz. Theta waves tend to appear during rapid eye movement (REM) sleep (i.e., dream sleep) and the **hypnagogic state** (the transitional state between wakefulness and sleep), and are thought to play a critical role in learning and memory (see Schacter [93] for a review). If learning is a process of connecting existing knowledge with new information in creative ways, it is reasonable to conclude that the brain is primed for this type of associative or lateral thinking when theta waves are present (28). Slower still are **delta waves**, with frequencies ranging between 1.0 to 3.9 Hz. Delta waves are primarily associated with periods of non-REM sleep and during increased sleepiness in certain fatigued states (59). See table 26.1 for an overview of brain waves and their associated states of consciousness.

Electroencephalogram (EEG) studies have also provided insight into event-associated changes in the brain related to skill level. Research in skill acquisition suggests that the process of acquiring expertise is in part due to the gradual shifting of attention from the internal world of thought to the external world of action and goal-directed behavior (32). In other words, the novice performer must deal with a significant cognitive load in the early stages of learning. However, as skill level increases—eventually to a state of automaticity—the cognitive burden is eased and more attention can be focused externally (see Bertram and colleagues [7] for a review). In support of this notion, Hatfield and coworkers (48) concluded that cortical changes resulting from progression in ability are indicative of decreases in attentional demand and cognitive interference in skilled individuals. As it pertains specifically to EEG analyses, many researchers have noted that success in skilled individuals is associated with greater theta and alpha activity (5, 28, 89) and decreased beta activity (3, 47). Furthermore, Katahira and colleagues (56) showed that increased theta and alpha activity in certain frontal regions of the brain were associated with self-reported flow state experiences.

The Chemistry of Flow

Flow is a sought-after state of consciousness for athletes, due to both its perceived impact on performance and the positive effects associated with enhanced mood and intrinsic motivation (37). Several lines of evidence point to a unique mix of key neurochemicals to partially explain many of the phenomenological experiences (rapt attention, joy, ecstasy, effortlessness) reported in flow.

A commonly reported dimension of flow state is a sense of effortless attention to the task at hand and a decoupling of action from conscious effort (103). Unlike other realms of achievement wherein success depends on intentional concentration, performance in flow is typically reported to be more autonomous and accompanied by a sense of confidence and ease (101). Given the role of the PFC in the modulation of attention, coupled with the demonstrated impact of norepinephrine and dopamine on these structures (112), it stands to reason that these two neurotransmitters play a significant role in the chemistry of flow. For example, Knöpfli and colleagues (58) found strong links between competitive performance and higher levels of norepinephrine and dopamine secretion. Studies of attention-deficit hyperactivity disorder (ADHD) have likewise supported the position that attentional mechanisms are strongly regulated by norepinephrine and dopamine systems (8, 86).

Along with dopamine's role in regulating attention, it has also long been known as a key driver in the brain's reward system (31, 41) and has been linked to the flow experience (44, 92). Given the pervasive reports of the positive affective experiences of flow state, it is perhaps not surprising that the striatal dopamine system has been shown to be associated with the emotional experiences of the flow state (23).

Beyond norepinephrine and dopamine, investigations of the experience of runner's high have also implicated the pain-dampening effects of endogenous

TABLE 26.1 Brain Wave Overview

Type	Frequency	Associated state of consciousness
Delta	1.0-3.9 Hz	Deep, non-REM sleep
Theta	4.0-7.9 Hz	REM sleep; hypnagogic state
Alpha	8.0-12.9 Hz	Daydreamy; meditative yet alert
Beta	13-30 Hz	Normal waking state; attentive
Gamma	>31 Hz	Insight; heightened focus

opioids (10, 40) as well as neurochemicals of the endocannabinoid system such as anandamide (27, 35, 100) as contributing mechanisms to flow state phenomenology. Anandamide, a neurotransmitter whose name is derived from the Sanskrit word for joy or bliss, is known more broadly to enhance pleasure responses in the brain (70).

Taken together, these results suggest that many of the typical characteristics of flow state can be attributed to neurochemicals associated with heightened focus, increased pleasure and well-being, and a decreased perception of pain that athletes so often experience during peak performances.

MENTAL FATIGUE AND ITS IMPACT ON PERFORMANCE

It is understood that fatigue, generally speaking, is a significant limiting factor for athletes and high-performing individuals across all domains. Within the physical domain specifically, the impact of conditions such as overtraining syndrome and nonfunctional overreaching on the well-being and physical performance of individuals is profound. Thus an extensive body of literature that has sought to better understand the mechanisms and phenomenology of excessive physical fatigue. Likewise, research has also provided better guidelines for the prevention, early intervention, and treatment of the signs and symptoms of overtraining (106). Considerably less attention, however, has been paid to the issue of mental fatigue and the deleterious effects it has on both cognitive and physical performance in sport. Given the ever-increasing demands placed specifically (but not exclusively) on elite-level athletes, it is somewhat surprising that the issue has not garnered more attention in the high-performance literature.

Mental Fatigue and Cognitive Function

Prolonged and excessive amounts of cognitive activity can often lead to mental fatigue and result in symptoms ranging from general tiredness to decreased motivation and decreased cognitive performance (105). For example, in the workplace, a more extreme example of this phenomenon is commonly referred to as **burnout**, and its rate of occurrence is high and troubling from both a mental health and a productivity perspective. Data suggest that 77% of employees report feeling burned out either sometimes or often

at work (22). Some of the main factors that have been identified as contributing to these high rates of mental fatigue are such things as unmanageable workloads, lack of role clarity, and poor communication with superiors (11). In the world of sport, the phenomenon of athlete burnout is also a growing concern, with some reports indicating that up to 12% of competitive athletes experience high levels of burnout (39). Importantly, statistics such as these are indicators of the prevalence at the highest levels of mental fatigue. Rates of lower, sub-burnout levels have been reported to be as high as 45% in elite-level athletes, resulting in higher levels of anxiety and depression (90), along with feelings of disengagement, decreased motivation, and declining enthusiasm (91). These factors, coupled with reports of decreased sleep quality in athletes (4) along with increasing pressure to perform, time constraints, and media obligations, can all contribute to the subjective weariness commonly experienced by athletes. Regardless of their cause, experiences of mental fatigue are commonplace in the world of sport, and its impact on the mental health of athletes is significant.

Mental Fatigue and Physical Performance

Beyond its deleterious impact on cognitive and emotional function, a growing body of evidence is now indicating that increasing mental fatigue leads directly to decreases in certain critical aspects of physical performance. Furthermore, it is becoming apparent that when the mind is tired—and all other things are equal—physical performance suffers.

The first place that mental fatigue shows up in physical performance is at the level of reaction time. The term reaction time is often misunderstood as an indicator of how quickly someone can physically react to a stimulus (e.g., the sound of a starter's gun). While it is true that slowed reaction time affects the overall speed of the physical response, the mechanism behind true reaction time actually precedes the overt physical movement. **Reaction time** per se is the time that elapses between the perception of a stimulus and when a response is initiated. Said another way, reaction is the time it takes for the brain to identify a signal and to formulate the plans for a response. It is, quite literally, how fast the brain can process information. Here, the impact of mental fatigue is readily quantifiable (60). It is important to note that while slowed reaction times indicate a decrease in the brain's ability to process information, again the impact of the slowing is most readily visible at the level of the physical response itself and often with tragic consequences. Data from studies of overtired drivers clearly demonstrate the level of the cognitive slowing as mental fatigue increases (115), as well as the massive toll on roadways, with an alarming number of accidents and fatalities being attributed to mental fatigue (85).

Reaction-time data from mentally fatigued athletes is harder to come by, but it stands to reason that slower responses are going to significantly affect athletes in sports in which fast starts are critical or when rapid information processing is vital for correcting positional errors detected via proprioceptive mechanisms (e.g., air awareness in diving or certain snowboard disciplines). Support for this notion was put forth by Van Cutsem and colleagues (104), who linked mental fatigue to decreased reaction times in trained cyclists along with a corresponding increase in response errors. In other words, it appears that mental fatigue negatively affects the efficiency of information processing in terms of both speed and accuracy. For an athlete, the impact of this slowing on performance can be costly. A further point has to do with errors; other studies have shown similar decrements in the decision-making ability of mentally fatigued skilled soccer players (98). From a cognitive standpoint, then, mentally taxed athletes are doubly impaired by virtue of the fact that they will respond more slowly to stimuli at the outset, and that when they do respond, they are more likely to make errors or devise less effective strategic decisions or both.

Mental fatigue has also been shown to have a consequential impact on performance in tasks requiring high levels of physical endurance. Marcora and colleagues (71) provided the initial evidence for this phenomenon. These authors discovered that performance on a cycling ergometer task dropped significantly in participants who completed 90 minutes of cognitively demanding work before their ride. Specifically, time to exhaustion was reached 18% earlier (with a mean difference of 114 s) in the mentally fatigued group. Interestingly, however, no significant differences were found between the groups in terms of musculoenergetic effects, cardiovascular strain, or even pretask motivation. Instead, Marcora and colleagues (71) found that participants in the mental fatigue group reached their maximal perceived exertion significantly earlier than controls, at which point they disengaged from the task and quit. The critical point here is that mental fatigue negatively affects output potential during endurance tasks, but the limiting factor does not appear to be physical. Rather, the declining results are due strictly to a

subjectively higher perception of effort in the mentally fatigued participants. In other words, when the mind is mentally fatigued, physical tasks just seem to be more difficult than they objectively are, and athletes quit sooner as a result. These findings have been shown to be robust and have been consistently replicated in the literature (see Van Cutsem and colleagues [104] for a review).

Beyond the impacts on cognitive performance and physical endurance already mentioned, mental fatigue has also been shown to have a negative effect on the actual technical abilities of athletes. In more outcome-based, physical-level studies, performance decrements in certain functional elements of soccer such as running, passing, and shooting proficiency have been reported in mentally fatigued athletes (96). Overall, it is clear that being mentally overloaded for chronic periods of time has far-reaching and detrimental repercussions for the athlete.

Mechanisms of Mental Fatigue

Mental fatigue is a psychobiological state that has been linked to declining cognitive and physical performance. In the physical realm, it is now known that the urge to give up during physically demanding tasks is tied strongly to the perceived difficulty of the task. Therefore, it is perhaps not surprising that mechanistic explanations for this state have largely focused on brain regions and processes associated with conscious attention, automaticity, and neurochemical reward systems.

Current evidence suggests that certain cortical regions of the brain are thought to be linked with mental fatigue. Specifically, increased activation of the PFC has been shown to accompany mental fatigue in cognitive tasks (17) and has also been implicated as a contributing factor in chronic fatigue syndrome (15). Other studies have implicated decreased activity in the anterior cingulate cortex (ACC) as an underlying factor in mental fatigue (67). The ACC has strong neural connections to various cognitive, emotional, and motor control centers of the brain and is thought to be involved in many higher-level brain functions, including action monitoring, reward anticipation, and decision making. Lorist and colleagues (67) note that the ACC's performance monitoring function is mediated by dopamine levels, suggesting that fatigue states may also involve disruption at the dopaminergic level. Indeed, it is not uncommon for patients with Parkinson's—a disease characterized by diminished striatal dopamine levels—to report higher than normal levels of mental fatigue (68). Given the unique structural and functional interplay in this region, it is not surprising that deactivation of the ACC has been associated with mental fatigue, and specifically the declines is physical performance related to increased perceived exertion.

Additional mechanistic explanations for mental fatigue have been investigated using EEG indices in fatigue tasks. A study by Brownsberger and colleagues (12) showed that elevated beta band activity corresponded with increased perceived sensation of fatigue and decreased power output in a cycling task. Likewise, Okogbaa and colleagues (80) showed increased beta activity in knowledge workers under mentally fatiguing conditions. In apparent contradiction to these findings, several studies have suggested that increased alpha and theta activity occur during periods of mental fatigue. For example, Smith and colleagues (97) analyzed EEG patterns of participants learning memory tasks and video game tasks. In this study, it was noted that as time progressed, alpha band and frontal midline theta activity became more prominent, suggesting a possible link with mental fatigue (104). However, a closer inspection of the methodology reveals that the study was not designed to induce fatigue, but rather to study EEG patterns as the skill level of the participants increased. The finding that these changes in EEG patterns corresponded with increased learning and performance is wholly consistent with studies described earlier showing increased alpha/theta activity associated with skilled performance and flow state (56). Related to this are the findings of Nakashima and Sato (76), who also reported increases in frontal midline theta in a variety of cognitive or video game tasks. Here again, however, there was no indication that subjects were fatigued at any point during the experiment, and the authors themselves interpreted the increased levels of theta activity as associated with increased challenge and higher interest in certain tasks, and indicative of changes related to practice and learning.

Other investigations of driver fatigue (59) and sleep-deprived pilots (14) have reported increases in alpha or theta band activity (or both) over extended periods of time-on-task; however, it is worth noting here that mental fatigue and sleepiness are not necessarily equivalent phenomena from the standpoint of the brain. Therefore, it is likely that these two states have different electrophysiological signatures, including an increased level of delta activity demonstrated in research on drowsiness (14), that is not seen in more strictly defined and controlled mental fatigue settings (12). More investigation in this area is warranted.

STRATEGIES FOR FINDING FLOW AND MANAGING MENTAL FATIGUE

As discussed throughout this chapter, flow state has been widely cited as a key driver of numerous aspects of peak human performance. Conversely, the discussion has also detailed the deleterious effects on performance that are brought on by mental fatigue. The nine subjective characteristics presented earlier that define the flow experience are typically derived from post hoc phenomenological descriptions of a flow state. Attention has turned from viewing these nine dimensions of flow simply as descriptors of the state such that instead they have been conceptualized as **triggers** for flow. In other words, questions are now being asked about whether the state of flow is something that can be intentionally induced through the careful introduction of certain flow triggers into the performance environment. Central to this concept is the idea that the primary mechanisms of flow (i.e., brain region activation or deactivation, EEG patterns, and related neurochemicals) can be switched on through purposeful design. What follows is a description of three of the more commonly investigated approaches that can align certain preconditions for flow state: the controlled manipulation of the challenge/skills ratio, the redirection of attention from internally to externally focused cues, and the use of neurofeedback interventions to train the self-regulation of more optimal brain states.

The Challenge:Skills Ratio

One of the more notable contributions from Csíkszentmihályi's wealth of research on flow was the notion that happiness or flow does not simply happen by random chance. Rather, he argued that a more optimal state of mind must be cultivated intentionally by setting challenges that are neither too demanding nor too simple for one's abilities. As he notes in his seminal 1990 book *Flow: The Psychology of Optimal Experience* (20), "The best moments usually occur when a person's body or mind is stretched to its limits in a voluntary effort to accomplish something difficult and worthwhile." The idea that challenge is a necessary precondition for flow has been consistently demonstrated in the literature across domains such as academic work (34), video game design (53), and therapeutic rehabilitation settings (113) and has been verified through meta-analysis (33).

Research from more skill- or sport-based activities has likewise demonstrated the importance of an appropriate balance between challenge and skill. Much of this work was amalgamated by Guadagnoli and Lee (43). In presenting their challenge point framework, these investigators connected several converging lines of evidence around the central premise that more optimal levels of performance occur when the conditions of the learning environment incorporate appropriate levels of challenge relative to the skill level of the performer. Support for their framework comes from studies showing distinct performance advantages in the sport or motor domain under conditions of increased variability or randomness in practice (42, 63), when reliance on external feedback is reduced (49, 82), and when warm-up conditions are made more challenging (6) (see figure 26.1; 43). As it pertains specifically to athletes, the key takeaway from these studies is that a significant degree of challenge is required during training if learning or progression is to be optimized. As an example, rote repetition or memorizing a task (the hallmark of blocked-practice methods), while at times suitable for the novice, is seldom optimal for the more skilled athlete. Instead, higher-performing individuals are more apt to learn faster when more challenging training conditions are brought to bear. Similar findings have been consistently reported in various cognitive domains,

noting that rates of learning can be greatly enhanced by embracing certain "desirable difficulties" (see Bjork and Bjork [9] for a review).

Given the apparent advantages of correctly managing the challenge/skills ratio, the question remains: How much challenge is optimal? Both Csíkszentmihályi's flow channel model (18, 19) and Guadagnoli and Lee's optimal challenge framework (43) clearly espouse the benefits of challenge in performance, yet neither is adequately prescriptive in terms of what the balance of perceived challenge to skill should be. To this point, it is instructive to consider whether the desired outcome is to increase learning or increase performance. A frequent finding in skill acquisition literature is a phenomenon known as the learning–performance paradox (see Soderstrom and Bjork [99] for a review). The essence of the paradox is that experiencing success during practice does not necessarily indicate the extent to which actual learning has occurred. The converse is also true in that struggle or failure during practice does not necessarily indicate an absence of learning. To this point, in terms of performance and the maintaining of a flow state, there is evidence to suggest that perceived challenge should closely match (45, 57) or, at most, slightly exceed the current level of skill (75, 83). Data from the learning literature, on the other hand, suggests that better outcomes occur when challenge routinely outstrips skill level. In terms of actual ratios, a study by Wilson and colleagues (107) looking at training algorithms in artificial intelligence systems demonstrated that optimal rates of learning occurred when there was a 15.87% error rate during training, therefore suggesting that 85% success during training is the sweet spot for learning. Data from human learning studies provide some support for this ratio (36). Importantly, however, despite these apparent goal-specific differences in optimal challenge/skills ratios, there is evidence to suggest that flow states can enhance not only performance outcomes, but also learning outcomes (5). In a related paper, Farrow and Robertson (30) have argued that coaches should adopt new skill acquisition approaches akin to the periodized frameworks more typically reserved for the strength and conditioning setting. These authors suggest that well-researched physical principles such as progressive overload can serve as a foundation for better models of skill learning and performance. The critical issue to recognize here is that intentionally incorporating appropriate and adaptable levels of challenge to the learning environment can create access points to flow states, expedite rates of progression, and elevate physical performance in pressure situations.

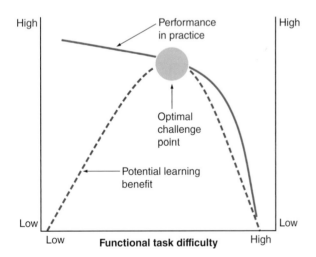

FIGURE 26.1 The relation between learning and performance curves and the optimal challenge point related to tasks of different levels of functional complexity. The point of functional task difficulty where learning is optimized is not the point at which practice performance is optimized.

Reprinted by permission from M.A. Guadagnoli and T.S. Lee (2004, pg. 212-224).

Focus of Attention

The perceived effortlessness, combined with the heightened focus of attention that occurs during a flow state, has been described throughout this chapter. Ashinoff and Abu-Akel (1) have described this aspect of flow state as a positive manifestation of **hyperfocus** characterized by both increases in sustained attention and a heightened perception of task-relevant information. Regarding the issue of attention and task relevance, an impressive body of evidence in the motor learning literature suggests that directing attention toward factors outside the body (i.e., externally) is far more effective than internal focus (e.g., toward a limb of the movement of a particular body part). Examples of experimental manipulations of attention focus include instructions such as "focus on the target" (external) versus "focus on your hands" (internal), or, "focus on the sound on the starting signal" (external) versus "focus on the movement of your feet" (internal) (see chapter 28 for more detail). Collectively, these findings have been discussed in the context of a constrained-action hypothesis whereby it is postulated that focusing attention externally allows for a greater degree of movement automaticity that is controlled by faster, more unconscious mechanisms (see Wulf [109] and chapter 28). Evidence in support of the constrained-action hypothesis has come from a host of performance domains. Research has consistently demonstrated that when participants are instructed to focus their attention externally, advantages are reported in terms of better reaction times (111), improved balance (16), and increased jump height (110), as well as improved accuracy in complex skills such as golf (84).

Beyond the motor domain, advantages of an external focus of attention have also been shown at the cognitive level in terms of perceived exertion. For example, Lohse and Sherwood (65) found that in a 90-degree wall sitting task, participants were not only better able to withstand fatigue when focusing their attention externally; they also reported decreased perceptions of exertion during these times of prolonged exertion.

In an important link between attentional focus and flow state, Harris, Vine, and Wilson (46) demonstrated, during a simulated driving task, that participants reported heightened flow state experiences and higher outcome expectancies when following external versus internal focusing instructions. These results, alongside the wider body of literature on the performance advantages of externally focused attention, point to an opportunity for interesting new lines of investigation for researchers, as well as potentially

impactful strategies for practitioners.

Collectively, these results indicate that intentionally employing relatively simple strategies—designed to focus attention externally—can increase the likelihood of generating flow states. Furthermore, it is suggested that flow could be mechanistically linked to the aforementioned array of desirable performance outcomes for athletes that result from shifting attention away from the self and onto external objects or locations. As has been discussed, not only does externally focused attention positively affect discrete tasks of accuracy, increased power output, and increased information-processing speed; it also appears to affect mental aspects of performance in that it lowers perceived levels of exertion in tasks requiring higher levels of sustained physical output.

Neurofeedback Approaches

The two previous sections have presented ideas for creating the preconditions for flow state and centered on strategies within the learning–performance environment in order to better align the challenge/skills ratio and more effectively allocate and focus attentional resources. Beyond these design- or intention-based approaches to performance, other research suggests that certain technologies can be leveraged to target and enhance brain activity, and thus performance more directly. **Neurofeedback** (NFB) is a type of biofeedback that allows users to view real-time EEG activity (or some representation of that activity) with a goal of training better awareness of, and self-regulation over, the electrical or functional output of the brain or both. Neurofeedback has been shown to be an effective clinical intervention for conditions such as posttraumatic stress disorder (81) and attention-deficit hyperactivity disorder (94), as well as an effective tool in mindfulness training (78). Within the high-performance realm, investigators have begun to ask questions about the utility of NFB as a tool to produce brain outputs commonly associated with expertise and flow state. Recall from earlier in this chapter that (a) when experts are performing at or near their best, and (b) when people are in a state of flow, brain activity appears to settle around the high-theta, low-alpha range (along with an associated decrease in beta activity). Neurofeedback training specifically designed to focus on the alpha-theta spectrum has been shown to significantly affect certain cognitive measures such as increases in relaxed concentration (61) as well as increased ratings of flow state coupled with decreased anxiety (95).

In terms of motor learning and performance, other studies looking at the effects of alpha/theta NFB training have shown significant improvements in the expert rating of technique and creativity in musical performance (28), as well as in the timing and overall execution of dancers (89). In a study looking at rates of learning in marksmanship, Berka and colleagues (5) combined alpha/theta NFB with heart rate data in a novel psychophysical training tool in a group of novice archers. The results showed the rate of learning in the psychophysical feedback group to be more than double that of controls.

Taken together, there is a growing body of evidence to support the idea that NFB training can be a useful tool for increasing awareness of more functionally optimal brain states that can lead to improved cognitive and physical outcomes. More research is certainly warranted in this area to further elucidate dose–response issues, as well as to provide better evidence-based parameters for applied settings.

SUMMARY OF PSYCHOBIOLOGY

The purpose of this chapter was twofold. First, an overview of the research and mechanistic explanations was provided for two opposing forces in cognitive and physical performance: the mentally fatigued state and flow state. Here, contrasts were drawn between the neurobiological states of fatigue and flow in several key brain regions and processes. Specifically, it was noted that key regions of the brain that increase in activation during fatigue (e.g., the prefrontal cortex) are the same regions that deactivate during flow. A case was also made that EEG patterns, shown to be prominent in flow state (increased alpha/theta; decreased beta) in certain instances, reversed under conditions of fatigue. Furthermore, evidence was presented that many of the neurochemical mechanisms shown to be diminished when people are mentally fatigued are the same substrates that come online during flow state.

The second purpose of the chapter was to present practical strategies for how learning and performance environments could be designed to help create the preconditions for flow. Specific recommendations were made around managing the challenge–skills balance during training, and how to more optimally focus attentional resources. Additional suggestions were made for how advances in NFB technology could be leveraged to help athletes self-regulate more optimal states of mind. Here again, each of these approaches has been shown empirically to positively affect the same performance outcomes (e.g., better reaction times, increased tolerance for physical exertion, improved technique, decreased anxiety) that have been shown to be deficient under conditions of high mental fatigue.

CONCLUSION

Future protocols aspiring to elicit flow states or reduce mental fatigue (or both) could potentially focus on other known flow triggers such as enhanced novelty, perceived risk, or purposeful creativity. Such approaches could be designed to test the viability of various flow triggers either independently or in conjunction with other factors known to simultaneously give rise to flow states and mitigate mental fatigue, such as exercise (26), meditation (29), or both.

RECOMMENDED READINGS

Benson, H, and Proctor, W. *The Breakout Principle: How to Activate the Natural Trigger That Maximizes Creativity, Athletic Performance, Productivity, and Personal Well-Being.* New York: Simon and Schuster, 2003.

Bertram, CP, Guadagnoli, MA, and Marteniuk, RG. The stages of learning and implications for optimized learning environments. In *Routledge International Handbook of Golf Science.* New York: Routledge, 119-128, 2017.

Csíkszentmihályi, M. *Flow: The Psychology of Optimal Experience.* New York: Harper Perennial, 1990.

Kotler, S. *The Rise of Superman: Decoding the Science of Ultimate Human Performance.* New York: Houghton Mifflin Harcourt, 2014.

Stulberg, B, and Magness, S. *Peak Performance: Elevate Your Game, Avoid Burnout, and Thrive With the New Science of Success.* New York: Rodale Wellness, 2017.

CHAPTER 27

Neuroscience Approach to Performance

Roman N. Fomin, PhD

Cassandra C. Collins, BS

The body of an athlete, like an orchestra, is composed of many different instruments—the heart, the muscles, and the lungs, to name just a few. The performance of each individual system is crucial to the performance of the whole; thus, athletes have always worked to adapt their muscular, cardiovascular, and respiratory systems for performance. However, the one system that athletes often neglect during training, the nervous system, is the system that drives and coordinates all other bodily systems like the conductor of an orchestra. It is the nervous system that determines how quickly athletes learn, whether their organism as a whole is ready to perform, how well they perform in the moment (stress resistance, psycho-emotional stability, adaptability, etc.), and how quickly they recover from injury. This chapter not only provides sport scientists with an understanding of the role of the nervous system in performance, but also provides information about modern neuroscience tools that can be incorporated into training routines to assess, monitor, and adapt the nervous system for performance.

NERVOUS SYSTEM AND THE BRAIN

The organism of an athlete is a living system that follows strict biological laws. The nervous system is responsible for transmitting signals around the body to direct and manage its actions according to these laws. The **central nervous system** (CNS), which consists of the brain and the spinal cord, receives and transmits signals via pathways outside the brain and spinal cord in the **peripheral nervous system** (PNS). Athletes can use an understanding of how training loads affect the physiological processes of the CNS to effectively achieve high results and avoid consequences such as overtraining, illness or injury, or both. In this regard, the diagnosis of the functional state of the CNS and the search for methods that increase its efficiency are a promising direction for sport science.

Structure of the Central Nervous System

Neurons are the primary structural and functional units of the CNS. A neuron consists of three main parts. The **cell body** contains the nucleus and organelles of the neuron that generate its energy. A single **axon** protrudes out from the cell body like a long wire. Bundles of these axons constitute the **nerves** that carry information in the PNS. Branch-like **dendrites** extend outward from the cell body of a neuron to connect with the axons of other neurons at gap junctions called **synapses**. A group of interconnected neurons that work together to carry out a specific function in the brain is called a **neural circuit**. Neural circuits can be further organized into **neural networks** that subserve distributed processes in the brain.

Neurons use electrochemical signals to transmit information from one area of the nervous system to another and exchange signals between the nervous system and other systems. These signals begin with a change in a neuron's **resting membrane potential**— the difference in electrical voltage between the inside and outside of a neuron at rest. At rest, neurons are **polarized**: Their resting membrane potential is a negative voltage due to the uneven distribution of **ions** (charged particles like sodium and potassium) inside and outside the cell. When a neuron's membrane becomes **depolarized** by a temporary positive spike in voltage, it releases or **fires** an electrical impulse called an **action potential**. This action potential travels down the length of the axon of the **presynaptic** (firing) **neuron**, triggering the release of chemicals called **neurotransmitters** into its synapses with the dendrites of other neurons (40) (see figure 27.1). The neurotransmitters are picked up by receptors on the **postsynaptic (**receiving) **neuron**, where they can trigger a **postsynaptic potential** (PSP)**,** which is a temporary change in the membrane potential of the postsynaptic neuron. A positive change in membrane potential (depolarization) produces an **excitatory PSP** that increases the likelihood that the receiving neuron will fire, whereas a negative change in membrane potential (hyperpolarization) produces an **inhibitory PSP** that decreases the likelihood the receiving neuron will release an action potential.

The neurons of the CNS constitute two types of tissue: **gray matter** and **white matter**. Gray matter is primarily made up of the cell bodies of neurons and accordingly is where most processing in the brain occurs. The outer layer of the brain (**cerebral cortex**) is made up of gray matter. As the leading department of the human CNS, it manages the most complex functions such as consciousness, thinking, speech, and memory. In contrast, white matter consists mostly of the axons that connect the cell bodies in the gray matter.

Functions of the Central Nervous System

The structure of the CNS allows it to sense, process, and respond to changes in the external and internal environments of athletes, working to connect, regulate, and optimize the athlete's body to perform a skill. More specifically, these are the main functions that the CNS fulfills:

- Perception and analysis of stimuli acting on the human body
- Regulation and coordination of all tissues and organs
- Integration of tissues and organs
- Organization of human movements
- Ensuring the adaptation of the body to changing environmental conditions
- Systemic organization of human behavior in accordance with current needs

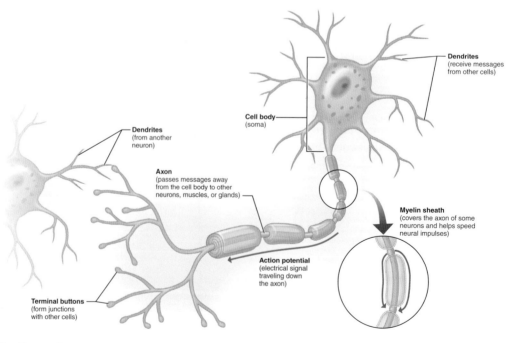

FIGURE 27.1 Parts of a neuron.

NEUROPLASTICITY

The human nervous system can significantly rearrange and change at all stages of a human's life according to experience. This innate ability of the nervous system to reorganize its structural and functional circuits in response to constantly changing environmental conditions is known as **neuroplasticity** (35). Neuroplastic changes in the brain include changes in the state, activity, and connections of neurons, nerves, and neural networks in response to various stimuli (new information, experiences, development, or training). These changes allow humans to create new or more efficient connections as they learn new skills or to restore lost connections after damage.

Neuroplasticity is based on the mechanisms of **synaptic potentiation** and **synaptic depression**. Synaptic potentiation refers to a temporary increase in the strength of synapses in response to their repeated activation. This potentiation can be induced by natural sources like the repeated voluntary muscle contraction involved in sport training or artificial sources like applied electrical stimulation. Synaptic potentiation can increase or decrease the amplitude of postsynaptic potentials, either of which can increase neuroplasticity depending on the specific skill. Synaptic potentiation can be expressed in two forms characterized by duration:

- **Short-term synaptic potentiation** (STP) refers to the temporary enhancement of synaptic transmission created by an increase in the rate of neurotransmitter release. Short-term synaptic potentiation can last from a few milliseconds to several minutes.

- **Long-term synaptic potentiation** (LTP) refers to the lasting enhancement of postsynaptic neuron excitation created by high-intensity, repeated activations of the presynaptic neuron. Long-term synaptic potentiation can be observed in all parts of the CNS, though it is especially prominent in the hippocampus, an important area of the brain for memory. Long-term synaptic potentiation can last from a few hours to days.

Synaptic depression (or synaptic fatigue) refers to a weakening of synaptic strength. Typically, synaptic depression is caused by the following factors:

- Neurotransmitter depletion
- Decreased sensitivity of postsynaptic neurons to the neurotransmitter resulting in a minimum level of postsynaptic depolarization

- Increased metabolism products (waste)
- pH changes (excessive excitation of the same neural pathways can create an acidic environment)

As the basis for neuroplasticity, synaptic depression and potentiation underlie the development of any skill, including an athlete's ability to adapt to training and achieve optimal performance.

COGNITIVE FUNCTION AND PERFORMANCE

Modern athletes go to great lengths to optimize their bodies, always searching for the next tool that will give them the performance edge they seek. Yet despite these technological leaps, experts assert that elite performance in most sports has stagnated: World records are being attained less frequently and represent smaller gains over past records (3). In order to escape this performance plateau, athletes need to start rethinking their training to focus less on their bodies and more on their brains.

Motor Cortex Control of Movement

In order for **skeletal muscles**—muscles like the biceps that are attached to the skeleton—to contract, they must be triggered by action potentials that are primarily released from an area of the brain called the **motor cortex**. Without these signals from the motor cortex, skeletal muscles are static bunches of protein fibers wrapped in connective tissue.

Motor neurons are the messengers that carry the electrical signals from the motor cortex to the muscle fibers, stimulating them to generate force by contracting. This pathway of neurons that runs down the brain and the spinal cord to the muscles is called the **corticospinal tract**. The brain sends signals along the motor neurons of this pathway to the muscles just as a power strip sends current through a charging cord to a computer. Together, a motor neuron and the muscle fiber it stimulates are called a **motor unit**. Many motor units tend to work together to stimulate all the muscle fibers in a muscle to make the entire muscle contract.

Neural Drive

The sum of all the stimulating action potentials a muscle receives from motor neurons is called **neural drive**. Neural drive determines whether a muscle contracts and the power with which it contracts. The brain regulates muscular endurance by adjusting neural drive over time according to feedback it receives from the muscle's sensory input. To increase or decrease neural drive, the brain can adjust how many motor units fire action potentials in a process known as **motor unit recruitment**. Alternatively, rather than recruit more motor units, the brain can increase neural drive by increasing the rate of motor unit firing. Of course, most sports require more than just sustained raw power: The brain also directs muscle control and coordination by adjusting the timing of motor unit recruitment. Importantly, the fact that the brain drives movement does not mean athletes can abandon their physical training altogether. Since neural drive involves activation of both the brain and the muscles, both must be trained in tandem.

Repetition and Motor Skill Acquisition

The best way to train the brain is with repetition. Repetition activates the mechanisms of synaptic potentiation and depression that allow for neuroplastic changes in the brain. As a result, when athletes practice a skill, they strengthen the neural pathways involved in that skill to make them as efficient as possible. Numerous studies show that motor skill training increases the volume of gray matter in the areas of the brain that control that skill (15). These plastic changes in the brain can increase the power, control, and endurance with which an athlete executes a skill.

As an athlete fine-tunes the execution of a skill with repetition, the skill shifts from being under **explicit** control, where the athlete has to actively think about and monitor the performance, to being under **implicit** control, where the athlete can automatically execute a skill with minimal thought. Subserving this shift is a change in brain activation from an explicit circuit involving the motor cortex to an implicit system controlled by deep structures in the brain called the **basal ganglia** (15). When a motor skill is under implicit control, athletes say that it is committed to **muscle memory**. It is a common misconception that muscle memory lives in muscles: It actually lies in the strength of neural connections in the brain. Muscles cannot learn or remember, but the brain can. This process by which skills become less consciously driven and more automatic over time is called **motor skill learning**.

Cognitive Control of Movement in Sport

Driving muscle firing is just the tip of the iceberg with respect to the role the brain plays in performance. While motor neurons may explain how athletes move, they fail to explain how athletes adaptively perform within the dynamic, stress-inducing, complex environment of a sport. Athletes draw upon a slew of other brain processes or **cognitive functions** to receive, process, store, and act on real-time feedback from the external world.

An area of the brain called the **prefrontal cortex** (PFC) maintains **cognitive control** in the brain by directing and monitoring cognitive functions including attention, inhibition, and memory. Located at the front of the brain, the PFC has extensive connections to other brain areas involved in sport performance, including the motor and sensory regions of the brain. Just as the brain of an athlete learns to direct muscle movement more effectively with repetition, so too can it learn to better direct these cognitive functions. Accordingly, athletes exhibit more connections between neurons and a higher proportion of gray matter in networks involving the PFC and other task-relevant brain areas (16, 42).

Attention, Inhibition, and Memory

Humans are simply incapable of directing their awareness or **attention** to all the information in the external environment. To be successful at a sport, athletes must learn how to quickly direct their attention to only the most relevant information while **inhibiting**, or suppressing, distractions. Two mechanisms subserve attention and inhibition: bottom-up and top-down processing.

Bottom-up processing quickly and automatically identifies objects that "stick out" in the environment, such as a ball that is moving when all other objects are stationary. In contrast, **top-down processing** deliberately directs attention to objects that are goal-relevant, such as a player who is stationary but open for a pass. Since sports are goal-driven, top-down processing ability can distinguish a novice athlete from an expert (2). The PFC works with other task-specific brain areas to direct top-down processing, determining what information is attended to and whether that information is stored temporarily in **working memory** (12).

From working memory, information can be further consolidated into **long-term memory**, where it can guide attention in the future.

Flow State

A state of total task attention that defines peak performance has become known as **flow state**. Psychologist Mihály Csíkszentmihályi was the first to explore the concept of flow, asserting that flow is characterized by nine dimensions: challenge–skill balance, action–awareness merging, clear goals, unambiguous feedback, total task concentration, sense of control, loss of self-consciousness, transformation of time, and intrinsically rewarding experience. These dimensions have since been validated as associated with peak performance in athletes by the work of Dr. Susan Jackson and colleagues (20). Entrance into a flow state is characterized by a shift in the location and type of brain activity that occurs during task performance. A brain in a flow state exhibits a phenomenon known as **transient hypofrontality**—a temporary decrease in activity in the frontal areas of the brain (15). This represents the automaticity of flow as control shifts away from the explicit systems of the brain run by the PFC and the motor cortex toward the implicit systems.

Flow in the brain is also associated with a change in how neurons communicate. When many neurons fire action potentials synchronously, the result is a pulsing of brain activity that looks like waves. Scientists divide these **brainwaves** into different frequency ranges (i.e., alpha, beta, delta, and theta) that are linked to different functions.

Individuals experiencing flow during skill execution have been shown to exhibit an increase in **sensorimotor rhythm** (SMR), a special pattern of brainwaves observed in the sensorimotor areas of the brain. A stronger SMR signal indicates less activity in the motor cortex, meaning the skill is under greater implicit control. This SMR shift thus reflects the automaticity and expertise that characterize a flow state (10, 11).

COGNITIVE TRAINING APPLICATIONS

Just as athletes use tools to understand, monitor, and train the performance of their cardiovascular, muscular, and respiratory systems (e.g., weights, heart rate monitors, cryotherapy, supplements), so too can they incorporate cognitive training tools into their routines. Today, athletes can use neuroscience tools and techniques to record their brain activity, stimulate their brain and muscles, train their visual attention, and construct mental training routines.

Electroencephalography and Neural Feedback

Athletes are unaware of many of the internal processes in their bodies that contribute to their performance. **Biofeedback** arose as a way of using technology to give athletes visibility into these processes, such as their heart rate and oxygen consumption. Athletes can use this insight to shape their internal processes for optimal performance. One type of biofeedback that athletes are increasingly using to enhance their performance is information about the neural activity in the brain, or **neurofeedback**.

Neurofeedback Training for Sports

Electroencephalogram (EEG) technology—covered in chapter 15—allows athletes to watch their brainwaves in real time on a computer. A technique called **neurofeedback training** (NFT) uses EEG to record athletes' brainwaves while they perform a basic mental task and provide them with feedback on what their brainwaves indicate about their task performance. This feedback typically takes the form of audio tones, visual feedback, or a combination of both. For example, when an athlete is exhibiting "optimal" brainwave patterns for performing the task, the athlete may hear pleasing audio tones (34) (see figure 27.2). With observation and expert coaching, the athlete learns to associate different internal states with their corresponding patterns of brainwaves and thus how to change the brainwave patterns to be more adaptive for task performance. The success of NFT should be measured by both a change in brainwave activity and task performance from baseline data recorded before the NFT intervention.

Efficacy of Neurofeedback Training

Research on the efficacy of NFT for sport performance has yielded mixed results. Studies have found that NFT of the SMR can significantly enhance golf putting and rifle shooting performance, but not gymnastics ability (9, 11, 34). Likewise, alpha wave NFT has been found to be beneficial for archery perfor-

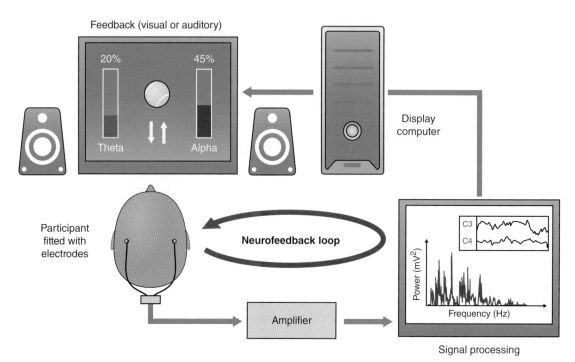

FIGURE 27.2   Example of neurofeedback training protocol.

Adapted by permission from J.L. Park et al. (2015, pg. 117-130).

mance, but not tennis (9, 11, 34). The variability of the results reflects the variety of NFT protocols, sports, and skill levels of the athletes involved in the studies conducted. Since every athlete has a different brain and every sport elicits different cognitive demands, the efficacy of NFT is bound to increase in the future as protocols are developed for specific sports and individual athletes (34).

Transcranial Magnetic Stimulation

While EEG allows athletes to observe the activity occurring in their brains, different types of **neurostimulation**—stimulation of the nervous system—can be used to change activity in the nervous system. **Magnetic stimulation** (MS) refers to the use of magnetic fields to noninvasively stimulate the CNS, PNS, or human skeletal muscles. Magnetic stimulation works through **electromagnetic induction**, in which a conductor (i.e., a coil) placed in a magnetic field generates an electrical current.

Transcranial magnetic stimulation (TMS) is a specific type of MS that uses magnetic pulses applied through the scalp to stimulate the brain and the corticospinal tract. The use of TMS for the human brain was pioneered by Barker and colleagues in 1985 at the University of Sheffield (1). Transcranial magnetic stimulation of the brain has proven to be an effective, painless, and safe tool for modulating processes in the human nervous system.

Transcranial magnetic stimulation works by exciting or inhibiting the neurons in the tissue underlying the area targeted by the magnetic pulses. As such, TMS is assessed by metrics of conductivity, excitability, and inhibition, which are discussed later in this section. Transcranial magnetic stimulation has broad diagnostic and therapeutic capabilities for scientific research and clinical applications in neurology, neurophysiology, and neuropsychiatry (19, 37). Despite the widespread application of TMS in medical science and research, a limited number of studies have been done on the application of TMS in sport and exercise sciences. The research that has been done on TMS in athletes has focused on investigating training-related changes in motor cortex excitability, the effect of fatigue on corticospinal pathways, the neural signatures of elite performance, and enhancing recovery from injuries such as concussions (32).

Most studies on movement involve the application of TMS to a specific part of the motor cortex to excite or inhibit motor neurons. Different parts of the motor cortex map to different parts of the body, meaning that specialists can cause a muscle to contract by using TMS to stimulate the part of the motor cortex that

5555

controls it. The effect of TMS can thus be assessed by measuring the muscle response as a **motor evoked potential** (MEP). An MEP is the summed bioelectrical activity (in the form of a wave) of the target skeletal muscle contraction in response to a single pulse of TMS to the corresponding region in the motor cortex (or spinal cord or peripheral nerve) (see figure 27.3; 21).

Transcranial Magnetic Stimulation: Basic Principles of Measurement

Transcranial magnetic stimulation requires equipment to produce the electromagnetic stimulation as well as equipment to measure the effect of the stimulation. The **magnetic stimulator** used in TMS includes a high electrical current (5 kA or more) **pulse generator** that is connected via a cable to a magnetic stimulation **coil**. The coil is placed over the scalp above the underlying target brain location in the

subject. The pulse generator then drives the current through the coil, generating a magnetic impulse with the strength of several **tesla**—units that measure the strength of magnetic induction. The magnetic field depolarizes the underlying neural tissue, activating neurons and neural networks in the nervous system. In motor studies, this activation can be measured via the MEPs produced. Motor evoked potentials can be detected and recorded by skin electrodes connected to **surface electromyography** (EMG), which records the electrical activity generated by muscle contractions. A computer monitor allows for the visualization and further analysis of the recorded MEPs.

Transcranial Magnetic Stimulation: Key Physiological Metrics

Transcranial magnetic stimulation of the motor cortex is used to assess the functioning of the corticospinal tract via measures of **conductivity**, **excitability**, and **inhibition**.

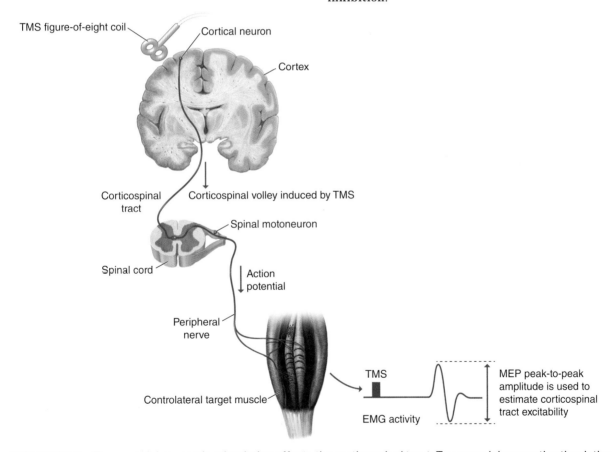

FIGURE 27.3 Transcranial magnetic stimulation affects the corticospinal tract. Transcranial magnetic stimulation (TMS) applied over the motor cortex preferentially activates interneurons oriented in a plane parallel to the brain surface. This placement leads to a transsynaptic activation of pyramidal cells evoking descending volleys in the pyramidal axons projecting on spinal motoneurons, also termed the corticospinal tract.

Adapted by permission from W. Klomjai, R. Katz, and A. Lackmy-Vallée (2015, pg. 208-213).

Conductivity   **Conductivity** of the corticospinal system refers to the flow of action potentials between the motor cortex and spinal cord. It is evaluated by the latency, amplitude, duration, and form of the target muscle's MEP in response to TMS and by central motor conduction time (see figure 27.4).

- **Latency** is the period of time from the application of TMS to the appearance of the MEP in the targeted muscle (recorded by EMG and measured in milliseconds).

- **Amplitude** is the maximum displacement from the equilibrium position of the wave of MEP. Peak-to-peak amplitude refers to the value between the highest MEP amplitude value and the lowest amplitude value.

- **Duration** is the period from the beginning (starting point) to the end of MEP.

- **Form** reflects different characteristics of the negative and positive phases of the MEP (i.e., double-phasic, triple-phasic, etc.).

In healthy individuals, TMS can be used to record an MEP from almost any skeletal muscle. In clinical practice, the wrist, arm, shin, and foot muscles are most commonly targeted. **Magnetic stimulus intensity** significantly affects the MEP amplitude, such that a higher magnetic intensity stimulates a higher MEP amplitude. Since MEPs can vary, it is standard practice for a specialist to record five or six MEPs and select the one with the largest amplitude and shortest latency as the measurement. Normally, this MEP amplitude is between 2 and 15 mV.

In general, MEP size reflects the number of corticospinal motor neurons activated by magnetic stimulation. In particular, the following physiological mechanisms determine the size of the MEP produced by the target muscle:

- Number of motor units recruited in the spinal cord in response to TMS

- Number of motor neurons that fire more than once in response to TMS

- Synchronization of the motor neurons that fire in response to TMS

Two factors that must be controlled because they can affect MEP size are the position of the subject (standing, sitting, or lying down) and the person's height (6).

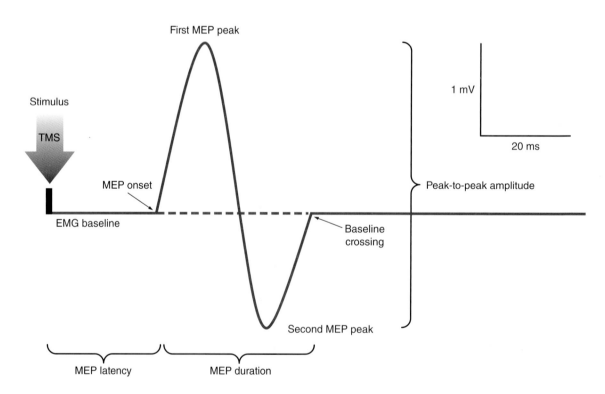

FIGURE 27.4   Key physiological characteristics of the motor evoked potential.

Studies show that athletes have a shorter MEP latency and higher MEP amplitude than non-athletes, which is associated with improved performance on measures such as reaction time (31). **Central motor conduction time** (CMCT) is the time it takes a neural impulse to travel from the motor cortex to the spinal roots. Central motor conduction time reflects connectivity in the corticospinal tract; faster conductance indicates higher connectivity. Measuring CMCT is especially useful because it is a stable and reproducible parameter that is not significantly influenced by intraindividual fluctuations. To obtain CMCT, a specialist first conducts cortical and segmental magnetic stimulation (i.e., stimulation of the brain and then different segments of the spinal cord) of the selected target muscle. After recording multiple MEPs from this stimulation, the specialist selects the cortical MEP with minimal latency and the segmental MEP with maximal latency. The CMCT is calculated by subtracting the segmental latent period from the cortical period. Normally, the range for CMCT for the arms is 4.3 to 10.6 ms while the CMCT for the legs is between 11 and 20.8 ms. Coaches and athletes can use changes in CMCT as a metric of training effectiveness. High-intensity interval training has been shown to be more effective at enhancing CMCT than moderate-intensity continuous training (27).

Excitability The **excitability** of the corticospinal tract, meaning the energy needed to activate it, can be evaluated by measuring the motor threshold in the brain.

Motor threshold (MT) is the lowest intensity of motor cortex magnetic stimulation required to produce a MEP of minimal amplitude in a target skeletal muscle in 50% of 10 to 20 trials. Motor threshold is clinically important because it is used to individually determine a safe dose of TMS. Additionally, MT recorded in the motor cortex can be used to estimate excitability of other brain regions.

Motor threshold can be measured when a muscle is at rest (**resting MT**) or when a muscle is performing a slight contraction (**active MT**) at approximately 20% of its **maximal voluntary isometric contraction** (MVIC)—the maximum amount of force athletes can produce to contract their muscles. For calculating resting MT, the minimal MEP amplitude is set at greater than 50 µV, whereas for measuring an active motor threshold the minimal MEP amplitude needed is 100 µV. Electromyography is used to measure the degree of skeletal muscle relaxation and contraction.

The first step in measuring MT is determining the optimal position and orientation of the magnetic coil above the head when the target muscle is relaxed. The optimal position will best target the "hot spot" (optimal location for stimulation) in the motor cortex that controls the targeted muscle. Specialists know they have accurately localized the hot spot for a target muscle in the motor cortex when they can reliably produce consistent MEPs with the minimum possible stimulation intensity. Starting at 35% of the maximum stimulator output, the intensity is incrementally increased and decreased until the stimulation intensity is reached at which fewer than 10 MEPs from 20 attempts at eliciting MEPs are recorded. At this point, the MT will be calculated as that current magnetic intensity plus 1%. The MT can fluctuate from 40% to 80% depending on TMS technical characteristics; however, it is always higher for leg muscles than for arm muscles. This is due to the anatomical and functional peculiarities of the motor cortex: The motor representation of the arms in the cortex is larger than the representation of the legs. Compared to non-athletes, athletes have been shown to demonstrate higher cortical excitability as measured by lower resting motor threshold (rMT). This increased excitability has been correlated with better performance as quantified by shorter reaction times (31). Assessing cortical excitability via MT can also be useful for understanding injury recovery in athletes. For example, athletes who received anterior cruciate ligament reconstruction surgery demonstrated higher rMT 2 weeks after surgery (46).

Inhibition Inhibition mechanisms in the CNS are evaluated by measuring a phenomenon known as the silent period of muscle contraction. After the initial spike in EMG activity generated by voluntary muscle contraction, there is a short silent period (100-300 ms) during which no bioelectrical activity is recorded despite the contraction being sustained. This period ends when EMG activity resumes. The first part of the silent period is believed to reflect inhibition mechanisms in the spinal cord, while the second part of the silent period reflects inhibition by the brain.

Transcranial magnetic stimulation can be used to produce this silent period. Silent period duration increases with magnetic induction intensity. A **cortical silent period** (CSP) is observed after stimulation of the motor cortex with TMS, whereas a **peripheral silent period** (PSP) is observed after stimulation of a peripheral nerve. Usually, the CSP is measured from the end of the TMS-generated MEP to the end of absolute bioelectric silence on the EMG, which is referred to as **isoline**, or a return to a constant EMG baseline.

A shorter silent period is interpreted as less inhibition whereas a longer silent period signals more inhibition. This makes cortical silent period an important marker to measure cortical inhibition after injury and exercise. Muscular fatigue, for example, has been shown to increase the silent period by 30% (29, 43). Additionally, TMS studies have demonstrated that athletes who have sustained a concussion demonstrate a longer CSP—indicative of elevated cortical inhibition—both immediately after sustaining a concussion and up to 30 years later (14). Inhibition measured by TMS-invoked CSPs has been correlated with underlying brainwave patterns using EEG. Specifically, the duration of CSP has been associated with the relative power of alpha oscillations in the brain. This provides further support for the inhibitory mechanisms underlying CSP given that alpha waves are generally associated with decreased excitability and increased inhibition (17).

Transcranial Magnetic Stimulation Parameters

Transcranial magnetic stimulation protocols and neuromodulatory effects can vary according to which of the following technical characteristics they use.

Transcranial Magnetic Stimulation Pulse Characteristics Transcranial magnetic stimulation is performed using different TMS patterns—**single stimuli** (single TMS), **paired stimuli** (paired TMS) or a series of pulses (**repetitive TMS** or **rTMS**). Single and paired TMS are primarily used for understanding corticospinal functioning. Repetitive

TMS can modulate cortical excitability so it is used for therapeutic purposes including the treatment of pain, diseases of the motor system, stroke, multiple sclerosis, epilepsy, depression, and schizophrenia. High-frequency rTMS can enhance the excitability of the stimulated region while low-frequency rTMS can inhibit it (22).

Transcranial magnetic stimulation pulses can also vary in temporal width (0.1-1.0 ms), frequency (**low-frequency TMS** is <1 Hz while **high-frequency TMS** is >60-100 Hz), and number (500 or more) (36). Pulses are delivered within different types of **waveforms** that vary in how many sine wave cycles there are per pulse (see figure 27.5). **Monophasic** waveforms (including only the peak of the sine cycle per pulse) are highly accurate at targeting the intended region and quiet, and they generate little heat but are difficult to use for recording a cortical response. Comparatively, **biphasic** (a full sine wave per pulse—two phases) and **polyphasic** (multiple full sine cycles per pulse) waveforms are better for cortical stimulation but less accurate and louder, and they generate more heat.

Transcranial Magnetic Stimulation Coils Different **TMS coil configurations** generate different magnetic field characteristics and thus are used for different purposes. The amplitude or strength of magnetic **field intensity** typically ranges from 1.0 to 2.5 tesla but can go up to 4 tesla. While there are more than 70 different configurations of TMS coils in use today, the 2 most common are the following (see figure 27.6):

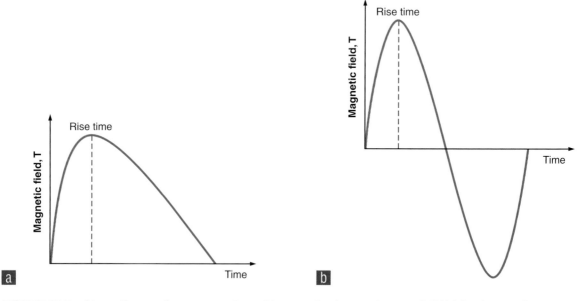

FIGURE 27.5 Magnetic waveform parameters: (a) monophasic waveform and (b) biphasic waveform.

- The **single coil** (i.e., round) is the original type of TMS coil. This coil is very popular and widely used for stimulating the motor cortex and spinal cord. The limitation of this coil is a lack of focality of activated structures. As the diameter of the coil decreases, stimulation accuracy increases but magnetic intensity tends to decrease, since coils will overheat.
- **Double coils** (i.e., butterfly or figure eight coil) consist of two windings placed side-by-side. Maximum magnetic intensity is localized in the center of this coil, where the windings cross. This coil is often used for brain mapping because it can more accurately define the area of stimulation and provide deeper brain stimulation than the single coil.

Benefits of Using Transcranial Magnetic Stimulation

There are several advantages of using TMS for diagnostics, recovery, and sport science research compared to other types of noninvasive neurostimulation. These benefits include the following:

- The magnetic field flows freely and unchanged through anatomical structures. This allows it to excite nervous tissue that is located in remote places, at a considerable depth, or tightly enclosed within bones or muscles.
- Transcranial magnetic stimulation is not accompanied by pain or discomfort as can be the case with noninvasive electrical stimulation.

- Transcranial magnetic stimulation does not require prior preparation of the skin for stimulation and can be applied at some distance from it.
- The magnetic coil used for TMS can move freely relative to the head, allowing for the rapid identification of the optimal point for stimulation.
- Transcranial magnetic stimulation allows for a more direct assessment of cortical excitability because it almost always induces an MEP from the target muscle in healthy individuals.
- Ongoing research points to great potential for TMS to be used in the future for the enhancement of physical qualities (strength and power) and improvements of neuromuscular characteristics of the motor system.

However, TMS requires the use of incredibly specialized and costly equipment and must be overseen by a trained specialist to ensure the safety of the subject.

Elements of Visual Skills in Performance

Athletes' movements are guided by the sensory information they choose to focus their attention on and how their brain interprets or **perceives** that information. Since most sports require precise control of body movement within a dynamic space, vision is the main sense athletes rely on to guide their performance. Through the process of **visuomotor integration** athletes use the visual processes in the brain to guide the motor systems in planning and executing movement.

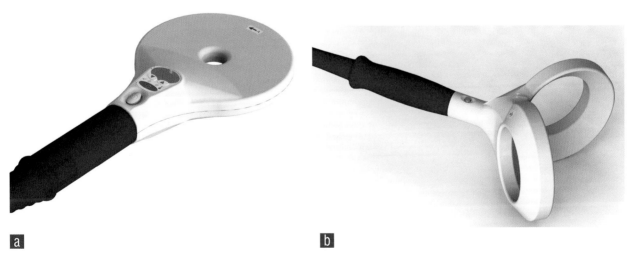

a   b

FIGURE 27.6   Transcranial magnetic stimulation coils: *(a)* single coil and *(b)* double cone coil.

Perception to Action: How Athletes Respond to Game Play

Processing of visual information proceeds in a hierarchical manner from very low-level, bottom-up processing of basic features to high-level, top-down processing by the PFC. Information from the retina is first transformed into electrical signals that are transmitted to the visual areas in the back part of the brain. Different groups of neurons in this area of the brain are tuned to respond strongly to different basic features of a visual stimulus, such as line orientation or color. After these basic visual features are extracted, the information diverges along two possible pathways that conduct more complex feature analysis.

The **ventral pathway** identifies what an object is by grouping basic features into coherent wholes. The term ventral in neuroscience refers to the lower part of the brain across which information in this pathway flows (see figure 27.7; 30). Comparatively, the **dorsal pathway** conducts information about where an object is in space along the upper part of the brain. Both pathways ultimately send the information back toward the PFC to guide attention, movement planning, and execution (30).

Action to Perception: How Athletes Anticipate Game Play

With many years of practice, the pathways in elite athletes' brains that associate **perceptual targets**— specific objects and locations—with their sport-

appropriate actions strengthen. The fact that these perception-action associations often occur in the same sequence in time for a given sport allows athletes to modulate their brain activity in anticipation of what they predict will happen next. The PFC can signal these attentional expectations before a perceptual target even appears by increasing the baseline activity of neurons tuned to an expected feature by up to 40%. Additionally, visual target anticipation is signaled by a change in alpha rhythms (specifically desynchronization) (30). In short, elite athletes' brains prepare them for action by deploying their visual attention according to the action that is most likely to occur next in the sequence of game play. This fine-tuning of visual attentional expectations is particularly evident in the play of elite tennis players. By observing the speed, angle, and direction of an opponent's swing relative to the ball, an elite tennis player like Serena Williams is able to predict the most likely location on the court where an opponent will hit the ball. Williams will immediately act upon this information—moving toward this predicted location before her opponent has even finished swinging her racket. As the opponent finishes her swing, Williams is then able to update her prediction as she tracks the trajectory of the ball through the air.

Coordination of Action and Perception

Athletes colloquially refer to visuomotor integration as coordination (i.e., hand–eye coordination). Cristiano

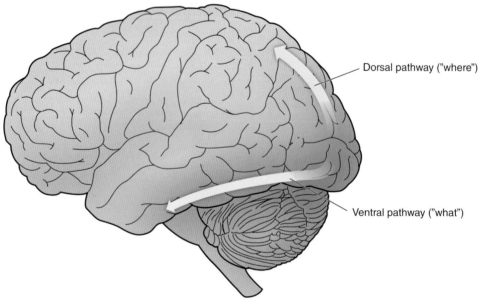

FIGURE 27.7 Ventral and dorsal pathways in the brain.

Reprinted by permission from M.T. Miller and W.C. Clapp (2011, pg. 131-139).

Ronaldo's bicycle kick goal in the UEFA Champions League quarter finals for Real Madrid against his current club Juventus is an excellent example of an elite athlete employing visuomotor integration to coordinate the movement of the body with the visual cues of game play. The goal was prefaced by Ronaldo's teammate dribbling up the side of the field and crossing the ball in the air to the center of the field where Ronaldo stood waiting, back toward the goal. The identification of the moving ball and player required the ventral "what" pathway of Ronaldo's brain to process basic features into coherent wholes. As the ball sailed through the air toward Ronaldo, his dorsal "where" pathway engaged to track its location in space. Finally, at just the right moment based on the location of the ball and his past experience, Ronaldo sent neural drive to his muscles to propel his body into a backward flip. This resulted in his right foot connecting with the ball to send it flying into the upper right corner of the goal. Rarely do the fans of the home sport team clap for a goal by the away team; however, the extreme degree of effortless coordination displayed in this feat elicited applause from fans of both teams.

Visual Attention Tracking as a Measure of Sporting Expertise

Neuroscientists are able to compare how novices and experts direct their visual attention by using eye-tracking tools to monitor where they look. When athletes survey a scene, their eyes quickly move around it like a spotlight, briefly stopping a few times to focus or **fixate** on points their attention identifies as salient. The timing, duration, and steadiness of an athlete's fixations before movement initiation have been shown to be a hallmark of expert performance across different types of sports.

The **quiet eye period** refers to the duration of athletes' last fixation point before they initiate a movement. For example, a quiet eye period occurs right before athletes hit a baseball as they fixate on the ball. This final fixation period has been shown to occur earlier and to last about 60% longer in elite athletes compared to novice athletes (26, 39). The earlier onset and longer duration of quiet eye gives elite athletes more time to organize their neural circuits for performance. This is crucial given the rapid pace of play and high-information demands elite athletes face (38). Roger Federer, for example, serves at an average speed of 130 mph. To be able to successfully return a serve of this speed, an athlete must be prepared to act within a third of a second.

The steadiness of **quiet eye dwell**, meaning the follow-through of an athlete's gaze from the quiet eye period to right before movement initiation, has also been shown to predict expertise. This suggests that experts have optimized their neural networks both for focusing and for sustaining visual attention (39). Athletes can use eye-tracking and video feedback to train their quiet eye abilities.

Motor Imagery and Performance

Physical visual skills are not the only visual skills that can enhance athletes' performance. **Motor imagery training** (MIT) refers to the mental process of imagining performing a movement without actually moving. Motor imagery training engages many of the same visual and motor areas of the brain areas that activate when an athlete physically performs a skill. This means that MIT can induce plastic changes in brain structure and function over time, accelerating learning and motor skill mastery (38). However, MIT is believed to be less effective than physical training since it is not modulated by feedback from the muscles and the senses. For example, MIT alone has been shown to increase the strength of an isometric contraction by 22% compared to a 30% increase with physical strength training (25). Additionally, MIT cannot replace physical training: physical practice is necessary to establish the neural representations of a skill that are activated and enhanced by mental practice (25).

Research during the second decade of this century revealed that athletes should use MIT for complex skill training because efficacy increases with task difficulty. Additionally, athletes should limit MIT to 60 imagined repetitions, since accuracy has been shown to decrease beyond this point. Alternatively, to prevent this accuracy drop, athletes can intersperse MIT with physical training: Training sessions consisting of 50% to 75% MIT and 25% to 50% physical training have been shown to yield the largest skill improvements for difficult tasks (38).

RELAXATION AND REGENERATION

Athletes know that rest is vital after high-intensity exercise to allow the muscles to repair themselves with stronger tissue. However, relaxation and regeneration are just as important for the brain to be able to continue to adaptively drive the muscles to sustain a high level of performance. Stress and fatigue can impair brain functioning on both a short-term and a long-term basis, resulting in overtraining and athlete burnout (8). These negative effects of stress and fatigue are both preventable and reversible with proper relaxation and recovery (28).

Stress and the Impairment of Brain Structure and Function

Athletes experience **stress** when they are presented with physical or psychological demands that disturb their ability to maintain homeostasis. The body's response to stress is carried out by what is known as the **hypothalamic-pituitary-adrenal axis** (HPA) in the body. As the name suggests, this axis involves a feedback loop between two areas of the brain—the hypothalamus and the pituitary—and the adrenal glands of the body. Activation of this axis results in the production of **stress hormones** that increase heart rate, respiration, and fuel breakdown in the body.

At low levels of stress, these changes can actually increase cognitive performance. However, sustained or **chronic** high levels of stress can result in negative changes in the architecture of the brain through a phenomenon known as **stress-induced neuroplasticity**. Stress-induced plasticity especially affects the PFC, decreasing neuronal firing and impairing connectivity (28).

Fatigue and Brain Function

Every athlete knows that fatigue—a reduced capacity for exercise—is the enemy of sustaining a high level of performance. While most athletes are familiar with **peripheral fatigue** of the muscles, few know that there are two other types of fatigue that prevent the brain from executing its role in sport performance.

Central fatigue refers to a decrease in performance stemming from exhaustion of the brain mechanisms for neural drive. Like peripheral fatigue, central fatigue stems from feedback that the body is no longer functioning optimally, such as decreased oxygen levels and depletion of fuel stores (see figure 27.8; 33). This feedback results in **inhibitory** "stop" signals getting sent to the motor cortex, which decreases neural drive to return the body to homeostasis. Central fatigue can be identified by a decrease in MVIC. Depending on exercise intensity, duration, and type, the brain can take anywhere from 30 seconds to 30 minutes to recover from central fatigue (7).

Even before central and peripheral fatigue cause an athlete's performance to drop, **mental fatigue** arising from the exhaustion of cognitive control processes can hinder performance. On a neural level, mentally fatigued individuals exhibit increased beta wave power, suggesting sustained attention, and increased theta power in their PFC, indicating reduced ability

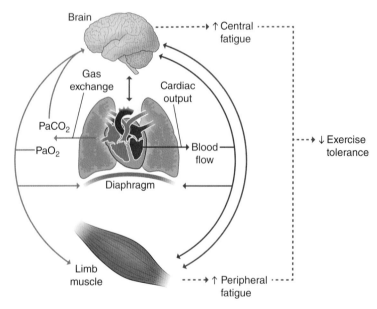

FIGURE 27.8 Central and peripheral fatigue.

Reprinted from M.F. Oliveira et al. (2015, pg. 514).

for top-down control. Additionally, mental fatigue is associated with decreased communication between the PFC and other areas of the brain (5, 24).

Relaxation and Regeneration Tools to Combat and Prevent Stress and Fatigue

Athletes today have a wealth of new tools available to help them recover from and protect against the effects of stress and fatigue so they can perform their best. Yet sufficient sleep and proper nutrition are arguably still the two most important performance tools in an athlete's toolbox.

Sleep

While the body may go offline during sleep, the brain is quite active, reorganizing its own circuits and directing the repair and enhancement of the body. **Rapid eye movement** (REM) sleep is a time for motor skills and visual learning to undergo **memory consolidation—** the process through which memories are solidified, enhanced, and integrated into long-term memory. The same pattern of brain activity observed during the performance of a motor task while one is awake can be reactivated during sleep, indicating that memories of that task are being replayed. During this time, the pattern of brain activity can change as the memories are enhanced to reflect learning. Some researchers are calling these functional and structural changes that occur in the brain **sleep-dependent plasticity** (41).

While REM sleep is particularly important for the reorganization of the brain, **nonrapid eye movement** (NREM) sleep is a crucial period for body regeneration. The brain prompts the muscles to grow and repair by releasing growth hormone from the pituitary gland—a pea-sized structure at the base of the brain. The brain also triggers the release of other hormones involved in metabolic processes such as fat burning (13).

For athletes, this means sleep is the time their hard work pays dividends. A few good nights of sleep after practice can translate into improved motor skill performance without any additional practice. Conversely, sleep deprivation can prevent this learning enhancement, impairing sport performance by accelerating the onset of fatigue, slowing cognitive functioning, and disrupting attention and memory processes (4, 13).

Since learning and body regeneration are crucial for athletes, experts recommend that athletes get more sleep than average individuals. Yet research shows that nearly a third to half of elite athletes report poor-quality sleep (44). Athletes can use an understanding of the factors that affect their sleep-wake cycles, or **circadian rhythm**, to improve their sleep quality.

Light is one of the biggest environmental determinants of circadian rhythm. The detection of light by the eye signals to the brain that it should be awake. As the eyes detect less light, an area in the brain called the pineal gland releases **melatonin**, an important hormone for prompting feelings of sleepiness. Since blue light inhibits melatonin production, athletes should limit blue-light exposure from electronics before sleep and strive to make their rooms as dark as possible. Body temperature also varies with the circadian rhythm. When people fall asleep, their hypothalamus decreases their body temperature by up to two degrees. To facilitate this drop in body temperature, athletes should sleep in an environment between 16 and 21°C (60-70 °F) and limit exercise right before bed since it raises body temperature.

Nutrition

Proper nutrition—the topic of chapter 24—is just as important for athletes' brains as it is for their body. Diet affects vital brain processes including the communication between neurons, the production of neurotransmitters, and synaptic plasticity (17). The brain will preferentially use carbohydrates as its primary source of fuel if enough glucose is present; however, when there is not enough glucose available, the brain will burn fat in the form of ketones for fuel. This is the basis for the popular low-carb, high-fat ketogenic diet.

While the best diet for athletes remains a topic for debate, experts agree that athletes should consume foods such as **antioxidants** that protect against **neurodegeneration**—damage to neuron structure or function. As their name suggests, antioxidants prevent molecules in the body from damage caused by oxidation, or the loss of an electron. Lipids, proteins, and the nucleic acids of DNA can all lose electrons to unstable molecules called **free radicals** that have unpaired electrons. Antioxidants prevent free radicals from stealing electrons by donating them one of their own electrons. When there are not enough antioxidants to buffer against the free radicals, a condition called **oxidative stress** results that can reduce plasticity in the brain (23). Since high-intensity exercise increases free radical production, athletes need to consume extra antioxidant-rich foods to protect against oxidative stress (45).

Assessment of Athlete Readiness

The balance between factors that decrease an athlete's ability to perform (i.e., stress and fatigue) and factors that help regenerate an athlete's performance ability (i.e., sleep and nutrition) determine the **functional state** of an athlete. The functional state is a highly sensitive and accurate physiological indicator that objectively describes individual short-term and long-term adaptations of the athlete's body to various stressors, including training loads. The goal of every coach should be to improve the management of an athlete's functional state by assessing that athlete's state of **readiness**.

Readiness is the current functional state of an athlete that determines subsequent behavior. An optimal state of readiness indicates that athletes have fully adapted to their environmental demands, allowing them to realize their full potential for performance. In contrast, a suboptimal state of readiness prevents athletes from reaching their full potential. Traditional approaches to assessing an athlete's functional state have failed because they do not take into account the specific body system that gave rise to the adaptational processes that created the current functional state. Measuring the readiness of the individual systems of the body can solve this issue. Biofeedback tools can be used to help athletes understand how the systems of their body reflect their performance.

Readiness of the cardiac system of the body, for example, can be assessed via **heart rate variability** (HRV)—the degree of variation in the time between an athlete's heartbeats (see chapter 14). Heart rate variability reflects the quality of the recuperative processes in the cardiac system. Heart rate variability

values that are too high or too low indicate that the cardiac system is functioning outside the optimal range, reflecting a state of high tension during adaptation to training loads and an incomplete recovery process. While fluctuations within the optimal zone are acceptable, a higher value within the optimal zone is indicative of a more efficient recovery process.

CONCLUSION

Traditionally, athletes have focused on training their muscles, lungs, and cardiovascular systems. Yet this conventional view of sport performance neglects the one part of the body that controls every movement of the body—the **brain**. Processes in the brain led by the prefrontal and motor cortices drive the muscles to adaptively control the power, precision, and duration of exercise for optimal performance. Since the brain is plastic, athletes can prime these processes by strengthening their underlying neural pathways through training. Accordingly, expert athletes can be identified by training-induced structural and functional changes in their neural circuits, including increased gray matter volume, faster motor conductance, and enhanced top-down regulation of visual attention. Cognitive training tools such as EEG, neurofeedback, and TMS can be used to optimize training programs according to an understanding of the activity occurring in the brain. For athletes to reap the full benefits of these training tools, they need to ensure they are giving their brains the fuel and rest needed to recover and learn from the demands of performance. The continued refinement of these brain-based tools in the coming years has great potential to help athletes break the glass ceiling that has materialized in elite sports.

RECOMMENDED READINGS

Asprey, D. *Game Changers: What Leaders, Innovators, and Mavericks Do to Win at Life*. New York: HarperCollins, 2018.

Hovey, C, and Jalinous, R. *The Guide to Magnetic Stimulation*. Wales: The Magstim Company Ltd, 2006.

Wang, XJ. Neurophysiological and computational principles of cortical rhythms in cognition. *Physiol Rev* 90:1195-1268, 2010.

Wassermann, E, Epstein, C, and Ziemann, U. *The Oxford Handbook of Transcranial Stimulation*. Oxford, England: Oxford Library of Psychology, 2008.

CHAPTER 28

Motor Performance

Gabriele Wulf, PhD

Skilled motor performance is essential for many activities in daily life, but perhaps more than anywhere else in sport, where optimal performance is often the goal. Skill is characterized by accuracy and consistency in achieving the desired movement outcome, as well as fluent and economical movements that require little physical and mental effort. The role of applied sport scientists, coaches, or physical trainers is to design tasks and practice schedules, provide instruction, and give athletes feedback with the goal of facilitating the learning of effective and efficient movement patterns, and ultimately optimizing performance. Understanding how various factors influence learning and performance is essential for the development of effective training methods.

KEY FACTORS IN LEARNING AND MOTOR PERFORMANCE

In general, an understanding of how the learning process and the performance of motor skills are influenced by practice conditions and instructional methods has significantly evolved. Specifically, three factors have been identified as key for both optimal motor learning and performance. These factors are central to the OPTIMAL (Optimizing Performance Through Intrinsic Motivation and Attention for Learning) theory of motor learning (see figure 28.1; 60). Two of the key variables are motivational, **enhanced expectancies** for performance and **autonomy support**, and one is related to the performers' attention, an **external focus of attention** (see figure 28.1). The importance of each factor is supported by extensive lines of research. While learning reflects relatively permanent changes in a person's capability to perform

a motor skill as a result of practice, performance refers to what is seen, or measured, at any given moment in time (42). Learning studies typically use a between-participants design, including two or more groups of participants who practice under different conditions (e.g., types of feedback or instruction, task order, challenge level), with learning measured by delayed (i.e., 24 hours or more) retention or transfer tests in which all groups perform under the same conditions. The knowledge generated through learning studies can help practitioners design effective practice conditions for longer-term changes in skill. In contrast, studies concerned with motor performance use a within-participants design, where all participants perform under all experimental conditions, typically in a counterbalanced order. Of interest here is how certain factors immediately affect performance. Such studies often have practical implications for enhancing performance, for example, in competitive situations. This chapter reviews findings related to each factor, based on both performance and learning studies, but with particular consideration for those relevant to applied sport scientists. The chapter also provides examples of how sport scientists and coaches may incorporate the three factors in their work with their athletes.

Enhancing Performance Expectancies

Being confident in one's ability to perform well—or having positive expectations for future performance—is critical for optimal motor performance. Providing individuals with a heightened sense of confidence, or enhancing their expectancies, is also important

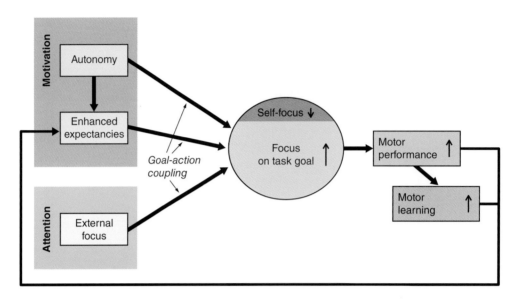

FIGURE 28.1 Schematic of the OPTIMAL theory.

Reprinted by permission from G. Wulf and R. Lewthwaite (2016, pg. 1391).

for effective long-term changes in performance (i.e., learning) and sustained performance at a higher level. Experimentally, performance expectancies have been enhanced in various ways. In several studies, feedback was provided to different groups on trials with relatively small errors versus larger errors (3, 5, 41). Intuitively, one might expect feedback to be more effective when it is provided after less successful trials. Yet in several studies, skill learning has been found to be facilitated when feedback is given on more accurate trials. Highlighting good performances increased performers' self-efficacy and therefore resulted in more effective learning than did feedback after poor performance.

Other types of positive feedback have been shown to be effective as well. These include feedback that involves favorable social comparisons. Studies have demonstrated interesting effects when participants were provided with (false) feedback indicating that they were performing above average (although such feedback is not recommended for direct practical application due to its deceptive nature). Relative to participants who received neutral or negative social-comparative feedback, these participants demonstrated enhanced performance and learning of tasks requiring balance, accuracy, sustained maximum force production, or endurance (2, 11, 18). In one such study, the authors used a handgrip dynamometer and found greater sustained maximum force production,

increased self-efficacy, and lower perceived exertion as a function of positive normative feedback compared with both negative feedback and control conditions (11). In another study, favorable feedback enhanced running efficiency (i.e., reduced oxygen consumption) in experienced runners (46). Stoate, Wulf, and Lewthwaite asked experienced runners to run on a treadmill, which was set at a speed that corresponded to 75% of their maximal oxygen consumption (46). The authors provided feedback to one group of participants that indicated they were performing more efficiently than others (e.g., "You look very relaxed. You are a very efficient runner."). Oxygen consumption significantly decreased across the run for that group while it remained the same in a control group. Moreover, participants who were given positive feedback reported greater ease of running and increased positive affect. Even maximum aerobic capacity ($\dot{V}O_2$max) has been shown to be increased when runners' expectations were enhanced (28). Participants in that study were experienced runners who completed two $\dot{V}O_2$max tests within 2 weeks. Before the second test, the experimenter made a casual remark to one group of participants, letting them know that their aerobic capacity on the first test was above the group average. Providing runners with this positive feedback resulted in a significant increase in $\dot{V}O_2$max (+3.28%) relative to their first test. The other group (control) showed a decrease in $\dot{V}O_2$max, presumably because participants were disinclined to run to exhaustion again within a relatively short period of time. Thus, even though maximal oxygen consumption is typically assumed to be an objective and reliable measure of physical fitness, findings showed that even maximal aerobic capacity can vary as a function of the individual's self-efficacy expectations.

Other studies have also demonstrated that simple statements can suffice to promote performance and learning. Information suggesting that peers typically do well on a given task or encouraging statements about the learner's performance or improvement resulted in more effective learning than no such information (54, 55). Increasing performers' perceptions of success can be achieved through other means as well. For example, setting criteria that purportedly indicate good performance, but that can be reached relatively easily, will raise learners' expectancies—with beneficial effects for performance and learning (31, 47, 67). In one study, participants performed a golf putting task in which the target was surrounded by two concentric circles (31). One group was informed that putting within the larger circle would constitute good putts, whereas another group was told that balls ending up in the smaller circles would be considered good. While one might expect the smaller circle to lead to more intense concentration and enhanced learning, the large-circle group actually putted more accurately during the practice phase than did the other group (small circle). Importantly, in delayed retention and transfer tests, with the circles removed, these group differences were maintained. Thus, making learners feel successful during practice resulted in more effective learning (47).

A study of professional golfers on the European Professional Golfers Association tour highlights the importance of expectancies for performance (40). The authors examined performance in subsequent tournaments 1 week after a golfer barely made or missed the prior tournament's cut. Uninfluenced by preexisting skill differences (scoring average), those golfers who had received a boost of confidence from making the cut outperformed those who just failed to make the cut in the next tournament.

Autonomy

Performer autonomy is another variable that appears to be indispensable for optimal performance and learning. Conditions that give performers a sense of autonomy, for example, by providing them with choices, are beneficial for motor performance and

learning. For instance, allowing learners to choose when to receive feedback about their performance (15), letting them decide when to use an assistive device (4), or letting them choose the amount of practice (38) has been shown to enhance learning.

The motivational underpinnings of the learner-controlled practice were first highlighted by Lewthwaite and Wulf (19). Interestingly, and in line with this view, even minor and seemingly insignificant choices have been found to facilitate learning and performance. For example, in one study (51), participants were asked to perform three different balance exercises. In one group, participants were able to choose the order in which they wanted to perform those tasks. In the control group, the order was chosen for them. In fact, each participant's order was determined, unbeknownst to them, by what an assigned counterpart in the choice group had selected. The choice group showed superior balance performance on all tasks, compared with the control group, throughout the practice phase. More importantly, a delayed retention test with a fixed order of tasks demonstrated that this minor choice also enhanced learning. In another study, using different exercises (lunges, jumping jacks, bear crawls, medicine ball throws) but a similar experimental design, participants were also able to choose the order of exercises (choice group) or not (control group) (58). Before performing the tasks, all participants were asked how many sets and repetitions they wanted to complete for each exercise. Participants in the choice group chose to perform a significantly greater number of sets (3.0) and repetitions (13.2), on average, than did the control group participants (2.3 sets, 10.8 repetitions). Autonomy-supportive climates have been found to be associated with persistence in activity engagement in other studies as well (64). Thus, an additional benefit of giving learners choices is that it can increase their motivation to practice—which might have additional indirect benefits for learning.

Choices as trivial as the color of objects or equipment to be used have been shown to lead to more effective motor learning. This includes one study (17) in which participants were able to choose the color of golf balls on a putting task. Specifically, in a choice group, learners had the opportunity to choose the ball color (white, orange, or yellow) six times during the practice phase. In the control group, learners were provided balls of the same color that an assigned counterpart in the choice group had used. The choice group demonstrated superior learning, as measured by putting accuracy on a retention test 1 day later, in which only white balls were used.

To see "how low one can go," Lewthwaite and colleagues conducted another experiment in which they gave one group of learners choices that were completely unrelated to the task they were about to learn (i.e., a balance task) (17). Participants were given a choice related to a different task they would practice afterward, and they were asked their opinion as to which of two pictures should be hung on the laboratory wall. Relative to a control group that was simply informed of the second task or the picture to be hung, the choice group demonstrated more effective learning of the balance task. These findings demonstrate that giving learners choices—even small ones or ones that are incidental to the task—have the capacity to facilitate motor skill learning.

Furthermore, the type of instructional language has been found to have an impact on motor learning. Hooyman and colleagues (10) varied the way in which instructions for performing a novel motor task, a cricket bowling action, were presented. Instructions that gave the learners a sense of choice (autonomy-supportive language) led to superior learning than instructions that offered little option for how to execute the skill (controlling language). On a delayed retention test without further instructions, the autonomy-supportive language group showed greater accuracy in hitting a target than did the controlling-language group.

Providing individuals choices has also been shown to have benefits for maximum force production and movement efficiency. For instance, in a study by Halperin and coworkers (9), kickboxers who competed at national and international levels performed standard punching performance tests across several days. Each test consisted of maximal-effort punches completed in a specific order: lead straight, rear straight, lead hook, and rear hook. This standard protocol served as the control condition. Each athlete also performed an additional test under a choice condition on each day. That is, the athlete delivered the same number and types of punches but was able to choose the order of those punches. The choice (A) and control (B) conditions were completed in a counterbalanced order across 6 days (AB-BA-AB-BA-AB-BA). Allowing the boxers to choose the order of punches generally led to greater punching velocity and higher impact forces than did an assigned order of punches. A relatively small choice resulted in athletes punching faster and harder, even though they were highly skilled

athletes who had extensive experience with the task. In a follow-up study with non-athletes, Iwatsuki and colleagues (12) asked participants to squeeze a hand dynamometer and perform several repeated maximum-effort trials. When participants were able to choose the order of their right and left hands, they were able to maintain maximum forces. In contrast, forces declined in control group participants (each of whom had the same order of hands as an assigned counterpart in the choice group). Thus, an increased sense of autonomy seemed to facilitate sustained maximal force production.

The production of maximum forces requires optimal motor unit recruitment as well as avoidance of unnecessary cocontractions of muscles. The studies by Halperin and colleagues (9) and Iwatsuki and colleagues (12) provided initial evidence that autonomy support may indeed facilitate neurophysiological efficiency. More direct evidence for this notion was sought in a study by Iwatsuki and colleagues (13). In their study, participants completed a 20-minute submaximal run (65% of $\dot{V}O_2$max) on a treadmill. Before the run, participants in one group were able to choose pictures that would be shown to them on a screen during the run. Throughout the run, this group ran with greater efficiency, as measured by oxygen consumption and heart rate, compared with performers viewing the same picture but without having a choice.

The most direct evidence for increased movement efficiency resulting from autonomy support comes from a study by Iwatsuki and colleagues (14) in which they examined the effects of performer autonomy on motor performance by measuring neuromuscular activity through the use of electromyography (EMG). Participants were asked to perform a motor task that involved the production of accurate forces through ankle plantar flexion. All participants performed three variations of the task (i.e., different target torques: 80%, 50%, 20% of maximum voluntary contractions) under both choice and control conditions. The results showed that EMG activity was lower in the choice relative to the control condition. That is, participants produced the same torques with less muscle activation when they had a small choice (task order). These findings highlight the importance of autonomy support for neuromuscular efficiency.

External Focus of Attention

A performer's focus of attention plays another key role with respect to the effectiveness and efficiency of movements. Since 1998, many studies have shown that adopting an external focus, that is, concentrating on the intended movement effect, enhances motor performance and learning compared with an internal focus on body movements (59). An external focus might be one that is directed at the motion of an implement (e.g., racquet, ball, skis, discus, kayak), even a sticker attached to the body (e.g., chest), a target to be hit, the force exerted against the ground, or an image such as the pendulum-like motion of a golf club. Compared with an internal focus (e.g., arms, shoulders, hips), an external focus enhances movement effectiveness (e.g., movement accuracy) and efficiency (e.g., muscle activation). This benefit to performance and learning has been demonstrated for a wide variety of skills, levels of expertise, age, or ability or disability. In essence, by adopting an external focus, a higher skill level is reached in less time (for reviews, see Wulf [50] and Wulf and Lewthwaite [60]).

This section highlights some findings related to the efficiency of movements as a function of an external versus internal focus. A movement pattern is considered more efficient or economical if the same movement outcome is achieved with less energy expended. Direct measures of efficiency include muscular (EMG) activity, oxygen consumption, and heart rate. Neuromuscular efficiency is also reflected in the production of forces and can therefore be seen in maximum force production, movement speed, or muscular endurance.

Several studies measured EMG activity in participants who performed motor tasks under external versus internal focus conditions. In the first study, by Vance and colleagues (48), participants performed biceps curls while concentrating on the weight bar (external focus) or their arms (internal focus). An external focus resulted in lower EMG activity in both agonist and antagonist muscles (see also Marchant and colleagues [24]). Greater efficiency with an external focus has also been found in studies involving an isometric force production task (22). The participants' task was to press against a force platform with their foot with 30% of their maximum force. Focusing on the calf muscles (internal) led to less accurate force production than did concentrating on the force platform (external), as well as higher degrees of muscle activation and increased cocontractions between agonists and antagonists. The authors also found indications of superfluous motor unit recruitment of larger motor units within the muscles when participants focused internally. Unnecessary

muscle activation—be it between muscles or within muscles—interferes with movement accuracy. Therefore, in target-oriented tasks such as basketball free throws (65) and dart throwing (21), higher degrees of muscle activation with an internal focus were associated with reduced accuracy. In contrast, an external focus on the hoop or dart trajectory, respectively, resulted in greater accuracy and lower activation of arm muscles.

Reduced muscular activity with an external relative to an internal focus is associated not only with more accurate force production, but also with the production of greater maximal forces. The production of maximum force requires an optimal activation of agonist and antagonist muscles, as well as optimal muscle fiber recruitment. Cocontractions, imperfect timing, or direction of forces (or more than one of these) would result in less than maximal force output. Marchant and colleagues (25) asked experienced exercisers to produce maximum voluntary isokinetic contractions of the elbow flexors while focusing on their arm muscles (internal) or the crank bar of the dynamometer (external). Participants produced significantly greater peak joint torque when they focused externally.

Maximum vertical jump height has also been also found to be increased with an external relative to an internal focus (and control conditions) (56, 63). Participants in those studies were instructed to concentrate on the tips of their fingers (internal) or on the rungs (external) of the measurement device (e.g., a Vertec) they attempted to displace during the jumps. Performers jumped significantly higher with the external focus. Furthermore, the vertical displacements of the center of mass, impulses, and joint moments about the ankle, knee, and hip joints were significantly greater—demonstrating that increased jump height with an external focus was achieved through greater force production (56). Moreover, greater jump height with an external focus was associated with reduced EMG activity, indicating increased neuromuscular efficiency (57). Standing long-jump performance has also been shown to be enhanced with an external focus (33, 35, 49). Also, the performance of other skills requiring maximum force production, such as discus throwing (66), has been shown to benefit from an external focus.

The greater efficiency with an external focus also manifests itself in increased movement fluidity, speed, and endurance. Porter and colleagues demonstrated the benefits of adopting an external focus for tasks involving running (34, 36). In one study, the authors found that an external focus reduced the time taken to complete a whole-body agility task (e.g., an L run) (34). Relative to internal focus instructions and control conditions, the same participants ran faster when given external focus instructions. In another study (36), 20-meter sprint times were significantly reduced with an external focus (i.e., clawing the floor with the shoes) compared with an internal focus (i.e., moving the legs and feet down and back as quickly as possible). Focus of attention also affects swim speed. Both intermediate swimmers (7) and expert swimmers (45) were found to swim faster when they were asked to focus on pushing the water back (external focus) relative to pulling their hands back (internal focus).

Greater neuromuscular efficiency with an external focus should also manifest itself in increased endurance since greater efficiency means less energy is consumed. In one study (43), oxygen consumption as a function of attentional focus was measured in skilled runners. For three 10-minute periods, they ran on a treadmill at a speed that corresponded to 75% of their $\dot{V}O_2$max under the respective focus conditions. For 10 minutes each, they were asked to concentrate on their running movement (internal focus), breathing (internal focus), or a video display that simulated running outdoors (external focus). The results showed that runners needed significantly less oxygen with an external focus of attention compared with either of the internal foci.

Another study examined muscular endurance in trained individuals performing exercise routines (23). The authors measured the number of repetitions to failure during various exercises (i.e., assisted bench press, free-weight bench press, free-weight back squat) with weights corresponding to 75% of each participant's repetition maximum. An external focus on the movement of the bar being lifted allowed for a significantly greater number of repetitions than an internal focus on the movements of the limbs involved (i.e., arms, legs) in all three exercises. In another study using an isometric force production task (e.g., a wall sit), Lohse and Sherwood (20) found increased time to failure with external focus (keeping imaginary lines between the hips and knees horizontal) versus internal focus (horizontal position of the thighs). Thus, there is converging evidence demonstrating greater movement efficiency when performers adopt an external focus of attention.

KEY MOTOR PERFORMANCE FACTORS AND PERFORMANCE OPTIMIZATION

High expectancies prepare the performer for movement success at various levels (e.g., cognitive, attentional, neuromuscular). They ensure that movement goals are effectively coupled with necessary actions. **Goal-action coupling** (see figure 28.1 on page 422) refers to the fluidity with which the intended movement goal is translated into action (60). An important feature of goal-action coupling is effective and efficient neuromuscular coordination (e.g., recruitment of motor units). Confidence protects the performer from thoughts that would interfere with optimal performance, such as distracting thoughts or self-referential thinking (26) that reduces attentional capacity and detracts from a goal focus. As indicated in figure 28.1, high performance expectancies have a dual role for goal-action coupling: maintaining a focus on the task goal and preventing a self-focus (or other distracting thoughts). Expectations of rewarding experiences elicit dopaminergic responses (44) that facilitate the establishment of functional neural connections necessary for successful motor performance. Dopamine, in conjunction with task practice, also facilitates the consolidation of memories (i.e., learning) and builds structural and functional connections that underlie skilled performance (e.g., Milton and colleagues [27]).

Autonomy-supportive conditions are rewarding (30) and thus increase individuals' anticipation or expectations for future reward or success. Thus, they enhance performance and learning through the enhanced expectancy route. Autonomy, or lack thereof, may also have a more direct impact on motor performance and learning (see arrow from autonomy to self-focus or focus on task goal in figure 28.1). Controlling conditions that deprive performers of a sense of autonomy tend to be stressful (39). The stress hormone cortisol has a downregulatory effect on the brain's reward network (29), which might contribute to degraded learning under those conditions (10). Autonomy-supportive conditions allow performers to focus their attention (externally) on the task goal, without the need for self-regulatory activity resulting from controlling environments.

An external focus directly contributes to goal-action coupling by helping the performer direct attention to the task goal and preventing disruptive body or self-related distractions from the task goal. That is, an external focus is assumed to facilitate neural connections that are critical for optimal performance. The result is greater automaticity (62) and neural efficiency (16) (for a review, see Wulf [50]). In addition, by consistently producing successful movement outcomes, an external focus likely enhances expectancies for future performance and goal-action coupling (see figure 28.1).

IMPLICATIONS FOR APPLIED SPORT SCIENCE

The findings reviewed in this chapter have important practical implications. This final section summarizes the main points made throughout this chapter and gives examples of how sport scientists might apply these principles. Table 28.1 provides an overview of the key factors for optimal performance, different means of implementation, and specific examples.

Enhancing Athletes' Performance Expectancies

Sport scientists can facilitate movement effectiveness and efficiency relatively easily by enhancing their athletes' performance expectancies. The ability to sustain effort, the ability to move efficiently and accurately, and the ability to maintain balance are all key attributes of successful performance. To this end, coaches may want to reconsider a number of factors that are considered standard practice in coaching. These include the predominance of offering feedback on unsuccessful trials instead of successful ones. Feedback that is mostly corrective or prescriptive (or both) tends to undermine the performer's confidence, with negative consequences for performance. In contrast, performance and learning benefit when performers feel competent and successful. Further, setting performance goals that are challenging but achievable can serve to provide athletes with a boost of confidence, which in turn will enhance their motivation, performance, and learning. Enhanced performance expectancies are also important during warm-up before a competition. Setting simple and attainable goals during the warm-up, or ending the warm-up with a successful trial, can help athletes enhance their expectancies for performance in the upcoming competition.

Providing Autonomy Support

The effects of autonomy support also have considerable implications for athletes and coaches. The findings reported here seem to contrast with approaches that are predominant in applied settings. Coaches often prescribe the task they want athletes to perform, or the order of different tasks, and they provide feedback or give demonstrations of the skill when they believe

TABLE 28.1   Key Factors for Optimal Performance and Learning

Key factors for optimal performance and learning	Ways of implementation	Examples
Enhanced expectancies	• Positive outcome expectations • Positive feedback, including after good trials • Liberal definitions of success • Task difficulty that allows for success with challenge • Proximal, measurable goals	Highlighting an athlete's improvement or providing feedback about positive aspects of performance
Autonomy	• Self-controlled feedback, assistive devices, amount of practice, and so on • Small and incidental choices • Autonomy-supportive instructions	Allowing an athlete to choose the order of exercises or the number of repetitions
External focus of attention	Instructions or feedback that directs concentration to the intended movement effect: • Implement (e.g., golf club, discus, skis, weights) • Environment (e.g., water, ground, target) • Images, analogies, metaphors	Giving instructions that direct the athlete's attention to the desired spin of a ball or the movement path of a barbell

it is necessary or helpful. Sport scientists can help their athletes move more effectively and efficiently by providing them with choices. Even small or incidental choices have been shown to result in more effective performance and learning, enhanced motivation, and positive affect. Instructional language that is autonomy-supportive rather than controlling has similar effects. Potential benefits include (competitive) performance advantages, experiences of movement fluidity and effortlessness, and longer practice durations.

Promoting an External Focus

Because of the consistency with which an external focus has been shown to facilitate performance and learning, it should be considered the default attentional focus. Subtle differences in the wording of instructions or feedback can have a significant impact on immediate performance and longer-term learning. Yet even experienced performers do not always adopt the optimal focus, which may be partly the result of histories of instruction (8). For example, in interviews with track and field competitors at national championships, the majority (84.6%) reported that their coaches gave instructions related to body movements (37). Instructors, coaches, and performers themselves should be aware of the strength of the evidence favoring an external focus and should develop strategies to identify and maintain external foci. These efforts may require creativity and experimentation in finding the right external focus, as well as include changes to those foci as the performer's skill level increases. The benefits for performance and learning are arguably among the most reliable with regard to supporting effective performance.

Additive Benefits

Practitioners might wonder whether it is necessary to include all three factors (enhanced expectancies, autonomy, external focus) in practice or training protocols. The importance of each factor for enhancing performance and learning has been demonstrated in numerous studies. While each of these variables plays an important role in and of itself, a series of studies has shown that these factors can have additive benefits.

Conditions that included combinations of two factors resulted in greater benefits than did those that included only one of these factors, or none (1, 32, 52, 53). Moreover, the presence of all three factors enhanced learning to an even greater extent than did combinations of two factors (61). One study addressed for the first time the question whether motor performance could be immediately enhanced by implementing all three factors in succession (6). Using a maximum vertical jump test, the authors indeed found additive benefits for performance. With each addition of a variable on successive blocks of trials in one group, jump height increased whereas it did not change in a control group. Thus, "maximum" jump height was further enhanced by each variable.

Performance Testing

These findings also have implications for performance testing. The fact that simple conditions promoting enhanced expectancies, performer autonomy, and an external focus of attention can enhance performance suggests that performance under neutral conditions does not necessarily represent the individual's optimal or maximal performance. That is, what is seen, even with maximal-effort instructions, is not necessarily all that can be produced. Using optimized performance conditions can help testers ensure that their measurements for a maximum neurophysiological or cardiovascular assessment are as close as possible to maximal performance when that is the desired outcome. Practitioners should be aware of these influences in their work when assessing athletes' capabilities.

CONCLUSION

Sport scientists can easily take advantage of the effects outlined in this chapter. These require little more than small changes in the way instructions or feedback is given—and, of course, some creativity. Giving their athletes choices, providing success experiences, and avoiding references to body movements and instead directing their attention externally can go a long way in terms of facilitating motor performance and learning. The resulting movement success may even create a "virtuous cycle" with overall positive consequences for learning, performance, and motivation.

RECOMMENDED READINGS

Halperin, I, Chapman, DT, Martin, DT, Lewthwaite, R, and Wulf, G. Choices enhance punching performance of competitive kickboxers. *Psychol Res* 81:1051-1058, 2017.

Kuhn, YA, Keller, M, Ruffieux, J, and Taube, W. Adopting an external focus of attention alters intracortical inhibition within the primary motor cortex. *Acta Physiologica* 220:289-299, 2017.

Lewthwaite, R, and Wulf, G. Social-comparative feedback affects motor skill learning. *Q J Exp Psychol* 63:738-749, 2010.

Wulf, G. Attentional focus and motor learning: a review of 15 years. *Int Rev Sport Exerc Psychol* 6:77-104, 2013.

Wulf, G, and Lewthwaite, R. Optimizing performance through intrinsic motivation and attention for learning: the OPTIMAL theory of motor learning. *Psychon Bull Rev* 23:1382-1414, 2016.

Sport Science of Injury

David Joyce, BPhty (Hons), MPhty (Sports), MSc
Kay Robinson, BSc (Hons)

Injury detracts from performance. At the most benign level it is a distractor, and at worst, injury precludes participation entirely, sometimes for a short period, and occasionally permanently. Therefore, it makes sense to be diligent in understanding the nature of injury as well as the healing process in a sporting context. Moreover, it is necessary to take time to explore how sport scientists can work collaboratively with sports medicine professionals to employ methods that facilitate effective recovery from injury, culminating in a successful return to sport. Success in this regard is exemplified not simply by a return to competition, but a return to performance. It is this performance model that is front of mind as this chapter explores the sport science of injury. The purpose of the chapter is not to instruct sport scientists so that they can be primary caregivers; that is not their role or responsibility. Rather, it is to educate them regarding the nature of pathology and recovery so that they may be better prepared to assist sports medicine professionals in providing performance-based solutions in a collaborative team environment.

Every injury since the dawn of time has occurred because the load imposed on a body tissue exceeded that tissue's load tolerance. This can occur in an acute incident (e.g., a direct hit onto the rib cage of a rugby player), or it can occur as the result of an accumulation of a multitude of subthreshold stresses that eventually overcome the tissue's tolerance (e.g., rib stress fracture in a rower). Although the healing processes of these two examples may have strong similarities given the nature of bone remodeling, the antecedent causes are discrete, reflecting a different set of predisposing risk factors. It is the aim of this chapter to explore these nuances, with reference to the causes and implications of muscle, tendon, bone, and ligament injuries and how

sport scientists can support sports medicine professionals in the management of injury and maximize the athlete's return to performance. The recovery from injury and the risk mitigation involved in seeking to intervene before an injury occurs cannot be thought of solely through the lens of a sports medicine professional. An interdisciplinary team involving sport scientists, data analysts, psychologists, and technical coaches, as well as sports medicine professionals, need to all bring their skills and knowledge to the table and work effectively together to optimize athlete health and performance. This chapter views injury through this interdisciplinary lens.

Rather than simply examining injury at the level of the peripheral tissue implicated, however, the chapter overlays a discussion of the neurophysiology of pain, since it is pain that is most often the complaint when an athlete presents with an injury. For some 400 years it has been assumed that pain is directly related to tissue damage, but modern pain science has refined understanding of this ancient alert system. In addition, the chapter examines elements of rehabilitation and retraining that are critical to consider when seeking to return an individual to a state of health and performance following an injury. Finally, the chapter presents a conceptual model for decision making when it comes to determining readiness to return to play following an injury; this model emphasizes the collaboration between sport scientists and sports medicine professionals.

MUSCLE INJURY

Muscle injuries account for the greatest proportion of sport injuries and have a significant reinjury rate (18). There is clearly a demonstrable need to understand sport injuries, their risk factors, and the best methods of rehabilitating them. Muscle injuries can be broadly categorized into contusions and strains, with a third category, lacerations, being uncommon in the sporting context (and as such, not discussed in detail here). **Contusions** are the result of a sudden, usually blunt compressive force such as a direct blow. These are most common in collision sports such as the football codes and ice hockey, striking sports such as boxing and martial arts, and sports in which athletes can be struck by rapidly moving projectiles such as baseball, softball, and cricket. Muscle **strains** are usually due to a rapid lengthening action of the muscle that exceeds the strain tolerance but can also result from a submaximal load application upon a fatigued muscle, as can be the case with a soleus calf strain. Strains can also result from overstretching, for example, hamstring strains occurring in a water skier whose leg is violently flexed overhead in a fall.

Of these causes, the contraction mechanism is the most common in a sporting context. These contraction mechanisms are the ones that readily come to mind when one thinks of a muscle strain such as in a sprinter who is in full flight and suddenly grabs the back of the thigh. These strains most commonly affect the region adjacent to the musculotendinous junction (MTJ) because it is at this point of the muscle that the tissue structure is at its relatively weakest (18, 23, 28).

Pathophysiology of Muscle Injury

Although skeletal muscle follows a consistent pattern of repair irrespective of the injurious mechanism (e.g., contusion, contraction strain, or overstretch), healing timelines are highly variable and depend on the nature, severity, and location of the injury. The healing process consists of three main phases, with considerable overlap between phases 2 and 3 (18, 23):

1. **Destruction** is characterized by the rupture and ensuing necrosis of myofibers. A hematoma is formed to bridge the gap between ruptured fibers. The inflammatory cell reaction commences as a means of beginning the healing process.

2. **Repair** is phagocytosis of the necrotized tissue by cells brought into the region courtesy of the inflammatory reaction. At the same time, regeneration of myofibers is witnessed alongside the formation of scar tissue and capillary ingrowth.

3. **Remodeling** consists of maturation and strengthening of the regenerated myofibers alongside scar reorganization and return of functional muscle capacity.

Assessment of Muscle Injury

Muscle injuries should be diagnosed by appropriate sports medicine professionals gathering a full history of the incident including **mechanism**, **symptoms**, and **previous injury**. Specific note should be made of the level of pain and dysfunction immediately following the incident, with the possibility of early insight into prognosis being gleaned as a result (35). It is also worthwhile to consider the nature of the onset of injury, noting whether fatigue is likely to be implicated, if there was a sudden loss of function, or whether the issue gradually evolved. The sport scientist can aid assessment collaboratively with clinicians by identifying data showing any antecedent training alterations over the previous month, making specific note of demonstrable peaks or troughs of relevant loading parameters. This information is important to gain in order to understand the underlying cause of the injury, and in order for any mistakes of the past to be avoided in the future. There is a clear and vital role for the sport scientist to capture, analyze, and communicate with the relevant stakeholders (e.g., sports medicine professionals, coaches, and other high-performance practitioners) about any unexpected loading patterns. This information is critical to allow the interdisciplinary team to optimize subsequent loading and recovery stimuli for individuals or an entire team. Finally, it is worthwhile to understand the athlete's previous injury history, because this may provide clues as to the underlying causes and may point the care team in the appropriate direction for a thorough management strategy.

Following a comprehensive history taking, a full clinical assessment should ensue, and this may be supported by imaging modalities such as ultrasound and magnetic resonance imaging (MRI). The primary reason for a radiological investigation is to give a clearer clinical picture if the diagnosis is uncertain. In addition, there is evidence that tendon involvement in muscle injuries can increase return-to-play time as well as the occurrence of reinjury (20, 28). Should there be an index of suspicion of tendon involvement, or if the clinical picture is somewhat unclear, the use of imaging is justified. This is a decision made by the sports medicine professional leading the care of the athlete rather than the sport scientist, but it is explained here for completeness of the discussion.

Grading of Muscle Injury

The traditional approach to muscle injury grading is to classify it as follows:

- *Grade 1:* Muscle fiber strain without any tissue discontinuity
- *Grade 2:* Muscle tear with some tissue discontinuity
- *Grade 3:* Complete muscle rupture

With the increasing use of radiological imaging techniques, the classification of muscle injuries is becoming more granular. This is evident in the British Athletics Muscle Injury Classification system (20, 28), which provides diagnostic guidelines for radiologists reporting on magnetic resonance images of muscle injuries and has the following ranges:

- *Grade 0:* Ranging from no injury to delayed-onset muscle soreness (DOMS)
- *Grade 1:* Minor muscle injury involving less than 10% of the cross-sectional area (CSA) of the muscle
- *Grade 2:* Moderate muscle injury involving 10% to 50% of the muscle's CSA
- *Grade 3:* Extensive tear involving greater than 50% of the muscle's CSA with marked loss of function
- *Grade 4:* Complete rupture

This grading system is further increased in granularity by an additional descriptor based on the subtype of tissue. Specifically, this is denoted by these descriptors (see figure 29.1; 20):

- *a:* Injury to the overlying myofascial tissue surrounding the peripheral aspect of the muscle
- *b:* Injury within the muscle itself, most commonly at the MTJ as stated previously
- *c:* Injury that extends into the tendon

According to this classification system, therefore, a minor calf injury to the MTJ of the gastrocnemius without tendon involvement would be classed as grade 1b, whereas a more extensive injury to the soleus involving around 40% of the muscle's CSA but also extending into the tendon would be classed as grade 2c.

Muscle Injury Retraining

Injury rehabilitation should always be led by a sports medicine team; however, it is important for sport scientists to have an understanding of the process and ways in which they can support the team. Acute muscle injury rehabilitation begins with the protection phase, in which the priorities are the stabilization of bleeding, support of healing, and reduction of tensile stresses that could exacerbate the injury. Measures to reduce pain and bleeding such as ice and compression

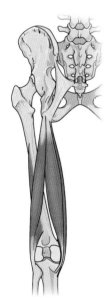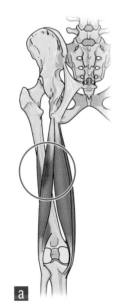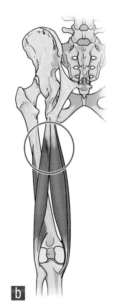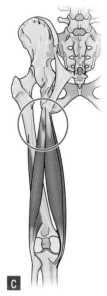

FIGURE 29.1 Examples of injury subtypes *(a, b, c)* compared to undamaged tissue according to the British Athletics Muscle Injury Classification system.

are advocated (15). Although evidence regarding the effectiveness of ice is lacking, consensus supports its use in combination with light movement (4).

Although one of the early goals of muscle injury retraining is the restoration of normalized movement, a short period of reduced loading and relative rest allows scar tissue to form and build sufficient tensile strength (18). Practical examples of load reduction are inserting a heel raise into the shoe after a calf strain or placing the arm in a sling after a biceps brachii rupture. Long-term immobilization past the early acute stage (2-3 days) should be avoided, however, due to the risk of muscle atrophy and excessive scar deposition. Early mobilization of the muscle stimulates tissue healing and revascularization and encourages a more parallel orientation of the regenerating myofibers, something considered important in the restoration of both strength and extensibility of the repairing scar (20).

Given the importance of the inflammatory response in the early stages of muscle healing, the use of anti-inflammatory medications is not advocated. Indeed, there is robust evidence to support the notion that their administration delays muscle repair (5).

In the case of a contusion from a direct blow, care must be taken to ensure that measures that enhance blood flow are limited in the initial 48 to 72 hours. These include massage, heat, alcohol, vigorous exercise, and anti-inflammatory (and other vasodilatory) medications. This is to accelerate the healing process, but also to limit the leakage of inflammatory cytokines that in some cases can lead to a condition known as **myositis ossificans traumatica**, in which bone is formed within the traumatized muscle (commonly quadriceps) due to an error in the differentiation of stem cells from fibroblasts to osteogenic (bone-forming) cells. Although relatively uncommon, **myositis ossificans** (MO) is characterized by pain and usually a significant loss of muscle extensibility that does not resolve over the usual timeline of 1 to 2 weeks. If MO is suspected, calcium deposits can sometimes be observed under ultrasound at around 14 days, whereas MO is not typically observed on plain film radiographs (x-ray) until 4 weeks. Although MO can typically be treated successfully with conservative (nonsurgical) management, it is often a lengthy process lasting months, and occasionally may require operative excision.

Following a short period of relative rest following a muscle strain, initial loading should commence once directed by the leader of the sports medicine team. In the simplest and lowest load form, some isometric

muscle actions may be the starting point. In the case of a lower-body muscle injury, encouragement of a normalized pain-free gait pattern is considered a vital early priority; depending on the extent of injury, this could commence in a pool.

The aims of load reintroduction at this stage are to restore neuromuscular function as soon as possible, to commence the remodeling phase of myofibrillar tension tolerance, and to get the athlete progressing on the path to physical and psychological recovery.

In order to progress rehabilitation, athletes should be pain-free during activities of daily living, have pain-free isometric contractions throughout muscle range, have no acute inflammatory signs, and have a pain-free range of motion greater than 75% of the contralateral side.

A strategic rehabilitation program begins with the end in mind. Specifically, this means that it is important to determine how the muscle will be expected to function when the athlete is back to competition. For example, will the muscle be subjected to high velocity or more endurance loads? Will it be acting over a single joint, or over two joints? Is its role primarily as a stabilizer or as a primary mover? Answering these questions will allow the practitioner to program the reloading appropriately, accounting for type of muscle contraction, plane of movement, and associated joints with particular consideration for injuries occurring in biarticular muscles (e.g., biceps femoris crossing hip and knee). It is at this juncture that the sport scientist has a critical role. As with any training stimulus planning, rehabilitation should commence with the end goal in mind. Frequently, the sports medicine staff will be concerned with the current state of the injury, but by analyzing athletes' likely training and competition loading requirements once they return to action, the sport scientist will facilitate the strategic rehabilitation loading parameters and ensure that all aspects of the planning have been accounted for.

Eccentric muscle action is the most common mechanism for injury and is therefore an essential component of muscle rehabilitation. An appropriately planned progression from bodyweight loading through to resistance with the addition of external load is necessary but not sufficient, since consideration must also be given to the volume, speed, and movement complexity specific to the expected sporting demands. The authors of this chapter also believe that restricting rehabilitation to the specific injured muscle is folly and thus advocate a whole-body approach that involves combined movements and trunk stability (31).

Following a lower-limb muscle injury, a return to running is often a key milestone for athletes. Timelines for when this can commence vary between specific injuries. However, they can be integrated into rehabilitation following a period of loading and when the athlete has demonstrated sufficient strength, rate of force production, and neuromuscular control required to tolerate running (33). Running should be progressed through graded exposure of volume and intensity, along with satisfying the necessary components of gait reeducation, always taking into account the athlete's response to these various elements. Tasks should then be incorporated with demands and conditions specific to the sport such as surface, acceleration, deceleration, pace variance, multidirectional change of direction, reactivity, and combination movements such as jumping and kicking as appropriate. Again, the sport scientist is a key player here. The sport scientist is best placed to plan, collect, analyze, and provide feedback (in many cases contemporaneously) to the athlete and the performance and sports medicine staff regarding the reloading plan. The sport scientist's knowledge of the demands of the sport can aid the rehabilitation plan and its integration into team training by monitoring accrued loads each session and advising on demands of each drill, which can then be carefully crafted into the periodized return-to-performance schedule.

As discussed in a later section on return to competition decision making, the rehabilitation planning process needs to take into account the various high-demand activities that an injured tissue will be exposed to. In most cases involving the lower body, this will involve heavy resistance work or high-velocity muscle actions such as sprinting. The authors of this chapter advocate continuing a rehabilitative process until the athlete has completed a body of work and given all stakeholders comfort that any competitive exposure would be appropriately handled. Specifically, practitioners should seek to expose athletes to high-speed running demands that equate to 120% of a normal competitive output, both in an acute dose and over the course of 7 to 14 days, with evidence that athletes are both competent and confident running at a velocity within 5% of their maximum. Developing and accessing a historical loading database that covers the various aspects of load (distance, high-velocity running, collisions, accelerations, decelerations, etc.) is a key responsibility of the sport scientist. This record can be built over time and allows the performance team access to valuable information upon which to base these overload considerations.

TENDON INJURY

Tendon injuries can be broadly classified into (a) lacerations and (b) tendinopathies. Tendon **lacerations** usually result from an acute incident involving a blade or other sharp object. Long finger and toe flexors are the most susceptible to laceration given their relatively superficial location in the forearm and foot, respectively. Tendon lacerations are uncommon in sport but may be seen in winter sports, in which an ice skate or snowboard may be involved. A tendon laceration is most often managed surgically and has a much longer healing time compared to other tissues in the body, owing to the fact that tendons have a high collagen content with low oxygen consumption (24, 30). Following the destruction and repair phases, the amount of collagen steadily increases with the fibers gradually orientating themselves longitudinally and the progression of cross-linkage strengthening enabling the tendon fibers to withstand the high tensile forces placed upon them. The site of injury within the tendon and associated amount of collagen should also be considered following injury, with the musculotendinous junction having a high density of collagen fibers to reduce tensile stress during muscle contraction.

Tendinopathies are a maladaptive tendon response to overload that results in pain, reduced function, and decreased tendon loading tolerance (9, 29). Since about the turn of the century there has been much debate as to the presence of inflammatory cells in tendon pathology. The suffix -*itis* (as in *tendinitis*) is suggestive of the presence of inflammatory markers, but this notion was challenged when biopsies taken from long-term tendon pain sufferers failed to reveal such cells (19). This was the stimulus for changing the term from tendinitis to the term tendinosis, with the suffix -*osis* being more suggestive of a degenerative pathology. Both of these terms rely upon laboratory assessment, so the umbrella term tendinopathy has been suggested as more apt; this term can be applied following a clinical examination. Tendinopathy, therefore, is a catch-all term that encompasses the entire spectrum of tendon disorders, ranging from acute proliferative tendon dysfunction through to chronic degenerative tendinosis. Certainly in a sporting context, tendinopathies are the most common form of tendon injuries and as such are the focus of the remainder of this section.

As is the case with all injuries, tendinopathies are the result of load imposition in excess of the load tolerance of the given structure. Acutely, this may be due to a direct blow (e.g., a soccer cleat rake along the length of an opponent's Achilles tendon in a soccer match) or a short-term application of training load (typically over the course of 1-7 days) that exceeds the tensile strength of the tendon. Over the longer term, tendon dysfunction may be the result of a more gradual tendon structure breakdown. Particularly in chronic tendon disorders, it is common to see interaction between factors that are intrinsic to the individual athlete's ability to absorb load (e.g., strength, biomechanics, or sporting technique), with extrinsic load application factors such as long-term application of stretch-shortening cycle loading. Overlying this may be systemic illnesses such as diabetes and ankylosing spondylitis, hormonal changes, and genetically predisposing factors; but knowledge of these factors is currently incomplete and beyond the scope of this chapter.

Pathophysiology of Tendon Injury

It has been proposed that a sequence of tendon dysfunction commences with an acute overload and progresses to the more common degenerative condition that will be familiar to millions of middle-aged runners and is seen in sports medicine clinics worldwide (9). This tendinopathy continuum is proposed to involve three broad stages of a tendon disorder: acute proliferative, subacute, and chronic degenerative, with each stage characterized by differences in

tendon cell (**tenocyte**) activity and subsequent protein production. According to this continuum, tendon dysfunction falls into any of these three stages, but it must pass through the early phases to get to the later stages. It should be noted, however, that the presence of pain is not a necessary condition in any stage, and indeed most commonly appears for the first time in the degenerative phase.

As mentioned earlier, there has long been a dispute regarding the presence or absence of inflammation in tendon pain. It appears that in the acute phase of a tendinopathy, cells resembling inflammatory cytokines are present, indicative of the fact that this is a stage of recent injury with an active healing response being mounted by the body. As the tendon pathology progresses, however, it moves along the continuum toward a true tendinosis, where degenerative changes are conspicuous and the acute inflammatory process less so (9, 19, 24).

As can be seen in table 29.1, tendinopathy follows a sequence of pathological responses that include tendon cell (tenocyte) upregulation, ground substance proliferation, and disorganization of collagen, which can lead to degeneration and ultimately vessel ingrowth. The etiology of tendinopathy remains unclear, with the cycle of events showing no direct relationship between structure, pain, and dysfunction (9); however, it is linked to stages of the tendinopathy continuum that has been developed for lower-limb tendinopathies.

TABLE 29.1 Stages of Tendinopathy Progression

Stage	Pathology	Clinical
Reactive (acute)	• Noninflammatory proliferative cell and matrix response • Result of tensile overload • Thickening (short-term) of tendon due to increased cross-sectional area • Collagen integrity mostly maintained	• Acute overload • Most commonly in younger people • Can be as a result of direct trauma • Common following period of decreased training (injury, off-season) • Able to reverse with load management
Disrepair (subacute)	• Matrix disorganization • Increase in cell number • Increased protein production resulting in collagen separation • Possible increased vascularity	• Chronic overload in the younger person • Can develop in older people who have stiffer tendons, with relatively low loads • Reversibility possible
Degenerative (chronic)	• Progression of matrix and cell changes • Large areas of disordered matrix with vascular ingrowth • Areas of cell death are apparent • Heterogeneity of matrix with areas of pathology interspersed with normal tendon	• Primarily older people • Athletes with chronic overload • History of repeated periods of tendon pain • If extensive, can lead to rupture • Cell structure not reversible but symptoms can be

Based on Cook and Purdam (2009).

Assessment of Tendon Injury

A thorough clinical assessment conducted by the appropriately qualified sports medicine professional is paramount for diagnosing not just the injury itself, but also the underlying intrinsic and extrinsic risk factors. Although tendon ruptures most often involve an antecedent degenerative weakness, generally speaking they involve a memorable specific rupturing event and need to be examined by a sports medicine specialist to guide the most appropriate management.

Tendinopathies are localized to a focal point in the tendon and are aggravated by dose-dependent tensile loading. The only exception to this rule is in the case of the postmenopausal woman, with changing estrogen levels implicated rather than mechanical tendon loading (14). In the acute phase, there may be some swelling and crepitus, thought to be in part due to an inflammatory response. As the tendon progresses along the continuum toward a more chronic state, a palpable thickening may be evident.

The most aggravating factors with respect to tendons tend to be when they undergo a stretch-shortening contraction at length, with the energy storage and release phase causing the greatest aggravation. Examples of such tasks include hopping and running loads applied to the Achilles tendon, jumping and deceleration tasks loading the patellar tendon, and hill running on the proximal hamstring tendon. Any assessment battery should replicate these tasks in order to aid with the differential diagnosis and assist in targeting the correct stage of reloading at which to intervene. It is also important to examine for any repetitive low-load friction or compressive tasks frequently undertaken by the athlete. A common example is proximal hamstring tendon pain exacerbated by prolonged sitting (e.g., on a bike or at a desk).

Tendon Injury Retraining

When strategizing a tendon retraining plan, it is helpful to return to the equation alluded to earlier in this chapter:

Tendon pain occurs when load applied > load tolerance

This means that a complete strategy would seek to intervene on both sides of the equation, namely, decreasing the injurious load and also increasing the tendon's load tolerance capacity.

Although in the past, tendons were considered largely passive structures designed for the sole purpose of connecting muscles to bones, it is now accepted that they are active structures that adapt to the loads to which they are exposed. That is to say, that like muscle and bone, they atrophy when deloaded for a long period of time and build when loaded. This does not necessarily correlate with pain, however. Frequently it is seen that deloading the tendon completely will substantially alleviate pain, if not ameliorate it altogether. Although superficially this seems desirable, it does not take into account the other side of the equation, which behooves the practitioner to increase the tendon's load tolerance capabilities. Thus, there is a balancing act to be performed here. What is required, therefore, is a strategy that reduces the symptoms but does not altogether stop loading the tendon. Indeed, the aim is to gradually increase the load to stimulate the tendon to adapt.

Examination of the modifiable risk factors is imperative, and interventions aimed at reducing their significance form the cornerstone of any successful management strategy. Examples may be technique modification (including gait retraining), equipment modification (including grip size on a racket or oar, and footwear), organization of training load, and targeted strength work. Progressive sport scientists will recognize their value in researching, understanding, and educating the appropriate stakeholders regarding all the current and potential factors contributing to an athlete's tendinopathic state.

In terms of the retraining strategies employed, much will depend on what exactly constitutes the aggravating load and at what stage of the tendinopathy continuum the athlete presents. In reactive tendons, load is initially reduced to allow time for tendon adaptation and the matrix to resume its normal structure. Identification of the cause of increased load such as a training spike (for example, a change in training program or following resumption of training after a period of time off), footwear, or altered technique should be done early. As discussed already, prolonged unloading is not thought to be beneficial to the tendon matrix, but certainly in the acute phase it is thought to be better to take an aggressive deload approach in order to maximize the tendon's capacity to heal. A gradual reload and exposure to previously symptom-inducing tasks should take place over the course of 4 to 6 weeks.

As the tendon progresses along the continuum, the more likely underlying strength or biomechanical faults will be seen that contributed to the breakdown, and these should be addressed as a priority.

Classification of Tendon Loading

As a general rule, it is the stretch-shortening cycle that maximally loads a tendon. Given the tenocyte's relatively slow adaptive response time (21), it is best to structure any tendon loading program conservatively. This is best considered in terms of high tendon load (HTL) days, medium tendon load (MTL) days, and low tendon load (LTL) days. In the authors' experience, a progression is appropriate not just for the injured tendon, but for athletes wishing to avoid such an inconvenience. The progression is as follows:

Day 1: HTL

Day 2: LTL

Day 3: MTL

Day 4: LTL

Day 5: HTL

Day 6: LTL

Day 7: LTL

Of course, what constitutes high tendon load will vary between individuals, and may indeed vary within the same individual across time. As an example, performing 50 box jumps may be considered medium load for a volleyball player, but it would likely be high load for a swimmer. Equally, the same 50 box jumps may be seen as low load for the same volleyball player as that player improves strength and jumping and landing technique. It cannot be overstressed that load programming, delivery, and analysis is a collaborative endeavor. Sport scientists are perhaps best placed to provide critical input with respect to normal loading data within their sport and to communicate this with sports medicine staff to ensure that rehabilitation is sport- and athlete-specific.

This structure provides the tendon with sufficient time to adapt following each loading stimulus, but care should be exercised in terms of ensuring that loading is applied in response to pain and that it progressively builds strength and speed, brings about regaining of elastic function, and allows return to sport.

BONE INJURY

Similar to tendon injuries, bone injuries tend to fall into one of two distinct categories: acute traumatic fractures and chronic maladaptation to load that results in stress leading to mechanical failure (more commonly known as **stress fracture**). Both mecha-nisms of injury are commonly seen in sport, although the type of sport has a significant bearing on the incidence of traumatic fractures; these are more common in invasion and contact pursuits.

Pathophysiology of Acute Fracture

In the sporting population, acute fractures are usually the result of trauma (e.g., a high-velocity tackle in football, a bicycle crash during a mountain descent, or a fall onto an outstretched arm in gymnastics). This usually results in immediate severe pain, swelling, and impaired function. When a fracture occurs, the normal architecture of the capsule surrounding the bone is disrupted, which stimulates the acute response. **Hemorrhage** (bleeding) is the most significant concern following long-bone fracture (e.g., femur fracture) due to the high vascularity. Stabilization of this blood loss is the immediate priority in these cases.

The acute healing phase commences with vasoconstriction and the activation of the coagulation cascade, leading to a platelet- and fibrin-rich clot around the fracture site (2). Inflammatory cells are then attracted to the hematoma, which allows for the removal of necrotic tissues and the laying down of the scaffolding for fracture healing. This is needed for bone ossification once bone has formed, enabling weight bearing and causing the callus bone to remodel in response to loading, forming stronger lamellar bone.

Pathophysiology of Stress and Pathological Fractures

Bone is an active, albeit slowly adapting, tissue. It is continually changing, maintaining a balance between bone resorption carried out by **osteoclasts** and new bone formation undertaken by **osteoblasts**. Osteoblastic activity is stimulated by loading with the aim of strengthening the bone in areas of high force. The role of the osteoclasts is just as vital, continually breaking down bone material to ensure that there is regular mineral turnover and to safeguard against excessive bone formation. It is evident, therefore, that there is a balance to be achieved here, and that bone health relies on the successful interaction of both osteoblasts and osteoclasts.

Should loading application exceed the mechanical strength of the bone, failure can result. This can be seen as part of a continuum extending from the bone marrow becoming edematous, but without trabecular disruption (known as **bone stress**), to a stress fracture, characterized by structural disruption within the bone, which, if left unchecked, can lead to a cortical breach (shown by a fracture line extending through the bone). Symptoms are usually pain that can often be pinpointed, and functional impairment.

It behooves the performance professional to examine both sides of the load equation here. Clearly, the extrinsic load applied needs to be reduced, but equally intrinsic factors that may possibly have led to bone weakness should be investigated.

When examining extrinsic load application, it is common to uncover training load errors such that insufficient time has been allowed for tissue remodeling following a training stimulus. Examples include tibial stress fracture after an overly zealous commencement of marathon training, or repetitive loading of aberrant biomechanics eventually leading to bone failure (e.g., lumbar stress fractures in young cricket fast bowlers). As such, it is important that the boney loading stresses be cycled in an appropriate manner, respecting the remodeling period before applying another stimulus. When working with younger athletes it is imperative that the sport scientist have an understanding of the athlete's training age (cumulative amount of time spent training for a sport). The programming for a young female who has spent 5 years on the junior cross country circuit would be very different, for example, than for a talented soccer player who has been identified as a potential middle-distance runner in order to avoid bone stress.

When examining intrinsic reasons for bone mineral incompetence, it is important that the interdisciplinary team consider a range of endocrine or metabolic disorders that may have contributed. This is particularly important in women who report bone pain. Insufficiency fractures are a subset of stress fractures occurring as a result of increased physiological stress (such as high repetitive training loads) on a background of osteoporosis in which bones have an abnormally low density. It is important to be aware of this in sport settings due to the link with **RED-S syndrome** (**relative energy deficiency in sport**, previously known as **female athlete triad**). Low energy availability contributes to impaired bone health particularly in combination with **oligomenorrhea** (irregular menses) or **amenorrhea** (absence of menses) (22).

Finally, fractures can also develop without significant load or trauma as a result of bone disease,

infection, or tumor. This is termed a **pathological fracture** and is always accompanied by a systemic illness, although the fracture may be the first symptom of an altogether more serious underlying condition. A high index of suspicion is warranted when a lack of mechanical reasons for bone failure cannot be uncovered, and specialized medical assessment should be sought.

Pathophysiology of Bone Injury in Young Athletes

Specific bone physiology should be understood when one is working with young athletes. The growing areas of the bone include the physis, or growth plate, and epiphyses (or apophyses) (6). The physis is the area primarily responsible for longitudinal growth and if injured can cause irreversible damage including growth disturbances. The decreased resistance to stress, shear, and torsion of the growth plate cartilage makes it more susceptible to injury, something thought to be further accentuated during periods of rapid growth.

Epiphyses are categorized into pressure and traction epiphyses (6, 11). **Traction epiphyses** are found at the attachment point of muscle tendons; these contribute to bone shape but not bone length. These are subjected to tensile forces resulting in pain and inflammation at the attachment site. Commonly, a traction apophysitis can result in time lost from sport; however, it rarely leads to long-term problems. Examples of this include Sever's disease at the attachment onto the heel of the Achilles tendon, and Osgood-Schlatter disease, which is due to traction of the patella tendon on its tibial tuberosity attachment. **Pressure epiphyses** are located adjacent to the physis at the end of long bones and are subjected to compressive forces; if not managed correctly with medical guidance, they can result in growth disturbances; examples include distal radius in gymnasts and proximal tibia in football (6).

Assessment of Bone Injury

The assessment of bone injuries varies depending on the mechanism, severity, and site of injury, but x-ray is the most common imaging modality used if a fracture is suspected. Factors that should be considered to lower the index of suspicion for bone injury include the following (7):

- Specific trauma
- Osteoporosis
- Bone tumor
- Age >70 years
- Age <30 years
- Prolonged corticosteroid use
- Low body mass index
- History of recent fall and prior fracture

Acute fractures are associated with trauma and develop sudden pain, swelling, and impaired function with or without deformity and skin laceration indicating displaced fracture or dislocation and open fracture, respectively. Stress fractures tend to have an insidious onset, commonly without any abnormalities other than pain on loading and direct palpation; therefore a thorough history should be taken to identify any recent alterations in load or any red flags indicating possible underlying pathological processes. Sports medicine professionals referring for imaging will request specific views depending on the injury mechanism and location.

Early diagnosis of stress factors is crucial, with any delay increasing morbidity. Initial x-rays of suspected stress fractures may be negative, but computed tomography (CT) and MRI can identify them earlier; a high index of suspicion is warranted particularly in athletes with change in training load, a gradual onset, and worsening pain with loading progressing into aching during rest.

Common stress fractures sites are associated with these sports (27):

- *Running:* Pubic rami, femur, tibia, fibula, navicular, metatarsals
- *Ballet:* Pubic rami, neck of femur, tibial shaft, fibula, metatarsals
- *Jumping sports:* Neck of femur, medial malleolus, navicular, fifth metatarsal
- *Throwing:* Humerus, olecranon, ribs
- *Gymnastics:* Ulna, pars interarticularis

Traumatic injuries occurring in children and growing athletes should result in a high degree of suspicion of physis or epiphyseal injuries that if incorrectly diagnosed could result in long-term growth deficiencies. Growth plate deformities can also be seen as a result of repetitive overuse and are most commonly seen in the distal radial physes of young gymnasts. These injuries should be managed by a specialist; surgery is sometimes required in more severe cases.

Bone Injury Retraining

Early immobilization and analgesia are important for suspected acute fractures, with the initial management determined by a physician depending on the specific type, location, and severity of injury as well as any associated soft tissue, vascular, or nerve injury sustained. More complex fractures resulting in displacement are likely to need surgery to realign or fixate the bone, which has an increased risk of postoperative complications such as infection (25). Nondisplaced fractures are commonly immobilized for a period of time using a cast, splint, or boot with immobilization above and below the area of injury; this provides protection and pain control and promotes healing (8).

Stress fractures are predominantly treated by rest and offloading to allow bone osteoblast formation and remodeling of bone prevail to supersede rate of reabsorption (27). A number of exceptions to this require specialized medical management, such as femoral neck, humerus, and tibial shaft stress fractures that are deemed high risk due to the increased likelihood of **nonunion** (failure to heal). Fitness can be maintained through this healing time through activities maintaining offload of the affected bone. Athletes should be medically cleared to return to activity with close attention to load monitoring and slow progressions, addressing any other external risk factors such as footwear and equipment, as well as psychological and nutritional risk factors that require additional intervention.

Fracture healing is indicated by lack of pain on loading and on palpation; therefore, return should be driven by symptoms. Loading should be resumed at half intensity with short bouts of loading separated by rest to enhance osteogenesis (34), beginning with low loads. The use of reduced weight-bearing treadmills is an approach commonly used in the progressive rehabilitation of lower-limb fractures. Progressive loading alongside a comprehensive conditioning program should then be programmed and closely supervised over a period of 4 to 6 weeks and adjusted according to any pain response. Education of athletes and coaches is key to prevent reinjury, with training plans needing to incorporate adequate time for recovery and bone adaptation specific to each individual.

LIGAMENT INJURY

Skeletal **ligaments** connect bones and are joint stabilizers, guiding movement between motion arms, and act as restraints to excessive motion. Although they appear as one structure, ligaments contain different interconnected fibrous bundles (80% type I collagen) that are taut at different joint angles and depending on the forces applied (13). Ligaments also play a critical role in the body's proprioceptive awareness system. This is achieved by providing the central nervous system with barrages of data packets regarding changes in position and tension, which is then interpolated as alterations in joint position. Significant injuries to ligaments can compromise joint stability and physical function, as well as proprioception. In turn, it is thought that this can combine to predispose an individual to early osteoarthritis due to decreased shearing restraint at the level of the joint (12).

Pathophysiology of Ligament Injury

Ligamentous injuries can present as a complete tear, a partial tear, or a stretch injury, or can be altered in function resulting from a fracture usually as a result of trauma. Similarly to other structures, injured ligaments go through distinct phases of healing. Following injury there is a retraction of disrupted ligament ends, causing hemorrhage (which is subsequently reabsorbed) and inflammation, and proliferation where scar tissue is formed, followed by reorganization of the collagen fibers and maturation. However, complete ligament healing continues to be elusive, with long-term changes seen in the makeup of the collagen matrix (13).

Assessment of Ligament Injury

The gold standard for assessment of ligament injuries is using MRI, which offers additional information regarding severity and exact location of injury. It is true, however, that an experienced clinician can diagnose many ligament strains using clinical assessment techniques, mostly aimed at feeling for joint motion restraint. It is important also to have suspicion regarding boney injury associated with high-grade ligament injuries due to the reduced structural support of the joint; for example, a "kissing injury" can occur during ankle inversion when compressive forces cause bone

bruising of the medial malleolus and talus. Dependent on the severity of an injury, the location, and the activity levels of the athlete, management should be determined using a patient-centered, interdisciplinary approach. Anterior cruciate ligament injury is the most commonly discussed in the sporting population due to the extended time loss from sport, although there is growing discussion around the conservative management of these injuries. The majority of athletes undergo surgical repair using grafts, most commonly taken from the hamstring tendon or patella tendon (advised in the younger population), with little difference apparent regarding long-term outcomes (10).

Ligament Injury Retraining

Following initial management of acute inflammation as described in the treatment of other soft tissue injuries, early controlled resumption of loading after injury has beneficial effects such as enhanced strength, matrix organization, and collagen content of ligaments, along with being linked to earlier return to sport (16). Grade 2 or 3 ligament injuries should be protected through the use of braces to allow for healing and reduce torsional stress placed on the injury site, which could lead to delayed healing or chronic laxity.

Rehabilitation of ligament injuries varies in length depending on the extent of injury and the demands of the sport to which the athlete is returning. Each rehabilitation program should be individualized and progression guided by a sports medicine professional. Since it is known that long-term healing of ligaments can be slow and the makeup of the collagen remains altered after injury, it is paramount to focus on strengthening musculature around the joint as well as on neuromuscular and proprioceptive training from an early phase; this improves joint position sense and has been shown to have a preventive effect on reinjury as well as initial injury (26).

PAIN

Any of the injuries described in the preceding sections can (and often do) result in pain. Equally, pain can present in the absence of any specific demonstrable structural abnormality. Pain is, however, almost always a performance detractor and is therefore of particular interest to any performance professional.

For approximately 400 years, it was thought that pain was an unpleasant experience that was an input from the periphery (e.g., pain messages would be sent to the brain from the ligaments damaged following an ankle sprain), and that the motor response (e.g., limping) would be coordinated by the brain. It is now understood, however, that pain is an **output**, meaning that information from the damaged ankle ligaments is sent along the central nervous system to the brain, where it is then interpreted along with weighted consideration being afforded to previous experiences, future expectations, and cultural norms. If, when considering the totality of this information, the brain is satisfied that the body is under threat, a multidimensional protective action will be instituted, of which pain is a part (other parts including alterations in motor output, e.g., limping or muscle spasm, and increases in sympathetic nervous system activity). The key lesson here is that pain does not always have a linear relationship to damage; rather, it has a linear relationship to the brain's interpretation of the threat it perceives the body is facing.

This provides the explanation for why a specific injury may be severe but the pain is rather insignificant (i.e., the brain may decide that the information it is receiving is of little consequence), and equally why the structural nature of an injury may be insignificant but the pain response is severe (the brain has decided that the body is under threat and issues strong messages that the individual must stop the activity and get help).

PLANNING THE REHABILITATION PROGRAM

Certain key decisions need to be made regarding an athlete's readiness to return to competition, irrespective of the tissue involved in an injury. The best framework upon which to base these decisions is outlined later and should always commence with the end in mind. Specifically, this refers to having a clear understanding of the functional requirements of athletes when they return to competition, a process that can be supported by sport scientists and their ability to monitor and direct extrinsic and intrinsic workload progressions (3). This will vary with the sport and indeed often with the position played in the sport, so a thorough needs analysis should be the starting point.

It is beyond the scope of this chapter to provide great detail on the needs analysis (see chapter 5), but the domains in which the sports medicine professional should seek collaboration with sport scientists to understand the expectations for acute and chronic dose exposure (both volumes and intensities) include these:

- Running loads (this may require further granularity with respect to total distance, velocity exposure, distance of high-velocity running exposure, acceleration, deceleration, and change of direction)
- Collision loads
- G-force exposure
- Jumping and landing loads
- Striking, kicking, throwing, paddling, lifting loads

It is the authors' strongly held view that the concept of returning to performance cannot be at the forefront of a rehabilitation program in the absence of input from sport scientists. Moreover, it cannot involve just a top-down approach. The athletes should also contribute to this decision making because they may have unique insights into the aspects of their sporting performance that they are most anxious about or find the most threatening.

From here, an appropriately periodized approach to retraining can be planned. Although program periodization is covered in more depth in chapters 3 and 4 of this book, it is important to note that it should be applied to injury rehabilitation as well. Essentially, **periodization** is the strategic placement of training stimuli into a cohesive plan to progress performance toward a predefined peak. In the case of an injury, the predefined competitive peak is the return to competition date. Periodization also relies on the premise that to progress the performance of an injured individual, training loads need to fluctuate in volume and intensity and need to be suitably structured so that athletes (and other key stakeholders) have confidence that the body of work undertaken, and the stresses athletes have been exposed to, are sufficient to demonstrate athletic competency.

RETURNING TO COMPETITION

Readiness for a return to performance following muscle injury should be assessed following the resolution of signs and symptoms, clinical assessment, and the use of objective measures of strength and movement proficiency, along with discussion with the multidisciplinary team supporting the athlete (17).

Following injury, the long-term goal is to return to performance, whether the individual is a recreational or an elite athlete. Deciding when to return to sport is a complex and multifactorial decision and should involve a collaborative approach between the athlete and the support network. Decisions should be based on objective, psychological, and sport-specific criteria relevant to the athlete's level of participation (1). Numerous models can aid in the decision-making process; these consistently consider the biological, psychological, and social factors that underpin readiness to perform and involve regular assessment and review of goals and performance indicators (1).

The **Strategic Assessment of Risk and Risk Tolerance** (StARRT) framework (32) describes how athletes should be cleared to return to sport when the risk assessment (health risk and activity risk) is below the acceptable risk tolerance threshold. Health risks described in the study included patient demographics, symptoms, previous injury, and physical examination; activity risks included specific sport and position, functional testing (such as triple hop), comparison to baseline strength, and psychological readiness. The modifiers that could affect risk tolerance include any conflict of interest, timing within the season, and pressures from the athlete, family, or coaching staff. This framework should be used alongside continuous assessment to monitor the athlete's readiness and highlight any risks that require addressing.

All injuries should involve a battery of specific tests, including closed skill tasks (e.g., strength testing, triple hop, star excursion balance testing) and sprints alongside open skills that are directly related to the sport; these should have a reactive element, use surface and equipment that the athlete will be returning to, and be position-specific. For example, gradual, sequential ability to return to contact and scrummaging in rugby should be replicated before return to competition, initially using equipment followed by nonreactive and finally reactive drills as they integrate into team training. In this scenario, the sport scientist should be able to provide baseline data to assess readiness as well as symmetry.

Historically, physical testing has been the primary focus for return to sport; however, it is important to gauge psychological readiness to identify any fear of reinjury, decreased motivation, or low self-confidence at a number of stages throughout rehabilitation. If identified, referral to a sport psychologist is recommended.

Education on the injury and subsequent rehabilitation is paramount to athletes and their support network, along with realistic expectations. Rehabilitation based on time frames is being superseded by objective-led progression criteria with athlete-specific, measurable, realistic, and timely goals being critical in the process.

CONCLUSION

This chapter has sought to bring to light key pathophysiological issues regarding tissue injuries in a sporting context, along with important assessment and retraining issues. Moreover, an aim has been to overlay this with a modern approach to pain as an indicator of threat as opposed to damage, something that the authors believe is of vital importance to the performance professional. Finally, the key philosophical underpinnings of rehabilitation planning and return to competition decision making were discussed.

The principles of rehabilitation largely follow those of training. Progressive, planned overloading with consideration given to the fitness–fatigue model is as key to the injured athlete as it is to the noninjured athlete. It should be evident to the reader that contemporary injury retraining is a collaborative endeavor, with input from multiple stakeholders. The sport scientist is a major player. Sport scientists are skilled in providing valuable services to the training athlete, and the authors of this chapter contend that the needs of injured athletes cannot be fully met without similar skilled interventions. Not only is there an imperative to analyze, interpret, and communicate regarding loading parameters; sport scientists are well trained in research methodology and thus have a pivotal role in the continuous improvement of injury risk modification processes.

It is inevitable that injuries will occur at some point, but a cohesive and team-oriented approach to rehabilitation and returning to performance will see outcomes enhanced. When the information in this chapter is absorbed in conjunction with the other key topics in this text, it is hoped that the reader will have a much-enhanced understanding of the sport science of injury and rehabilitation.

RECOMMENDED READINGS

Ardern, CL, Glasgow, P, Schneiders, A, Witvrouw, E, Clarsen, B, Cools, A, Gojanovic, B, Griffin, S, Khan, KM, Moksnes, H, and Mutch, SA. Consensus statement on return to sport from the First World Congress in Sports Physical Therapy, Bern. *Br J Sports Med* 50:853-864, 2016.

Cook, JL, Rio, E, Purdam, CR, and Docking, SI. Revisiting the continuum model of tendon pathology: what is its merit in clinical practice and research? *Br J Sports Med* 50:1187-1191, 2016.

Joyce, D, and Butler, D. Pain and performance. In *Sports Injury Prevention and Rehabilitation.* Oxford: Routledge, 2016.

Macdonald, B, McAleer, S, Kelly, S, Chakraverty, R, Johnston, M, and Pollock, N. Hamstring rehabilitation in elite track and field athletes: applying the British Athletics Muscle Injury Classification in clinical practice. *Br J Sports Med* 53:1464-1473, 2019.

Nielsen, RO, Bertelsen, ML, Ramskov, D, Møller, M, Hulme, A, Theisen, D, Finch, CF, Fortington, LV, Mansournia, MA, and Parner, ET. Time-to-event analysis for sports injury research part 1: Time-varying exposures. *Br J Sports Med* 53:61-68, 2019.

PART VII

Education and Communication

CHAPTER 30

Interdisciplinary Support

Duncan N. French, PhD

When people observe sport, interrogate athletic performance, or analyze competition, it quickly becomes apparent that sporting activity is a highly complex interaction of many different technical, tactical, physical, physiological, and psychological components. Whether considering an individual sport in a controlled environment, a race event against the clock, or the chaos of invasion games and team sports, it is possible to evaluate how each of these respective components directly influences the likelihood of success. By understanding that sport is a complex interaction of many different factors, each of which is upregulated and downregulated throughout the course of competition, it becomes possible to acknowledge the importance that each component has in affecting the outcome of competition. Sport performance is truly **multidisciplinary**. However, to consider sport performance merely through a multidisciplinary lens does not convey the important and complex interplay between the different components (i.e., multidisciplinary reflects a construct with many parts, but does not necessarily indicate relationships between those parts); only when all the factors come together in an integrated or **interdisciplinary** fashion can true optimal performances be achieved. It is therefore critical that sport scientists, coaches, and performance specialists alike consider training, athlete development, and competition as an interdisciplinary construct.

HOLISTIC APPROACH TO SPORT PERFORMANCE

Supporting athletes to maximize their performance has not always been interdisciplinary. Indeed, as the performance sciences (e.g., physiology, medical services, strength and conditioning, dietetics) have

evolved over roughly the past century, technical disciplines have matured at different rates (i.e., the world's first sports medicine establishment took shape in the early 1900s, whereas strength and conditioning coaching became popular only in the late 1960s), and as a consequence the foresight to integrate and collaborate has not always been apparent. In addition, a degree of professional bias, ego, lack of willingness to interact, or the absence of respect for other professions, as well as technical disciplines that operate independently from one another (i.e., siloed), have been the norm for many years. Traditionally, a linear continuum from the start of a performance-based problem to the end point (e.g., return to play following injury, or the improvement in body composition) was thought of as a singular approach to managing a strategic process within the confines of a single technical discipline (i.e., medical management of return to play, or nutrition-only interventions to improve body composition). The consequence of this is that technical areas end up working on the same performance issues simultaneously, in a parallel fashion, independent of one another. Looking for a single cause or approach is indeed common, largely due to professional biases, and it is perhaps considered a simplification that seems necessary within the fast-paced environment of sport (16). However, this often misses the importance of the confluence of several factors or circumstances that might best influence a performance outcome (e.g., medical services engaging with psychologists during the management of a rehabilitation, or nutritionists, physiologists, and strength and conditioning coaches all collaborating to improve an athlete's body composition). As a result, the implementation of discipline-specific silos may in fact create greater problems, and certainly presents the risk of less than optimal performance impact (see figure 30.1). Instead, thinking in more holistic multifactorial

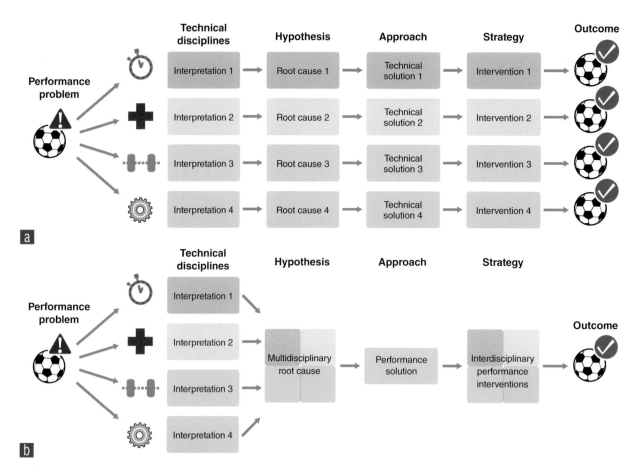

FIGURE 30.1 Approaches to problem solving in sport performance: *(a)* linear or siloed and *(b)* complex or interdisciplinary.

terms gives a significantly different perspective, which, while potentially more complex initially, likely poses a wider range of possible solutions both in the intermediate and in the longer term (16).

Thanks to our current understanding of basic science, training theory, and performance insights, it is difficult to endorse a siloed approach to performance support as optimal. For example, it is hard to rationalize that postsurgical rehabilitation would be better without the addition of nutritional interventions that reduce systemic inflammation, or that player movement and field position during a match could be comprehended accurately without video feedback from performance analysts, or that training for muscular power could be maximized without an objective understanding of force–velocity characteristics gained through diagnostic monitoring using sport science technologies. Instead, as one evaluates sport and its various components, it becomes more and more apparent that the interplay between technical or tactical and physical or physiological components is symbiotic within the competitive arena.

It is impossible to identify where one component stops and another one starts. Instead, the **determinants of performance** that influence a motor task work synergistically, upregulating and downregulating, in a synchronized fashion and therefore must be considered holistically. Different components are prioritized over others at various times within a sporting activity (e.g., striking with high-velocity actions during combat sports, reducing inflammation following injury, or demonstrating physiological regulation of breathing while shooting during a biathlon), but one cannot view the optimization of sport performance through a polarized lens that suggests any single technical discipline is more important than another. Instead, to truly maximize performance potential, all components of sport performance must be considered holistically as individual cogs that play a critical role as part of a larger machine. Only then can the interplay of technical disciplines (i.e., interdisciplinary) be viewed as the most effective way to maximize the performance, recovery and regeneration, or rehabilitation of athletes (see figure 30.2).

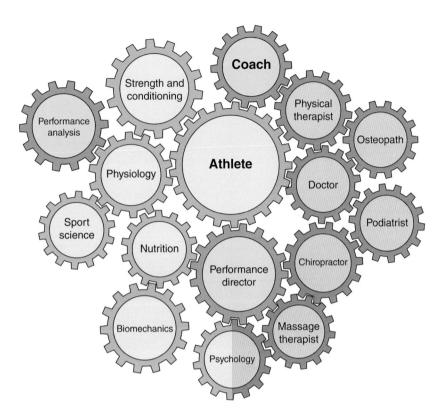

FIGURE 30.2   The performance-support "machine." The athlete is at the center of the machine, but each technical discipline represents an individual cog within the machine, each helping the machine to function optimally.

Systems-Based Approach to Performance

In order to better align the performance sciences with the specific needs of an athlete, to maximize any performance interventions, and to adhere to our current multifactorial understanding of basic science, a multicausal, multidimensional, and reciprocal approach to athlete support must be adopted. This is in stark contrast to a reductionist or linear methodology in which little collaboration is seen and where technical disciplines operate in parallel to one another. Instead, an **athlete-centered approach** must be adopted as a means to focus all the coaching and technical staff's efforts on the singular objective of achieving success for the athlete or team.

Philosophically, all support staff are required to elevate the rewards of success above their personal biases and those of their technical discipline. One of the key concepts in a systems-based approach to performance is **circular causality**, which creates a shift in how people understand and view professional relationships and interactions. Within any high-performance team or sporting organization, the concept of circular

causality allows complex operational structures to move away from a traditional linear approach and instead focus on reciprocal relationships between multiple technical disciplines. Of course, there needs to be a conscious decision to operate in such a fashion, but when there is the desire to interact in this way the potential to create collaborative solutions to the same performance-based problems increases exponentially. Furthermore, there is also a greater likelihood of increased efficiency relative to performance strategy (i.e., a reduced risk of having multiple departments trying to address the same performance problem at the same time, independently). **Reciprocal relationships** stem from the foundations of organizational cybernetics (i.e., a transdisciplinary approach for exploring regulatory systems), and move away from a mechanical way of viewing systems (i.e., individualized supply chains) toward a more relational approach (i.e., complex system) with a focus on interactional patterns of influence between contextual factors that exist within the same group or organization (9).

Circular causality is a concept that creates a shift in how organizational interactions are considered. Central to the paradigm of circular causality is an understanding of the impact that all internal and external factors have on a team or a unified system. By shifting our thinking away from a linear or reductionist approach toward a more circular or emergent thought process, the focus is no longer on single factors and individual root causes (e.g., training for muscle hypertrophy without considering the value that nutrition might have in augmenting muscle protein synthesis). Rather, by conceptualizing performance through the expanded perspective of circular causation, it becomes evident that all regulatory systems can be perceived as continually evolving, and that performance itself is affected by a myriad of external and internal factors (9). Applying this systems-based approach to sport science makes it possible to acknowledge the importance that each technical or tactical and physical or physiological factor might have on global performance standards.

Athlete-Centered Model

Every athlete has an innate genetic potential that represents a threshold in that athlete's maximum performance capabilities (i.e., a **genetic ceiling**) (see figure 30.3). Within any sporting ecosystem, sport scientists, practitioners, and coaches alike expose athletes to a host of external and internal stimuli (i.e., training, nutrition, recovery, mental coaching) with the objective of elevating their performance standards and maximizing their potential. These interventions are considered the process of training, through which multidisciplinary teams work to realize the performance potential of their athletes (23). Figure 30.3 indicates that innate potential and ability are different for all athletes based on their genetics (i.e., nature) (21). Perhaps more critical, however, is the understanding that any training intervention can fundamentally determine the extent to which performance potential is achieved or not (i.e., through nurture). Effective training allows athletes to harness all their genetic potential, while suboptimal training does little to promote athletes' ability to express their full capabilities. This theoretical model provides valuable insight into how performance enhancement occurs. Indeed, all athletes have a different physiological makeup, different motor skills, and different genetic potential, and every athlete responds differently according to the training stimulus. Owing to the complexity of

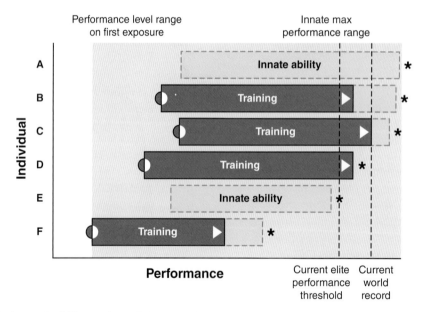

FIGURE 30.3 A theoretical illustration of the combined effects of nature (blue rectangles) and nurture (gray rectangles) on the actual and potential sporting performance level of six injury-free, healthy sub-elite and elite individuals (A to F). In this model, training is defined as the process by which genetic potential is realized. Two individuals (A and E) are not athletes or have not participated in the sport, while the remaining four individuals (B, C, D, and F) actively train and participate in the sport. The initial performance level on the first exposure to the sport and the current performance of the four athletes are indicated by blue-white circles and white triangles, respectively. The asterisk indicates the maximal performance threshold of the individuals.

Based on Tucker and Collins (2012).

human physiology and motor skill acquisition, athlete development is truly individual in nature. Even within the constructs of a team sport, exposure to the same training sessions likely induces a multitude of responses for each athlete on the team.

By acknowledging that every athlete is different, and that athletes respond to internal and external factors such as diet or training load in a heterogeneous fashion, one can suggest that performance potential can be maximized only when the specific needs of each individual athlete are met. Athlete-centric or athlete-centered training paradigms target the specific physical, physiological, psychological, and motor learning requirements of the individual. Such athlete-centered philosophies advocate that the development of any athlete is specific to that athlete's discrete individual needs and requirements. Indeed, only through an athlete-centered model in which training interventions, performance strategies, and any performance enhancement activity are aligned to the specific needs of the individual, can optimal capabilities be achieved. This is one of the major challenges within team sports, since determining how best to elevate the standards of many individuals simultaneously while training as a collective group can be challenging.

INTERDISCIPLINARY TEAMS

When all the practitioners involved in influencing an athlete or team recognize that high performance requires many different technical, physical, and psychosocial factors, and that these factors are individual to each athlete, it is possible to employ an interdisciplinary approach to performance optimization. **Interdisciplinary teams** (IDTs) comprise a host of different professions (e.g., coaches, physicians, psychologists, physiologists, sport scientists, dietitians) all working to help an individual athlete or group of athletes. The existence of an IDT that affects the planning and delivery of performance services should be considered fundamental for maximizing sport performance. Indeed, the previous sections established that optimal performance requires that a host of different factors be functioning concomitantly. However, one of the primary lessons learned over several decades in human service industries is that for IDTs to be effective, and for them to be a positive influence on performance, a climate of cooperation and collaboration must be actively fostered in what is potentially an environment that can foster competition, professional bias, and conflict (2, 10, 16).

With respect to the operational characteristics of IDTs within sport, several factors should be considered especially relevant:

- The need for clearly defined technical and tactical goals and objectives that are visible to all IDT members
- A structured training and competition schedule that is adhered to by all stakeholders
- An interdisciplinary sport science and medicine team that offers expertise in all the technical disciplines pertinent to the determinants of performance in a sport
- Endorsement of a holacracy framework (discussed in more detail later)
- An operational culture directed by the need to solve discrete performance-based problems (i.e., gap intervention strategies)
- The necessary infrastructure to promote communication and knowledge sharing, and a culture of candor and transparency through which cross-discipline interactions are promoted
- An organizational structure in which no discipline is perceived as more or less important than the next

The concept of IDTs involves a host of professionals across a wide variety of disciplines integrating their work while at the same time considering individual (i.e., discipline-specific) treatment plans or courses of action (20). An IDT in sport is formed by coaches, medical personnel, health care professionals, and practitioners from a variety of allied sport science disciplines who should be seen to collaborate in the formulation of specific strategies, recommendations, and interventions that ultimately facilitate the potential for success (i.e., winning). With the ongoing growth of different sport science disciplines, data analysts, and health care providers, the IDT in today's world of high-performance sport can be highly diverse and eclectic.

Performance Stakeholders

Conceptually, the IDT should work together to help manage the athletes' preparation and competitive performance. Through this support, athletes can leverage various expertise from a host of technical disciplines in order to optimize their preparedness or performance potential. Due to their respective roles in contributing to the athletes' success, all members of the IDT, including sport scientists, are considered **stakeholders** in their performance. With the emergence of technical specialists, acknowledgement that performance is a multifactorial construct, and understanding that increasing financial rewards in sport allow for larger investments in performance interventions (e.g., mental coaching, physical preparation, data analysis, recovery), the number of performance stakeholders, be they internal or external to the team, can become quite large.

The structure of an IDT greatly depends on the needs and resources in each situation, and IDTs should be constructed according to objective goals, targets, or finances (or more than one of these). Some IDTs are small and include only two or three key practitioners, while others, as previously discussed, can be very large and have a host of different technical experts. Holistically, most IDTs include professional expertise in common technical domains including technical or tactical coaches; medical and allied health professionals; physical preparation specialists, including dieticians, sport scientists, and data analysts; and equipment, resources, and operations staff (5, 13) (see figure 30.4; 5). The operational management of the IDT can depend on the specifics of the sport. Traditionally, a medical model has largely been adopted, whereby a chief medical officer (CMO) or team doctor leads the other technical disciplines. Later, IDTs evolved from this hierarchical medical model, and the interdisciplinary nature of team expertise is now recognized, with leadership distributed throughout the IDT. Indeed, there has been an increasing shift toward the inclusion of a performance director who has an umbrella role above all the performance services, including medical and science, and is positioned alongside the head coach in an effort to provide a bridge between the various IDT professionals and the technical or tactical coaches (5, 14). As with all IDTs, the greatest risk to organizational effectiveness lies in individual disciplines continuing to emphasize a reductionist approach, with each discipline potentially operating in its own silo and little focus on holistic athlete health and performance management, effective communication, integration, and an understanding of how to facilitate better decision making (5). From this perspective, high-performance interdisciplinary support can actually be viewed as a mindset rather than an organizational structure. Indeed, there needs to be a collective desire to adopt an integrated approach to solving performance-based problems.

The Role of the Sport Scientist in the Interdisciplinary Team

Sport scientists are often unique within the construct of the IDT, since they play an integral role in merging the productivity of other technical disciplines. The fundamental role of the sport scientist is to develop an evidence base to help answer questions from coaching staff in order to better inform decision making around an athlete's preparation and competition. In addition, sport scientists often possess technical skills and scientific expertise that can be leveraged by other technical disciplines, including technological expertise and data collection and analytics skills. Within the ecosystem of the IDT, establishing evidence in support of an athlete's preparedness to train or compete means that rather than operating in a reductionist fashion within a sport science silo, the sport scientist must instead operate horizontally across all departments of the IDT structure, capturing pertinent information from all stakeholders. From there, the sport scientist can manage the information or data flow (or both) in the most appropriate fashion in order to forecast an athlete's progression, regression, or performance potential to the coaching staff and the wider IDT.

The sport scientist is often a bridge between the various professions within the IDT and the technical coaching staff. The sport scientist's role is to understand basic science, undertake applied research (e.g., literature searches, primary research investigations), and work to aggregate information that can then be used to influence decision making and performance strategy, either within the individual technical areas or more holistically within the whole IDT. Within their work, sport scientists must adopt scientific methodology and critical thinking in order to study and investigate any concept potentially relating to athletic performance that might be of interest to the athlete, coaching staff, or other members of the IDT. Indeed, the sport scientist role should embrace scientific methodology within the paradigm of sport in order to question, observe, hypothesize, test, analyze, and theorize as to how best to maximize the likelihood of winning. Within the IDT, sport scientists, perhaps more than any other team member, are the individuals who should use the fundamental components of scientific methodology and critical thinking to influence performance outcomes. These components are as follows:

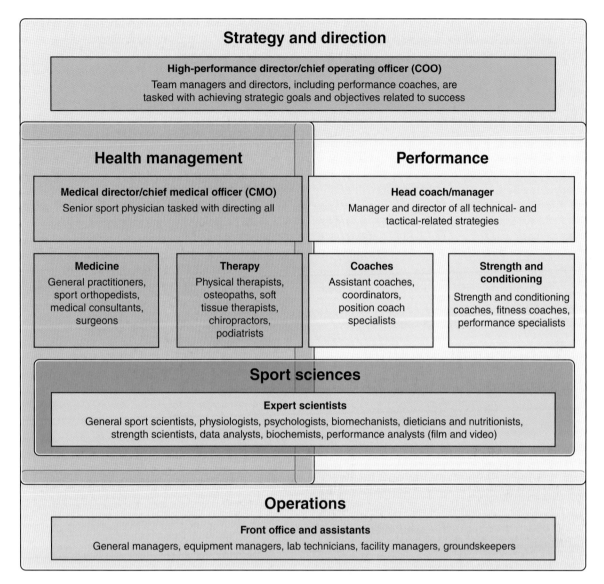

FIGURE 30.4 Interdisciplinary performance team model. All technical areas are defined according to themes (namely, strategy and direction, health management, performance, sport sciences, and operations). The whole performance model is directed by a high-performance director.

The health management and performance domains are managed by a medical director and a head coach, respectively. Performance sciences straddle both health management and performance. At its foundation, the model has operations that affect all the technical domains. Throughout the model are overlap and integration between specialist technical areas.

Adapted from Dijkstra et al. (2014).

- **Empiricism** is the use of empirical evidence, which is repeatable, in order to make vital decisions and reach sound conclusions.
- **Rationalism** refers to the use of critical thinking and logical reasoning, rather than emotional or wishful thinking, to evaluate what are true and what are false beliefs.

- **Skepticism** means possessing a skeptical attitude and constantly questioning accepted beliefs and conclusions in order to examine the evidence, arguments, and reasons for those beliefs.

External to the IDT, sport scientists can also take on additional roles facilitating partnerships with external stakeholders. This can include, for example, academic institutions with which teams, organizations, or other institutions are collaborating on research initiatives. Often, teams and organizations engage academic institutions to conduct investigations because they themselves may be limited in their research capabilities, expertise, or human resources. Consequently, since sport scientists possess knowledge of scientific methodology and investigation, they often become facilitators for data acquisition, as well as the conduit for interpreting high-level research findings, disseminating information, and upskilling coaching staff as to the best ways to operationalize scientific findings. Elsewhere, sport scientists can also play a significant role in communicating with vendors and suppliers, often filtering the latest technology, equipment, and software by evaluating their validity and reliability and then aligning hardware and software acquisitions to specific performance solution needs.

INTERDISCIPLINARY MODELS VERSUS MULTIDISCIPLINARY MODELS

As sporting organizations continue to embrace a diverse structure of different medical and technical experts, the **interdisciplinary high-performance model** has become the norm for optimal service delivery (21, 24). Indeed, bringing many different technical disciplines together, each drawing on its own disciplinary knowledge, has the potential to create collaborations that could maximize an athlete's preparedness and competitive performance. Organizations are beginning to embrace the establishment of a diverse group of technical experts as the way to improve all the factors that affect these performances, including injury prevention or rehabilitation, development of physical capacities, enhancement of technical

skills, and many other factors pertaining to optimal performance. As illustrated in figure 30.5, a multidisciplinary philosophy does not necessarily guarantee the desired circular causality previously discussed (26). Indeed, multidisciplinary structures still run the risk of becoming reductionist or individualized in their approach, whereby technical disciplines continue to work in parallel to one another (26). Although it is all well and good to bring different technical areas together in a multidisciplinary fashion, simply having a multidisciplinary structure does not guarantee that integrated knowledge sharing, collaborative workflow, and alignment of unified goals will occur.

Although use of the term multidisciplinary is certainly in vogue across the high-performance sporting landscape, instead of embracing a multidisciplinary paradigm, true high-performing support teams operate in an interdisciplinary fashion. Despite semantics, multidisciplinary reflects only the aggregation of many different technical disciplines together (see figure 30.5), while interdisciplinary refers to the cross-collaboration of individual disciplines, the integration of knowledge and methods, and the synthesis of unified approaches. Multidisciplinary simply refers to team members from different specialist areas who work together but remain in their discipline, whereas interdisciplinary systems bring those team members together and place their expertise and scientific knowledge collectively into an integrated plan. As a consequence, services become more condensed, more specific, more integrated, and more goal-directed from one single track.

Within high-performance sport it is not uncommon for many practitioners to believe that they work in an interdisciplinary fashion, when in fact they more commonly work in a multidisciplinary manner (22). Central to the paradigm of interdisciplinary services is the ability to create an **athlete-centered approach**, whereby collective expertise is aligned for the bet-

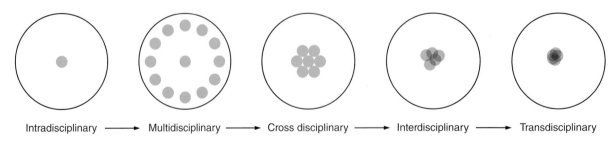

Intradisciplinary ⟶ Multidisciplinary ⟶ Cross disciplinary ⟶ Interdisciplinary ⟶ Transdisciplinary

FIGURE 30.5   The different disciplinaries.

Adapted by permission from E. Zeigler (1990, pg. 40-44).

terment of the team or athlete or both, and this can be achieved only when a unified strategy is adopted. Interdisciplinary services represent the panacea for sport science; a truly high-functioning, innovative, and performance-affecting structure that includes all the respective technical disciplines collaborating in an interdisciplinary way (i.e., sharing, challenging, innovating). For this reason, respective team members must recognize their role and how it aligns to the greater mission (i.e., how to achieve success), as well as acknowledge the importance that other technical areas have in this process. No one discipline has all the answers needed to solve the whole performance puzzle. Therefore, the lowering of discipline-specific barriers and the removal of siloed approaches is fundamental in order to optimize sport performance. Gone are the days when a scientific or medical discipline is considered subservient to another; in situations in which this remains, it is the ability to optimize performance that truly suffers.

Organizational Structure

Within professional teams, universities, and sporting institutions, either interdisciplinary services are constructed using an organizational framework, or they evolve organically into a particular way of functioning without a defined structure. Regardless of how they have been established, it is possible to categorize all interdisciplinary structures into one of four types: (a) a functional top-down organization, (b) a divisional organization, (c) a matrix organization, or (d) a flat organization. When considering the best way to create IDTs that have the greatest potential to affect performance, one can evaluate how an IDT would operate using these next four frameworks.

Firstly, a functional **top-down hierarchy** is an organizational structure in which technical disciplines are tiered in a hierarchical fashion, with disciplines considered the most important at the top of the organizational structure and those considered least important at the bottom. Within this tiered approach is hierarchical leadership and management whereby one technical discipline (e.g., sport medicine) is responsible for directing all the other technical areas below it. An example of top-down hierarchy is the traditional medical model, often employed in professional soccer (5, 13), in which a physician, team doctor, or CMO oversees all the other technical disciplines, including sports medicine, nutrition, physiology, strength and conditioning, performance analysis, and sport science. In this scenario, medical expertise (i.e., the CMO) is perceived as the most influential, and therefore the other disciplines become subservient in a structure led by medical personnel. In this type of structure, there is a high risk that professional bias will skew the operational approach, that technical services lack influence and visibility, that experts can become disengaged due to their lack of impact, and that communication with other departments can suffer.

Secondly, a **divisional organization** reflects a classic multidiscipline team structure in which disciplines are organized according to their technical area of expertise. Technical areas are aligned alongside each other, but each division is sufficiently independent from one another, often led by a performance director or head coach at the top of the whole structure. Such a divisional organization reflects vertical silos of expertise, and as previously discussed, this is often the most common representation of a support team (i.e., backroom staff) today. The greatest risk with this type of structure is that at its core it is a reductionist approach, and due to the vertical silos, it actively promotes technical expertise that works independently in parallel to other technical expertise. For this reason, collaboration and knowledge sharing are often minimized, paranoia between disciplines that do not communicate and interact can grow, and the system as a whole includes high levels of redundancy as multiple technical disciplines work to solve similar performance problems independently from each other.

Thirdly, a **matrix organization** represents a framework in which staff from different technical disciplines are divided into teams by project or specific focus (e.g., staff allocated to work with specific playing positions, or multidisciplinary groups working on injury prevention strategies) that are led by a project manager, who then reports to a functional manager or director. This approach can be considered a more interdisciplinary approach because it can operate using blended cross-discipline units instead of vertical silos. A matrix approach to IDTs can help to facilitate better, more open communication. It allows resources to be easily shifted to where they are most needed, and it promotes collaboration between different technical areas of expertise in order to provide solutions to specific tasks or performance-based questions. However, the matrix approach is at risk of creating confusion and frustration as a result of dueling priorities and many supervisors or managers moving their individual units or teams in different directions.

Finally, a **flat organization** structure shows few or no levels of priority between IDT members from different technical disciplines. Expertise is considered equal throughout, and all technical areas report to an agnostic performance director who sets goals and objectives that are universal for all. This flattened organizational structure empowers self-management and greater decision-making ability (i.e., innovation) for every team member. The framework reflects decentralized management, in which authority and decision making can be distributed throughout groups of self-organizing teams within the IDT, rather than being vested in a technical discipline hierarchy. It is possible within a flattened structure for specific technical areas to take a **situational lead** at appropriate times or under certain circumstances (e.g., a medical lead in the early phase of return to play), but the structure can then flex back to a flat framework once a solution to a given performance problem has been achieved or the issue is no longer prioritized (e.g., inclusion of sport scientists and strength and conditioning to elevate workload as an athlete transitions from clinical care to reconditioning). A flattened IDT model means that all technical disciplines are acknowledged as equal to one another, thereby befitting the concept that sport performance is a construct of many factors all working symbiotically together (see figure 30.2 on page 449). The flattened structure means that rather than seeking solutions to performance problems only within vertical silos (i.e., within a technical area of expertise), the model promotes horizontal interactions between IDT members in order to create performance solutions using a unified approach. Professional bias is minimized, objective targets are aligned for all team members rather than being different for each technical area, and collaboration and interdisciplinary or transdisciplinary activities become the norm. The flattened organization approach represents **holacracy**, a term given to team structures and processes that are aligned to operational needs (i.e., athlete-centered) and where team members work efficiently and effectively together (18, 25).

Holacracy

The paradigm of holacracy is an approach that best defines flattened interdisciplinary structures with the potential to have a significant impact on athletic performance standards. Holacracy can be defined as a way of structuring and running an organization that replaces conventional hierarchical management models and instead promotes the distribution of power throughout an organization, thereby giving individuals and teams freedom while staying aligned to the organizational mission (9). Holacracy promotes the following (25):

1. *Lean and adaptable organizations:* Within the fast-paced world of sport where decision making, monitoring, and evaluation are very transient, the ability of a group of support staff to be agile and dynamic is crucial for IDTs to be effective.

2. *Highly effective collaboration and communication:* As discussed throughout this chapter, the construct of sport is multifactorial. It is therefore critical that organizations promote collaboration between various technical disciplines as a means to formulate integrated solutions to the same performance-based problems.

3. *Clearly distributed authority:* Each medical service and sport science discipline has a role to play at different times along the pathway of sport mastery. For this reason, no one area of expertise can be perceived as more or less important than the next. Indeed, the requirement for each technical discipline is upregulated and downregulated at different times throughout training and competition. Distribution of authority is fundamental to an effective interdisciplinary approach to performance support.

4. *Purpose-driven work:* In order to influence performance standards, support services must be targeted in their approach and must directly affect the determinants of performance. By aligning performance services to the same purpose and performance objectives, work can be efficient, intentional, and impactful.

A holacratic approach to interdisciplinary support is advantageous in that it distributes leadership and authority throughout the IDT. This inspires a more open system whereby team members are better connected within the ever-changing environment of sport. The IDT becomes more agile and responsive. By energizing staff through the removal of top-down hierarchies and promoting integration and collaboration between technical areas that have traditionally worked independently of one another, individuals can better sense opportunities, called **tensions**, to improve

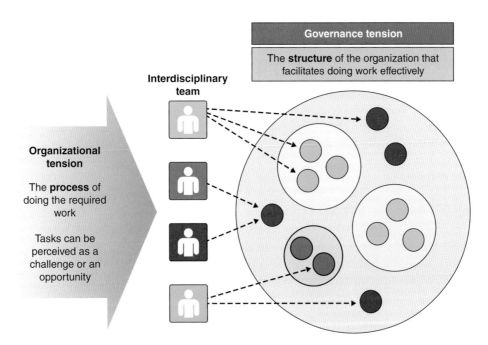

FIGURE 30.6 The Holacracy process. A representation of the "tensions" within a holacratic organizational structure; including organizational tension, or the specific *processes* that need to be performed, and governance tension, which defines the organizational *structure* adopted to facilitate these processes.

Small colored circles = individual roles; medium colored circles = teams or subdivisions; large circle = organization.

Interdisciplinary team: Yellow and green = one team member can have multiple roles; gray and red = one role can be filled by multiple team members.

service delivery and to better align with the specific needs of athletes (25). Holacracy divides these tensions into two categories: **operations tension** (i.e., the process of doing the required work), and **governance tension** (i.e., the structure of the organization that facilitates doing the work) (9, 19) (see figure 30.6).

To facilitate the execution of interventions that address these tensions within IDT operations, the various team members work together to evolve operations and governance processes and agree upon the situational roles that are needed at the specific stages of training and competition. As previously discussed, these roles will upregulate and downregulate based on the changing needs of the athlete or team. Each technical expert can synchronize discipline-specific information with the whole team and promote rapid decision making using transferable data to enable rapid feedback and action through dynamic steering techniques (19). Elsewhere, dynamic steering of governance tensions allows the quality of the IDT structure

to continually evolve and adapt by acknowledging and noting the various IDT experiences (i.e., responses to training interventions, competition performances). Tension is indeed critical within a high-functioning team. Tension that is well managed and not allowed to grow into a negative influence promotes positive actions such as intrinsic evaluation, questioning, and innovation. Indeed, from tension comes **emergence**, in which novel and coherent structures arise, and effective patterns and procedures become apparent during the process of self-organization of complex systems (i.e., problem solving) (3, 8).

Instead of a traditional top-down hierarchy that has a tendency to negate true interdisciplinary work, IDTs that adopt a holacratic approach to organization consist of self-organizing personnel who work in an innovative and collaborative fashion on unified goals and targets. Each role has a defined purpose, with explicit description of the work to be done and the necessary responsibilities and authority to fulfill the role (25), and this is agreed upon by the whole team. Decision making and the opportunity to act on tensions that team members feel at their level of the organization are then passed on to all members to address using their own professional expertise and skill sets. The team then self-organizes by addressing the energizing tensions that influence athletic performance. Information flows throughout all levels of the IDT and therefore provides a framework for efficient and highly targeted interdisciplinary solutions.

EVIDENCE-BASED PRACTICE

At the foundation of interdisciplinary support is the need for systematic **decision making**. All members of the IDT, including sport scientists, must develop an approach to making sound decisions with respect to assessment, diagnosis, intervention strategy, and the goals of their respective technical service (12). At the heart of decision making is **critical thinking**. Gambrill (7) defined critical thinking as "a unique kind of purposeful thinking in which we use standards such as clarity and fairness. It involves the careful examination and evaluation of beliefs and actions in order to arrive at well-reasoned decisions."

Critical thinking is a fundamental component of the scientific process, and sport science is no different. The process of science involves decision making and can be seen as a way of thinking about and actively investigating the world around us. The scientific method can be summarized as using four discreet steps: (a) selecting a problem, (b) defining questions about the problem by proposing a theory, (c) critically discussing and testing the theory, and (d) responding to flaws in the theory or new information by going back to the previous step and then working forward again (15). In contrast, **pseudoscience** can be defined as offering science-like claims and failing to provide evidence in support of those claims (11). Owing to things like tradition, "coaching eye," and coaching intuition, an overreliance on anecdotal evidence, a lack of critical skepticism, and a tendency to ignore data that is unsupportive of commonly held beliefs are commonplace in sport, even at the most elite levels. Coaches and athletes can hold on to well-established ideologies, rightly or wrongly, and this can present a significant challenge to overcome for the sport scientist and other IDT members. Indeed, these ingrained beliefs present barriers to critical thinking, logic, and scientific process, and they can ultimately suppress

valuable performance interventions that are backed by objective research findings and evidence.

In an effort to navigate around misconstrued information and anecdotal evidence, sport scientists and other members of the IDT are tasked with demonstrating that their insights and theories are based on sound evidence and that they have an impact on desired outcome goals and targets (6). By adopting scientific methods, IDTs should use critical thinking to engage in **evidence-based practice**, whereby they facilitate well-reasoned decisions through scientific research findings, including review of the literature, in order to create a clear understanding of how to best answer performance-based questions. Adopting evidence-based practice is a systematic method of reviewing the best evidence, combining it with art and intuition, and making informed choices to influence performance (1). Coutts (4) has perhaps given the most current definition of evidence-based practice relating to sport as "the integration of coaching expertise, athlete values, and the best relevant scientific and research evidence into the decision-making process for day-to-day service delivery to athletes."

Evidence-based practice should be considered nonnegotiable for IDT members in today's world of high-performance sport. It can help staff improve training and performance, reduce training errors (e.g., injuries and inappropriate training loads), help to balance known beliefs with risks in decision making, challenge belief-based views with appropriate evidence, and integrate athlete and coach preferences into decision making around approaches to training and performance (4). All of these things represent both operational and governance tensions that can be experienced by the IDT. Developing evidence-based practice within the IDT often involves many key stakeholders and follows an iterative process that includes the following:

- Identifying relevant performance-based questions to research
- Searching and critically evaluating any available evidence for its validity, impact, and applicability
- Developing strategies to implement the best available evidence into contemporary applied practice
- Assessing the effectiveness of the new practice in athletes
- Continuing to reevaluate and challenge the evidence and assess current practices

Evidence-based practice is essential for the sport scientist, as well as other medicine and allied science professionals within the IDT. The gap between research and practice inevitably culminates either in training methods that are well behind the most current state of scientific knowledge, or in outpacing research findings from laboratory-based research studies because innovative developments in training or competition mean that research cannot keep up with ever-changing innovations in sport. Evidence-based approaches to scientific investigation are vital in both these situations. Appropriate scientific evidence can be used either to minimize the disparity between existing scientific research and the practical application of research findings or to provide evidence that either confirms or dismisses an established anecdotal approach as valuable or not. This latter scenario is often referred to as **practice-based evidence**, whereby scientific investigation is used to corroborate that an exercise, drill, or technique is valuable or not—after it has already been put into use in an applied setting before any evidence attesting to worth. While much innovation in sport performance has evolved from a practice-based evidence approach, this strategy also risks a significant time investment in training interventions that are later proven by science to be ineffective.

To be truly impactful, interdisciplinary support structures should embrace a conscious choice to move away from professional practice that is based simply on tradition, ease of execution, or appeal to authority. Where this approach is the norm, professional decision making is typically based solely on expert testimonial, consensus, and habit (12). These approaches are at risk of modifying or misusing evidentiary findings that contradict practice styles, and justify the continuation of long-held yet questionable techniques and strategies. Instead, wherever possible, practitioners should seek to provide evidence that justifies and supports their theories and hypotheses through critical thinking and scientific processes of investigation. Evidence can be gathered through a host of appropriate methods; including literature searches, applied research projects, epidemiological data analysis, and larger controlled research studies in partnership with academic institutions.

CONCLUSION

For many athletes, coaches, clinicians, and performance science practitioners, an integrated and performance-focused approach to service provision remains a difficult concept. This is largely a consequence of historical discipline-specific perceptions, working environments that are not conducive to collaboration, and professional bias. Within such ecological constructs, which can be multidisciplinary but can lack an interdisciplinary approach, practitioners from different technical disciplines tend to work in silos, and each discipline focuses on its own evidence in order to have the final say on how best to create solutions to performance-based problems. Often the same problems are being addressed by many team members at the same time, independent of one another, thereby creating high levels of redundancy in the system. Indeed, multidisciplinary team members overlook the potential performance and psychological consequences when making decisions in isolation, with the preferences of athletes, coaches, and other team members excluded from consideration (5).

The most impactful, innovative, and efficient way to support an athlete or team is through an interdisciplinary athlete-centered organizational approach. Performance services that work in an interdisciplinary fashion demonstrate a holacratic or flattened organizational structure, in which leadership and authority are distributed throughout an IDT, and team members are better connected—thereby becoming more agile and innovative in their ability to respond to issues relating to performance. Hierarchy of services is largely removed, and all technical disciplines are perceived as having the same importance and impact. Within the interdisciplinary structure, technical disciplines collaborate to answer performance-based questions together, thereby increasing efficiency and focus but also stimulating innovation and unified goal setting. Through the use of evidence-based approaches to their work, in which anecdotal evidence and pseudoscience are replaced by theory, rationale, and supporting data as evidence, interdisciplinary teams can offer the highest level of influence on performance potential and the process of achieving success.

RECOMMENDED READINGS

Arnold, B, and Schilling, B. *Evidence-Based Practice in Sport and Exercise: A Guide to Using Research.* Philadelphia: F.A. Davis Company, 2016.

Coutts, A. Challenges in developing evidence-based practice in high-performance sport. *Int J Sport Physiol Perform* 12:717-718, 2017.

Dijkstra, H, Pollock, N, Chakraverty, R, and Alonso, J. Managing the health of the elite athlete: a new integrated performance health management and coaching model. *Br J Sports Med* 48:523-531, 2014.

Moreau, W, and Nabhan, D. Organizational and multidisciplinary work in Olympic high-performance centers in USA. *Rev Med Clin Condes* 23:337-342, 2012.

Reid, C, Stewart, E, and Thorne, G. Multidisciplinary sport science teams in elite sport: comprehension servicing or conflict and confusion? *Sport Psychol* 18:204-217, 2004.

CHAPTER 31

Information Dissemination

Yann Le Meur, PhD

Sport science has demonstrated a rapid growth since approximately 2010. During this period, the quantity of information available and the related ramifications (e.g., training methodology, motor skill learning, sport psychology, nutrition, recovery) increased exponentially. For instance, the number of scientific publications dedicated to team sports on the PubMed search engine increased from 104 in 1998 to 320 in 2009 and 1,253 in 2020. Many factors seem to be at play to explain such a trend. First, most scientific journals in sport science are reporting a sharp increase in the number of manuscripts they are receiving for publication. This increasing number of submissions seems to be associated with the increase in sport scientists and students within the field, but also due to easier access to technology that facilitates data collection. Secondly, a growing number of scientific journals dedicated to sport sciences are now available, offering more places to publish scientific research. Although this increase in the quantity of information available in sport sciences has some clear positive benefits, it is also associated with some limitations and drawbacks. It is important to address the issue of keeping the findings digestible and impactful for stakeholders operating in applied settings. This point is addressed in the first part of this chapter.

In a fashion similar to the way it has influenced the number of publications in sport science in this century, the sharp increase in technology available to sporting organizations had also had a strong impact on the quantity of information available for people working with athletes, especially at the highest level. Based on both subjective and objective data collection using multiple tools (e.g., apps, tracking systems, sensors), the sport scientist can now potentially provide significant amounts of information to coaches. When appropriately collected and interpreted, these reports should inform decision-making processes regarding the planning and manipulation of training. The appropriate use of analysis, visualization, and communication remains a real challenge, however, which is discussed later in this chapter.

MAXIMIZING THE IMPACT OF RESEARCH

One of the main aims of sport science research is to positively affect the decisions and practices of coaches and to support staff by challenging their methods and beliefs. Peer-reviewed journals serve as an anchor to centralize this knowledge, but evidence demonstrates that sport scientists can considerably maximize the impact of their research findings by dedicating time to disseminate them through more accessible and easy-to-digest media.

Traditionally the establishment of knowledge and scientific communication has been completed through peer-reviewed journal articles and publications. Publishing a study in an internationally peer-reviewed scientific journal can be considered the final step in a long process that characterizes research methodology. That includes the following steps:

- Identifying a solid and potentially impactful research question to address
- Developing hypotheses relating to the research question
- Designing the experimental protocol
- Conducting the experiment and analyzing the results
- Writing a scientific report
- Addressing the concerns raised during the peer-review process

- Publishing the findings and contributing to the scientific body of knowledge

When the final scientific manuscript has been accepted, the research process could be considered done. Nevertheless, publishing in a scientific journal clearly does not ensure that an article will be impactful, and most of the time research findings do not result in rapid, efficient changes of applied practice. While such a process has been important in ensuring scientific robustness, subscription-based publishing models and peer-review processes can take considerable time and can hinder the dissemination of research outputs to wider audiences. For instance, a study estimated that there is a 17-year lag between the completion of a research study and translation of this new evidence into the practices of medical professionals. Even then, the translation may be only partial at best (15).

Traditionally, the impact of a researcher's work is measured solely by publications (number of published articles and their impact factor) and citations (e.g., h-index, i10 index). Even if these metrics are good indicators of acceptance and uptake by the scientific community, they fail to capture the value of the research to nonacademic stakeholders involved in sport performance (e.g., coaches, physicians, physiotherapists, athletes). Most of the time, academic research takes years to reach publication, having before remained largely inaccessible to most coaches, athletes, and practitioners. In a study published in 2015, Stoszkowski and Collins (19) reported that most coaches do not particularly like or ascribe much importance to formal learning. The results indicated that academic journals were classified as the worst method for acquiring coaching knowledge, with only ~2% reporting that academic journals were their preferred method of acquiring such knowledge in a cohort of 320 participants (versus 42%, 12%, and 11% for peer discussion, books, and watching other coaches, respectively).

These findings bring into question whether the suggestion that coaches do not like formal learning is much less a comment about its effectiveness than about its quality or the way in which it is offered to coaches, or both. For example, when reporting reasons for their learning preferences, coaches clearly value the opportunity for social interaction and discussion. This is perhaps unsurprising, especially if one considers the convenience and ease of access indicated by the participants in the study (both common criticisms of formal methods of acquiring knowledge) (19). After all, coaches can get information relatively quickly and

efficiently from the other coaches that they interact with. Furthermore, such communication is likely to be more clearly applied (e.g., "If I were you, I would do this . . ." [i.e., procedural]) rather than more global (e.g., "You might like to consider . . ." [i.e., declarative]). Similarly, participants clearly attached more value to modes of learning that they viewed as being immediately relatable to the realities of their own coaching practice—another common criticism of academic journals or formal education courses (12, 21, 22).

In addition to the lack of transferability between scientific manuscripts and applied practices within sport, several other reasons can also be considered:

- When available, applied studies are diluted by research of lower practical interest, which does not address questions that practitioners have and contributes to disconnect with sport sciences from the field (3). It indeed appears that sport scientists often research what is relevant to their personal interests rather than those of the key stakeholders—defined as interesting rather than useful (10).

- Practitioners do not always understand all the information in academic journal articles due to the use of scientific jargon and complex terminology (14).

- The paper format is inappropriate and unengaging. Practitioners complain that most articles have long, dense blocks of text with minimal images (1), and more engaging formats like video remain extremely rare.

- Conducting a scientific survey and reading articles are time-consuming, and the key stakeholders involved in the performance process do not have enough time to perform this type of work.

- Many peer-reviewed scientific articles are protected by expensive subscriptions and memberships.

COMMUNICATING POTENTIAL SOLUTIONS

Theoretically, applied sport science research aims to produce an outcome that is relevant to sport for the purpose of enhancing performance. For this to be achieved, relevant information generated from applied studies must be communicated effectively to the key stakeholders involved in the performance process (14). There are opportunities for a more creative, dialogue-based relationship between sport scientists and the public, which would help overcome the knowledge gap and transform the deficit model of conducting and communicating science. As Grand and colleagues (8) argue, practicing science in the open can contribute to a more engaged, informed, and critical culture.

The Internet has also created new opportunities for open science and for the dissemination of research findings in more interactive ways, which could help overcome the knowledge gap and transform the traditional academic approach to conducting and communicating science. A larger variety of interactive media are now available, including social media, blogs, infographics, podcasts, videos, and audio abstracts, to name but a few. As indicated by Purdam and Zhu (18), there is clearly a link between these different approaches to communicating research, and therefore multiple formats and channels could potentially be used as part of an integrated communication process, with publication of journal articles as the anchor.

Open-Access Journals

Because one of the barriers that limits science dissemination is related to the ability to easily access scientific manuscripts, publishing in open-access journals can represent a good alternative that can maximize the visibility of a scientific article, simply because more people have access to it. In comparing the level of citations between open-access and subscription-based articles in journals from different disciplines, Norris (17) showed that full-text downloads of open-access papers were 89% higher, PDF downloads were 42% higher, and unique visitors were 23% higher than those for subscription-based articles. Publishing in open-access journals also seems to have a positive impact on the growth of citations and is associated with a more rapid communication process (2). Nevertheless, the cost associated with subscription-based publication can be prohibitive (with costs reaching $1,500-$5,000). Instead, some totally free access alternatives (e.g., *Sport Performance and Science Reports*) may represent a more appropriate solution that facilitates the dissemination of sport science to a broader audience. However, such initiatives remain in their infancy, and the near future will reveal if this kind of platform can succeed in building a solid reputation and finding its place next to well-established open-access and subscription-based journals.

Academic Social Networking Platforms

In the same way that open-access journals can facilitate access to academic publications, academic social networking platforms may also represent an interesting option for sport scientists wishing to disseminate their work in its academic format. Sites such as ResearchGate, Academia.edu, or Mendeley offer a valuable place to share papers, ask questions, receive answers, and interact with potential collaborators. A study by Niyazov and colleagues (16) showed that papers uploaded to Academia.edu received a 69% boost in citations in 5 years between 2009 and 2014. Nevertheless, while these platforms are likely to facilitate networking between academic and research scientists, the presence of practitioners involved in sport performance (e.g., coaches, physicians, physiotherapists) remains highly unlikely, suggesting that complementary methods should be investigated in order to better reach a nonacademic audience.

Social Media

Social media tools such as Facebook, Twitter, and Instagram have fundamentally affected the way people communicate since roughly 2010. The scientific community is no different, and these media provide new opportunities for open scientific communication, especially targeting nonacademic audiences. Among the different social media, Twitter in particular has emerged as the preferred social media platform for scientific communications and correspondence.

Using social media to leverage scientific communication also has the potential to lead to opportunities, exposure, and impact beyond scientific circles. Indeed, a study by Côté and Darling (6) showed that scientists with more than 1,000 Twitter followers reach a broad audience, including educational organizations, media, and members of the public—people who are unlikely to access research articles in scientific journals. However, presenting oneself as a scientist on social media can present some challenges, discussed in more detail by Burke (5):

- *Connectivity 24/7:* Relentless input from email, social media, and other sources with the expectation of an immediate response can promote a reactive rather than a proactive approach to scientific communication, with impulsive rather than considered outputs becoming the norm. This approach does not allow scientists to promote or defend theories and findings with appropriate depth and discussion.

- *Complex scientific issues reduced to sound bites:* The brevity of the communication styles enforced (e.g., 280 characters on Twitter at the time of this publication), or culturally determined by many platforms, leads to an oversimplification of issues and general support for black-and-white thinking and universal truths.

- *Celebrities assuming the role of science educators:* Actors, chefs, fitness trainers, and other individuals who have no scientific training have been allowed to exploit their fame, or create fame, to actively promote their opinions on health, diet, and exercise. These individuals are often judged to be the most powerful sources of information on complicated topics.

- *Celebrity scientists:* Television and social media have created opportunities for some scientists to become household names or to develop a huge following on social media platforms. While some of these scientists are outstanding researchers who can promote their fields and science in general, others do not represent mainstream views and promote their own ideologies and agendas. Audiences may have little appreciation of their professional biases.

- *Public distrust of industry-supported research:* Disclosure of anomalies or bias in some industry-funded research has caused a general backlash against funding sources, despite the research having been conducted with ethical rigor and impartiality. This is particularly difficult for sport science since its low-priority status within competitive grant agencies and academic funding bodies makes it more reliant on industry funding. Outcomes then include a reduction in research outputs and unfair dismissal of projects that have received industry support.

Tips for sport scientists to make good use of social media as a mechanism to disseminate scientific material are presented in figure 31.1 (5).

Infographics and Animations

Indirectly connected to social media is the use of another emerging method for distributing scientific information: the creation and dissemination, through social media, of so-called infographics and animations. Infographics are graphical visual representations of information, data, or knowledge with the intention to present content in a clear and succinct fashion (see figure 31.2). Animations are a form of video that uses text and moving images to enhance visual learning. Animations essentially serve as a dynamic version of infographics.

The concise format of infographics and animations is engaging and facilitates ease of knowledge transfer and retention. In fact, people are 6.5 times more likely to remember new information from an infographic or animation compared to reading the same information in text only (1). Malone and colleagues (13) confirmed that practitioners reported a preference toward this kind of media as a method of dissemination. Indeed, such methods are useful for simplifying the overall message to key stakeholders (e.g., coaches and athletes). The following list outlines some guidelines that people should adhere to in order to build an engaging and fair infographic:

1. Pick a topic by starting with the questions that coaches and support staffs are asking. Design an infographic for the audience.

2. Critique the original research before feeding it forward, and do not consider that the audience will necessarily do so.

3. Indicate the level of evidence within the article that the infographic is presenting, or at least be cautious with respect to the conclusions.

4. Cite all sources and encourage the audience to consult them.

5. Limit scientific jargon and adopt a vocabulary that end users will understand.

6. Limit highly mechanistic and basic science aspects.

7. Highlight the potential practical implications of what is being reported.

8. Invest energy in the style and design: Choose a template that fits with the organization of the ideas in the infographic, for example, the compilation of isolated arguments, logical sequence of ideas, and presentation of different points of view.

9. Choose illustrations to favor the reader's understanding and not only for visual embellishment; every element should actively contribute to the reader's understanding.

10. Use charts to highlight the key results when possible.

11. Limit the text length as much as possible.

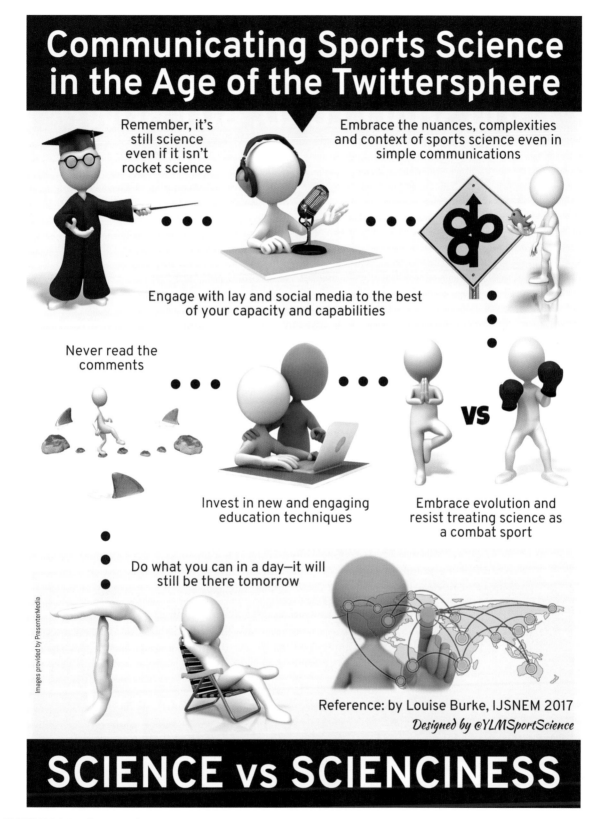

FIGURE 31.1 Communicating sport science in the age of the Twittersphere.

Data from LM Burke. (2017, pg. 1-5); designed by @YLMSportScience; provided with permission.

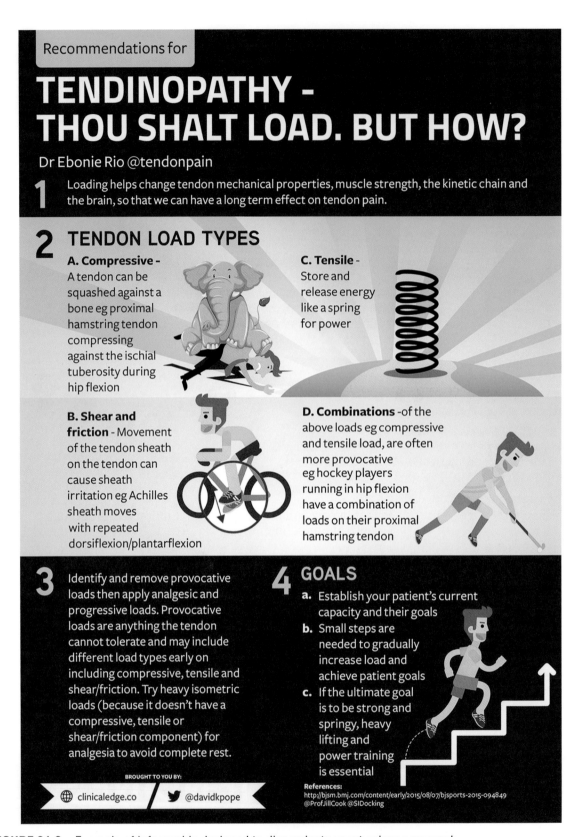

FIGURE 31.2 Example of infographic designed to disseminate sport science research.

Designed by @davidkpope; provided with permission.

12. Highlight the potential practical implications of what is being reported.

13. When finished with steps 1 through 12, take a 24-hour break from working on the infographic, then reevaluate to determine if all the components of the infographic are needed. If so, make refinements if possible.

As discussed by Impellizzeri (9), there is an inherent risk of oversimplification or misinterpretation, especially on the part of an audience not educated in science, with use of infographics and animations to disseminate scientific information. For this reason, it is important to take the following steps:

- Acknowledge that infographics and animations are a simplification of studies that are already adopting a simplified way to share the complex phenomena that scientists are trying to better understand.

- Encourage the reader to approach infographics and animations with a good degree of skepticism (infographics do not always highlight the biases and the limitations of the research that they are presenting, which may potentially give the findings an overemphasis that is not always commensurate to the real strength of the data and design).

- Encourage people not to infer too much from a single infographic or animation, and educate them on how to evaluate the level of evidence behind the scientific research being presented (some conclusions are robust, others less so; some conclusions can be generalized, others should not be).

- Balance the debate by designing infographics or animations on pros and cons on hot topics to help readers build their own opinion.

- Systematically encourage people to explore the scientific articles on which the infographics and animations are based by indicating the source on the infographic and adding a link to the original article in social media posts and blogs (i.e., the infographics should be viewed as a complement to and not a substitute for scientific articles—similar to the use of a trailer for promoting the launch of a movie).

Blogs and Vlogs

Blogs (usually <600 words) or **vlogs** (blogs based on video content) serve as an outlet for original thinking, promoting conversations around hot topics or summarizing key articles, and they can be an effective method for sharing information with the wider sport-performance community. Maintaining a blog, however, requires time, especially when compared to microblogging platforms like Twitter; but blogging does allow sport scientists to share more in-depth information than social media. As indicated by Dunleavy (7), blog posts represent a way to build knowledge of academic work, to increase the readership of useful articles and research reports, to build up citations, and to foster debate. Blogs generally make formal learning more palatable and applicable to sport scientists working in applied settings, perhaps by creating the opportunity to draw more effectively on examples and practical implications.

Eleven key points support the writing of blog articles (7)*:

1. Assume that a journal article is 8,000 words long. The task is to get to a decent version of it in 600 to 1,000 words, as quickly and painlessly as possible.

2. Begin by cutting out the whole of the methodology section—it may matter, but most readers will not care. If the methods are innovative, people will probably need to read the original article to make detailed sense of them. So briefly sum up the methods in intuitive terms within the post (and even then, more toward the end), and then link to the article, using an open-access version when possible.

3. Get rid of the long literature review at the beginning. In the blog context, no one cares about academic credentialing or point scoring. Also cut most of any closing discussion of how the results agree with or diverge from other people's work. A line or two somewhere near the start, and then two lines of closing thoughts or pointers at the end of the post, normally suffices.

4. Write a narrative heading that gives the essential message substantively. Try to tell readers very

---

*The eleven key points are adapted from (7) (Dunleavy P. How to write a blogpost from your journal article in eleven easy steps. https://blogs.lse.ac.uk/impactofsocialsciences/2016/01/25/how-to-write-a-blogpost-from-your-journal-article. January 2016.)

clearly and simply what was discovered. A meaningful message is needed, but it should be less than 280 characters; that way, the blog title can also be the tweet. Do not try just a single heading; experiment with 6 to 10 different variants to find one that really works.

5. Always try to include a "trailer" paragraph in the blog post that spells out, in no more than three or four lines, why the post is interesting and provides another take on what the key message is (without repeating the title wording). The task here is to evoke interest and give readers a good narrative steer that attracts them to the post and assures them that they will understand it.

6. Now comes the part in which the key findings and arguments are taken from the journal article to form the text body of the blog. What did the researchers discover or conclude? What points can be made about the key findings or conclusions? If the blog presents an argument, integrates ideas, or develops a theme, it is still important to have a clear and substantive summation of the central message. It is vital here to frontload the material, putting it into a very different sequence from the conventional article (which is end-loaded):

   - Start off in a high-impact way, ideally trying to begin with something motivating for readers: either a startling fact, a paradox resolved, a key summary statistic, or a great quote. For blog readers, something topical linking to a recent development is often a good start. Alternatively, promising readers a change in our knowledge, or other new things, is a great motivator. Once readers are hooked, it is acceptable to have a small amount of context here (3 or 4 lines) that draws out the salience of the issue. It is worthwhile writing a high-impact starting section carefully and trying to keep it punchy.

   - Explain early in the body text the core of the findings or argument from the journal version. Move straight to what worked in the research study, experiment, and archive search, for example, and tell readers clearly what was found or concluded. In a blog post, the best bits arrive early on, not just at the end. Cut any text from the article covering intermediate stages, or earlier models, or avenues taken that did not lead to results.

   - Once that is done, unpack the message a little, perhaps highlighting no more than three

specific aspects—ideally the aspects with the widest interest or appeal to readers, or the greatest claim to advance our knowledge.

7. Wherever possible, include at least one table or chart, maybe two or three, but try to avoid ever having more than four exhibits.

   - Explain tables or charts properly, label them very clearly, and simplify them if they are overly complex. Include a short explanatory note under each chart or table that explains what is being shown and helps readers to understand it. Make sure column or row headings in tables, as well as both the axis labels in charts, are crystal clear.

   - Look carefully at any chart or table that is being considered for inclusion and determine if all its components are really needed (e.g., are all the columns of the table needed, or could some intermediate ones be cut out to just show the columns with the final results?). Similarly, try to have simple charts, in which every bar or line is needed because it actively helps build readers' understanding; otherwise it gets cut.

   - The acid test for any exhibit is, "What do readers really need to know?"

8. Do not assume that readers know what is meant without explanation.

   - If specialist vocabulary ("jargon") is needed (e.g., in academic work), keep it to a minimum and explain all terms at first use that are likely to be unfamiliar.

   - Be especially careful with acronyms and initials and formulas. Do not explain the acronym or formula once and then use it 20 or 50 times. Explain once; then use the full expression (or refresh the explanation) every five or six times the acronym or formula is subsequently deployed.

   - Write shorter paragraphs than in a journal, say 150 words. But do not write text in which every sentence is its own paragraph. That style may work for press releases, but ordinary readers will quickly find it disorganizing. Proper paragraphs are units of thought; when written well, they give the blog text a subtle substructure that makes it far more understandable.

- In blog posts, all references are unobtrusive hyperlinks. The URL sits behind a relevant highlighted term or a short phrase. Of course, digital links go just to the top of the source cited.

9. Try to end the blog post in a decisive and interesting fashion, an ending that sums up and encapsulates the argument in a new and neat way, perhaps opening out to next steps or future developments. Again, try for a very well-written finish that leaves a good lasting impression with readers.

10. Below the post, give the title of the long article and a clear link to it, ideally a hyperlink to an open-access, full-text version.

11. Lastly, include a few (4 or 5) lines of bio-related information about the blog writer. Ideally this should include the writer's organizational position, a link to the writer's Twitter, Facebook, or email accounts, and perhaps a brief mention of recent books (hyperlink the titles) or other key works.

Podcasts

Whether they work in an academic environment or in a club, team, or federation, sport scientists are often engaged in multiple tasks and face busy schedules. These time constraints often make it difficult to find extra time to write blog articles or design infographics. In the same way, sport practitioners may not always have the time to actively follow many sources of information, especially when they can be time-consuming to digest (e.g., reading long blog articles or watching long videos). In this context, podcasts may represent an effective solution that allows sport scientists to share their ideas without dedicating significant amounts of time, while also allowing sport practitioners to consume them efficiently as they exercise (e.g., running, biking) or travel (e.g., in the car, a bus, a train, a plane). Like a blog article, podcasts allow experts to share their opinions and to provide anecdotes while adopting a more personalized tone than in academic journals. They can range from informal discussions on a broad topic to a deep dive into a specific research paper or topic.

DISSEMINATING INFORMATION TO THE PERFORMANCE TEAM

Due to the significant importance of effective information dissemination, this section repeats and reinforces concepts explained in chapter 21.

Thornton and colleagues (20) identified three sequential procedures:

1. Selecting what information is important to present
2. Identifying the most appropriate ways to present data
3. Communicating and delivering information effectively

The appreciation for and application of sport science support has grown exponentially beginning in the 1990s, especially in team sports. Despite the fact that the role of the sport scientists may differ between organizations, one of their main responsibilities is to monitor athletes' fitness and training. Monitoring data provides useful information to determine whether an athlete is responding appropriately to the demands of training and competition. Evaluating monitoring data is essential to ensure that athletes are training appropriately to face the requirements of competition, while also ensuring that they are appropriately adapting to the workload (20). This process should assist in maximizing the performance potential of athletes while minimizing the risk of overreaching or injury. From this perspective, sport scientists and support staff often collect a wide range of data reflecting the external and internal workloads that their athletes have undergone, as well as the physiological and psychological assessments of fatigue and physical performance. When appropriately collected and interpreted, these data should inform the decision-making process relating to the planning and manipulation of training.

Thornton and colleagues (20) provided a methodological outline that can help practitioners to develop and employ simple and effective feedback methods for coaches and athletes (see figure 31.3; 19). Their framework is composed of four steps:

1. Considerations for athlete monitoring
2. Methods of analyzing data
3. Determining meaningful changes in data
4. Establishing effective methods to present and communicate important information

Selecting Important Information for Presentation

As previously mentioned, the more data collected, the harder it often becomes to keep information succinct, straight to the point, and easy to digest. Sport scientists seek to explore and understand phenomena that are complex and multifaceted (e.g., fatigue, injury prevention); however, it is often difficult to restrict the number of key variables to report without making the report too simplistic. At the same time, the role of the sport scientist is to provide information to members of the coaching and medical staff in order to optimize their decision making, but not to make the decisions for them unless a decision is a part of the sport scientist's responsibilities. In this regard, workloads and wellness monitoring, for example, can be a primary concern for the sport scientist; but the medical staff can have different issues, such as an injured starting player, while elsewhere the coaches have a game to prepare for. Thus, it is necessary to reconsider how to simplify the reports and the key information shared during both meetings and informal discussions by concentrating on the information the audience needs to know. Producing straight-to-the-point and easy-to-digest reports requires time and effort and should encourage the sport scientist to frequently challenge the way various staff members interpret the reports and use them effectively to decide.

Identifying the Most Appropriate Ways to Present Data

Data and results can be presented in many different ways (4). Once the relevant questions have been identified, the best variables have been selected, and the appropriate statistics applied, the greatest challenge for sport scientists then becomes understanding the most efficient type of data visualization and reporting to get their message across. This is particularly important to

- help the staff to understand information quickly;
- tell a story;
- hold the audience's interest longer;
- ensure the retention of important information; and
- identify the outliers, which will often represent key information to consider (except when they are related to technical errors).

Three steps can be followed to achieve this goal:

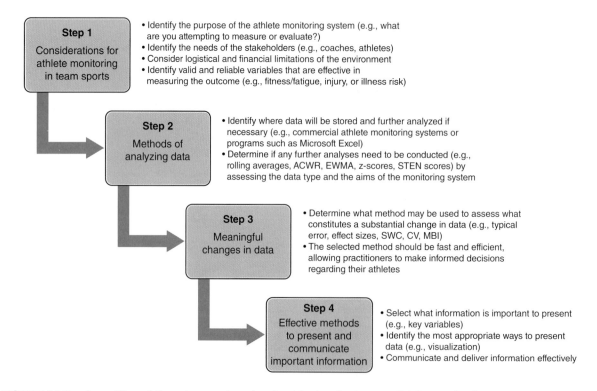

FIGURE 31.3   An outline of the primary steps involved in developing an athlete monitoring system.

ACWR, acute-to-chronic-workload ratio; EWMA, exponentially weighted moving averages; STEN, standard tens; SWC, smallest worthwhile change; CV, coefficient of variation; MBI, magnitude-based inferences.

Based on Thornton and colleagues (2019).

1. Select the starting point and develop technical skills.

   - Measure what matters most and evolve and improve the process from there.

   - Have three or four key bullet points highlighting the main information the report is intended to share, since some people may not take the time to read the report in full.

   - Use machine learning to identify the parameters that should be highlighted in reports, without losing too much information (e.g., principal component analysis, clustering).

   - Keep learning about metrics and potential new metrics, and about how to use them in reports.

   - Develop skills using resources that help to make the data analysis more time-efficient and the presentation effective. Examples include reports based on spreadsheets; software or environments based on programming language, focusing on statistical analysis (e.g., R, Python); and platforms for analysis and visual presentation (e.g., dashboards on PowerBI or Tableau). The idea is to make reports interactive and easy to share on different tools (PCs, tablets, smartphones).

   - If possible, ask for support from a data scientist to help with these challenges.

2. Know your audience and adapt your reports accordingly.

   - Narrow your target audience. Create different communications for different audiences. The more you know about your audience, the better.

   - Have discussions with the people who will receive the information and make sure that they think the reports are easy to digest and eye-catching. Constantly challenge reports being shared with staff members: Are they using a report? If they are not or only partially making use of it, make every attempt to understand why. Keep working hard to remedy the situation if the response is not satisfying. Finding the optimal option is often a rocky road requiring setting up a trial-and-error approach.

   - Match the message to coach and athlete expectations, preferences, and habits: visual versus verbal information, paper versus digital reports, quantitative versus qualitative interpretation, tables versus graphs (and types of graphs [e.g., bars versus radars]).

3. Reports should be as simple and as informative as possible ("simple but powerful").

   - Frequently, less is more. Even when collecting a great amount of data, focus on reporting only a few important data points (those that can be used to answer the questions that coaches and athletes have asked and can have an impact on the program).

   - Consider implementing traffic light systems in your tables. They convey athlete monitoring information in an easily interpretable manner.

   - Ensure that unnecessary noise is removed (such as decimal places).

   - Write all text horizontally for readability.

   - Add labels to graphs so that exact values can be seen too (graph for patterns, numbers for details, if required).

   - Highlight meaningful changes or differences to be seen at a glance (with different possible levels of data analysis).

   - Include error bars where possible to acknowledge uncertainty (typical error of the measurement and confidence intervals for individual and average values, respectively).

   - Univariate scatterplots or dot plots are recommended, showing the raw data when the sample size is small, or use box plots with interquartile ranges (25th and 75th percentile of the sample); whiskers may be included to demonstrate outliers.

   - Violin plots are effective in demonstrating the distribution of the data in medium and large sample sizes.

   - Bar graphs should be avoided in presenting continuous data, particularly with small sample sizes.

   - Be aware that compiling simple reports can become complex. To solve this, consider building interactive dashboards telling a story, rather than rigid reports.

Communicating and Delivering Information Effectively

As explained by Buchheit (4), the usefulness of sport scientists' work within a performance support team is strongly determined by their influence on the decisions made by the other stakeholders. Within this perspective, the ability of sport scientists to communicate with coaches, as well as members of the medical staff, is paramount. If they cannot create positive interest and interactions with the coaches and players, they will be challenged to get their message across (i.e., deliver), and their fancy reports with high-quality stats will largely be rendered worthless and likely end up in the trash. In the same way, the athletes are the most important piece of the puzzle when it comes to sport performance. An organization can have the best facilities, the latest technology, or the coolest wearables, but if the players do not want to use these resources and the technology is in a storage room gathering dust, that will also be of no help (11).

Understanding the culture of a sport or a very specific community of athletes takes many years. Having the respect and trust of high-profile athletes is often more a matter of personality and behavior than scientific knowledge and skills. Here are a few tips that may help create bridges (11):

- Understand and respect the work of others.
- Learn from the expertise and experience of others. Share personal experience and expertise.
- Do what is needed to be viewed as a resource, not as a constraint. Ask people how to best help them or how to work in a way that is complementary to theirs.
- Identify the best ambassadors on the staff and those who are less interested or reluctant. Drive projects with the former while remaining ready to collaborate with the latter.
- Be empathic with other staff members when the aim is to implement something new and suggest accordingly. Understanding is the most important step in communication.
- Accept and support the staff decision, including instances when they do not follow suggestions in a report.
- Work on patience and tolerance of frustration. The information is only one piece of the puzzle.
- Demonstrate emotional stability and keep smiling. Circumstances are never perfect, but one's attitude can be.

- Be fair and reliable, including (especially) in the bad moments.
- Recognize when a communication contains a mistake or when no answer to a question has emerged.
- Share reports quickly but double-check before sending them.

EVOLUTION OF INFORMATION DISSEMINATION

The media and software available to disseminate information are constantly evolving. Who could have said back in the day that social media, podcasts, blogs, and infographics would play such a role in disseminating sport science today? It is unlikely that the reality of tomorrow will be exactly the same as today. Within this perspective, being curious and open-minded, without compromising ideas because of trends in fashion, is probably a key to staying innovative and proactive at sharing sport science. Since it is not possible to invest in each new medium of communication, the best solution is probably to estimate the potential of each platform to connect with the targeted audience, the time required to build a solid community on that platform, and the time required to produce content appropriate to the platform. The mediums demonstrating the best balance of these three factors will probably represent the best options in which to invest time and energy.

CONCLUSION

Whether sport scientists are involved in an academic environment or part of an applied high-performance team, their role should always be to maximize their efforts to support improved decision making and practices of the audience (i.e., students, staff members, athletes). Within this perspective, publishing scientific articles or producing generic monitoring reports is very likely to be insufficient, when the intention is to have a real impact. This should push sport scientists to go further with regard to the implementation of effective methods of dissemination to connect with the world around them. Identifying the barriers that are limiting dissemination of the information and the buy-in of the targeted audience is certainly the first step to identify appropriate strategies and to build a plan. It requires observation and empathy, but also a certain ability to question oneself and to recognize what one could improve to communicate better. Whether it is about highlighting novelties in sport science research or sharing a training report, information dissemination is about psychology and about understanding the way the targeted stakeholders behave, and think, and about identifying which solution may push them to benefit from the information that sport science can provide. Since the initial academic education that most sport scientists receive does not deal with this dimension, it appears essential that sport scientists stay curious and creative and keep challenging themselves in order to develop their ability to communicate effectively. This is true especially when they observe that their impact remains limited. Being aware that this aspect is critical if sport scientists want to have an opinion about what matters.

RECOMMENDED RESOURCES

Type	Source	Focus
Blogs	https://complementarytraining.net/	Physical preparation and sport science
	https://martin-buchheit.net/	Training and sport science
	https://jbmorin.net/	Training and sport science
	https://hiitscience.com/	Training and sport science
	http://sportsdiscovery.net/journal/	Training and sport science
	www.clinicaledge.co	Physiotherapy
Infographics	https://ylmsportscience.com	Sport science
	http://adamvirgile.com/	Sport science
	https://mysportscience.com	Sport nutrition
	www.clinicaledge.co	Physiotherapy
	www.strengthandconditioningresearch.com/	Strength and conditioning
Videos	www.youtube.com/user/ExcelTricksforSports	Training monitoring
	www.clinicaledge.co	Physiotherapy
	https://footballscienceinstitute.com/	Training and sport science in football
Podcasts	https://paceyperformancepodcast.podbean.com/	High performance
	www.supportingchampions.co.uk/podcast	High performance
	http://feeds.bmj.com/bjsm/podcasts	Sport medicine
	https://guruperformance.com/podcasts/	Sport nutrition

REFERENCES

Preface

1. Bishop, D. An applied research model for the sport sciences. *Sports Med* 38:253-263, 2008.

2. Bishop, D, Burnett, A, Farrow, D, Gabbett, T, and Newton, R. Sports-science roundtable: does sport-science research influence practice? *Int J Sports Physiol Perform* 1:161-168, 2006.

3. Haff, GG. Sport science. *Strength Cond J* 32:33-45, 2010.

4. Masic, I, Miokovic, M, and Muhamedagic, B. Evidence based medicine: new approaches and challenges. *Acta Inform Med* 16:219-225, 2008.

5. Messersmith, LL. A study of the distance traveled by basketball players. *Res Q* 15:29-37, 1944.

6. Messersmith, LL, and Fay, P. Distances traversed by football players. *Res Q* 1:78-80, 1932.

7. Swisher, A. Practice-based evidence. *Cardiopul Phys Ther J* 21:4, 2010.

8. Ward, P, Windt, J, and Kempton, T. Business intelligence: how sport scientists can support organization decision making in professional sport. *Int J Sports Physiol Perform* 14:544-546, 2019.

Chapter 1

1. Coutts, AJ. Working fast and working slow: the benefits of embedding research in high performance sport. *Int J Sport Physiol Perform* 11:1-2, 2016.

2. Dellaserra, CL, Gao, Y, and Ransdell, L. Use of integrated technology in team sports: a review of opportunities, challenges, and future directions for athletes. *J Strength Cond Res* 28:556-573, 2014.

3. Diebold, FX, Doherty, NA, and Herring, RJ. *The Known, the Unknown, and the Unknowable in Financial Risk Management: Measurement and Theory Advancing Practice*. Princeton, NJ: Princeton University Press, 59-73, 2010.

4. Kahneman, D. *Thinking, Fast and Slow*. New York: Farrar, Strauss and Giroux, 115-199, 2011.

5. Le Meur, Y, and Torres-Ronda, L. 10 Challenges facing today's applied sport scientist. *Sport Perform Sci Rep* 57:v1, 2019. https://sportperfsci.com/10-challenges-facing-todays-applied-sport-scientist/.

6. Nancarrow, SA, Booth, A, Ariss, S, Smith, T, Enderby, P, and Roots, A. Ten principles of good interdisciplinary team work. *Hum Resour Health* 11:19, 2013.

7. Senge, PM. *The Fifth Discipline: The Art & Practice of the Learning Organization*. Broadway Business, 174-204, 2006.

8. Torres-Ronda, L, and Schelling, X. Critical process for the implementation of technology in sport organizations. *Strength Cond J* 39:54-59, 2017.

Chapter 2

1. Abbis, CR, and Laursen, PB. Models to explain fatigue during prolonged endurance cycling. *Sports Med* 35:865-898, 2005.

2. Akenhead, R, and Nassis, GP. Training load and player monitoring in high-level football: current practice and perceptions. *Int J Sports Physiol Perform* 11:587-593, 2016.

3. Akubat, I, Barrett, S, and Abt, G. Integrating the internal and external training loads in soccer. *Int J Sports Physiol Perform* 9:457-462, 2014.

4. Appleby, BB, Cormack, SJ, and Newton, RU. Reliability of squat kinetics in well-trained rugby players: implications for monitoring training. *J Strength Cond Res* 33:2635-2640, 2019.

5. Aubry, A, Hausswirth, C, Louis, J, Coutts, AJ, and Le Meur, Y. Functional overreaching: the key to peak performance during the taper? *Med Sci Sports Exerc* 46:1769-1777, 2014.

6. Aughey, RJ, and Falloon, C. Real-time versus post-game GPS data in team sports. *J Sci Med Sport* 13:348-349, 2010.

7. Badin, OO, Smith, MR, Conte, D, and Coutts, AJ. Mental fatigue: impairment of technical performance in small-sided soccer games. *Int J Sports Physiol Perform* 11:1100-1105, 2016.

8. Banister, E, Calvert, T, Savage, M, and Bach, T. A systems model of training for athletic performance. *Aust J Sports Med* 7:57-61, 1975.

9. Banyard, HG, Nosaka, K, Sato, K, and Haff, GG. Validity of various methods for determining velocity, force, and power in the back squat. *Int J Sports Physiol Perform* 12:1170-1176, 2017.

10. Barrett, S, Midgley, A, Reeves, M, Joel, T, Franklin, E, Heyworth, R, Garrett, A, and Lovell, R. The within-match patterns of locomotor efficiency during professional soccer match play: implications for injury risk? *J Sci Med Sport* 19:810-815, 2016.

11. Bellenger, CR, Fuller, JT, Thomson, RL, Davison, K, Robertson, EY, and Buckley, JD. Monitoring athletic training status through autonomic heart rate regulation: a systematic review and meta-analysis. *Sports Med* 46:1461-1486, 2016.

12. Bompa, TO, and Haff, GG. *Periodization: Theory & Methodology of Training*. Champaign, IL: Human Kinetics, 14, 2009.

13. Borresen, J, and Lambert, MI. The quantification of training load, the training response and the effect on performance. *Sports Med* 39:779-795, 2009.

14. Bourdon, PC, Cardinale, M, Murray, A, Gastin, P, Kellmann, M, Varley, MC, Gabbett, TJ, Coutts, AJ, Burgess, DJ, and Gregson, W. Monitoring athlete training loads: consensus statement. *Int J Sports Physiol Perform* 12:S2161-S2170, 2017.

15. Boyd, LJ, Ball, K, and Aughey, RJ. The reliability of MinimaxX accelerometers for measuring physical activity in Australian football. *Int J Sports Physiol Perform* 6:311-321, 2011.

16. Brown, DM, Dwyer, DB, Robertson, SJ, and Gastin, PB. Metabolic power method: underestimation of energy expenditure in field-sport movements using a global positioning system tracking system. *Int J Sports Physiol Perform* 11:1067-1073, 2016.

17. Buchheit, M. Monitoring training status with HR measures: do all roads lead to Rome? *Front Physiol* 5(73):1-19, 2014.

18. Buchheit, M. Want to see my report, coach? *Aspetar Sports Med J* 6:36-43, 2017.

19. Buchheit, M, Al Haddad, H, Simpson, BM, Palazzi, D, Bourdon, PC, Di Salvo, V, and Mendez-Villanueva, A. Monitoring accelerations with GPS in football: time to slow down? *Int J Sports Physiol Perform* 9:442-445, 2014.

20. Buchheit, M, Gray, A, and Morin, J-B. Assessing stride variables and vertical stiffness with GPS-embedded accelerometers: preliminary insights for the monitoring of neuromuscular fatigue on the field. *J Sports Sci Med* 14:698, 2015.

21. Buchheit, M, and Simpson, BM. Player-tracking technology: half-full or half-empty glass? *Int J Sports Physiol Perform* 12:S235-S241, 2017.

22. Budgett, R, Newsholme, E, Lehmann, M, Sharp, C, Jones, D, Jones, T, Peto, T, Collins, D, Nerurkar, R, and White, P. Redefining the overtraining syndrome as the unexplained underperformance syndrome. *Br J Sports Med* 34:67-68, 2000.

23. Busso, T. Variable dose-response relationship between exercise training and performance. *Med Sci Sports Exerc* 35:1188-1195, 2003.

24. Canfield, AA. The "sten" scale-a modified C-Scale. *Educ Psychol Meas* 11:295-297, 1951.

25. Cardinale, M, Newton, R, and Nosaka, K. *Strength and Conditioning: Biological Principles and Practical Applications.* Hoboken, NJ: John Wiley & Sons, 338-339, 2011.

26. Chiu, LZF, and Barnes, JL. The fitness-fatigue model revisited: implications for planning short- and long-term training. *Strength Cond J* 25:42-51, 2003.

27. Claudino, JG, Cronin, J, Mezêncio, B, McMaster, DT, McGuigan, M, Tricoli, V, Amadio, AC, and Serrão, JC. The countermovement jump to monitor neuromuscular status: a meta-analysis. *J Sci Med Sport* 20:397-402, 2017.

28. Claudino, J, Mezêncio, B, Soncin, R, Ferreira, J, Couto, B, and Szmuchrowski, L. Pre vertical jump performance to regulate the training volume. *Int J Sports Med* 33:101-107, 2012.

29. Colby, MJ, Dawson, B, Peeling, P, Heasman, J, Rogalski, B, Drew, MK, and Stares, J. Improvement of prediction of noncontact injury in elite Australian footballers with repeated exposure to established high-risk workload scenarios. *Int J Sports Physiol Perform* 13:1130-1135, 2018.

30. Cormack, SJ, Mooney, MG, Morgan, W, and McGuigan, MR. Influence of neuromuscular fatigue on accelerometer load in elite Australian football players. *Int J Sports Physiol Perform* 8:373-378, 2013.

31. Cormack, SJ, Newton, RU, and McGuigan, MR. Neuromuscular and endocrine responses to an elite Australian Rules football match. *Int J Sports Physiol Perform* 3:359-374, 2008.

32. Cormack, SJ, Newton, RU, McGuigan, MR, and Cormie, P. Neuromuscular and endocrine responses of elite players during an Australian Rules football season. *Int J Sports Physiol Perform* 3:439-453, 2008.

33. Cormack, SJ, Newton, RU, and McGuigan, MR. Neuromuscular and endocrine responses of elite players to an Australian Rules football match. *Int J Sports Physiol Perform* 3:359-374, 2008.

34. Cormack, SJ, Smith, RL, Mooney, MM, Young, WB, and O'Brien, BJ. Accelerometer load as a measure of activity profile in different standards of netball match play. *Int J Sports Physiol Perform* 9:283-291, 2014.

35. Coutts, AJ, Crowcroft, S, and Kempton, T. Developing athlete monitoring systems: theoretical basis and practical applications. In: *Sport, Recovery and Performance: Interdisciplinary Insights.* Kellmann, M and Beckmann, J, eds. Abingdon, UK: Routledge, 19-32, 2018.

36. Coutts, AJ, and Duffield, R. Validity and reliability of GPS devices for measuring movement demands of team sports. *J Sci Med Sport* 13:133-135, 2010.

37. Coutts, AJ, Kempton, T, Sullivan, C, Bilsborough, J, Cordy, J, and Rampinini, E. Metabolic power and energetic costs of professional Australian football match-play. *J Sci Med Sport* 18:219-224, 2015.

38. Crowcroft, S, McCleave, E, Slattery, K, and Coutts, AJ. Assessing the measurement sensitivity and diagnostic characteristics of athlete-monitoring tools in national swimmers. *Int J Sports Physiol Perform* 12:S295-S2100, 2017.

39. Cunanan, AJ, DeWeese, BH, Wagle, JP, Carroll, KM, Sausaman, R, Hornsby, WG, Haff, GG, Triplett, NT, Pierce, KC, and Stone, MH. The general adaptation syndrome: a foundation for the concept of periodization. *Sports Med* 48:787-797, 2018.

40. Delaney, JA, Duthie, GM, Thornton, HR, and Pyne, DB. Quantifying the relationship between internal and external work in team sports: development of a novel training efficiency index. *Sci Med Football* 2:149-156, 2018.

41. Delaney, JA, Scott, TJ, Thornton, HR, Bennett, KJ, Gay, D, Duthie, GM, and Dascombe, B. Establishing duration-specific running intensities from match-play analysis in rugby league. *Int J Sports Physiol Perform* 10:725-731, 2015.

42. di Prampero, PE, and Osgnach, C. Metabolic power in team sports-part 1: an update. *Int J Sports Med* 39:581-587, 2018.

43. Drew, MK, and Finch, CF. The relationship between training load and injury, illness and soreness: a systematic and literature review. *Sports Med* 46:861-883, 2016.

44. Driller, MW, Mah, CD, and Halson, SL. Development of the athlete sleep behavior questionnaire: a tool for identifying maladaptive sleep practices in elite athletes. *Sleep Sci* 11:37, 2018.

45. Eckard, TG, Padua, DA, Hearn, DW, Pexa, BS, and Frank, BS. The relationship between training load and injury in athletes: a systematic review. *Sports Med* 48:1929-1961, 2018.

46. Edwards, S, White, S, Humphreys, S, Robergs, R, and O'Dwyer, N. Caution using data from triaxial accelerometers housed in player tracking units during running. *J Sports Sci* 37:810-818, 2019.

47. Enoka, RM, and Duchateau, J. Muscle fatigue: what, why and how it influences muscle function. *J Physiol* 586:11-23, 2008.

48. Enoka, RM, and Duchateau, J. Translating fatigue to human performance. *Med Sci Sports Exerc* 48:2228, 2016.

49. Falbriard, M, Meyer, F, Mariani, B, Millet, GP, and Aminian, K. Accurate estimation of running temporal parameters using foot-worn inertial sensors. *Front Physiol* 9:610, 2018.

50. Fanchini, M, Rampinini, E, Riggio, M, Coutts, AJ, Pecci, C, and McCall, A. Despite association, the acute: chronic work load ratio does not predict non-contact injury in elite footballers. *Sci Med Football* 2:108-114, 2018.

51. Fowles, JR. Technical issues in quantifying low-frequency fatigue in athletes. *Int J Sports Physiol Perform* 1:169-171, 2006.

52. Fox, JL, Stanton, R, Sargent, C, Wintour S-A, and Scanlan, AT. The association between training load and performance in team sports: a systematic review. *Sports Med* 48:2743-2774, 2018.

53. Gallo, TF, Cormack, SJ, Gabbett, TJ, and Lorenzen, CH. Pre-training perceived wellness impacts training output in Australian football players. *J Sports Sci* 34:1445-1451, 2016.

54. Garrett, J, Graham, SR, Eston, RC, Burgess, DJ, Garrett, LJ, Jakeman, J, and Norton, K. Comparison of a countermovement jump test and submaximal run test to quantify the sensitivity for detecting practically important changes within high-performance Australian Rules football. *Int J Sports Physiol Perform* 15(1):68-72, 2020.

55. Garrett, J, Graham, SR, Eston, RC, Burgess, DJ, Garrett, LJ, Jakeman, J, and Norton, K. A novel method of assessment for monitoring neuromuscular fatigue within Australian Rules football players. *Int J Sports Physiol Perform* 14(5):598-605, 2019.

56. Gastin, PB, McLean, O, Spittle, M, and Breed, RV. Quantification of tackling demands in professional Australian football using integrated wearable athlete tracking technology. *J Sci Med Sport* 16:589-593, 2013.

57. Gathercole, R, Sporer, B, Stellingwerff, T, and Sleivert, G. Alternative countermovement-jump analysis to quantify

acute neuromuscular fatigue. *Int J Sports Physiol Perform* 10:84-92, 2015.

58. Gathercole, RJ, Sporer, BC, Stellingwerff, T, and Sleivert, GG. Comparison of the capacity of different jump and sprint field tests to detect neuromuscular fatigue. *J Strength Cond Res* 29:2522-2531, 2015.

59. Gescheit, DT, Cormack, SJ, Duffield, R, Kovalchik, S, Wood, TO, Omizzolo, M, and Reid, M. A multi-year injury epidemiology analysis of an elite national junior tennis program. *J Sci Med Sport* 22:11-15, 2019.

60. Gibson, NE, Boyd, AJ, and Murray, AM. Countermovement jump is not affected during final competition preparation periods in elite rugby sevens players. *J Strength Cond Res* 30:777-783, 2016.

61. Graham, SR, Cormack, S, Parfitt, G, and Eston, R. Relationships between model estimates and actual match-performance indices in professional Australian footballers during an in-season macrocycle. *Int J Sports Physiol Perform* 13:339-346, 2018.

62. Graham, SR, Cormack, S, Parfitt, G, and Eston R. Relationships between model-predicted and actual match-play exercise-intensity performance in professional Australian footballers during a preseason training macrocycle. *Int J Sports Physiol Perform* 14:232-238, 2019.

63. Haff, GG, and Triplett, NT. *Essentials of Strength Training and Conditioning.* 4th ed. Champaign, IL: Human Kinetics, 249-316, 2016.

64. Halson, SL. Monitoring training load to understand fatigue in athletes. *Sports Med* 44:139-147, 2014.

65. Halson, SL, and Jeukendrup, AE. Does overtraining exist?: an analysis of overreaching and overtraining research. *Sports Med* 34:967-981, 2004.

66. Heidari, J, Beckmann, J, Bertollo, M, Brink, M, Kallus, KW, Robazza, C, and Kellmann, M. Multidimensional monitoring of recovery status and implications for performance. *Int J Sports Physiol Perform* 14:2-8, 2019.

67. Hellard, P, Avalos, M, Lacoste, L, Barale, F, Chatard, JC, and Millet, GP. Assessing the limitations of the Banister model in monitoring training. *J Sports Sci* 24:509-520, 2006.

68. Hoffman, DT, Dwyer, DB, Bowe, SJ, Clifton, P, and Gastin, PB. Is injury associated with team performance in elite Australian football? 20 years of player injury and team performance data that include measures of individual player value. *Br J Sports Med* 54:475-479, 2020.

69. Hopkins, WG. A new view of statistics. Internet Society for Sport Science, 2000. www.sportsci.org/resource/stats.

70. Houghton, L, and Dawson, B. Recovery of jump performance after a simulated cricket batting innings. *J Sports Sci* 30:1069-1072, 2012.

71. Hulin, BT, Gabbett, TJ, Johnston, RD, and Jenkins, DG. Wearable microtechnology can accurately identify collision events during professional rugby league match-play. *J Sci Med Sport* 20:638-642, 2017.

72. Impellizzeri, FM, Marcora, SM, and Coutts, AJ. Internal and external training load: 15 years on. *Int J Sports Physiol Perform* 14:270-273, 2019.

73. Impellizzeri, FM, Rampinini, E, and Marcora, SM. Physiological assessment of aerobic training in soccer. *J Sports Sci* 23:583-592, 2005.

74. Impellizzeri, F, Woodcock, S, Coutts, AJ, Fanchini, M, McCall, A, and Vigotsky, A. Acute to random workload ratio is "as" associated with injury as acute to actual chronic workload ratio: time to dismiss ACWR and its components. 2020. [e-pub ahead of print].

75. Jennings, D, Cormack, S, Coutts, AJ, Boyd, LJ, and Aughey, RJ. The validity and reliability of GPS units for measuring distance in team sport running patterns. *Int J Sports Physiol Perform* 5:328-341, 2010.

76. Johnston, RD, Gabbett, TJ, Jenkins, DG, and Hulin, BT. Influence of physical qualities on post-match fatigue in rugby league players. *J Sci Med Sport* 18:209-213, 2015.

77. Johnston, RJ, Watsford, ML, Pine, MJ, Spurrs, RW, Murphy, AJ, and Pruyn, EC. The validity and reliability of 5-Hz global positioning system units to measure team sport movement demands. *J Strength Cond Res* 26:758-765, 2012.

78. Kallus, K, and Kellmann, M. *The Recovery-Stress-Questionnaire for Athletes User Manual.* Champaign, IL: Human Kinetics, 92-96, 2001.

79. Kellmann, M. Preventing overtraining in athletes in high-intensity sports and stress/recovery monitoring. *Scand J Med Sci Sports* 20:95-102, 2010.

80. Kempton, T, Sirotic, AC, Rampinini, E, and Coutts, AJ. Metabolic power demands of rugby league match play. *Int J Sports Physiol Perform* 10:23-28, 2015.

81. Lamberts, RP, Lemmink, K, Durandt, JJ, and Lambert, MI. Variation in heart rate during submaximal exercise: implications for monitoring training. *J Strength Cond Res* 18:641-645, 2004.

82. Lamberts, RP, Maskell, S, Borresen, J, and Lambert, MI. Adapting workload improves the measurement of heart rate recovery. *Int J Sports Med* 32:698-702, 2011.

83. Lamberts, R, Swart, J, Capostagno, B, Noakes, T, and Lambert, M. Heart rate recovery as a guide to monitor fatigue and predict changes in performance parameters. *Scand J Med Sci Sports* 20:449-457, 2010.

84. Lee, JB, Sutter, KJ, Askew, CD, and Burkett, BJ. Identifying symmetry in running gait using a single inertial sensor. *J Sci Med Sport* 13:559-563, 2010.

85. Le Meur, Y, Louis, J, Aubry, A, Guéneron, J, Pichon, A, Schaal, K, Corcuff, J-B, Hatem, SN, Isnard, R, and Hausswirth, C. Maximal exercise limitation in functionally overreached triathletes: role of cardiac adrenergic stimulation. *J Appl Physiol* 117:214-222, 2014.

86. Lolli, L, Batterham, AM, Hawkins, R, Kelly, DM, Strudwick, AJ, Thorpe, R, Gregson, W, and Atkinson, G. Mathematical coupling causes spurious correlation within the conventional acute-to-chronic workload ratio calculations. *Br J Sports Med* 53:921-922, 2019.

87. Main, L, and Robert, GJ. A multi-component assessment model for monitoring training distress among athletes. *Eur J Sport Sci* 9:195-202, 2009.

88. Malone, JJ, Murtagh, CF, Morgans, R, Burgess, DJ, Morton, JP, and Drust, B. Countermovement jump performance is not affected during an in-season training microcycle in elite youth soccer players. *J Strength Cond Res* 29:752-757, 2015.

89. Marcora, SM. Do we really need a central governor to explain brain regulation of exercise performance? *Eur J Appl Physiol* 104:929, 2008.

90. Marcora, SM, and Staiano W. The limit to exercise tolerance in humans: mind over muscle? *Eur J Appl Physiol* 109:763-770, 2010.

91. Marcora, SM, Staiano, W, and Manning, V. Mental fatigue impairs physical performance in humans. *J Appl Physiol* 106:857-864, 2009.

92. Marrier, B, Le Meur, Y, Robineau, J, Lacome, M, Couderc, A, Hausswirth, C, Piscione, J, and Morin, J-B. Quantifying neuromuscular fatigue induced by an intense training session in rugby sevens. *Int J Sports Physiol Perform* 12:218-223, 2017.

93. McLean, BD, Coutts, AJ, Kelly, V, McGuigan, MR, and Cormack, SJ. Neuromuscular, endocrine, and perceptual fatigue responses during different length between-match microcycles in professional rugby league players. *Int J Sports Physiol Perform* 5:367-383, 2010.

94. McNair, DM, Lorr, M, and Droppleman, LF. *EITS Manual for the Profile of Mood States.* San Diego: Educational and Industrial Testing Services, 1-27, 1971.

95. McNamara, DJ, Gabbett, TJ, Chapman, P, Naughton, G, and Farhart, P. The validity of microsensors to automatically detect bowling events and counts in cricket fast bowlers. *Int J Sports Physiol Perform* 10:71-75, 2015.

96. Mooney, M, Cormack, S, O'Brien, B, Morgan, W, and McGuigan, M. Impact of neuromuscular fatigue on match exercise intensity in elite Australian football. *J Strength Cond Res* 27:166-173, 2013.

97. Mooney, MG, Cormack, S, O'Brien, BJ, Morgan, WM, and McGuigan, M. Impact of neuromuscular fatigue on match exercise intensity and performance in elite Australian football. 27:166-173, 2013.

98. Mooney, M, O'Brien, B, Cormack, S, Coutts, A, Berry, J, and Young, W. The relationship between physical capacity and match performance in elite Australian football: a mediation approach. *J Sci Med Sport* 14:447-452, 2011.

99. Morton, R, Fitz-Clarke, J, and Banister, E. Modeling human performance in running. *J Appl Physiol* 69:1171-1177, 1990.

100. Mujika, I. Quantification of training and competition loads in endurance sports: methods and applications. *Int J Sports Physiol Perform* 12:S29-S217, 2017.

101. Murray, A, Buttfield, A, Simpkin, A, Sproule, J, and Turner, AP. Variability of within-step acceleration and daily wellness monitoring in collegiate American football. *J Sci Med Sport* 22:488-493, 2019.

102. Murray, NB, Gabbett, TJ, and Townshend, AD. Relationship between preseason training load and in-season availability in elite Australian football players. *Int J Sports Physiol Perform* 12:749-755, 2017.

103. Neupert, EC, Cotterill, ST, and Jobson, SA. Training-monitoring engagement: an evidence-based approach in elite sport. *Int J Sports Physiol Perform* 14:99-104, 2019.

104. Nicol, C, Avela, J, and Komi, PV. The stretch-shortening cycle. *Sports Med* 36:977-999, 2006.

105. Noakes, TD, Gibson, ASC, and Lambert, EV. From catastrophe to complexity: a novel model of integrative central neural regulation of effort and fatigue during exercise in humans: summary and conclusions. *Br J Sports Med* 39:120-124, 2005.

106. Norris, D, Joyce, D, Siegler, J, Clock, J, and Lovell, R. Recovery of force–time characteristics after Australian Rules football matches: examining the utility of the isometric midthigh pull. *Int J Sports Physiol Perform* 1-6, 2019.

107. O'Keeffe, S, O'Connor, S, and Ní Chéilleachair, N. Are internal load measures associated with injuries in male adolescent Gaelic football players? *Eur J Sport Sci*:1-12, 2019.

108. Osgnach, C, Poser, S, Bernardini, R, Rinaldo, R, and Di Prampero, PE. Energy cost and metabolic power in elite soccer: a new match analysis approach. *Med Sci Sports Exerc* 42:170-178, 2010.

109. Panebianco, GP, Bisi, MC, Stagni, R, and Fantozzi, S. Analysis of the performance of 17 algorithms from a systematic review: influence of sensor position, analysed variable and computational approach in gait timing estimation from IMU measurements. *Gait Posture* 66:76-82, 2018.

110. Peterson, M, Rhea, M, and Alvar, B. Maximizing strength development in athletes: a meta-analysis to determine the dose response relationship. *J Strength Cond Res* 18:377-382, 2004.

111. Pettit, RW. The standard difference score: a new statistic for evaluating strength and conditioning programs. *J Strength Cond Res* 24:287-291, 2010.

112. Rhea, MR. Determining the magnitude of treatment effects in strength training research through the use of the effect size. *J Strength Cond Res* 18:918-920, 2004.

113. Robertson, S, Bartlett, JD, and Gastin, PB. Red, amber, or green? Athlete monitoring in team sport: the need for decision-support systems. *Int J Sports Physiol Perform* 12:S273-S279, 2017.

114. Rowell, AE, Aughey, RJ, Clubb, J, and Cormack, SJ. A standardized small sided game can be used to monitor neuromuscular fatigue in professional A-league football players. *Front Physiol* 9:1011, 2018.

115. Rowell, AE, Aughey, RJ, Hopkins, WG, Esmaeili, A, Lazarus, BH, and Cormack, SJ. Effects of training and competition load on neuromuscular recovery, testosterone, cortisol, and match performance during a season of professional football. *Front Physiol* 9:668, 2018.

116. Rowell, AE, Aughey, RJ, Hopkins, WG, Stewart, AM, and Cormack, SJ. Identification of sensitive measures of recovery after external load from football match play. *Int J Sports Physiol Perform* 12:969-976, 2017.

117. Ruddy, JD, Cormack, SJ, Whiteley, R, Williams, MD, Timmins, RG, and Opar, DA. Modeling the risk of team sport injuries: a narrative review of different statistical approaches. *Front Physiol* 10:829, 2019.

118. Ruddy, JD, Pietsch, S, Maniar, N, Cormack, SJ, Timmins, RG, Williams, MA, Carey, DL, and Opar, DA. Session availability as a result of prior injury impacts the risk of subsequent non-contact lower limb injury in elite male Australian footballers. *Front Physiol* 10:737, 2019.

119. Rushall, BS. A tool for measuring stress tolerance in elite athletes. *J Appl Sport Psychol* 2:51-66, 1990.

120. Russell, S, Jenkins, D, Rynne, S, Halson, SL, and Kelly, V. What is mental fatigue in elite sport? Perceptions from athletes and staff. *Eur J Sport Sci* 19:1367-1376, 2019.

121. Ryan, S, Kempton, T, Impellizzeri, FM, and Coutts, AJ. Training monitoring in professional Australian football: theoretical basis and recommendations for coaches and scientists. *Sci Med Football* 1-7, 2019.

122. Saw, AE, Kellmann, M, Main, LC, and Gastin, PB. Athlete self-report measures in research and practice: considerations for the discerning reader and fastidious practitioner. *Int J Sports Physiol Perform* 12:S2127-S2135, 2017.

123. Schwellnus, M, Soligard, T, Alonso, J-M, Bahr, R, Clarsen, B, Dijkstra, HP, Gabbett, TJ, Gleeson, M, Hägglund, M, and Hutchinson, MR. How much is too much? (Part 2) International Olympic Committee consensus statement on load in sport and risk of illness. *Br J Sports Med* 50:1043-1052, 2016.

124. Scott, BR, Duthie, GM, Thornton, HR, and Dascombe, BJ. Training monitoring for resistance exercise: theory and applications. *Sports Med* 46:687-698, 2016.

125. Selye, H. *The Stress of Life.* New York: McGraw-Hill, 25-47, 1956.

126. Skorski, S, Mujika, I, Bosquet, L, Meeusen, R, Coutts, AJ, and Meyer, T. The temporal relationship between exercise, recovery processes, and changes in performance. *Int J Sports Physiol Perform* 14:1015-1021, 2019.

127. Smith, MR, Coutts, AJ, Merlini, M, Deprez, D, Lenoir, M, and Marcora, SM. Mental fatigue impairs soccer-specific physical and technical performance. *Med Sci Sports Exerc* 48:267-276, 2016.

128. Smith, MR, Thompson, C, Marcora, SM, Skorski, S, Meyer, T, and Coutts, AJ. Mental fatigue and soccer: current knowledge and future directions. *Sports Med* 48:1525-1532, 2018.

129. Soligard, T, Schwellnus, M, Alonso, J-M, Bahr, R, Clarsen, B, Dijkstra, HP, Gabbett, T, Gleeson, M, Hägglund, M, and Hutchinson, MR. How much is too much? (Part 1) International Olympic Committee consensus statement on load in sport and risk of injury. *Br J Sports Med* 50:1030-1041, 2016.

130. St Clair Gibson, A, Swart, J, and Tucker, R. The interaction of psychological and physiological homeostatic drives and role of general control principles in the regulation of physiological systems, exercise and the fatigue process–the Integrative Governor theory. *Eur J Sport Sci* 18:25-36, 2018.

131. Stevens, TG, de Ruiter, CJ, van Niel, C, van de Rhee, R, Beek, PJ, and Savelsbergh, GJ. Measuring acceleration and deceleration in soccer-specific movements using a local position measurement (LPM) system. *Int J Sports Physiol Perform* 9:446-456, 2014.

132. Sullivan, C, Bilsborough, JC, Cianciosi, M, Hocking, J, Cordy, JT, and Coutts, AJ. Factors affecting match performance in professional Australian football. *Int J Sports Physiol Perform* 9:561-566, 2014.

133. Sweeting, AJ, Aughey, RJ, Cormack, SJ, and Morgan, S. Discovering frequently recurring movement sequences in team-sport athlete spatiotemporal data. *J Sports Sci* 35:2439-2445, 2017.

134. Sweeting, AJ, Cormack, SJ, Morgan, S, and Aughey, RJ. When is a sprint a sprint? A review of the analysis of Team-Sport Athlete Activity Profile. *Front Physiol* 8:432, 2017.

135. Tanner, R, and Gore, C. *Physiological Tests for Elite Athletes.* Champaign, IL: Human Kinetics, 165-497, 2012.

136. Taylor, JL, Amann, M, Duchateau, J, Meeusen, R, and Rice, CL. Neural contributions to muscle fatigue: from the brain to the muscle and back again. *Med Sci Sports Exerc* 48:2294, 2016.

137. Thornton, HR, Nelson, AR, Delaney, JA, Serpiello, FR, and Duthie, GM. Interunit reliability and effect of data-processing methods of global positioning systems. *Int J Sports Physiol Perform* 14:432-438, 2019.

138. Thorpe, RT, Atkinson, G, Drust, B, and Gregson, W. Monitoring fatigue status in elite team-sport athletes: implications for practice. *Int J Sports Physiol Perform* 12:S227-S234, 2017.

139. Tofari, PJ, Kemp, JG, and Cormack, SJ. Self-paced team-sport match simulation results in reductions in voluntary activation and modifications to biological, perceptual, and performance measures at halftime and for up to 96 hours postmatch. *J Strength Cond Res* 32:3552-3563, 2018.

140. Van Cutsem, J, Marcora, S, De Pauw, K, Bailey, S, Meeusen, R, and Roelands, B. The effects of mental fatigue on physical performance: a systematic review. *Sports Med* 47:1569-1588, 2017.

141. Vanrenterghem, J, Nedergaard, NJ, Robinson, MA, and Drust, B. Training load monitoring in team sports: a novel framework separating physiological and biomechanical load-adaptation pathways. *Sports Med* 47:2135-2142, 2017.

142. Ward, P, Coutts, AJ, Pruna, R, and McCall, A. Putting the "I" back in team. *Int J Sports Physiol Perform* 13:1107-1111, 2018.

143. Watkins, CM, Barillas, SR, Wong, MA, Archer, DC, Dobbs, IJ, Lockie, RG, Coburn, JW, Tran, TT, and Brown, LE.

Determination of vertical jump as a measure of neuromuscular readiness and fatigue. *J Strength Cond Res* 31:3305-3310, 2017.

144. Weaving, D, Dalton, NE, Black, C, Darrall-Jones, J, Phibbs, PJ, Gray, M, Jones, B, and Roe, GA. The same story or a unique novel? Within-participant principal-component analysis of measures of training load in professional rugby union skills training. *Int J Sports Physiol Perform* 13:1175-1181, 2018.

145. Weaving, D, Jones, B, Till, K, Abt, G, and Beggs, C. The case for adopting a multivariate approach to optimize training load quantification in team sports. *Front Physiol* 8:1024, 2017.

146. Weaving, D, Marshall, P, Earle, K, Nevill, A, and Abt, G. Combining internal-and external-training-load measures in professional rugby league. *Int J Sports Physiol Perform* 9:905-912, 2014.

147. Wehbe, G, Gabbett, T, Dwyer, D, McLellan, C, and Coad, S. Monitoring neuromuscular fatigue in team-sport athletes using a cycle-ergometer test. *Int J Sports Physiol Perform* 10:292-297, 2015.

148. Weir, JP, Beck, TW, Cramer, JT, and Housh, TJ. Is fatigue all in your head? A critical review of the central governor model. *Br J Sports Med* 40:573-586, 2005.

149. Weiss, KJ, Allen, SV, McGuigan, MR, and Whatman, CS. The relationship between training load and injury in men's professional basketball. *Int J Sports Physiol Perform* 12:1238-1242, 2017.

150. Williams, S, Trewartha, G, Kemp, SP, Brooks, JH, Fuller, CW, Taylor, AE, Cross, MJ, and Stokes, KA. Time loss injuries compromise team success in elite rugby union: a 7-year prospective study. *Br J Sports Med* 50:651-656, 2016.

151. Williams, S, West, S, Cross, MJ, and Stokes, KA. Better way to determine the acute:chronic workload ratio? *Br J Sports Med* 51:209-210, 2017.

152. Winter, EM, Abt, GA, and Nevill, AM. Metrics of meaningfulness as opposed to sleights of significance. *J Sports Sci* 32:901-902, 2014.

Chapter 3

1. Afonso, J, Nikolaidis, PT, Sousa, P, and Mesquita, I. Is empirical research on periodization trustworthy? A comprehensive review of conceptual and methodological issues. *J Sports Sci Med* 16:27-34, 2017.

2. Alhadad, SB, Tan, PMS, and Lee, JKW. Efficacy of heat mitigation strategies on core temperature and endurance exercise: a meta-analysis. *Front Physiol* 10:71, 2019.

3. Banister, EW, Carter, JB, and Zarkadas, PC. Training theory and taper: validation in triathlon athletes. *Eur J Appl Physiol Occup Physiol* 79:182-191, 1999.

4. Bartlett, JD, O'Connor, F, Pitchford, N, Torres-Ronda, L, and Robertson, SJ. Relationships between internal and external training load in team-sport athletes: evidence for an individualized approach. *Int J Sports Physiol Perform* 12:230-234, 2017.

5. Belval, LN, Hosokawa, Y, Casa, DJ, Adams, WM, Armstrong, LE, Baker, LB, Burke, L, Cheuvront, S, Chiampas, G, and González-Alonso, J. Practical hydration solutions for sports. *Nutrients* 11:1550, 2019.

6. Blythe, DA, and Kiraly, FJ. Prediction and quantification of individual athletic performance of runners. *PLoS One* 11:e0157257, 2016.

7. Böhlke, N, and Robinson, L. Benchmarking of elite sport systems. *Management Decision* 47:67-84, 2009.

8. Bompa, TO, Blumenstein, B, Orbach, I, and Hoffman, J. Present state of the art. In *Integrated Periodization in Sports Training &*

Athletic Development. Bompa, TO, Blumenstein, B, Hoffman, J, Howell, S and Orbach, I, eds. Ann Arbor, MI: Meyer & Meyer Sport, 12-22, 2019.

9. Bompa, TO, and Buzzichelli, CA. Periodization as planning and programming of sport training. In *Periodization Training for Sports.* Champaign, IL: Human Kinetics, 87-98, 2015.

10. Bompa, TO, and Buzzichelli, CA. Periodization of the annual plan. In *Periodization: Theory and Methodology of Training,* sixth edition. Champaign, IL: Human Kinetics, 165-206, 2019.

11. Bompa, TO, and Haff, GG. Annual training plan. In *Periodization: Theory and Methodology of Training,* fifth edition. Champaign, IL: Human Kinetics, 125-185, 2009.

12. Bompa, TO, and Haff, GG. Basis for training. In *Periodization: Theory and Methodology of Training,* fifth edition. Champaign, IL: Human Kinetics, 3-30, 2009.

13. Bompa, TO, Hoffman, J, Blumenstein, B, and Orbach, I. Tapering and peaking for competitions. In *Integrated Periodization in Sports Training & Athletic Development.* Bompa, TO, Blumenstein, B, Hoffman, J, Howell, S, and Orbach, I, eds. Ann Arbor, MI: Meyer & Meyer Sport, 174-197, 2019.

14. Bourdon, PC, Cardinale, M, Murray, A, Gastin, P, Kellmann, M, Varley, MC, Gabbett, TJ, Coutts, AJ, Burgess, DJ, Gregson, W, and Cable, NT. Monitoring athlete training loads: Consensus Statement. *Int J Sports Physiol Perform* 12:S2161-S2170, 2017.

15. Caparros, T, Casals, M, Solana, A, and Pena, J. Low external workloads are related to higher injury risk in professional male basketball games. *J Sports Sci Med* 17:289-297, 2018.

16. Casadio, JR, Kilding, AE, Siegel, R, Cotter, JD, and Laursen, PB. Periodizing heat acclimation in elite Laser sailors preparing for a world championship event in hot conditions. *Temperature (Austin)* 3:437-443, 2016.

17. Chow, JW, and Knudson, DV. Use of deterministic models in sports and exercise biomechanics research. *Sports Biomech* 10:219-233, 2011.

18. Claudino, JG, Capanema, DO, de Souza, TV, Serrao, JC, Machado Pereira, AC, and Nassis, GP. Current approaches to the use of artificial intelligence for injury risk assessment and performance prediction in team sports: a systematic review. *Sports Med Open* 5:28, 2019.

19. Connolly, F, and White, P. The evolution of preparation. In *Game Changer.* Canada: Victory Belt Publishing Inc, 247-264, 2017.

20. Cormack, SJ, Newton, RU, McGuigan, MR, and Cormie, P. Neuromuscular and endocrine responses of elite players during an Australian rules football season. *Int J Sports Physiol Perform* 3:439-453, 2008.

21. Counsilman, JE, and Counsilman, BE. Advanced theories in the planning of training. In *The New Science of Swimming.* Englewood Cliffs, NJ: Prentice Hall, 229-255, 1994.

22. Cunanan, AJ, DeWeese, BH, Wagle, JP, Carroll, KM, Sausaman, R, Hornsby, WG III, Haff, GG, Triplett, NT, Pierce, KC, and Stone, MH. The general adaptation syndrome: a foundation for the concept of periodization. *Sports Med* 48:787-797, 2018.

23. DeWeese, BH, Gray, HS, Sams, ML, Scruggs, SK, and Serrano, AJ. Revising the definition of periodization: merging historical principles with modern concerns. *Olympic Coach Magazine* 24:5-19, 2015.

24. Evans, M. Strength and conditioning for cycling. In *Strength and Conditioning for Sports Performance.* Jeffreys, I and Moody, J, eds. Abingdon, Oxon: Routledge, 642-646, 2016.

25. Fleck, SJ. Periodized strength training: a critical review. *J Strength Cond Res* 13:82-89, 1999.

26. Francis, C. Structure of training for speed. Charlie Francis. COM, 1-72, 2008.

27. Gamble, P. Planning and scheduling: periodisation of training. In *Strength and Conditioning for Team Sports: Sport-Specific Physical Preparation for High Performance.* London: Routledge, 204-220, 2013.

28. Geurkink, Y, Vandewiele, G, Lievens, M, de Turck, F, Ongenae, F, Matthys, SPJ, Boone, J, and Bourgois, JG. Modeling the prediction of the session rating of perceived exertion in soccer: unraveling the puzzle of predictive indicators. *Int J Sports Physiol Perform* 14:841-846, 2019.

29. Haff, GG. The essentials of periodisation. In *Strength and Conditioning for Sports Performance.* Jeffreys, I and Moody, J, eds. Abingdon, Oxon: Routledge, 404-448, 2016.

30. Haff, GG. Peaking for competition in individual sports. In *High-Performance Training for Sports.* Joyce, D and Lewindon, D, eds. Champaign, IL: Human Kinetics, 524-540, 2014.

31. Haff, GG. Periodization and power integration. In *Developing Power.* McGuigan, M, ed. Champaign, IL: Human Kinetics, 33-62, 2017.

32. Haff, GG. Periodization for tactical populations. In *NSCA's Essentials of Tactical Strength and Conditioning.* Alvar, BA, Sell, K, and Deuster, PA, eds. Champaign, IL: Human Kinetics, 181-204, 2017.

33. Haff, GG. Periodization of training. In *Conditioning for Strength and Human Performance.* Brown, LE and Chandler, J, eds. Philadelphia: Wolters Kluwer, Lippincott, Williams & Wilkins, 2012, 326-345, 2012.

34. Haff, GG. Periodization strategies for youth development. In *Strength and Conditioning for Young Athletes: Science and Application.* Lloyd, RS and Oliver, JL, eds. London: Routledge, Taylor & Francis Group, 149-168, 2014.

35. Haff, GG, and Haff, EE. Training integration and periodization. In *Strength and Conditioning Program Design.* Hoffman, J, ed. Champaign, IL: Human Kinetics, 209-254, 2012.

36. Haff, GG, Kraemer, WJ, O'Bryant, HS, Pendlay, G, Plisk, S, and Stone, MH. Roundtable discussion: periodization of training-part 1. *NSCA J* 26:50-69, 2004.

37. Halson, SL. Monitoring training load to understand fatigue in athletes. *Sports Med* 44(suppl 2):139-147, 2014.

38. Herda, TJ, and Cramer, JT. Bioenergetics of exercise and training. In *Essentials of Strength Training and Conditioning.* Haff, GG and Triplett, N, eds. Champaign, IL: Human Kinetics, 43-63, 2016.

39. Hopkins, WG. Competitive performance of elite track-and-field athletes: variability and smallest worthwhile enhancements. *Sportscience* 9:17-20, 2005.

40. Ingham, S. The big goal. In *How to Support a Champion.* UK: Simply Said LTD, 40-63, 2016.

41. Ingham, S. How do you know? In *How to Support a Champion.* UK: Simply Said LTD, 64-85, 2016.

42. Ingham, S. Seven spinning plates. In *How to Support a Champion.* UK: Simply Said LTD, 86-119, 2016.

43. Issurin, VB. Benefits and limitations of block periodized training approaches to athletes' preparation: a review. *Sports Med* 46:329-338, 2016.

44. Issurin, VB. Biological background of block periodized endurance training: a review. *Sports Med* 49:31-39, 2019.

45. Issurin, VB. New horizons for the methodology and physiology of training periodization. *Sports Med* 40:189-206, 2010.

46. Jeffreys, I. Quadrennial planning for the high school athlete. *Strength Cond J* 30:74-83, 2008.

47. Kelly, VG, and Coutts, AJ. Planning and monitoring training loads during the competition phase in team sports. *Strength Cond J* 29:32-37, 2007.

48. Kiely, J. New horizons for the methodology and physiology of training periodization: block periodization: new horizon or a false dawn? *Sports Med* 40:803-805; author reply 805-807, 2010.

49. Kiely, J. Periodization paradigms in the 21st century: evidence-led or tradition-driven? *Int J Sports Physiol Perform* 7:242-250, 2012.

50. Kiely, J. Periodization theory: confronting an inconvenient truth. *Sports Med* 48:753-764, 2018.

51. Kipp, K, Krzyszkowski, J, and Kant-Hull, D. Use of machine learning to model volume load effects on changes in jump performance. *Int J Sports Physiol Perform* 1-13, 2019. [e-pub ahead of print].

52. Lee, EC, Fragala, MS, Kavouras, SA, Queen, RM, Pryor, JL, and Casa, DJ. Biomarkers in sports and exercise: tracking health, performance, and recovery in athletes. *J Strength Cond Res* 31:2920-2937, 2017.

53. Malisoux, L, Gette, P, Urhausen, A, Bomfim, J, and Theisen, D. Influence of sports flooring and shoes on impact forces and performance during jump tasks. *PLoS One* 12:e0186297, 2017.

54. Mattocks, KT, Dankel, SJ, Buckner, SL, Jessee, MB, Counts, BR, Mouser, JG, Laurentino, GC, and Loenneke, JP. Periodization: what is it good for? *J Trainol* 5:6-12, 2016.

55. Mendes, B, Palao, JM, Silverio, A, Owen, A, Carrico, S, Calvete, F, and Clemente, FM. Daily and weekly training load and wellness status in preparatory, regular and congested weeks: a season-long study in elite volleyball players. *Res Sports Med* 26:462-473, 2018.

56. Moore, CA, and Fry, AC. Nonfunctional overreaching during off-season training for skill position players in collegiate American football. *J Strength Cond Res* 21:793-800, 2007.

57. Mujika, I, Halson, S, Burke, L, Balagué, G, and Farrow, D. An integrated, multifactorial approach to periodization for optimal performance in individual and team sports. *Int J Sports Physiol Perform* 13:538-561, 2018.

58. Mujika, I, and Padilla, S. Detraining: loss of training-induced physiological and performance adaptations. Part I: Short term insufficient training stimulus. *Sports Med* 30:79-87, 2000.

59. Mujika, I, and Padilla, S. Scientific bases for precompetition tapering strategies. *Med Sci Sports Exerc* 35:1182-1187, 2003.

60. Mujika, I, Padilla, S, and Pyne, D. Swimming performance changes during the final 3 weeks of training leading to the Sydney 2000 Olympic Games. *Int J Sports Med* 23:582-587, 2002.

61. Mujika, I, Villanueva, L, Welvaert, M, and Pyne, DB. Swimming fast when it counts: a 7-year analysis of Olympic and World Championships performance. *Int J Sports Physiol Perform* 14:1132-1139, 2019.

62. Munroe, L, and Haff, GG. Sprint cycling. In *Routledge Handbook of Strength and Conditioning*. Turner, A, ed. New York: Routledge, 506-525, 2018.

63. Norris, SR, and Smith, DJ. Planning, periodization, and sequencing training and competition: the rationale for a competently planned, optimally executed training and competition program, supported by a multidisiplinary team. In *Enhancing Recovery: Preventing Underperformance in Athletes*. Kellmann, M, ed. Champaign, IL: Human Kinetics, 121-141, 2002.

64. Olbrect, J. Basics of training planning. In *The Science of Winning: Planning, Periodizing, and Optimizing Swim Training*. Luton, England: Swimshop, 171-192, 2000.

65. Painter, K, Haff, G, Ramsey, M, McBride, J, Triplett, T, Sands, W, Lamont, H, Stone, M, and Stone, M. Strength gains: block versus daily undulating periodization weight training among track and field athletes. *Int J Sports Physiol Perform* 7:161-169, 2012.

66. Peltonen, H, Walker, S, Lahitie, A, Hakkinen, K, and Avela, J. Isometric parameters in the monitoring of maximal strength, power and hypertrophic resistance-training. *Appl Physiol Nutr Metab* 43:145-153, 2018.

67. Plisk, SS, and Stone, MH. Periodization strategies. *Strength Cond J* 25:19-37, 2003.

68. Pritchard, HJ, Barnes, MJ, Stewart, RJ, Keogh, JW, and McGuigan, MR. Higher- versus lower-intensity strength-training taper: effects on neuromuscular performance. *Int J Sports Physiol Perform* 14:458-463, 2019.

69. Rein, R, and Memmert, D. Big data and tactical analysis in elite soccer: future challenges and opportunities for sports science. *Springerplus* 5:1410, 2016.

70. Robertson, S, and Joyce, D. Evaluating strategic periodisation in team sport. *J Sports Sci* 36:279-285, 2018.

71. Robertson, SJ, and Joyce, DG. Informing in-season tactical periodisation in team sport: development of a match difficulty index for Super Rugby. *J Sports Sci* 33:99-107, 2015.

72. Rønnestad, BR, Hansen, J, and Ellefsen, S. Block periodization of high-intensity aerobic intervals provides superior training effects in trained cyclists. *Scand J Med Sci Sports* 24:34-42, 2014.

73. Ronnestad, BR, Ofsteng, SJ, and Ellefsen, S. Block periodization of strength and endurance training is superior to traditional periodization in ice hockey players. *Scand J Med Sci Sports* 29:180-188, 2019.

74. Rowbottom, DG. Periodization of training. In *Exercise and Sport Science*. Garrett, WE and Kirkendall, DT, eds. Philadelphia: Lippincott Williams and Wilkins, 499-512, 2000.

75. Schwellnus, M, Soligard, T, Alonso, J-M, Bahr, R, Clarsen, B, Dijkstra, HP, Gabbett, TJ, Gleeson, M, Hägglund, M, Hutchinson, MR, Janse Van Rensburg, C, Meeusen, R, Orchard, JW, Pluim, BM, Raftery, M, Budgett, R, and Engebretsen, L. How much is too much? (Part 2) International Olympic Committee consensus statement on load in sport and risk of illness. *Br J Sports Med* 50:1043-1052, 2016.

76. Siewe, J, Rudat, J, Zarghooni, K, Sobottke, R, Eysel, P, Herren, C, Knoll, P, Illgner, U, and Michael, J. Injuries in competitive boxing. A prospective study. *Int J Sports Med* 36:249-253, 2015.

77. Soligard, T, Schwellnus, M, Alonso, J-M, Bahr, R, Clarsen, B, Dijkstra, HP, Gabbett, T, Gleeson, M, Hägglund, M, Hutchinson, MR, Janse van Rensburg, C, Khan, KM, Meeusen, R, Orchard, JW, Pluim, BM, Raftery, M, Budgett, R, and Engebretsen, L. How much is too much? (Part 1) International Olympic Committee consensus statement on load in sport and risk of injury. *Br J Sports Med* 50:1030-1041, 2016.

78. Solli, GS, Tonnessen, E, and Sandbakk, O. Block vs. traditional periodization of HIT: two different paths to success for the world's best cross-country skier. *Front Physiol* 10:375, 2019.

79. Suarez, DG, Mizuguchi, S, Hornsby, WG, Cunanan, AJ, Marsh, DJ, and Stone, MH. Phase-specific changes in rate of force development and muscle morphology throughout a block periodized training cycle in weightlifters. *Sports* 7:129, 2019.

80. Viru, A. Some facts about microcycles. *Mod Athlete Coach* 28:29-32, 1990.

81. Zatsiorsky, VM, and Kraemer, WJ. Timing in strength training. In *Science and Practice of Strength Training*. Champaign, IL: Human Kinetics, 89-108, 2006.

Chapter 4

1. Buchheit, M. The 30-15 Intermittent Fitness Test: accuracy for individualizing interval training of young intermittent sport players. *J Strength Cond Res* 22:365-374, 2008.

2. Buchheit, M. Applying the acute:chronic workload ratio in elite football: worth the effort? *Br J Sports Med* 51:1325-1327, 2017.

3. Buchheit, M. Individualizing high-intensity interval training in intermittent sport athletes with the 30-15 Intermittent Fitness Test. *NSCA Hot Topic Series* November, 2011. https://30-15ift.com/wp-content/uploads/2013/07/buchheit-30-15ift-hottopic-nsca.pdf.

4. Buchheit, M. Managing high-speed running load in professional soccer players: the benefit of high-intensity interval training supplementation. *Sport Perform Sci Rep* 53:v1, 2019.

5. Buchheit, M. Programming high-intensity training in handball. *Aspetar Sports Med J* 3:120-128, 2014.

6. Buchheit, M. Programming high-speed running and mechanical work in relation to technical contents and match schedule in professional soccer. *Sport Perform Sci Rep* 69:v1, 2019.

7. Buchheit, M, Allen, A, Poon, TK, Modonutti, M, Gregson, W, and Di Salvo, V. Integrating different tracking systems in football: multiple camera semi-automatic system, local position measurement and GPS technologies. *J Sports Sci* 32:1844-1857, 2014.

8. Buchheit, M, and Laursen, PB. High-intensity interval training, solutions to the programming puzzle: part I: cardiopulmonary emphasis. *Sports Med* 43:313-338, 2013.

9. Buchheit, M, Laursen, PB, Kuhnle, J, Ruch, D, Renaud, C, and Ahmaidi, S. Game-based training in young elite handball players. *Int J Sports Med* 30:251-258, 2009.

10. Buchheit, M, Leblond, F, Renaud, C, Kuhnle, J, and Ahmaidi, S. Effect of complex vs. specific aerobic training in young handball players. *Coach Sport Sci* 3:22, 2008.

11. Buchheit, M, and Mayer, N. Restoring players' specific fitness and performance capacity in relation to match physical and technical demands. In *Muscle Injury Guide: Prevention of and Return to Play From Muscle Injuries.* Barca Innovation Hub 29-35, 2019. https://static.capabiliaserver.com/frontend/clients/barca/wp/wp-content/uploads/2019/03/105e3b07-muscle-guide-general-principles-of-return-to-play-from-muscle-injury.pdf.

12. Buchheit, M, and Simpson, BM. Player tracking technology: half-full or half-empty glass? *Int J Sports Physiol Perform* 12:S235-S241, 2017.

13. Cunningham, DJ, Shearer, DA, Carter, N, Drawer, S, Pollard, B, Bennett, M, Eager, R, Cook, CJ, Farrell, J, Russell, M, and Kilduff, LP. Assessing worst case scenarios in movement demands derived from global positioning systems during international rugby union matches: rolling averages versus fixed length epochs. *PLoS One* 13:e0195197, 2018.

14. Delgado-Bordonau, JL, and Mendez-Villanueva, A. The tactical periodization model. In *Fitness in Soccer: The Science and Practical Application.* Moveo Ergo Sum/Klein-Gelman, 46-53.2014.

15. Dellal, A, Varliette, C, Owen, A, Chirico, EN, and Pialoux, V. Small-sided games versus interval training in amateur soccer players: effects on the aerobic capacity and the ability to perform intermittent exercises with changes of direction. *J Strength Cond Res* 26:2712-2720, 2012.

16. Duhig, S, Shield, AJ, Opar, D, Gabbett, TJ, Ferguson, C, and Williams, M. Effect of high-speed running on hamstring strain injury risk. *Br J Sports Med* 50:1536-1540, 2016.

17. Edouard, P, Mendiguchia, J, Guex, K, Lahti, J, Samozino, P, and Morin, JB. Sprinting: a potential vaccine for hamstring injury? *Sport Perform Sci Rep* 48:v1, 2019.

18. Fanchini, M, Pons, E, Impellizzeri, F, Dupont, G, Buchheit, M, and McCall, A. Exercise-based strategies to prevent muscle injuries. In *Muscle Injury Guide: Prevention of and Return to Play From Muscle Injuries.* Barca Innovation Hub 34-41, 2019. https://static.capabiliaserver.com/frontend/clients/barca/wp/wp-content/uploads/2019/03/105e3b07-muscle-guide-general-principles-of-return-to-play-from-muscle-injury.pdf.

19. Fanchini, M, Rampinini, E, Riggio, M, Coutts, A, Pecci, C, and McCall, A. Despite association, the acute:chronic work load ratio does not predict non-contact injury in elite footballers. *Sci Med Football* 2:109-114, 2018. https://doi.org/10.1080/2473393 8.2018.1429014.

20. Gabbett, TJ. The training-injury prevention paradox: should athletes be training smarter and harder? *Br J Sports Med* 50:273-280, 2016.

21. Hader, K, Mendez-Villanueva, A, Williams, B, Ahmaidi, S, and Buchheit, M. Changes of direction during high-intensity intermittent runs: neuromuscular and metabolic responses. *BMC Sports Sci Med Rehabil* 6:2, 2014.

22. Iaia, FM, Rampinini, E, and Bangsbo, J. High-intensity training in football. *Int J Sports Physiol Perform* 4:291-306, 2009.

23. Impellizzeri, FM, Marcora, SM, Castagna, C, Reilly, T, Sassi, A, Iaia, FM, and Rampinini, E. Physiological and performance effects of generic versus specific aerobic training in soccer players. *Int J Sports Med* 27:483-492, 2006.

24. Lacome, M, Simpson, BM, Cholley, Y, Lambert, P, and Buchheit, M. Small sided games in elite soccer: does one size fits all? *Int J Sports Physiol Perform* 13:1-24, 2017.

25. Laursen, PB, and Buchheit, M. *Science and Application of High-Intensity Interval Training (HIIT): Solutions to the Programming Puzzle.* Human Kinetics; First edition (December 28, 2018), 2018.

26. Laursen, PB, Buchheit, M, eds. *Science and Application of High-Intensity Interval Training: Solutions to the Programming Puzzle.* 1st ed. Champaign, IL: Human Kinetics, 3-661, 2018.

27. Lolli, L, Batterham, AM, Hawkins, R, Kelly, DM, Strudwick, AJ, Thorpe, RT, Gregson, W, and Atkinson, G. The acute-to-chronic workload ratio: an inaccurate scaling index for an unnecessary normalisation process? *Br J Sports Med* 53, 2018. http://dx.doi.org/10.1136/bjsports-2017-098884.

28. Malone, S, Roe, M, Doran, DA, Gabbett, TJ, and Collins, K. High chronic training loads and exposure to bouts of maximal velocity running reduce injury risk in elite Gaelic football. *J Sci Med Sport* 20:250-254, 2017.

29. van den Tillaar, R, Solheim, JAB, and Bencke, J. Comparison of hamstring muscle activation during high-speed running and various hamstring strengthening exercises. *Int J Sports Phys Ther* 12:718-727, 2017.

Chapter 5

1. Ali, A. Measuring soccer skill performance: a review. *Scand J Med Sci Sports* 21:170-183, 2011.

2. Barbosa, TM, Costa, MJ, and Marinho, DA. Proposal of a deterministic model to explain swimming performance. *Int J Swim Kinet* 2:1-54, 2013.

3. Barbosa, LP, Sousa, CV, Sales, MM, Olher, RDR, Aguiar, SS, Santos, PA, Tiozzo, E, Simoes, HG, Nikolaidis, PT, and Knechtle, B. Celebrating 40 years of ironman: how the champions perform. *Int J Environ Res Public Health* 16:1019, 2019.

4. Bennell, KL, and Crossley, K. Musculoskeletal injuries in track and field: incidence, distribution and risk factors. *Aust J Sci Med Sport* 28:69-75, 1996.

5. Berthelot, G, Sedeaud, A, Marck, A, Antero-Jacquemin, J, Schipman, J, Saulière, G, Marc, A, Desgorces, F-D, and

Toussaint, J-F. Has athletic performance reached its peak? *Sports Med* 45:1263-1271, 2015.

6. Berthelot, G, Thibault, V, Tafflet, M, Escolano, S, El Helou, N, Jouven, X, Hermine, O, and Toussaint, J-F. The citius end: world records progression announces the completion of a brief ultra-physiological quest. *PLoS One* 3:e1552, 2008.

7. Boccia, G, Moisè, P, Franceschi, A, Trova, F, Panero, D, La Torre, A, Rainoldi, A, Schena, F, and Cardinale, M. Career performance trajectories in track and field jumping events from youth to senior success: the importance of learning and development. *PLoS One* 12:e0170744, 2017.

8. Boccia, G, Riccardo, PR, Moisè, P, Franceschi, A, La Torre, A, Schena, F, Rainoldi, A, and Cardinale, M. Elite national athletes reach their peak performance later than non-elite in sprints and throwing events. *J Sci Med Sport* 22:342-347, 2019.

9. Brandon, LJ. Physiological factors associated with middle distance running performance. *Sports Med* 19:268-277, 1995.

10. British Triathlon. Olympic World Class Programme Selection Process 2019–2020. 2019. www.britishtriathlon.org/britain/documents/gb-teams/selection-policies/2019--selection-policies/2020-selection-policies/2019-20-olympic-wcp-selection-policy---final.pdf. Accessed September 8, 2020.11.

11. Cardinale, M. Developing young talent to Olympic champions in athletics: understanding realistic progressions. *Aspetar Sports Med J* 250-255, 2019. Available online at: https://www.aspetar.com/journal/viewarticle.aspx?id=469#.XxM-b55KhPY. Accessed September 8, 2020.

12. Carlsen, KH. Asthma in Olympians. *Paediatr Respir Rev* 17:34-35, 2016.

13. Chow, JW, and Knudson, DV. Use of deterministic models in sports and exercise biomechanics research. *Sports Biomech* 10:219-233, 2011.

14. Daoud, AI, Geissler, GJ, Wang, F, Saretsky, J, Daoud, YA, and Lieberman, DE. Foot strike and injury rates in endurance runners: a retrospective study. *Med Sci Sports Exerc* 44:1325-1334, 2012.

15. Farrow, D, and Robertson, S. Development of a skill acquisition periodisation framework for high-performance sport. *Sports Med* 47:1043-1054, 2017.

16. Federation Internationale de Gymnastique. Rules. www.gymnastics.sport/site/rules/rules.php. Accessed September 8, 2020.

17. Glazier, PS, and Mehdizadeh, S. Challenging conventional paradigms in applied sports biomechanics research. *Sports Med* 49:171-176. 2019.

18. Glazier, PS, and Robins, MT. Comment on "Use of deterministic models in sports and exercise biomechanics research" by Chow and Knudson (2011). *Sport Biomech* 11:120-122, author reply 123-124, 2012.

19. Gonzalo-Skok, O, Tous-Fajardo, J, Suarez-Arrones, L, Arjol-Serrano, JL, Casajús, JA, and Mendez-Villanueva, A. Validity of the V-cut test for young basketball players. *Int J Sports Med* 36:893-899, 2015.

20. Hay, JG,. *The biomechanics of Sports Technique. 4th Edition.* Englewood Cliffs, NJ: Prentice-Hall, 424-429, 1993.

21. Helenius, I, and Haahtela, T. Allergy and asthma in elite summer sport athletes. *J Allergy Clin Immunol* 106:444-452, 2000.

22. Hiley, MJ, Zuevsky, VV, and Yeadon, MR. Is skilled technique characterized by high or low variability? An analysis of high bar giant circles. *Hum Mov Sci* 32:171-180, 2013.

23. Hughes, M, Caudrelier, T, James, N, Redwood-Brown, A, Donnelly, I, Kirkbride, A, and Duschesne, C. Moneyball and soccer - an analysis of the key performance indicators of elite male soccer players by position. *J Hum Sport Exerc* 7:402-412, 2012.

24. Iino, Y, and Kojima, T. Kinematics of table tennis topspin forehands: effects of performance level and ball spin. *J Sports Sci* 27:1311-1321, 2009.

25. Ingham, SA, Whyte, GP, Pedlar, C, Bailey, DM, Dunman, N, and Nevill, AM. Determinants of 800-m and 1500-m running performance using allometric models. *Med Sci Sports Exerc* 40:345-350, 2008.

26. Karkazis, K, and Fishman, JR. Tracking U.S. professional athletes: the ethics of biometric technologies. *Am J Bioeth* 17, 45-60, 2017.

27. Krause, LM, Buszard, T, Reid, M, Pinder, R, and Farrow, D. Assessment of elite junior tennis serve and return practice: a cross-sectional observation. *J Sports Sci* 37:2818-2825, 2019.

28. Longmuir, PE, Boyer, C, Lloyd, M, Borghese, MM, Knight, E, Saunders, TJ, Boiarskaia, E, Weimo, Z, and Tremblay, MS. Canadian Agility and Movement Skill Assessment (CAMSA): validity, objectivity, and reliability evidence for children 8–12 years of age. *J Sport Health Sci* 6:231-240, 2017.

29. Martínez-Silván, D, Díaz-Ocejo, J, and Murray, A. Predictive indicators of overuse injuries in adolescent endurance athletes. *Int J Sports Physiol Perform* 12:153-156, 2017.

30. McLean, SG, Lipfert, SW, and Van Den Bogert, AJ. Effect of gender and defensive opponent on the biomechanics of sidestep cutting. *Med Sci Sports Exerc* 36:1008-1016, 2004.

31. MLB Stats. http://m.mlb.com/stats\. Accessed September 8, 2020.

32. National Hockey League. Statistics. www.nhl.com/stats\. Accessed September 8, 2020.

33. NBA Advanced Stats. Players Tracking Speed & Distance. https://stats.nba.com/players/speed-distance. Accessed September 8, 2020.

34. Nevill, AM, Whyte, GP, Holder, RL, and Peyrebrune, M. Are there limits to swimming world records? *Int J Sports Med* 28:1012-1017, 2007.

35. Nieman, DC. Exercise, upper respiratory tract infection, and the immune system. *Med Sci Sports Exerc* 26:128-139, 1994.

36. Official ISU Judging System. ISU Updates. www.isujudgingsystem.com/news/. Accessed September 8, 2020.

37. Ofoghi, B, Zeleznikow, J, Macmahon, C, Rehula, J, and Dwyer, DB. Performance analysis and prediction in triathlon. *J Sports Sci* 34:607-612, 2016.

38. Sampaio, J, and Maças, V. Measuring tactical behavior in football. *Int J Sports Med* 33:395-401, 2012.

39. Sampaio, J, McGarry, T, Calleja-González, J, Jiménez Sáiz, S, Schelling, I, Del Alcázar, X, and Balciunas, M. Exploring game performance in the National Basketball Association using player tracking data. *PLoS One* 10:e0132894, 2015.

40. Sandford, GN, Kilding, AE, Ross, A, and Laursen, PB. Maximal sprint speed and the anaerobic speed reserve domain: the untapped tools that differentiate the world's best male 800 m runners. *Sports Med* 49:843-852, 2019.

41. Sandford, GN, Laursen, PB, Kilding, AE, and Ross, A. Defining the role of the anaerobic speed reserve in middle distance running. *NZ J Sports Med* 2017.

42. Sandford, GN, Rogers, SA, Sharma, AP, Kilding, AE, Ross, A, and Laursen PB. Implementing anaerobic speed reserve testing in the field: validation of vVO2max prediction from 1500m race performance in elite middle-distance runners. *Int J Sports Physiol Perform* 14:1147-1150, 2019.

43. Saxon, LA. Athletic performance monitoring, pseudo science and metaphysics meet ethics. *Am J Bioeth* 17:61-62, 2017.

44. Schabort, EJ, Killian, SC, St Clair Gibson, A, Hawley, JA, and Noakes, TD. Prediction of triathlon race time from laboratory testing in national triathletes. *Med Sci Sports Exerc* 32:844-849, 2000.

45. Sigward, S, and Powers, CM. The influence of experience on knee mechanics during side-step cutting in females. *Clin Biomech (Bristol, Avon)* 21:740-747, 2006.

46. Suchomel, TJ, Lamont, HS, and Moir, GL. Understanding vertical jump potentiation: a deterministic model. *Sports Med* 46:809-828, 2016.

47. Tønnessen, E, Svendsen, IS, Olsen, IC, Guttormsen, A, and Haugen, T. Performance development in adolescent track and field athletes according to age, sex and sport discipline. *PLoS One* 10:e0129014, 2015.

48. United Kingdom Athletics. Performance Funnels. www.uka.org.uk/performance/performance-funnels/. Accessed September 8, 2020.

49. Valter, DS, Adam, C, Barry, M, and Marco, C. Validation of Prozone ®: a new video-based performance analysis system. *Int J Perform Anal Sport* 6:108-119, 2006.

50. Van Schuylenbergh, R, Vanden Eynde, B, and Hespel P. Prediction of sprint triathlon performance from laboratory tests. *Eur J Appl Physiol* 91:94-99, 2004.

51. Williams, LR, and Walmsley, A. Response timing and muscular coordination in fencing: a comparison of elite and novice fencers. *J Sci Med Sport* 3:460-475, 2000.

52. Zebis, MK, Andersen, LL, Bencke, J, Kjaer, M, and Aagaard, P. Identification of athletes at future risk of anterior cruciate ligament ruptures by neuromuscular screening. *Am J Sports Med* 37:1967-1973, 2009.

Chapter 6

1. Argus, CK, Gill, ND, and Keogh, JW. Characterization of the differences in strength and power between different levels of competition in rugby union athletes. *J Strength Cond Res* 26:2698-2704, 2012.

2. Baker, DG. 10-year changes in upper body strength and power in elite professional rugby league players--the effect of training age, stage, and content. *J Strength Cond Res* 27:285-292, 2013.

3. Baker, DG. Comparison of strength levels between players from within the same club who were selected vs. not selected to play in the Grand Final of the National Rugby League competition. *J Strength Cond Res* 31:1461-1467, 2017.

4. Barbosa, AC, Valadao, PF, Wilke, CF, Martins, F, Silva, DCP, Volkers, SA, Lima, COV, Riberio, JRC, Bittencourt, NF, and Barroso, R. The road to 21 seconds: a case report of a 2016 Olympic swimming sprinter. *Int J Sports Sci Coach* 14:393-405, 2019.

5. Bazyler, CD, Mizuguchi, S, Zourdos, MC, Sato, K, Kavanaugh, AA, DeWeese, BH, Breuel, KF, and Stone, MH. Characteristics of a national level female weightlifter peaking for competition: a case study. *J Strength Cond Res* 32:3029-3038, 2018.

6. Bishop, PA, Williams, TD, Heldman, AN, and Vanderburgh, PM. System for evaluating powerlifting and other multievent performances. *J Strength Cond Res* 32:201-204, 2018.

7. Bourne, MN, Bruder, AM, Mentiplay, BF, Carey, DL, Patterson, BE, and Crossley, KM. Eccentric knee flexor weakness in elite female footballers 1-10 years following anterior cruciate ligament reconstruction. *Phys Ther Sport* 37:144-149, 2019.

8. Comfort, P, and Pearson, SJ. Scaling--which methods best predict performance? *J Strength Cond Res* 28:1565-1572, 2014.

9. Comfort, P, Thomas, C, Dos'Santos, T, Suchomel, TJ, Jones, PA, and McMahon, JJ. Changes in dynamic strength index in response to strength training. *Sports (Basel)* 6:4, 2018.

10. Crewther, BT, McGuigan, MR, and Gill, ND. The ratio and allometric scaling of speed, power, and strength in elite male rugby union players. *J Strength Cond Res* 25:1968-1975, 2011.

11. Gillen, ZM, Shoemaker, ME, McKay, BD, and Cramer, JT. Performance differences between National Football League and high school American football combine participants. *Res Q Exerc Sport* 90:227-233, 2019.

11a. Haff, GG and Triplett, NT, eds. *Essentials of strength training and conditioning.* Champaign, IL: Human Kinetics, 292, 2016.

12. Hakkinen, K, Pakarinen, A, Alen, M, Kauhanen, H, and Komi, PV. Neuromuscular and hormonal adaptations in athletes to strength training in two years. *J Appl Physiol (1985)* 65:2406-2412, 1988.

13. Halperin, I. Case studies in exercise and sport sciences: a powerful tool to bridge the science-practice gap. *Int J Sports Physiol Perform* 13:824-825, 2018.

14. Halperin, I, Hughes, S, and Chapman, DW. Physiological profile of a professional boxer preparing for Title Bout: a case study. *J Sports Sci* 34:1949-1956, 2016.

15. Harden, M, Wolf, A, Haff, GG, Hicks, KM, and Howatson, G. Repeatability and specificity of eccentric force output and the implications for eccentric training load prescription. *J Strength Cond Res* 33:676-683, 2019.

16. Harper, LD, and McCunn, R. "Hand in glove": using qualitative methods to connect research and practice. *Int J Sports Physiol Perform* 12:990-993, 2017.

17. Haugen, TA, Breitschadel, F, and Seiler, S. Sprint mechanical variables in elite athletes: are force-velocity profiles sport specific or individual? *PLoS One* 14:e0215551, 2019.

18. Haugen, T, and Buchheit, M. Sprint running performance monitoring: methodological and practical considerations. *Sports Med* 46:641-656, 2016.

19. Haugen, TA, Solberg, PA, Foster, C, Moran-Navarro, R, Breitschadel, F, and Hopkins, WG. Peak age and performance progression in world-class track-and-field athletes. *Int J Sports Physiol Perform* 13:1122-1129, 2018.

20. Haugen, T, Tønnessen, E, and Seiler, S. Speed and countermovement jump characteristics of elite female soccer players, 1995-2010. *Int J Sports Physiol Perform* 7:340-349, 2012.

21. Hoffman, JR, Ratamess, NA, and Kang, J. Performance changes during a college playing career in NCAA division III football athletes. *J Strength Cond Res* 25:2351-2357, 2011.

22. Hortobagyi, T, Katch, FI, and LaChance, PF. Interrelationships among various measures of upper body strength assessed by different contraction modes. Evidence for a general strength component. *Eur J Appl Physiol Occup Physiol* 58:749-755, 1989.

23. Jimenez-Reyes, P, Samozino, P, Brughelli, M, and Morin, JB. Effectiveness of an individualized training based on force-velocity profiling during jumping. *Front Physiol* 7:677, 2016.

24. Jimenez-Reyes, P, Samozino, P, and Morin, JB. Optimized training for jumping performance using the force-velocity imbalance: individual adaptation kinetics. *PLoS One* 14:e0216681, 2019.

24a. Joyce, D, and Lewindon, D. *High-performance training for sports.* 10, 2014.

25. Khamis, HJ, and Roche, AF. Predicting adult stature without using skeletal age: the Khamis-Roche method. *Pediatrics* 94:504-507, 1994.

26. Lloyd, RS, Cronin, JB, Faigenbaum, AD, Haff, GG, Howard, R, Kraemer, WJ, Micheli, LJ, Myer, GD, and Oliver, JL. National Strength and Conditioning Association position statement on long-term athletic development. *J Strength Cond Res* 30:1491-1509, 2016.

27. Maffiuletti, NA, Aagaard, P, Blazevich, AJ, Folland, J, Tillin, N, and Duchateau, J. Rate of force development: physiological and methodological considerations. *Eur J Appl Physiol* 116:1091-1116, 2016.

28. Malina, RM, Eisenmann, JC, Cumming, SP, Ribeiro, B, and Aroso, J. Maturity-associated variation in the growth and functional capacities of youth football (soccer) players 13-15 years. *Eur J Appl Physiol* 91:555-562, 2004.

29. Malina, RM, Rogol, AD, Cumming, SP, Coelho e Silva, MJ, and Figueiredo, AJ. Biological maturation of youth athletes: assessment and implications. *Br J Sports Med* 49:852-859, 2015.

30. McGuigan, MR. Administration, scoring, and interpretation of selected tests. In *Essentials of Strength Training and Conditioning*. Haff, GG and Triplett, NT, eds. Champaign, IL: Human Kinetics, 259-316, 2016.

31. McGuigan, MR, Cormack, S, and Gill, ND. Strength and power profiling of athletes. *Strength Cond J* 35:7-14, 2013.

32. McIntosh, S, Kovalchik, S, and Robertson, S. Multifactorial benchmarking of longitudinal player performance in the Australian Football League. *Front Psychol* 10:1283, 2019.

33. McMaster, DT, Gill, ND, Cronin, JB, and McGuigan, MR. Force-velocity-power assessment in semiprofessional rugby union players. *J Strength Cond Res* 30:1118-1126, 2016.

34. Mirwald, RL, Baxter-Jones, AD, Bailey, DA, and Beunen, GP. An assessment of maturity from anthropometric measurements. *Med Sci Sports Exerc* 34:689-694, 2002.

35. Newton, RU, and Dugan, E. Application of strength diagnosis. *Strength Cond J* 24:50-59, 2002.

36. Perez-Castilla, A, Piepoli, A, Delgado-Garcia, G, Garrido-Blanca, G, and Garcia-Ramos, A. Reliability and concurrent validity of seven commercially available devices for the assessment of movement velocity at different intensities during the bench press. *J Strength Cond Res* 33:1258-1265, 2019.

37. Porter, JM, Anton, PM, and Wu, WF. Increasing the distance of an external focus of attention enhances standing long jump performance. *J Strength Cond Res* 26:2389-2393, 2012.

38. Robertson, S, Bartlett, JD, and Gastin, PB. Red, amber, or breen? Athlete monitoring in team sport: the need for decision-support systems. *Int J Sports Physiol Perform* 12:S273-S279, 2017.

39. Ruddock, AD, Boyd, C, Winter, EM, and Ranchordas, M. Considerations for the scientific support process and applications to case studies. *Int J Sports Physiol Perform* 1-5, 2018.

40. Shaw, G, Scrpell, B, and Baar, K. Rehabilitation and nutrition protocols for optimising return to play from traditional ACL reconstruction in elite rugby union players: a case study. *J Sports Sci* 15:1794-1803, 2019.

41. Sheppard, J, Chapman, D, and Taylor, KL. An evaluation of a strength qualities assessment method for the lower body. *J Aust Strength Cond* 19:4-10, 2011.

42. Shurley, JP, and Todd, JS. "The strength of Nebraska": Boyd Epley, Husker Power, and the formation of the strength coaching profession. *J Strength Cond Res* 26:3177-3188, 2012.

43. Simpson, MJ, Jenkins, DG, Leveritt, MD, and Kelly, VG. Physical profiles of elite, sub-elite, regional and age-group netballers. *J Sports Sci* 37:1212-1219, 2019.

44. Sinclair, RG. Normalizing the performances of athletes in Olympic weightlifting. *Can J Appl Sport Sci* 10:94-98, 1985.

45. Solberg, PA, Hopkins, WG, Paulsen, G, and Haugen, TA. Peak age and performance progression in world-class weightlifting and powerlifting athletes. *Int J Sports Physiol Perform* 1-24, 2019.

46. Suchomel, TJ, Nimphius, S, and Stone, MH. Scaling isometric mid-thigh pull maximum strength in division I athletes: are we meeting the assumptions? *Sports Biomech* 19:532-546, 2020.

47. Thornton, HR, Delaney, JA, Duthie, GM, and Dascombe, BJ. Developing athlete monitoring systems in team sports: data analysis and visualization. *Int J Sports Physiol Perform* 6:698-705, 2019.

48. Tonnessen, E, Haugen, TA, Hem, E, Leirstein, S, and Seiler, S. Maximal aerobic capacity in the winter-Olympics endurance disciplines: Olympic-medal benchmarks for the time period 1990-2013. *Int J Sports Physiol Perform* 10:835-839, 2015.

49. Vanderburgh, PM, and Batterham, AM. Validation of the Wilks powerlifting formula. *Med Sci Sports Exerc* 31:1869-1875, 1999.

50. Young, KP, Haff, GG, Newton, RU, Gabbett, TJ, and Sheppard, JM. Assessment and monitoring of ballistic and maximal upper-body strength qualities in athletes. *Int J Sports Physiol Perform* 10:232-237, 2015.

51. Young, W, Newton RU, Doyle TL, Chapman D, Cormack S, Stewart G, and Dawson, B. Physiological and anthropometric characteristics of starters and non-starters and playing positions in elite Australian rules football: a case study. *J Sci Med Sport* 8:333-345, 2005.

Chapter 7

1. Ardern, CL, Glasgow, P, Schneiders, A, Witvrouw, E, Clarsen, B, Cools, A, Gojanovic, B, Griffin, S, Khan, KM, Moksnes, H, Mutch, SA, Phillips, N, Reurink, G, Sadler, R, Silbernagel, KG, Thorborg, K, Wangensteen, A, Wilk, KE, and Bizzini, M. 2016 Consensus statement on return to sport from the First World Congress in Sports Physical Therapy, Bern. *Br J Sports Med* 50:853-864, 2016.

1a. Arthur WB, Polak W. The evolution of technology within a simple computer model. *Complexity* 11, 23–31. 2006.

2. Christensen, CM. *The Innovator's Dilemma: When New Technologies Cause Great Firms to Fail.* 1st ed. Boston: Harvard Business Review Press, 1997.

3. Ellapen, T, and Paul, Y. Innovative sport technology through cross-disciplinary research: future of sport science. *South African Journal for Research in Sport, Physical Education and Recreation* 38:51-59, 2016.

4. Kevin, K. *The Inevitable: Understanding the 12 Technological Forces That Will Shape Our Future.* New York: Viking Press, 2016.

5. Le Meur, Y, and Torres-Ronda, L. 10 Challenges facing today's applied sport scientist. *Sport Perform Sci Rep* 57:v1, 2019. https://sportperfsci.com/10-challenges-facing-todays-applied-sport-scientist.

6. Lewis, M. *The Undoing Project: A Friendship That Changed Our Minds.* US: W.W. Norton & Company, 2016.

7. Muller, JZ. *The Tyranny of Metrics.* Princeton, NJ: Princeton University Press, 3, 2018.

8. Peake, JM, Kerr, G, and Sullivan, JP. A critical review of consumer wearables, mobile applications, and equipment for providing biofeedback, monitoring stress, and sleep in physically active populations. *Front Physiol* 9:743, 2018.

9. Ringuet-Riot, C, and James, D. How innovative are you? High performance sport training centers. *Aspetar Sport Med J* 2:290-295, 2013.

10. Ringuet-Riot, CJ, Hahn, A, and James, DA. A structured approach for technology innovation in sport. *Sports Technol* 6:137-149, 2013.

11. Silver, N. *The Signal and the Noise: Why Most Predictions Fail–but Some Don't.* New York: Penguin Group, 17, 2012.

12. Torres-Ronda, L, and Schelling, X. Critical process for the implementation of technology in sport organizations. *Strength Cond J* 39:54-59, 2017.

13. Youn, H, Bettencourt, L, Strumsky, D, and Lobo, J. Invention as a combinatorial process: evidence from US patents. *J R Soc Interface* 12, 2014. https://doi.org/10.1098/rsif.2015.0272.

Chapter 8

1. Alexiou, H, and Coutts, AJ. A comparison of methods used for quantifying internal training load in women soccer players. *Int J Sports Physiol Perform* 3:320-330, 2008.

2. Batterham, AM, and Hopkins, WG. Making meaningful inferences about magnitudes. *Int J Sports Physiol Perform* 1:50-57, 2006.

3. Berthoin, S, Gerbeaux, M, Turpin, E, Guerrin, F, Lensel-Corbeil, G, and Vandendorpe, F. Comparison of two field tests to estimate maximum aerobic speed. *J Sports Sci* 12:355-362, 1994.

4. Bland, JM, and Altman, DG. Measuring agreement in method comparison studies. *Stat Methods Med Res* 8:135-160, 1999.

5. Borg, GA. Psychophysical bases of perceived exertion. *Med Sci Sports Exerc* 14:377-381, 1982.

6. Borg, E, and Kaijser, L. A comparison between three rating scales for perceived exertion and two different work tests. *Scand J Med Sci Sports* 16:57-69, 2006.

7. Broman, KW, and Woo, KH. Data organization in spreadsheets. *Am Stat* 72:2-10, 2018.

8. Buchheit, M, Al Haddad, H, Simpson, B, Palazzi, D, Bourdon, P, Di Salvo, V, and Mendez-Villanueva, A. Monitoring accelerations with GPS in football: time to slow down? *Int J Sports Physiol Perform* 9:442-445, 2014.

9. Cardinale, M, and Varley, MC. Wearable training-monitoring technology: applications, challenges, and opportunities. *Int J Sports Physiol Perform* 12:S255-S262, 2017.

10. Chadwick, D. Stop that subversive spreadsheet! In *Integrity and Internal Control in Information Systems V IICIS 2002 IFIP – The International Federation for Information Processing.* Gertz, M, ed. Boston: Springer, 205-211, 2003.

11. Coutts, AJ. In the age of technology, Occam's razor still applies. *Int J Sports Physiol Perform* 9:741, 2014.

12. Ellis, SE, and Leek, JT. How to share data for collaboration. *Am Stat* 72:53-57, 2018.

13. Foster, C, Florhaug, JA, Franklin, J, Gottschall, L, Hrovatin, LA, Parker, S, Doleshal, P, and Dodge, C. A new approach to monitoring exercise training. *J Strength Cond Res* 15:109-115, 2001.

14. Gregson, W, Drust, B, Atkinson, G, and Salvo, VD. Match-to-match variability of high-speed activities in premier league soccer. *Int J Sports Med* 31:237-242, 2010.

15. Hooper, SL, Mackinnon, LT, Howard, A, Gordon, RD, and Bachmann, AW. Markers for monitoring overtraining and recovery. *Med Sci Sports Exerc* 27:106-112, 1995.

16. Hopkins, WG. How to interpret changes in an athletic performance test. *Sportscience* 8:1-7, 2004. www.sportsci.org/jour/04/wghtests.htm.

17. Impellizzeri, FM, Rampinini, E, Coutts, AJ, Sassi, A, and Marcora, SM. Use of RPE-based training load in soccer. *Med Sci Sports Exerc* 36:1042-1047, 2004.

18. Kleppner, D. Ensuring the integrity, accessibility, and stewardship of research data in the digital age. International Association of Scientific and Technological University Libraries, 31st Annual Conference, Paper 10, June 21, 2010.

19. Kyprianou, E, Lolli, L, Haddad, HA, Di Salvo, V, Varley, MC, Mendez Villanueva, A, Gregson, W, and Weston, M. A novel approach to assessing validity in sports performance research: integrating expert practitioner opinion into the statistical analysis. *Sci Med Football* 3:333-338, 2019.

20. Leger, L, and Boucher, R. An indirect continuous running multistage field test: the Université de Montréal track test. *Can J Appl Sport Sci* 5:77-84, 1980.

21. Leger, LA, Mercier, D, Gadoury, C, and Lambert, J. The multistage 20 metre shuttle run test for aerobic fitness. *J Sports Sci* 6:93-101, 1988.

22. Lovell, R., Halley, S., Seigler, J., Wignell, T., Coutts, A., Massard, T. (2020). Numerically blinded rating of perceived exertion in soccer: Assessing concurrent and construct validity. *Int J Sports Physiol Perform.* In Press.

22a. Malone, JJ, Lovell, R, Varley, MC, and Coutts, AJ. Unpacking the black box: applications and considerations for using GPS devices in sport. *Int J Sports Physiol Perform* 12:S218-S226, 2017.

23. Nisbet, R, Miner, G, and Yale, K. *Handbook of Statistical Analysis and Data Mining Application.* London, UK: Elsevier, 69, 2018.

24. Noble, BJ, Borg, GA, Jacobs, I, Ceci, R, and Kaiser, P. A category-ratio perceived exertion scale: relationship to blood and muscle lactates and heart rate. *Med Sci Sports Exerc* 15:523-528, 1983.

25. Pageaux, B. Perception of effort in exercise science: definition, measurement and perspectives. *Eur J Sport Sci* 16:885-894, 2016.

26. Peng, RD. Reproducible research in computational science. *Science* 334:1226, 2011.

27. Rahm, E, and Hai Do, H. Data cleaning: problems and current approaches. *IEEE Data Eng Bull* 23:3-13, 2000.

28. Rajalingham, K, Chadwick, D, Knight, B, and Edwards, D. Quality control in spreadsheets: a software engineering-based approach to spreadsheet development. Presented at Proceedings of the 33rd Annual Hawaii International Conference on System Sciences, 2000.

29. Sandve, GK, Nekrutenko, A, Taylor, J, and Hovig, E. Ten simple rules for reproducible computational research. *PLoS Comput Biol* 9:e1003285, 2013.

30. Thomas, JR, Nelson, JK, and Silverman, SJ. *Research Methods in Physical Activity.* Champaign, IL: Human Kinetics, 360-367, 2015.

31. Varley, MC, Jaspers, A, Helsen, WF, and Malone, JJ. Methodological considerations when quantifying high-intensity efforts in team sport using Global Positioning System technology. *Int J Sports Physiol Perform* 12:1059-1068, 2017.

32. Vincent, WJ, and Weir, J. *Statistics in Kinesiology.* Champaign, IL: Human Kinetics, 165-176, 1994.

33. Wang, W, Guo, Y, Huang, B, Zhao, G, Liu, B, and Wang, L. Analysis of filtering methods for 3D acceleration signals in body sensor network. Presented at International Symposium on Bioelectronics and Bioinformatics 2011, 2011.

34. Watt, A, and Eng, N. *Database Design.* Victoria, BC: BCcampus, 10-14, 2014.

35. Weston, M. Difficulties in determining the dose-response nature of competitive soccer matches. *J Athl Enhanc* 2, 2012.

Chapter 9

1. Akenhead, R, and Nassis, GP. Training load and player monitoring in high-level football: current practice and perceptions. *Int J Sports Physiol Perform* 11:587-593, 2016.

2. Alarifi, A, Al-Salman, A, Alsaleh, M, Alnafessah, A, Al-Hadhrami, S, Al-Ammar, M, and Al-Khalifa, HS. Ultra wideband indoor positioning technologies: analysis and recent advances. *Sensors* 16:707, 2016.

3. Andreoni, G, Standoli, C, and Perego, P. Defining requirements and related methods for designing sensorized garments. *Sensors (Basel)* 16:769, 2016.

4. Barrett, S, Midgley, A, and Lovell, R. PlayerLoad™: reliability, convergent validity, and influence of unit position during treadmill running. *Int J Sports Physiol Perform* 9:945-952, 2014.

5. Barrett, S, Midgley, A, Reeves, M, Joel, T, Franklin, E, Heyworth, R, Garrett, A, and Lovell, R. The within-match patterns of locomotor efficiency during professional soccer match play: implications for injury risk? *J Sci Med Sport* 19:810-815, 2016.

6. Beato, M, De Keijzer, KL, Carty, B, and Connor, M. Monitoring fatigue during intermittent exercise with accelerometer-derived metrics. *Front Physiol* 10:780, 2019.

7. Boyd, L. A new way of using accelerometers in Australian rules football: assessing external loads. 1-260, 2011. Available from: http://vuir.vu.edu.au/21297/

8. Boyd, LJ, Ball, K, and Aughey, RJ. Quantifying external load in Australian football matches and training using accelerometers. *Int J Sports Physiol Perform* 8:44-51, 2013.

9. Bradshaw, EJ, Rice, V, and Landeo, R. Impact load monitoring using inertial measurement units on different viscoelastic sport surfaces: a technical report. In ISBS *Proceedings Archive*, vol. 36. Auckland, 2018.

10. Brown, DM, Dwyer, DB, Robertson, SJ, and Gastin, PB. Metabolic power method: underestimation of energy expenditure in field-sport movements using a Global Positioning System tracking system. *Int J Sports Physiol Perform* 11:1067-1073, 2016.

11. Buchheit, M, Gray, A, and Morin, J. Assessing stride variables and vertical stiffness with GPS-embedded accelerometers: preliminary insights for the monitoring of neuromuscular fatigue on the field. *J Sports Sci Med* 14:698-701, 2015.

12. Buchheit, M, and Simpson, BM. Player-tracking technology: half-full or half-empty glass? *Int J Sports Physiol Perform* 12:S235-S241, 2017.

13. Carling, C, Bloomfield, J, Nelsen, L, and Reilly, T. The role of motion analysis in elite soccer. *Sports Med* 38:839-862, 2008.

14. Carling, C, Williams, A, and Reilly, T. *Handbook of Soccer Match Analysis: A Systematic Approach to Improving Performance*. Abington, Oxon: Routledge, 148-160, 2007.

15. Chambers, R, Gabbett, T, Cole, MH, and Beard, A. The use of wearable microsensors to quantify sport-specific movements. *Sports Med* 45:1065-1081, 2015.

16. Cummins, C, Orr, R, O'Connor, H, and West, C. Global Positioning Systems (GPS) and microtechnology sensors in team sports: a systematic review. *Sports Med* 43:1025-1042, 2013.

17. Delaney, JA, Cummins, CJ, Thornton, HR, and Duthie, GM. Importance, reliability and usefulness of acceleration measures in team sports. *J Strength Cond Res* 32:1, 2017.

18. Dines, JS, Tubbs, T, Fleisig, GS, Dines, JS, Dines, DM, Altchek, DW, and Dowling, B. The relationship of throwing arm mechanics and elbow varus torque: within-subject variation for professional baseball pitchers across 81,999 throws. *Am J Sports Med* 45:3030-3035, 2017.

19. DiSalvo, V, Collins, A, McNeill, B, and Cardinale, M. Validation of Prozone ®: a new video-based performance analysis system. *Int J Perform Anal Sport* 6:108-119, 2006.

20. Edgecomb, SJ, and Norton, KI. Comparison of global positioning and computer-based tracking systems for measuring player movement distance during Australian football. *J Sci Med Sport* 9:25-32, 2006.

21. Gabbett, T. Relationship between accelerometer load, collisions, and repeated high-intensity effort activity in rugby league players. *J Strength Cond Res* 29:3424-3431, 2015.

22. Gabbett, T, Jenkins, D, and Abernethy, B. Physical collisions and injury during professional rugby league skills training. *J Sci Med Sport* 13:578-583, 2010.

23. Gastin, P, McLean, O, Spittle, M, and Breed, RV. Quantification of tackling demands in professional Australian football using integrated wearable athlete tracking technology. *J Sci Med Sport* 16:589-593, 2013.

24. Harper, DJ, Carling, C, and Kiely, J. High-intensity acceleration and deceleration demands in elite team sports competitive match play: a systematic review and meta-analysis of observational studies. *Sports Med* 49:1923-1947, 2019.

25. Hummel, O, Fehr, U, and Ferger, K. Beyond ibeer – exploring the potential of smartphone sensors for performance diagnostics in sports. *Int J Comput Sci Sport* 12:46-60, 2013.

26. Kelley, J, Choppin, SB, Goodwill, SR, and Haake, SJ. Validation of a live, automatic ball velocity and spin rate finder in tennis. *Procedia Eng* 2:2967-2972, 2010.

27. Kelly, SJ, Murphy, AJ, Watsford, ML, Austin, D, and Rennie, M. Reliability and validity of sports accelerometers during static and dynamic testing. *Int J Sports Physiol Perform* 10:106-111, 2015.

28. King, GA, Torres, N, Potter, C, Brooks, TJ, and Coleman, KJ. Comparison of activity monitors to estimate energy cost of treadmill exercise. *Med Sci Sport Exerc* 36:1244-1251, 2004.

29. Lacome, M, Simpson, BM, and Buchheit, M. Monitoring training status with with player tracking technology: still on the road to Rome. Part 1. *Aspetar Sports Med J* 7: 54-64, 2018.

30. Larsson, P. Global Positioning System and sport-specific testing. *Sports Med* 33:1093-1101, 2003.

31. Lee, JB, Mellifont, RB, and Burkett, BJ. The use of a single inertial sensor to identify stride, step, and stance durations of running gait. *J Sci Med Sport* 13:270-273, 2010.

32. Lee, JB, Sutter, KJ, Askew, CD, and Burkett, BJ. Identifying symmetry in running gait using a single inertial sensor. *J Sci Med Sport* 13:559-563, 2010.

33. Li, RT, Kling, SR, Salata, MJ, Cupp, SA, Sheehan, J, and Voos, JE. Wearable performance devices in sports medicine. *Sport Health* 8:74-78, 2016.

34. Little, C, Lee, JB, James, DA, and Davison, K. An evaluation of inertial sensor technology in the discrimination of human gait. *J Sports Sci* 31:1312-1318, 2013.

35. Luteberget, LS, Holme, BR, and Spencer, M. Reliability of wearable inertial measurement units to measure physical activity in team handball. *Int J Sports Physiol Perform* 13:467-473, 2018.

36. Malone, JJ, Lovell, R, Varley, MC, and Coutts, AJ. Unpacking the black box: applications and considerations for using GPS devices in sport. *Int J Sports Physiol Perform* 12:S218-S226, 2017.

37. McLean, BD, Strack, D, Russell, J, and Coutts, AJ. Quantifying physical demands in the National Basketball Association (NBA): challenges in developing best-practice models for athlete care and performance. *Int J Sports Physiol Perform* 14:414-420, 2019.

38. Mitchell, E, Monaghan, D, and O'Connor, N. Classification of sporting activities using smartphone accelerometers. *Sensors* 13:5317-5337, 2013.

39. Montgomery, PG, Pyne, DB, and Minahan, CL. The physical and physiological demands of basketball training and competition. *Int J Sports Physiol Perform* 5:75-86, 2010.

40. Murray, A, Buttfield, A, Simpkin, A, Sproule, J, and Turner, AP. Variability of within-step acceleration and daily wellness monitoring in collegiate American football. *J Sci Med Sport* 22:488-493, 2019.

41. Neville, J, Wixted, A, Rowlands, D, and James, D. Accelerometers: an underutilized resource in sports monitoring. *2010 Sixth International Conference on Intelligent Sensors, Sensor Networks Information Processing,* Brisbane, QLD, pp. 287-290.

42. Park, LAF, Scott, D, and Lovell, R. Velocity zone classification in elite women's football: where do we draw the lines? *Sci Med Football* 3:21-28, 2019.

43. Polglaze, T, Dawson, B, and Peeling, P. Gold standard or fool's gold? The efficacy of displacement variables as indicators of energy expenditure in team sports. *Sports Med* 46:657-670, 2016.

44. Rantalainen, T, Gastin, PB, Spangler, R, and Wundersitz, D. Concurrent validity and reliability of torso-worn inertial measurement unit for jump power and height estimation. *J Sports Sci* 36:1937-1942, 2018.

45. Reilly, T, and Thomas, V. A motion analysis of work-rate in different positional roles in professional football match-play. *J Hum Mov Stud* 2:87-97, 1976.

46. Sabatini, A, Martelloni, C, Scapellato, S, and Cavallo, F. Assessment of walking features from foot inertial sensing. *IEEE Trans Biomed Eng* 52:486-494, 2005.

47. Sathyan, T, Shuttleworth, R, Hedley, M, and Davids, K. Validity and reliability of a radio positioning system for tracking athletes in indoor and outdoor team sports. *Behav Res Methods* 44:1108-1114, 2012.

48. Schelling, X, and Torres, L. Accelerometer load profiles for basketball-specific drills in elite players. *J Sports Sci Med* 15:585-591, 2016.

49. Schutz, Y, and Chambaz, A. Could a satellite-based navigation system (GPS) be used to assess the physical activity of individuals on earth? *Eur J Clin Nutr* 51:338-339, 1997.

50. Seidl, T, Czyz, T, Spandler, D, Franke, N, and Lochmann, M. Validation of football's velocity provided by a radio-based tracking system. *Procedia Eng* 147:584-589, 2016.

51. Sheerin, KR, Reid, D, and Besier, TF. The measurement of tibial acceleration in runners—a review of the factors that can affect tibial acceleration during running and evidence-based guidelines for its use. *Gait Posture* 67:12-24, 2019.

52. Sweeting, AJ, Cormack, S, Morgan, S, and Aughey, RJ. When is a sprint a sprint? A review of the analysis of team-sport athlete activity profile. *Front Physiol* 8:1-12, 2017.

53. Vanrenterghem, J, Nedergaard, NJ, Robinson, MA, and Drust, B. Training load monitoring in team sports: a novel framework separating physiological and biomechanical load-adaptation pathways. *Sports Med* 47:2135-2142, 2017.

54. Witte, TH, and Wilson, AM. Accuracy of non-differential GPS for the determination of speed over ground. *J Biomech* 37:1891-1898, 2004.

55. Woellik, H, Mueller, A, and Herriger, J. Permanent RFID timing system in a track and field athletic stadium for training and analysing purposes. *Procedia Eng* 72:202-207, 2014.

56. Wong, P, Chamari, K, and Wisløff, U. Effects of 12-week on-field combined strength and power training on physical performance among U-14 young soccer players. *J Strength Cond Res* 24:644-652, 2010.

57. Wundersitz, D, Josman, C, Gupta, R, Netto, KJ, Gastin, PB, and Robertson, SJ. Classification of team sport activities using a single wearable tracking device. *J Biomech* 48:3975-3981, 2015.

Chapter 10

1. Akenhead, R, French, D, Thompson, KG, and Hayes, PR. The acceleration dependent validity and reliability of 10Hz GPS. *J Sci Med Sport* 17:562-566, 2014.

2. Alexander, JP, Spencer, B, Mara, JK, and Robertson, S. Collective team behaviour of Australian rules football during phases of match play. *J Sports Sci* 37:237-243, 2019.

3. Aughey, RJ. Applications of GPS technologies to field sports. *Int J Sports Physiol Perform* 6:295-310, 2011.

4. Aughey, RJ, and Falloon, C. Real-time versus post-game GPS data in team sports. *J Sci Med Sport* 13:348-349, 2010.

5. Barnes, C, Archer, D, Hogg, B, Bush, M, and Bradley, P. The evolution of physical and technical performance parameters in the English Premier League. *Int J Sports Med* 35:1095-1100, 2014.

6. Barrett, S. Monitoring elite soccer players' external loads using real-time data. *Int J Sports Physiol Perform* 12:1285-1287, 2017.

7. Barrett, S, Midgley, A, Reeves, M, Joel, T, Franklin, E, Heyworth, R, Garrett, A, and Lovell, R. The within-match patterns of locomotor efficiency during professional soccer match play: implications for injury risk? *J Sci Med Sport* 19:810-815, 2016.

8. Barrett, S, Midgley, AW, Towlson, C, Garrett, A, Portas, M, and Lovell, R. Within-match PlayerLoad™ patterns during a simulated soccer match: potential implications for unit positioning and fatigue management. *Int J Sports Physiol Perform* 11:135-140, 2016.

9. Barris, S, and Button, C. A review of vision-based motion analysis in sport. *Sports Med* 38:1025-1043, 2008.

10. Beato, M, Coratella, G, Stiff, A, and Iacono, and Dello Iacono, A. The validity and between-unit variability of GNSS units (STATSports Apex 10 and 18 Hz) for measuring distance and peak speed in team sports. *Front Physiol* 9:1-8, 2018.

11. Boyd, LJ, Ball, K, and Aughey, RJ. The reliability of MinimaxX accelerometers for measuring physical activity in Australian football. *Int J Sports Physiol Perform* 6:311-321, 2011.

12. Bradley, PS, and Ade, JD. Are current physical match performance metrics in elite soccer fit for purpose or is the adoption of an integrated approach needed? *Int J Sports Physiol Perform* 13:656-664, 2018.

13. Bradley, PS, Sheldon, W, Wooster, B, Olsen, P, Boanas, P, and Krustrup, P. High-intensity running in English FA Premier League soccer matches. *J Sports Sci* 27:159-168, 2009.

14. Buchheit, M, Allen, A, Poon, TK, Modonutti, M, Gregson, W, and Di Salvo, V. Integrating different tracking systems in football: multiple camera semi-automatic system, local position measurement and GPS technologies. *J Sports Sci* 32:1844-1857, 2014.

15. Buchheit, M, Gray, A, and Morin, J. Assessing stride variables and vertical stiffness with GPS-embedded accelerometers: preliminary insights for the monitoring of neuromuscular fatigue on the field. *J Sports Sci Med* 14:698-701, 2015.

16. Buchheit, M, Al Haddad, H, Simpson, BM, Palazzi, D, Bourdon, PC, Di Salvo, V, and Mendez-Villaneuva, A. Monitoring accelerations with GPS in football: time to slow down? *Int J Sports Physiol Perform* 9:442-445, 2014.

17. Buchheit, M, and Simpson, BM. Player-tracking technology: half-full or half-empty glass? *Int J Sports Physiol Perform* 12:S235-S241, 2017.

18. Burgess, DJ. The research doesn't always apply: practical solutions to evidence-based training-load monitoring in elite team sports. *Int J Sports Physiol Perform* 12:S2136-S2141, 2017.

19. Carey, DL, Crossley, KM, Whiteley, R, Mosler, A, Ong, K-L, Crow, J, and Morris, ME. Modeling training loads and injuries. *Med Sci Sports Exerc* 50:2267-2276, 2018.

20. Carling, C, Bloomfield, J, Nelsen, L, and Reilly, T. The role of motion analysis in elite soccer. *Sports Med* 38:839-862, 2008.

21. Chen, KY, and Bassett, DR. The technology of accelerometry-based activity monitors: current and future. *Med Sci Sports Exerc* 37:S490-S500, 2005.

22. Corbett, DM, Bartlett, JD, O'Connor, F, Back, N, Torres-Ronda, L, and Robertson, S. Development of physical and skill training drill prescription systems for elite Australian rules football. *Sci Med Football* 2:51-57, 2018.

23. Cormack, S, Mooney, MG, Morgan, W, and McGuigan, MR. Influence of neuromuscular fatigue on accelerometer load in elite Australian football players. *Int J Sports Physiol Perform* 87:373-378, 2013.

24. Cormack, SJ, Smith, RL, Mooney, MM, Young, WB, and O'Brien, BJ. Accelerometer load as a measure of activity profile in different standards of netball match play. *Int J Sports Physiol Perform* 9:283-291, 2014.

25. Cummins, C, Orr, R, O'Connor, H, and West, C. Global Positioning Systems (GPS) and microtechnology sensors in team sports: a systematic review. *Sports Med* 43:1025-1042, 2013.

26. Delaney, JA, Duthie, GM, Thornton, HR, Scott, TJ, Gay, D, and Dascombe, BJ. Acceleration-based running intensities of professional rugby league match play. *Int J Sports Physiol Perform* 11:802-809, 2016.

27. DiSalvo, V, Collins, A, McNeill, B, and Cardinale, M. Validation of Prozone ®: a new video-based performance analysis system. *Int J Perform Anal Sport* 6:108-119, 2006.

28. Duran, A, and Earleywine, M. GPS data filtration method for drive cycle analysis applications. In: SAE Technical Paper Series 1, 2012.

28a. Dwyer, DB, and Gabbett, TJ. Global positioning system data analysis: Velocity ranges and a new definition of sprinting for field sport athletes. *Journal of Strength and Conditioning Research*, 26(3), 818–824, 2012.

29. Edwards, S, White, S, Humphreys, S, Robergs, R, and O'Dwyer, N. Caution using data from triaxial accelerometers housed in player tracking units during running. *J Sports Sci* 37:810-818, 2019.

30. Farrow, D, and Robertson, S. Development of a skill acquisition periodisation framework for high-performance sport. *Sports Med* 47:1043-1054, 2017.

31. Frencken, WGP, Lemmink, KAPM, and Delleman, NJ. Soccer-specific accuracy and validity of the local position measurement (LPM) system. *J Sci Med Sport* 13:641-645, 2010.

32. Gregson, W, Drust, B, Atkinson, G, and Salvo, VD. Match-to-match variability of high-speed activities in Premier League soccer. *Int J Sports Med* 31:237-242, 2010.

33. Halsey, LG, Shepard, ELC, and Wilson, RP. Assessing the development and application of the accelerometry technique for estimating energy expenditure. *Comp Biochem Physiol A Mol Integr Physiol* 158:305-314, 2011.

34. Halson, S. Monitoring training load to understand fatigue in athletes. *Sports Med* 44:139-147, 2014.

35. Halson, S, Peake, JM, and Sullivan, JP. Wearable technology for athletes: information overload and pseudoscience? *Int J Sports Physiol Perform* 11:705-706, 2016.

36. Henderson, MJ, Fransen, J, McGrath, JJ, Harries, SK, Poulos, N, and Coutts, AJ. Situational factors affecting rugby sevens match performance. *Sci Med Football* 1-6, 2019.

37. Hoppe, MW, Baumgart, C, Polglaze, T, and Freiwald, J. Validity and reliability of GPS and LPS for measuring distances covered and sprint mechanical properties in team sports. *PLoS One* 13:e0192708, 2018.

38. James, DA. The application of inertial sensors in elite sports monitoring. In: *The Engineering of Sport 6*. New York: Springer, 289-294, 2006.

39. Jennings, D, Cormack, S, Coutts, AJ, Boyd, LJ, and Aughey, RJ. Variability of GPS units for measuring distance in team sport movements. *Int J Sports Physiol Perform* 5:565-569, 2010.

40. Keller, TS, Weisberger, AM, Ray, JL, Hasan, SS, Shiavi, RG, and Spengler, DM. Relationship between vertical ground reaction force and speed during walking, slow jogging, and running. *Clin Biomech* 11:253-259, 1996.

41. Lacome, M, Peeters, A, Mathieu, B, Bruno, M, Christopher, C, and Piscione, J. Can we use GPS for assessing sprinting performance in rugby sevens? A concurrent validity and between-device reliability study. *Biol Sport* 36:25-29, 2019.

42. Ladin, Z, Flowers, WC, and Messner, W. A quantitative comparison of a position measurement system and accelerometry. *J Biomech* 22:295-308, 1989.

43. Linke, D, and Lames, M. Impact of sensor/reference position on player tracking variables: center of scapulae vs center of pelvis. *J Biomech* 83:319-323, 2019.

44. Linke, D, Link, D, and Lames, M. Validation of electronic performance and tracking systems EPTS under field conditions. *PLoS One* 13:e0199519, 2018.

45. Luteberget, LS, Spencer, M, and Gilgien, M. Validity of the Catapult ClearSky T6 Local Positioning System for team sports specific drills, in indoor conditions. *Front Physiol* 9:1-10, 2018.

46. Malone, JJ, Lovell, R, Varley, MC, and Coutts, AJ. Unpacking the black box: applications and considerations for using GPS devices in sport. *Int J Sports Physiol Perform* 12:S218-S226, 2017.

47. Mara, J, Morgan, S, Pumpa, K, and Thompson, K. The accuracy and reliability of a new optical player tracking system for measuring displacement of soccer players. *Int J Comput Sci Sport* 16:175-184, 2017.

48. McLean, BD, Strack, D, Russell, J, and Coutts, AJ. Quantifying physical demands in the National Basketball Association (NBA)–challenges in developing best-practice models for athlete care and performance. *Int J Sports Physiol Perform* 14:414-420, 2019.

49. Minne, K, Macoir, N, Rossey, J, Van den Brande, Q, Lemey, S, Hoebeke, J, and Di Poorter, E. Experimental evaluation of UWB indoor positioning for indoor track cycling. *Sensors (Basel)* 19:2041, 2019.

50. Montgomery, PG, Pyne, DB, and Minahan, CL. The performance and physiological demands of basketball competition and training. *Int J Sports Physiol Perform* 5:75-86, 2010.

51. Murray, NB, Gabbett, TJ, and Townshend, AD. The use of relative speed zones in Australian football: are we really measuring what we think we are? *Int J Sports Physiol Perform* 13:442-451, 2018.

52. Murray, A, and Varley, MC. Activity profile of international rugby sevens: effect of score line, opponent, and substitutes. *Int J Sports Physiol Perform* 10:791-801, 2015.

53. Nistala, A, and Guttag, J. Using deep learning to understand patterns of player movement in the NBA. *Sloan Anal Conf*, 2019.

54. O'Connor, F, Thornton, HR, Ritchie, D, Anderson, J, Bull, L, Rigby, A, Leonard, Z, Stern, S, and Bartlett, JD. Greater association of relative thresholds than absolute thresholds with noncontact lower-body injury in professional Australian rules footballers: implications for sprint monitoring. *Int J Sports Physiol Perform* 1-9, 2019. [e-pub ahead of print].

55. Ogris, G, Leser, R, Horsak, B, Kornfeind, P, Heller, M, and Baca, A. Accuracy of the LPM tracking system considering dynamic position changes. *J Sports Sci* 30:1503-1511, 2012.

56. Pezzack, JC, Norman, RW, and Winter, DA. An assessment of derivative determining techniques used for motion analysis. *J Biomech* 10:377-382, 1977.

57. Polglaze, T, Dawson, B, Hiscock, DJ, and Peeling, P. A comparative analysis of accelerometer and time–motion data in elite men's hockey training and competition. *Int J Sports Physiol Perform* 10:446-451, 2015.

58. Randers, MB, Mujika, I, Hewitt, A, Santisteban, J, Bischoff, R, Solano, R, Zubillaga, A, Peltola, E, Krustrup, P, and Mohr, M. Application of four different football match analysis systems: a comparative study. *J Sports Sci* 28:171-182, 2010.

59. Reilly, T, and Thomas, V. A motion analysis of work-rate in different positional roles in professional football match-play. *J Hum Mov Stud* 2:87-97, 1976.

60. Roe, G, Darrall-Jones, J, Black, C, Shaw, W, Till, K, and Jones, B. Validity of 10-HZ GPS and timing gates for assessing maximum velocity in professional rugby union players. *Int J Sports Physiol Perform* 12:836-839, 2017.

61. Roewer, BD, Ford, KR, Myer, GD, and Hewett, TE. The "impact" of force filtering cut-off frequency on the peak knee abduction moment during landing: artefact or "artifiction"? *Br J Sports Med* 48:464-468, 2014.

62. Rowell, AE, Aughey, RJ, Clubb, J, and Cormack, S. A standardized small sided game can be used to monitor neuromuscular fatigue in professional A-league football players. *Front Physiol* 9:1-13, 2018.

63. Sampaio, J, McGarry, T, Calleja-González, J, Jiménez Sáiz, S, Schelling I, Del Alcázar, X, and Balciunas, M. Exploring game performance in the National Basketball Association using player tracking data. *PLoS One* 10:1-14, 2015.

64. Sathyan, T, Shuttleworth, R, Hedley, M, and Davids, K. Validity and reliability of a radio positioning system for tracking athletes in indoor and outdoor team sports. *Behav Res Methods* 44:1108-1114, 2012.

65. Scott, BR, Lockie, RG, Knight, TJ, Clark, AC, and Janse de Jonge, XAK. A comparison of methods to quantify the in-season training load of professional soccer players. *Int J Sports Physiol Perform* 8:195-202, 2013.

66. Stevens, TGA, de Ruiter, CJ, van Niel, C, van de Rhee, R, Beek, PJ, and Savelsbergh, GJP. Measuring acceleration and deceleration in soccer-specific movements using a Local Position Measurement (LPM) System. *Int J Sports Physiol Perform* 9:446-456, 2014.

66a. Suárez-Arrones, LJ, Portillo, LJ, González-Ravé, JM, Muoz, VE, and Sanchez, F. Match running performance in Spanish elite male rugby union using global positioning system. *Isokinetics and Exercise Science.* https://doi.org/10.3233/IES-2012-0444, 2012.

67. Sweeting, AJ, Cormack, S, Morgan, S, and Aughey, RJ. When is a sprint a sprint? A review of the analysis of team-sport athlete activity profile. *Front Physiol* 8:1-12, 2017.

68. Taberner, M, O'Keefe, J, Flower, D, Phillips, J, Close, G, Cohen, DD, Richter, C, and Carling, C. Interchangeability of position tracking technologies;

can we merge the data? *Sci Med Football* 4:1, 76-81, DOI: 10.1080/24733938.2019.1634279, 2020.

69. Thornton, HR, Delaney, JA, Bartlett, JD, and Duthie, GM. No meaningful difference between absolute and relative speed thresholds when converted to a standard-ten score within a load monitoring system. *Sport Perform Sci Rep* 58:v1, 2019.

70. Thornton, HR, Nelson, AR, Delaney, JA, Serpiello, FR, and Duthie, GM. Interunit reliability and effect of data-processing methods of Global Positioning Systems. *Int J Sports Physiol Perform* 14:432-438, 2019.

71. Vales-Alonso, J, Chaves-Dieguez, D, Lopez-Matencio, P, Alcaraz, JJ, Parrado-Garcia, FJ, and Gonzalez-Castano, FJ. SAETA: a smart coaching assistant for professional volleyball training. *IEEE Trans Syst Man Cybern Syst* 45:1138-1150, 2015.

72. Varley, MC, and Aughey, RJ. Acceleration profiles in elite Australian soccer. *Int J Sports Med* 34:34-39, 2013.

73. Varley, MC, Di Salvo, V, Modonutti, M, Gregson, W, and Mendez-Villanueva, A. The influence of successive matches on match-running performance during an under-23 international soccer tournament: the necessity of individual analysis. *J Sports Sci* 36:585-591, 2018.

74. Varley, MC, Fairweather, IH, and Aughey, RJ. Validity and reliability of GPS for measuring instantaneous velocity during acceleration, deceleration, and constant motion. *J Sports Sci* 30:121-127, 2012.

75. Varley, MC, Jaspers, A, Helsen, WF, and Malone, JJ. Methodological considerations when quantifying high-intensity efforts in team sport using Global Positioning System technology. *Int J Sports Physiol Perform* 12:1059-1068, 2017.

76. Warman, GE, Cole, MH, Johnston, RD, Chalkley, D, and Pepping, G-J. Using microtechnology to quantify torso angle during match-play in field hockey. *J Strength Cond Res* 33:2648-2654, 2019.

77. Weaving, D, Jones, B, Ireton, M, Whitehead, S, Till, K, and Beggs, CB. Overcoming the problem of multicollinearity in sports performance data: a novel application of partial least squares correlation analysis. *PLoS One* 14:e0211776, 2019.

78. Weaving, D, Jones, B, Marshall, P, Till, K, and Abt, G. Multiple measures are needed to quantify training loads in professional rugby league. *Int J Sports Med* 38:735-740, 2017.

79. Weaving, D, Jones, B, Till, K, Marshall, P, Earle, K, and Abt, G. Quantifying the external and internal loads of professional rugby league training modes. *J Strength Cond Res*, 2017. [e-pub ahead of print].

80. Weston, M, Siegler, J, Bahnert, A, McBrien, J, and Lovell, R. The application of differential ratings of perceived exertion to Australian Football League matches. *J Sci Med Sport* 18:704-708, 2015.

81. Winter, DA. Kinematics In: *Biomechanics and Motor Control of Human Movement.* Hoboken, NJ: John Wiley & Sons, 66-67, 2009.

82. Witte, TH, and Wilson, AM. Accuracy of non-differential GPS for the determination of speed over ground. *J Biomech* 37:1891-1898, 2004.

83. Woellik, H. RFID timing antenna for open water swimming competitions. *Proceedings* 2:300, 2018.

84. Woellik, H, Mueller, A, and Herriger, J. Permanent RFID timing system in a track and field athletic stadium for training and analysing purposes. *Procedia Eng* 72:202-207, 2014.

85. Wundersitz, D, Gastin, PB, Richter, C, Robertson, SJ, and Netto, KJ. Validity of a trunk-mounted accelerometer to assess peak accelerations during walking, jogging and running. *Eur J Sport Sci* 15:382-390, 2015.

Chapter 11

1. Abdelsattar, M, Konrad, A, and Tilp, M. Relationship between Achilles tendon stiffness and ground contact time during drop jumps. *J Sports Sci Med* 17:223-228, 2018.

2. Al-Amri, M, Nicholas, K, Button, K, Sparkes, V, Sheeran, L, and Davies, JL. Inertial measurement units for clinical movement analysis: reliability and concurrent validity. *Sensors (Basel)* 18:719, 2018.

3. Alenezi, F, Herrington, L, Jones, P, and Jones, R. How reliable are lower limb biomechanical variables during running and cutting tasks. *J Electromyogr Kinesiol* 30:137-142, 2016.

4. Attia, A, Dhahbi, W, Chaouachi, A, Padulo, J, Wong, DP, and Chamari, K. Measurement errors when estimating the vertical jump height with flight time using photocell devices: the example of Optojump. *Biol Sport* 34:63-70, 2017.

5. Azevedo, LB, Lambert, MI, Vaughan, CL, O'Connor, CM, and Schwellnus, MP. Biomechanical variables associated with Achilles tendinopathy in runners. *Br J Sports Med* 43:288-292, 2009.

6. Barton, CJ, Bonanno, DR, Carr, J, Neal, BS, Malliaras, P, Franklyn-Miller, A, and Menz, HB. Running retraining to treat lower limb injuries: a mixed-methods study of current evidence synthesised with expert opinion. *Br J Sports Med* 50:513-526, 2016.

7. Bishop, C, Read, P, McCubbine, J, and Turner, A. Vertical and horizontal asymmetries are related to slower sprinting and jump performance in elite youth female soccer players. *J Strength Cond Res,* 2018. [e pub ahead of print].

8. Breen, DT, Foster, J, Falvey, E, and Franklyn-Miller, A. Gait re-training to alleviate the symptoms of anterior exertional lower leg pain: a case series. *Int J Sports Phys Ther* 10:85-94, 2015.

9. Brown, CN, Padua, DA, Marshall, SW, and Guskiewicz, KM. Hip kinematics during a stop-jump task in patients with chronic ankle instability. *J Athl Train* 46:461-467, 2011.

10. Brughelli, M, Cronin, J, and Chaouachi, A. Effects of running velocity on running kinetics and kinematics. *J Strength Cond Res* 25:933-939, 2011.

11. Ceseracciu, E, Sawacha, Z, and Cobelli, C. Comparison of markerless and marker-based motion capture technologies through simultaneous data collection during gait: proof of concept. *PLoS One* 9:e87640, 2014.

12. Chau, T. A review of analytical techniques for gait data. Part 1: Fuzzy, statistical and fractal methods. *Gait Posture* 13:49-66, 2001.

13. Chau, T. A review of analytical techniques for gait data. Part 2: Neural network and wavelet methods. *Gait Posture* 13:102-120, 2001.

14. Chinn, L, Dicharry, J, and Hertel, J. Ankle kinematics of individuals with chronic ankle instability while walking and jogging on a treadmill in shoes. *Phys Ther Sport* 14:232-239, 2013.

15. Daly, C, Persson, UM, Twycross-Lewis, R, Woledge, RC, and Morrissey, D. The biomechanics of running in athletes with previous hamstring injury: a case-control study. *Scand J Med Sci Sports* 26:413-420, 2016.

16. Dempsey, AR, Lloyd, DG, Elliott, BC, Steele, JR, and Munro, BJ. Changing sidestep cutting technique reduces knee valgus loading. *Am J Sports Med* 37:2194-2200, 2009.

17. Dempsey, AR, Lloyd, DG, Elliott, BC, Steele, JR, Munro, BJ, and Russo, KA. The effect of technique change on knee loads during sidestep cutting. *Med Sci Sports Exerc* 39:1765-1773, 2007.

18. Diebal, AR, Gregory, R, Alitz, C, and Gerber, JP. Forefoot running improves pain and disability associated with chronic exertional compartment syndrome. *Am J Sports Med* 40:1060-1067, 2012.

19. Dierks, TA, Manal, KT, Hamill, J, and Davis, IS. Proximal and distal influences on hip and knee kinematics in runners with patellofemoral pain during a prolonged run. *J Orthop Sports Phys Ther* 38:448-456, 2008.

20. Dixon, PC, Stebbins, J, Theologis, T, and Zavatsky, AB. Spatio-temporal parameters and lower-limb kinematics of turning gait in typically developing children. *Gait Posture* 38:870-875, 2013.

21. Dona, G, Preatoni, E, Cobelli, C, Rodano, R, and Harrison, AJ. Application of functional principal component analysis in race walking: an emerging methodology. *Sports Biomech* 8:284-301, 2009.

22. Donnelly, CJ, Lloyd, DG, Elliott, BC, and Reinbolt, JA. Optimizing whole-body kinematics to minimize valgus knee loading during sidestepping: implications for ACL injury risk. *J Biomech* 45:1491-1497, 2012.

23. Donoghue, OA, Harrison, AJ, Coffey, N, and Hayes, K. Functional data analysis of running kinematics in chronic Achilles tendon injury. *Med Sci Sports Exerc* 40:1323-1335, 2008.

24. Dos'Santos, T, Thomas, C, Comfort, P, and Jones, PA. The effect of angle and velocity on change of direction biomechanics: an angle-velocity trade-off. *Sports Med (Auckland, NZ)* 48:2235-2253, 2018.

25. Dos'Santos, T, Thomas, C, Jones, PA, and Comfort, P. Mechanical determinants of faster change of direction speed performance in male athletes. *J Strength Cond Res* 31:696-705, 2017.

26. Dos'Santos, T, Thomas, C, Jones, PA, and Comfort, P. Assessing asymmetries in change of direction speed performance; application of change of direction deficit. *J Strength Cond Res* 33:2953-2961, 2018.

27. Franklyn-Miller, A, Richter, C, King, E, Gore, S, Moran, K, Strike, S, and Falvey, EC. Athletic groin pain (part 2): a prospective cohort study on the biomechanical evaluation of change of direction identifies three clusters of movement patterns. *Br J Sports Med* 51:460-468, 2017.

28. Fuerst, P, Gollhofer, A, Lohrer, H, and Gehring, D. Ankle joint control in people with chronic ankle instability during run-and-cut movements. *Int J Sports Med* 39:853-859, 2018.

29. Furlan, L, and Sterr, A. The applicability of standard error of measurement and minimal detectable change to motor learning research-a behavioral study. *Front Hum Neurosci* 12:95, 2018.

30. Golenia, L, Schoemaker, MM, Otten, E, Mouton, LJ, and Bongers, RM. What the dynamic systems approach can offer for understanding development: an example of mid-childhood reaching. *Front Psychol* 8:1774, 2017.

31. Gore, SJ, Franklyn-Miller, A, Richter, C, Falvey, EC, King, E, and Moran, K. Is stiffness related to athletic groin pain? *Scand J Med Sci Sports* 28:1681-1690, 2018.

32. Grau, S, Maiwald, C, Krauss, I, Axmann, D, Janssen, P, and Horstmann, T. What are causes and treatment strategies for patellar-tendinopathy in female runners? *J Biomech* 41:2042-2046, 2008.

33. Grimaldi, A, Mellor, R, Hodges, P, Bennell, K, Wajswelner, H, and Vicenzino, B. Gluteal tendinopathy: a review of mechanisms, assessment and management. *Sports Med* 45:1107-1119, 2015.

34. Harrison, AJ, Ryan, W, and Hayes, K. Functional data analysis of joint coordination in the development of vertical jump performance. *Sports Biomech* 6:199-214, 2007.

35. Hewett, TE, Myer, GD, Ford, KR, Heidt, RS Jr, Colosimo, AJ, McLean, SG, van den Bogert, AJ, Paterno, MV, and Succop, P. Biomechanical measures of neuromuscular control and valgus loading of the knee predict anterior cruciate ligament injury risk in female athletes: a prospective study. *Am J Sports Med* 33:492-501, 2005.

36. Higashihara, A, Nagano, Y, Takahashi, K, and Fukubayashi, T. Effects of forward trunk lean on hamstring muscle kinematics during sprinting. *J Sports Sci* 33:1366-1375, 2015.

37. Hopper, DM, Goh, SC, Wentworth, LA, Chan, DYK, Chau, JHW, Wootton, GJ, Strauss, GR, and Boyle, JJW. Test–retest reliability of knee rating scales and functional hop tests one year following anterior cruciate ligament reconstruction. *Phys Ther Sport* 3:10-18, 2002.

38. Ishida, K, Murata, M, and Hirano, Y. Shoulder and elbow kinematics in throwing of young baseball players. *Sports Biomech* 5:183-196, 2006.

39. Jones, PA, Herrington, LC, Munro, AG, and Graham-Smith, P. Is there a relationship between landing, cutting, and pivoting tasks in terms of the characteristics of dynamic valgus? *Am J Sports Med* 42:2095-2102, 2014.

40. Kadaba, MP, Ramakrishnan, HK, and Wootten, ME. Measurement of lower extremity kinematics during level walking. *J Orthop Res* 8:383-392, 1990.

41. Kellis, E, and Katis, A. Biomechanical characteristics and determinants of instep soccer kick. *J Sports Sci Med* 6:154-165, 2007.

42. Kenneally-Dabrowski, C, Brown, NAT, Warmenhoven, J, Serpell, BG, Perriman, D, Lai, AKM, and Spratford, W. Late swing running mechanics influence hamstring injury susceptibility in elite rugby athletes: a prospective exploratory analysis. *J Biomech* 92:112-119, 2019.

43. King, E, Franklyn-Miller, A, Richter, C, O'Reilly, E, Doolan, M, Moran, K, Strike, S, and Falvey, E. Clinical and biomechanical outcomes of rehabilitation targeting intersegmental control in athletic groin pain: prospective cohort of 205 patients. *Br J Sports Med* 52:1054-1062, 2018.

44. King, E, Richter, C, Franklyn-Miller A, Daniels, K., Wadey, R, Moran, R., and Strike, S. Biomechanical but not timed performance asymmetries persist between limbs 9 months after ACL reconstruction during planned and unplanned change of direction. *J Biomech* 81:93-103, 2018.

45. King, E, Richter, C, Franklyn-Miller, A, Daniels, K, Wadey, R, Moran, R, and Strike, S. Whole-body biomechanical differences between limbs exist 9 months after ACL reconstruction across jump/landing tasks. *Scand J Med Sci Sports* 28:2567-2578, 2018.

46. King, E, Richter, C, Franklyn-Miller, A, Wadey, R, Moran, R, and Strike, S. Back to normal symmetry? Biomechanical variables remain more asymmetrical than normal during jump and change-of-direction testing 9 months after anterior cruciate ligament reconstruction. *Am J Sports Med* 47:1175-1185, 2019.

47. Knudson, D. *Fundamentals of Biomechanics*. New York: Springer Science+Business Media, 128-130, 2007.

48. Kristianslund, E, Bahr, R, and Krosshaug, T. Kinematics and kinetics of an accidental lateral ankle sprain. *J Biomech* 44:2576-2578, 2011.

49. Kristianslund, E, Faul, O, Bahr, R, Myklebust, G, and Krosshaug, T. Sidestep cutting technique and knee abduction loading: implications for ACL prevention exercises. *Br J Sports Med* 48:779-783, 2014.

50. Kristianslund, E, and Krosshaug, T. Comparison of drop jumps and sport-specific sidestep cutting: implications for anterior cruciate ligament injury risk screening. *Am J Sports Med* 41:684-688, 2013.

51. Krzysztof, M, and Mero, A. A kinematics analysis of three best 100 m performances ever. *J Hum Kinet* 36:149-160, 2013.

52. Langhout, R, Tak, I, van der Westen, R, and Lenssen, T. Range of motion of body segments is larger during the maximal instep kick than during the submaximal kick in experienced football players. *J Sports Med Phys Fitness* 57:388-395, 2017.

53. Mai, P, Mählich, D, Fohrmann, D, Kurz, M, Trudeau, MB, Hamill, J, Jessie Weir, G, and Willwacher, S. Cut-off frequencies matter: the effects of filtering strategies and footwear on internal knee abduction moments in running. *Footwear Sci* 11:S44-S46, 2019.

54. Maloney, SJ, Richards, J, Nixon, DGD, Harvey, LJ, and Fletcher, IM. Vertical stiffness asymmetries during drop jumping are related to ankle stiffness asymmetries. *Scand J Med Sci Sports* 27:661-669, 2017.

55. Mann, R, and Herman, J. Kinematic analysis of Olympic sprint performance: men's 200 meters. *Int J Sport Biomech* 1:151-162, 1985.

56. Marshall, BM, Franklyn-Miller, AD, King, EA, Moran, KA, Strike, SC, and Falvey, EC. Biomechanical factors associated with time to complete a change of direction cutting maneuver. *J Strength Cond Res* 28:2845-2851, 2014.

57. Marshall, BM, Franklyn-Miller, AD, Moran, KA, King, EA, Strike, SC, and Falvey, EC. Can a single-legged squat provide insight into movement control and loading during dynamic sporting actions in patients with athletic groin pain? *J Sport Rehabil* 25:117-125, 2015.

58. Merriaux, P, Dupuis, Y, Boutteau, R, Vasseur, P, and Savatier, X. A study of Vicon system positioning performance. *Sensors (Basel)* 17:1591, 2017.

59. Mohammadi, F, Salavati, M, Akhbari, B, Mazaheri, M, Mohsen Mir, S, and Etemadi, Y. Comparison of functional outcome measures after ACL reconstruction in competitive soccer players: a randomized trial. *J Bone Joint Surg Am* 95:1271-1277, 2013.

60. Moisan, G, Descarreaux, M, and Cantin, V. Effects of chronic ankle instability on kinetics, kinematics and muscle activity during walking and running: a systematic review. *Gait Posture* 52:381-399, 2017.

61. Morin, J-B, Bourdin, M, Edouard, P, Peyrot, N, Samozino, P, and Lacour, J-R. Mechanical determinants of 100-m sprint running performance. *Eur J Appl Physiol* 112:3921-3930, 2012.

62. Morin, JB, Jimenez-Reyes, P, Brughelli, M, and Samozino, P. When jump height is not a good indicator of lower limb maximal power output: theoretical demonstration, experimental evidence and practical solutions. *Sports Med* 49:999-1006, 2019.

63. Moudy, S, Richter, C, and Strike, S. Landmark registering waveform data improves the ability to predict performance measures. *J Biomech* 78:109-117, 2018.

64. Mousavi, SH, Hijmans, JM, Rajabi, R, Diercks, R, Zwerver, J, and van der Worp, H. Kinematic risk factors for lower limb tendinopathy in distance runners: a systematic review and meta-analysis. *Gait Posture* 69:13-24, 2019.

65. Murphy, AJ, Lockie, RG, and Coutts, AJ. Kinematic determinants of early acceleration in field sport athletes. *J Sports Sci Med* 2:144-150, 2003.

66. Nimphius, S, Callaghan, SJ, Bezodis, NE, and Lockie, RG. Change of direction and agility tests: challenging our current measures of performance. *Strength Cond J* 40:26-38, 2018.

67. Nimphius, S, McGuigan, MR, and Newton, RU. Relationship between strength, power, speed, and change of direction performance of female softball players. *J Strength Cond Res* 24:885-895, 2010.

68. Noehren, B, Scholz, J, and Davis, I. The effect of real-time gait retraining on hip kinematics, pain and function in subjects with patellofemoral pain syndrome. *Br J Sports Med* 45:691-696, 2011.

69. Opar, DA, Williams, MD, and Shield, AJ. Hamstring strain injuries: factors that lead to injury and re-injury. *Sports Med* 42:209-226, 2012.

70. Pairot-de-Fontenay, B, Willy, RW, Elias, ARC, Mizner, RL, Dube, MO, and Roy, JS. Running biomechanics in individuals with anterior cruciate ligament reconstruction: a systematic review. *Sports Med* 49:1411-1424, 2019.

71. Panagiotakis, E, Mok, KM, Fong, DT, and Bull, AMJ. Biomechanical analysis of ankle ligamentous sprain injury cases from televised basketball games: understanding when, how and why ligament failure occurs. *J Sci Med Sport* 20:1057-1061, 2017.

72. Pataky, TC, Robinson, MA, and Vanrenterghem, J. Vector field statistical analysis of kinematic and force trajectories. *J Biomech* 46:2394-2401, 2013.

73. Paterno, MV, Schmitt, LC, Ford, KR, Rauh, MJ, Myer, GD, Huang, B, and Hewett, TE. Biomechanical measures during landing and postural stability predict second anterior cruciate ligament injury after anterior cruciate ligament reconstruction and return to sport. *Am J Sports Med* 38:1968-1978, 2010.

74. Pereira, LA, Nimphius, S, Kobal, R, Kitamura, K, Turisco, LAL, Orsi, RC, Cal Abad, CC, and Loturco, I. Relationship between change of direction, speed, and power in male and female national Olympic team handball athletes. *J Strength Cond Res* 32:2987-2994, 2018.

75. Perrott, MA, Pizzari, T, Cook, J, and McClelland, JA. Comparison of lower limb and trunk kinematics between markerless and marker-based motion capture systems. *Gait Posture* 52:57-61, 2017.

76. Powell, HC, Silbernagel, KG, Brorsson, A, Tranberg, R, and Willy, RW. Individuals post Achilles tendon rupture exhibit asymmetrical knee and ankle kinetics and loading rates during a drop countermovement jump. *J Orthop Sports Phys Ther* 48:34-43, 2018.

77. Powers, CM. The influence of abnormal hip mechanics on knee injury: a biomechanical perspective. *J Orthop Sports Phys Ther* 40:42-51, 2010.

78. Reis, ACd, Correa, JCF, Bley, AS, Rabelo, NDA, Fukuda, TY, and Lucareli, PRG. Kinematic and kinetic analysis of the single-leg triple hop test in women with and without patellofemoral pain. *J Orthop Sports Phys Ther* 45:799-807, 2015.

79. Richards, J. *Biomechanics in Clinic and Research*. Philadelphia: Churchill Livingstone, 123-124, 187-197 and 254-256, 2008.

80. Richter, C, O'Connor, NE, Marshall, B, and Moran, K. Comparison of discrete-point vs. dimensionality-reduction techniques for describing performance-related aspects of maximal vertical jumping. *J Biomech* 47:3012-3017, 2014.

81. Rosen, AB, Ko, J, Simpson, KJ, Kim, S-H, and Brown, CN. Lower extremity kinematics during a drop jump in individuals with patellar tendinopathy. *Orthop J Sports Med*, 2015. [e-pub ahead of print].

82. Ross, GB, Dowling, B, Troje, NF, Fischer, SL, and Graham, RB. Objectively differentiating movement patterns between elite and novice athletes. *Med Sci Sports Exerc* 50:1457-1464, 2018.

83. Sadeghi, H, Allard, P, Shafie, K, Mathieu, PA, Sadeghi, S, Prince, F, and Ramsay, J. Reduction of gait data variability using curve registration. *Gait Posture* 12:257-264, 2000.

84. Schuermans, J, Van Tiggelen, D, Palmans, T, Danneels, L, and Witvrouw, E. Deviating running kinematics and hamstring injury susceptibility in male soccer players: cause or consequence? *Gait Posture* 57:270-277, 2017.

85. Seay, JF, Van Emmerik, RE, and Hamill, J. Trunk bend and twist coordination is affected by low back pain status during running. *Eur J Sport Sci* 14:563-568, 2014.

86. Serner, A, Mosler, AB, Tol, JL, Bahr, R, and Weir, A. Mechanisms of acute adductor longus injuries in male football players: a systematic visual video analysis. *Br J Sports Med* 53:158-164, 2019.

87. Seroyer, ST, Nho, SJ, Bach, BR, Bush-Joseph, CA, Nicholson, GP, and Romeo, AA. The kinetic chain in overhand pitching: its potential role for performance enhancement and injury prevention. *Sports Health* 2:135-146, 2010.

88. Sheikhhoseini, R, Alizadeh, M-H, Salavati, M, O'Sullivan, K, Shirzad, E, and Movahed, M. Altered lower limb kinematics during jumping among athletes with persistent low back pain. *Ann Appl Sport Sci* 6:23-30, 2018.

89. Silbernagel, KG, Gustavsson, A, Thomee, R, and Karlsson, J. Evaluation of lower leg function in patients with Achilles tendinopathy. *Knee Surg Sports Traumatol Arthrosc* 14:1207-1217, 2006.

90. Sinclair, J, Currigan, G, Fewtrell, DJ, and Taylor, PJ. Biomechanical correlates of club-head velocity during the golf swing. *Int J Perform Anal Sport* 14:54-63, 2014.

91. Stojanovic, E, Ristic, V, McMaster, DT, and Milanovic, Z. Effect of plyometric training on vertical jump performance in female athletes: a systematic review and meta-analysis. *Sports Med* 47:975-986, 2017.

92. Terada, M, Pietrosimone, B, and Gribble, PA. Individuals with chronic ankle instability exhibit altered landing knee kinematics: potential link with the mechanism of loading for the anterior cruciate ligament. *Clin Biomech (Bristol, Avon)* 29:1125-1130, 2014.

93. Theisen, A, and Day, J. Chronic ankle instability leads to lower extremity kinematic changes during landing tasks: a systematic review. *Int J Exerc Sci* 12:24-33, 2019.

94. Thomee, R, Kaplan, Y, Kvist, J, Myklebust, G, Risberg, MA, Theisen, D, Tsepis, E, Werner, S, Wondrasch, B, and Witvrouw, E. Muscle strength and hop performance criteria prior to return to sports after ACL reconstruction. *Knee Surg Sports Traumatol Arthrosc* 19:1798-1805, 2011.

95. van der Kruk, E, and Reijne, MM. Accuracy of human motion capture systems for sport applications; state-of-the-art review. *Eur J Sport Sci* 18:806-819, 2018.

96. Van der Worp, H, de Poel, HJ, Diercks, RL, van den Akker-Scheek, I, and Zwerver, J. Jumper's knee or lander's knee? A systematic review of the relation between jump biomechanics and patellar tendinopathy. *Int J Sports Med* 35:714-722, 2014.

97. van Emmerik, REA, Ducharme, SW, Amado, AC, and Hamill, J. Comparing dynamical systems concepts and techniques for biomechanical analysis. *J Sport Health Sci* 5:3-13, 2016.

98. Van Hooren, B, and Zolotarjova, J. The difference between countermovement and squat jump performances: a review of underlying mechanisms with practical applications. *J Strength Cond Res* 31:2011-2020, 2017.

99. Vanrenterghem, J, Venables, E, Pataky, T, and Robinson, MA. The effect of running speed on knee mechanical loading in females during side cutting. *J Biomech* 45:2444-2449, 2012.

100. Warmenhoven, J, Cobley, S, Draper, C, Harrison, A, Bargary, N, and Smith, R. Considerations for the use of functional principal components analysis in sports biomechanics: examples from on-water rowing. *Sports Biomech* 18:317-341, 2019.

101. Weir, JP. Quantifying test-retest reliability using the intraclass

correlation coefficient and the SEM. *J Strength Cond Res* 19:231-240, 2005.

102. Welch, N, Richter, C, Franklyn-Miller, A, and Moran, K. Principal component analysis of the biomechanical factors associated with performance during cutting. *J Strength Cond Res*, 2019. [e-pub ahead of print].

103. Wild, JJ, Bezodis, IN, North, JS, and Bezodis, NE. Differences in step characteristics and linear kinematics between rugby players and sprinters during initial sprint acceleration. *Eur J Sport Sci* 18:1327-1337, 2018.

104. Willson, JD, Sharpee, R, Meardon, SA, and Kernozek, TW. Effects of step length on patellofemoral joint stress in female runners with and without patellofemoral pain. *Clin Biomech (Bristol, Avon)* 29:243-247, 2014.

105. Willy, RW, Scholz, JP, and Davis, IS. Mirror gait retraining for the treatment of patellofemoral pain in female runners. *Clin Biomech (Bristol, Avon)* 27:1045-1051, 2012.

106. Winter, DA. *Biomechanics and Motor Control of Human Movement.* Hoboken, NJ: John Wiley & Sons, 82-106 and 176-187, 2009.

107. Young, WB, Dawson, B, and Henry, GJ. Agility and change-of-direction speed are independent skills: implications for training for agility in invasion sports. *Int J Sports Sci Coach* 10:159-169, 2015.

108. Zatsiorsky, VM. *Kinetics of Human Motion.* Champaign, IL: Human Kinetics, 266-345 and 365-435, 2002.

Chapter 12

1. Andersen, LL, Andersen, JL, Zebis, MK, and Aagaard, P. Early and late rate of force development: differential adaptive responses to resistance training? *Scand J Med Sci Sports* 20:e162-e169, 2010.

2. Angelozzi, M, Madama, M, Corsica, C, Calvisi, V, Properzi, G, McCaw, ST, and Caccio, A. Rate of force development as an adjunctive outcome measure for return-to-sport decisions after anterior cruciate ligament reconstruction. *J Orthop Sports Phys Ther* 42:772-780, 2012.

3. Appleby, BB, Cormack, SJ, and Newton, RU. Reliability of squat kinetics in well-trained rugby players: implications for monitoring training. *J Strength Cond Res* 33:2635-2640, 2019.

4. Ashworth, B, Hogben, P, Singh, N, Tulloch, L, and Cohen, DD. The athletic shoulder (ASH) test: reliability of a novel upper body isometric strength test in elite rugby players. *BMJ Open Sport Exerc Med* 4:e000365, 2018.

5. Barker, LA, Harry, JR, and Mercer, JA. Relationships between countermovement jump ground reaction forces and jump height, reactive strength index, and jump time. *J Strength Cond Res* 32:248-254, 2018.

6. Baumgart, C, Hoppe, MW, and Freiwald, J. Phase-specific ground reaction force analyses of bilateral and unilateral jumps in patients with ACL reconstruction. *Orthop J Sports Med* 5:2325967117710912, 2017.

7. Baumgart, C, Schubert, M, Hoppe, MW, Gokeler, A, Freiwald, J. Do ground reaction forces during unilateral and bilateral movements exhibit compensation strategies following ACL reconstruction? *Knee Surg Sports Traumatol Arthrosc* 25, 1385–1394, 2017.

8. Beckham, GK, Sato, K, Santana, HA, Mizuguchi, S, Haff, GG, and Stone, MH. Effect of body position on force production during the isometric midthigh pull. *J Strength Cond Res* 32:48-56, 2018.

9. Bishop, C, Brashill, C, Abbott, W, Read, P, Lake, J, and Turner, A. Jumping asymmetries are associated with speed, change of direction speed, and jump performance in elite academy soccer players. *J Strength Cond Res*, 2019. [e-pub ahead of print].

10. Blazevich, AJ, Gill, N, and Newton, RU. Reliability and validity of two isometric squat tests. *J Strength Cond Res* 16:298-304, 2002.

11. Bosco, C, Luhtanen, P, and Komi, PV. A simple method for measurement of mechanical power in jumping. *Eur J Appl Physiol Occup Physiol* 50:273-282, 1983.

12. Bourdon, PC, Cardinale, M, Murray, A, Gastin, P, Kellmann, M, Varley, MC, Gabbett, TJ, Coutts, AJ, Burgess, DJ, Gregson, W, and Cable, NT. Monitoring athlete training loads: consensus statement. *Int J Sports Physiol Perform* 12:S2161-S2170, 2017.

13. Brady, CJ, Harrison, AJ, Flanagan, EP, Haff, GG, and Comyns, TM. A comparison of the isometric midthigh pull and isometric squat: intraday reliability, usefulness, and the magnitude of difference between tests. *Int J Sports Physiol Perform* 13:844-852, 2018.

14. Buckthorpe, M, Gimpel, M, Wright, S, Sturdy, T, and Stride, M. Hamstring muscle injuries in elite football: translating research into practice. *Br J Sports Med* 52:628-629, 2018.

15. Chan, M-S, and Sigward, SM. Loading behaviors do not match loading abilities postanterior cruciate ligament reconstruction. *Med Sci Sports Exerc* 51:1626-1634, 2019.

16. Chiu, LZ, and Barnes, JL. The fitness-fatigue model revisited: implications for planning short-and long-term training. *Strength Cond J* 25:42-51, 2003.

17. Claudino, JG, Cronin, J, Mezêncio, B, McMaster, DT, McGuigan, M, Tricoli, V, Amadio, AC, and Serrao, JC. The countermovement jump to monitor neuromuscular status: a meta-analysis. *J Sci Med Sport* 20:397-402, 2017.

18. Claudino, JG, Cronin, JB, Mezêncio, B, Pinho, JP, Pereira, C, Mochizuki, L, Amadio, AC, and Serrao, JC. Autoregulating jump performance to induce functional overreaching. *J Strength Cond Res* 30:2242-2249, 2016.

19. Claudino, JG, Mezêncio, B, Soncin, R, Ferreira, JC, Couto, BP, and Szmuchrowski, LA. Pre vertical jump performance to regulate the training volume. *Int J Sports Med* 33:101-107, 2012.

19a. Cohen, D, Burton, A, Wells, C, Taberner, M, Diaz, MA, and Graham-Smith, P. Single v double leg countermovement jump tests: not half an apple! *Aspetar Sports Med J* 9:34-41, 2020.

19b. Cohen, D, Clarke, N, Harland, S, Lewin, C. Are force asymmetries measured in jump tests associated with previous injury in professional footballers? *Br J Sports Med.* 48 (7):579-580, 2014.

20. Comfort, P, Jones, PA, McMahon, JJ, and Newton, R. Effect of knee and trunk angle on kinetic variables during the isometric midthigh pull: test–retest reliability. *Int J Sports Physiol Perform* 10:58-63, 2015.

21. Constantine, E, Taberner, M, Richter, C, Willett, M, and Cohen, DD. Isometric posterior chain peak force recovery response following match-play in elite youth soccer players: associations with relative posterior chain strength. *Sports (Basel)* 7:218, 2019.

22. Cormack, SJ, Mooney, MG, Morgan, W, and McGuigan, MR. Influence of neuromuscular fatigue on accelerometer load in elite Australian football players. *Int J Sports Physiol Perform* 8:373-378, 2013.

23. Cormack, SJ, Newton, RU, and McGuigan, MR. Neuromuscular and endocrine responses of elite players to an Australian rules football match. *Int J Sports Physiol Perform* 3:359-374, 2008.

24. Cormack, SJ, Newton, RU, McGuigan, MR, and Cormie, P. Neuromuscular and endocrine responses of elite players during an Australian rules football season. *Int J Sports Physiol Perform* 3:439-453, 2008.

25. Cormie, P, McBride, JM, and McCaulley, GO. Power-time, force-time, and velocity-time curve analysis of the countermovement jump: impact of training. *J Strength Cond Res* 23:177-186, 2009.

26. De Witt, JK, English, KL, Crowell, JB, Kalogera, KL, Guilliams, ME, Nieschwitz, BE, Hanson, AM, and Ploutz-Snyder, LL. Isometric midthigh pull reliability and relationship to deadlift one repetition maximum. *J Strength Cond Res* 32:528-533, 2018.

27. Douglas, J, Pearson, S, Ross, A, and McGuigan, M. Kinetic determinants of reactive strength in highly trained sprint athletes. *J Strength Cond Res* 32:1562-1570, 2018.

28. Drinkwater, E. Applications of confidence limits and effect sizes in sport research. *Open Sports Sci J* 1:3-4, 2008.

29. Gathercole, R, Sporer, B, and Stellingwerff, T. Countermovement jump performance with increased training loads in elite female rugby athletes. *Int J Sports Med* 36:722-728, 2015.

30. Gathercole, R, Sporer, B, Stellingwerff, T, and Sleivert, G. Alternative countermovement-jump analysis to quantify acute neuromuscular fatigue. *Int J Sports Physiol Perform* 10:84-92, 2015.

31. Gathercole, RJ, Sporer, BC, Stellingwerff, T, and Sleivert, GG. Comparison of the capacity of different jump and sprint field tests to detect neuromuscular fatigue. *J Strength Cond Res* 29:2522-2531, 2015.

32. Gonzalo-Skok, O, Moreno-Azze, A, Arjol-Serrano, JL, Tous-Fajardo, J, and Bishop, C. A comparison of 3 different unilateral strength training strategies to enhance jumping performance and decrease interlimb asymmetries in soccer players. *Int J Sports Physiol Perform* 14:1256-1264, 2019.

33. Grindem, H, Snyder-Mackler, L, Moksnes, H, Engebretsen, L, and Risberg, MA. Simple decision rules can reduce reinjury risk by 84% after ACL reconstruction: the Delaware-Oslo ACL cohort study. *Br J Sports Med* 50:804-808, 2016.

34. Harry, JR, Paquette, MR, Schilling, BK, Barker, LA, James, CR, and Dufek, JS. Kinetic and electromyographic subphase characteristics with relation to countermovement vertical jump performance. *J Appl Biomech* 34:291-297, 2018.

35. Hart, LM, Cohen, DD, Patterson, SD, Springham, M, Reynolds, J, and Read, P. Previous injury is associated with heightened countermovement jump force-time asymmetries in professional soccer players. *Transl Sports Med* 2:256-262, 2019.

36. Heishman, A, Daub, B, Miller, R, Brown, B, Freitas, E, and Bemben, M. Countermovement jump inter-limb asymmetries in collegiate basketball players. *Sports (Basel)* 7:103, 2019.

37. Hewett, TE, Myer, GD, Ford, KR, Heidt, RS, Colosimo, AJ, McLean, SG, van den Bogert, AJ, Paterno, MV, and Succop, P. Biomechanical measures of neuromuscular control and valgus loading of the knee predict anterior cruciate ligament injury risk in female athletes: a prospective study. *Am J Sports Med* 33:492-501, 2005.

38. Hornsby, W, Gentles, J, MacDonald, C, Mizuguchi, S, Ramsey, M, and Stone, M. Maximum strength, rate of force development, jump height, and peak power alterations in weightlifters across five months of training. *Sports (Basel)* 5:78, 2017.

39. Hughes, S, Chapman, DW, Haff, GG, and Nimphius, S. The use of a functional test battery as a non-invasive method of fatigue assessment. *PLoS One* 14:e0212870, 2019.

40. Jiménez-Reyes, P, Pareja-Blanco, F, Cuadrado-Peñafiel, V, Ortega-Becerra, M, Párraga, J, and González-Badillo, JJ. Jump height loss as an indicator of fatigue during sprint training. *J Sports Sci* 37:1029-1037, 2019.

41. Jiménez-Reyes, P, Samozino, P, Brughelli, M, and Morin, J-B.

42. Jiménez-Reyes, P, Samozino, P, Pareja-Blanco, F, Conceição, F, Cuadrado-Peñafiel, V, González-Badillo, JJ, and Morin, J-B. Validity of a simple method for measuring force-velocity-power profile in countermovement jump. *Int J Sports Physiol Perform* 12:36-43, 2017.

43. Jordan, MJ, Aagaard, P, and Herzog, W. Lower limb asymmetry in mechanical muscle function: a comparison between ski racers with and without ACL reconstruction. *Scand J Med Sci Sports* 25:e301-e309, 2015.

44. Kipp, K, Kiely, MT, and Geiser, CF. Reactive strength index modified is a valid measure of explosiveness in collegiate female volleyball players. *J Strength Cond Res* 30:1341-1347, 2016.

45. Kirby, TJ, McBride, JM, Haines, TL, and Dayne, AM. Relative net vertical impulse determines jumping performance. *J Appl Biomech* 27:207-214, 2011.

46. Koch, J, Riemann, BL, and Davies, GJ. Ground reaction force patterns in plyometric push-ups. *J Strength Cond Res* 26:2220-2227, 2012.

47. Komi, P. *Strength and Power in Sport*. Hoboken, NJ: John Wiley & Sons, 203-228, 2008.

48. Kotsifaki, A, Korakakis, V, Whiteley, R, Van Rossom, S, and Jonkers, I. Measuring only hop distance during single leg hop testing is insufficient to detect deficits in knee function after ACL reconstruction: a systematic review and meta-analysis. *Br J Sports Med* 54:139-153, 2020.

49. Layer, JS, Grenz, C, Hinshaw, TJ, Smith, DT, Barrett, SF, and Dai, B. Kinetic analysis of isometric back squats and isometric belt squats. *J Strength Cond Res* 32:3301-3309, 2018.

50. Leary, BK, Statler, J, Hopkins, B, Fitzwater, R, Kesling, T, Lyon, J, Phillips, B, Bryner, RW, Cormie, P, and Haff, GG. The relationship between isometric force-time curve characteristics and club head speed in recreational golfers. *J Strength Cond Res* 26:2685-2697, 2012.

51. Linthorne, NP. Analysis of standing vertical jumps using a force platform. *Am J Physics* 69:1198-1204, 2001.

52. Maffiuletti, NA, Aagaard, P, Blazevich, AJ, Folland, J, Tillin, N, and Duchateau, J. Rate of force development: physiological and methodological considerations. *Eur J Appl Physiol* 116:1091-1116, 2016.

52a. Malaver, JR, Cubides, JR, Argothy, R, and Cohen, DD. Risk factors associated with medial tibial stress syndrome in military cadets during basic training: 1019: Board# 253 May 29 3:30 PM-5:00 PM. *Med Sci Sports Exerc* 51:268, 2019.

53. Malone, S, Hughes, B, Roe, M, Collins, K, and Buchheit, M. Monitoring player fitness, fatigue status and running performance during an in-season training camp in elite Gaelic football. *Sci Med Football* 1:229-236, 2017.

54. Matinlauri, A, Alcaraz, PE, Freitas, TT, Mendiguchia, J, Abedin-Maghanaki, A, Castillo, A, Martinez-Ruiz, E, Carlos-Vivas, J, and Cohen, DD. A comparison of the isometric force fatigue-recovery profile in two posterior chain lower limb tests following simulated soccer competition. *PLoS One* 14:e0206561, 2019.

55. McMahon, J, Lake, J, and Comfort, P. Reliability of and relationship between flight time to contraction time ratio and reactive strength index modified. *Sports (Basel)* 6:81, 2018.

56. Myer, GD, Martin Jr, L, Ford, KR, Paterno, MV, Schmitt, LC, Heidt Jr, RS, Colosimo, A, and Hewett, TE. No association of time from surgery with functional deficits in athletes after anterior cruciate ligament reconstruction: evidence for objective return-to-sport criteria. *Am J Sports Med* 40:2256-2263, 2012.

Effectiveness of an individualized training based on force-velocity profiling during jumping. *Front Physiol* 7:677, 2017.

57. Nagahara, R, Mizutani, M, Matsuo, A, Kanehisa, H, and Fukunaga, T. Association of sprint performance with ground reaction forces during acceleration and maximal speed phases in a single sprint. *J Appl Biomech* 34:104-110, 2018.

58. Newham, DJ, Mills, KR, Quigley, BM, and Edwards, RHT. Pain and fatigue after concentric and eccentric muscle contractions. *Clin Sci* 64:55-62, 1983.

59. Norris, D, Joyce, D, Siegler, J, Clock, J, and Lovell, R. Recovery of force–time characteristics after Australian rules football matches: examining the utility of the isometric midthigh pull. *Int J Sports Physiol Perform* 14:765-770, 2019.

59a. Read, PJ, Oliver, JL, De Ste Croix, MBA, Myer, GD, and Lloyd, RS. A prospective investigation to evaluate risk factors for lower extremity injury risk in male youth soccer players. *Scand J Med Sci Sport* 28:1244-1251, 2018.

60. Read, PJ, Turner, AN, Clarke, R, Applebee, S, and Hughes, J. Knee angle affects posterior chain muscle activation during an isometric test used in soccer players. *Sports (Basel)* 7:13, 2019.

61. Richter, C, O'Connor, NE, Marshall, B, and Moran, K. Analysis of characterizing phases on waveforms: an application to vertical jumps. *J Appl Biomech* 30:316-321, 2014.

62. Robertson, S, Bartlett, JD, and Gastin, PB. Red, amber, or green? Athlete monitoring in team sport: the need for decision-support systems. *Int J Sports Physiol Perform* 12:S273-S279, 2017.

63. Roos, PE, Button, K, and van Deursen, RW. Motor control strategies during double leg squat following anterior cruciate ligament rupture and reconstruction: an observational study. *J Neuroeng Rehabil* 11:19, 2014.

64. Sanchez-Medina, L, and González-Badillo, JJ. Velocity loss as an indicator of neuromuscular fatigue during resistance training. *Med Sci Sports Exerc* 43:1725-1734, 2011.

65. Skein, M, Duffield, R, Minett, GM, Snape, A, and Murphy, A. The effect of overnight sleep deprivation after competitive rugby league matches on postmatch physiological and perceptual recovery. *Int J Sports Physiol Perform* 8:556-564, 2013.

66. Suarez, DG, Mizuguchi, S, Hornsby, WG, Cunanan, AJ, Marsh, DJ, and Stone, MH. Phase-specific changes in rate of force development and muscle morphology throughout a block periodized training cycle in weightlifters. *Sports (Basel)* 7:129, 2019.

67. Suchomel, TJ, Nimphius, S, and Stone, MH. Scaling isometric mid-thigh pull maximum strength in division I athletes: are we meeting the assumptions? *Sports Biomech* 19:532-546, 2020.

68. Taberner, M, van Dyk, N, Allen, T, Richter, C, Howarth, C, Scott, S, and Cohen, DD. Physical preparation and return to sport of the football player with a tibia-fibula fracture: applying the "control-chaos continuum." *BMJ Open Sport Exerc Med* 5:e000639, 2019.

69. Taylor, KL. Monitoring neuromuscular fatigue in high performance athletes (doctoral dissertation, Edith Cowan University), 2012.

70. Taylor, KL, Cronin, J, Gill, ND, Chapman, DW, and Sheppard, J. Sources of variability in iso-inertial jump assessments. *Int J Sports Physiol Perform* 5:546-558, 2010.

71. Thorpe, RT, Atkinson, G, Drust, B, and Gregson, W. Monitoring fatigue status in elite team-sport athletes: implications for practice. *Int J Sports Physiol Perform* 12:S2-S27, 2017.

72. Van der Does, HTD, Brink, MS, Benjaminse, A, Visscher, C, and Lemmink, K. Jump landing characteristics predict lower extremity injuries in indoor team sports. *Int J Sports Med* 37:251-256, 2016.

73. Welsh, TT, Alemany, JA, Montain, SJ, Frykman, PN, Tuckow, AP, Young, AJ, and Nindl, BC. Effects of intensified military field training on jumping performance. *Int J Sports Med* 29:45-52, 2008.

74. West, DJ, Owen, NJ, Jones, MR, Bracken, RM, Cook, CJ, Cunningham, DJ, Shearer, DA, Finn, CV, Newton, RU, Crewther, BT, and Kilduff, LP. Relationships between force–time characteristics of the isometric midthigh pull and dynamic performance in professional rugby league players. *J Strength Cond Res* 25:3070-3075, 2011.

75. Wu, PP-Y, Sterkenburg, N, Everett, K, Chapman, DW, White, N, and Mengersen, K. Predicting fatigue using countermovement jump force-time signatures: PCA can distinguish neuromuscular versus metabolic fatigue. *PLoS One* 14:e0219295, 2019.

Chapter 13

1. Arsac, LM, Belli, A, and Lacour, JR. Muscle function during brief maximal exercise: accurate measurements on a friction-loaded cycle ergometer. *Eur J Appl Physiol Occup Physiol* 74:100-106, 1996.

2. Balsalobre-Fernández, C, Glaister, M, and Lockey, RA. The validity and reliability of an iPhone app for measuring vertical jump performance. *J Sports Sci* 33:1574-1579, 2015.

3. Bobbert, MF. Why is the force-velocity relationship in leg press tasks quasi-linear rather than hyperbolic? *J Appl Physiol* 112:1975-1983, 2012.

4. Bosco, C, Belli, A, Astrua, M, Tihanyi, J, Pozzo, R, Kellis, S, Tsarpela, O, Foti, C, Manno, R, and Tranquilli, C. A dynamometer for evaluation of dynamic muscle work. *Eur J Appl Physiol Occup Physiol* 70:379-386, 1995.

5. Cross, MR, Brughelli, M, Samozino, P, Brown, SR, and Morin, J-B. Optimal loading for maximizing power during sled-resisted sprinting. *Int J Sports Physiol Perform* 12:1069-1077, 2017.

6. Cross, MR, Brughelli, M, Samozino, P, and Morin, J-B. Methods of power-force-velocity profiling during sprint running: a narrative review. *Sports Med* 47:1255-1269, 2017.

7. Cross, MR, Tinwala, F, Lenetsky, S, Samozino, P, Brughelli, M, and Morin, J-B. Determining friction and effective loading for sled sprinting. *J Sports Sci* 35:2198-2203, 2017.

8. Dorel, S, Couturier, A, Lacour, JR, Vandewalle, H, Hautier, C, and Hug, F. Force-velocity relationship in cycling revisited: benefit of two-dimensional pedal forces analysis. *Med Sci Sports Exerc* 42:1174-1183, 2010.

9. Driss, T, and Vandewalle, H. The measurement of maximal (anaerobic) power output on a cycle ergometer: a critical review. *Biomed Res Int* 2013:589361, 2013.

10. Frost, DM, Cronin, JB, and Newton, RU. A comparison of the kinematics, kinetics and muscle activity between pneumatic and free weight resistance. *Eur J Appl Physiol* 104:937-956, 2008.

11. García-Ramos, A, Pérez-Castilla, A, and Jaric, S. Optimisation of applied loads when using the two-point method for assessing the force-velocity relationship during vertical jumps. *Sport Biomech* 12:1-16, 2018.

12. Giroux, C, Rabita, G, Chollet, D, and Guilhem, G. What is the best method for assessing lower limb force-velocity relationship? *Int J Sports Med* 36:143-149, 2015.

13. Haugen, TA, Breitschädel, F, and Samozino, P. Power-force-velocity profiling of sprinting athletes. *J Strength Cond Res* 34:1769-1773, 2020.

14. Haugen, TA, Breitschädel, F, and Seiler, S. Sprint mechanical variables in elite athletes: are force-velocity profiles sport specific or individual? *PLoS One* 14:e0215551, 2019.

15. Hill, AJ. The heat of shortening and the dynamic constants of muscle. *Proc R Soc London Ser B Biol Sci* 126:136-195, 1938.

16. Janicijevic, D, Knezevic, O, Mirkov, D, Pérez-Castilla, A, Petrovic, M, Samozino, P, and Garcia-Ramos, A. Assessment of the force-velocity relationship during vertical jumps: influence of the starting position, analysis procedures and number of loads. *Eur J Sport Sci*, 2019. [e-pub ahead of print].

17. Jaric, S. Force-velocity relationship of muscles performing multi-joint maximum performance tasks. *Int J Sports Med* 36:699-704, 2015.

18. Jaskolska, A, Goossens, P, Veentra, B, Jaskolski, A, and Skinner, JS. Treadmill measurement of the force-velocity relationship and power output in subjects with different maximal running velocities. *Sports Med* 8:347-358, 1998.

19. Jiménez-Reyes, P, Samozino, P, Brughelli, M, and Morin, J-B. Effectiveness of an individualized training based on force-velocity profiling during jumping. *Front Physiol* 7:677, 2017.

20. Jiménez-Reyes, P, Samozino, P, Cuadrado-Peñafiel, V, Conceição, F, González-Badillo, JJ, and Morin, J-B. Validity of a simple method for measuring force-velocity-power profile in countermovement jump. *Int J Sport Physiol Perform* 12:36-43, 2017.

21. Jiménez-Reyes, P, Samozino, P, García-Ramos, A, Cuadrado-Peñafiel, V, Brughelli, M, and Morin, J-B. Relationship between vertical and horizontal force-velocity-power profiles in various sports and levels of practice. *Peer J* 6:e5937, 2018.

22. Jiménez-Reyes, P, Samozino, P, and Morin, J-B. Optimized training for jumping performance using the force-velocity imbalance: individual adaptation kinetics. *PLoS One* 14:e0216681, 2019.

23. Maffiuletti, NA, Aagaard, P, Blazevich, AJ, Folland, J, Tillin, N, and Duchateau, J. Rate of force development: physiological and methodological considerations. *Eur J Appl Physiol* 116:1091-1116, 2016.

24. Markovic, G, Vuk, S, and Jaric, S. Effects of jump training with negative versus positive loading on jumping mechanics. *Int J Sports Med* 32:365-372, 2011.

25. Martin, JA, Brandon, SCE, Keuler, EM, Hermus, JR, Ehlers, AC, Segalman, DJ, Allen, MS, and Thelen, DG. Gauging force by tapping tendons. *Nat Commun* 9:1592, 2018.

26. Morin, J-B, Edouard, P, and Samozino, P. Technical ability of force application as a determinant factor of sprint performance. *Med Sci Sport Exerc* 43:1680-1688, 2011.

27. Morin, J-B, Jiménez-Reyes, P, Brughelli, M, and Samozino, P. When jump height is not a good indicator of lower limb maximal power output: theoretical demonstration, experimental evidence and practical solutions. *Sport Med* 49:999-1006, 2019.

28. Morin, J-B, and Samozino, P. Interpreting power-force-velocity profiles for individualized and specific training. *Int J Sports Physiol Perform* 11:267-272, 2016.

29. Morin, J-B, Samozino, P, eds. *Biomechanics of Training and Testing: Innovative Concepts and Simple Field Methods.* Cham, Switzerland: Springer International Publishing, 65-237, 2018.

30. Morin, J-B, Samozino, P, Bonnefoy, R, Edouard, P, and Belli, A. Direct measurement of power during one single sprint on treadmill. *J Biomech* 43:1970-1975, 2010.

31. Morin, J-B, Samozino, P, Edouard, P, and Tomazin, K. Effect of fatigue on force production and force application technique during repeated sprints. *J Biomech* 44:2719-2723, 2011.

32. Morin, J-B, Samozino, P, Murata, M, Cross, MR, and Nagahara, R. A simple method for computing sprint acceleration kinetics from running velocity data: replication study with improved design. *J Biomech* 94:82-87, 2019.

33. Nagahara, R, Mizutani, M, Matsuo, A, Kanehisa, H, and Fukunaga, T. Association of step width with accelerated sprinting performance and ground reaction force. *Int J Sports Med* 38:534-540, 2017.

34. Padulo, J, Migliaccio, G, Ardigò, L, Leban, B, Cosso, M, and Samozino, P. Lower limb force, velocity, power capabilities during leg press and squat movements. *Int J Sports Med* 38:1083-1089, 2017.

35. Palmieri, G, Callegari, M, and Fioretti, S. Analytical and multibody modeling for the power analysis of standing jumps. *Comput Methods Biomech Biomed Eng* 18:1564-1573, 2015.

36. Rabita, G, Dorel, S, Slawinski, J, Sàez-de-Villarreal, E, Couturier, A, Samozino, P, and Morin, J-B. Sprint mechanics in world-class athletes: a new insight into the limits of human locomotion. *Scand J Med Sci Sport* 25:583-594, 2015.

37. Rivière, JR. Effect of velocity on lower limb force production capacities during single and repeated high-intensity exercises [PhD thesis]. University Savoie Mont Blanc, Chambéry (France); 2020.

38. Rivière, JR, Rossi, J, Jimenez-Reyes, P, Morin, J-B, and Samozino, P. Where does the one-repetition maximum exist on the force-velocity relationship in squat? *Int J Sports Med* 38:1035-1043, 2017.

39. Romero-Franco, N, Jiménez-Reyes, P, Castaño-Zambudio, A, Capelo-Ramírez, F, Rodríguez-Juan, JJ, González-Hernández, J, Toscano-Bendala, FJ, Cuadrado-Peñafiel, V, and Balsalobre-Fernández, C. Sprint performance and mechanical outputs computed with an iPhone app: comparison with existing reference methods. *Eur J Sport Sci* 17:386-392, 2017.

40. Samozino, P, Edouard, P, Sangnier, S, Brughelli, M, Gimenez, P, and Morin, J-B. Force-velocity profile: imbalance determination and effect on lower limb ballistic performance. *Int J Sports Med* 35:505-510, 2014.

41. Samozino, P, Morin, J-B, Hintzy, F, and Belli, A. A simple method for measuring force, velocity and power output during squat jump. *J Biomech* 41:2940-2945, 2008.

42. Samozino, P, Rabita, G, Dorel, S, Slawinski, J, Peyrot, N, Saez de Villarreal, E, and Morin J-B. A simple method for measuring power, force, velocity properties, and mechanical effectiveness in sprint running. *Scand J Med Sci Sports* 26:648-658, 2016.

43. Samozino, P, Rejc, E, Di Prampero, PE, Belli, A, and Morin, J-B. Optimal force-velocity profile in ballistic movements--altius: citius or fortius? *Med Sci Sports Exerc* 44:313-322, 2012.

44. Samozino, P, Rivière, JR, Rossi, J, Morin, J-B, and Jimenez-Reyes, P. How fast is a horizontal squat jump? *Int J Sports Physiol Perform* 13:910-916, 2018.

45. Suzovic, D, Markovic, G, Pasic, M, and Jaric, S. Optimum load in various vertical jumps support the maximum dynamic output hypothesis. *Int J Sports Med* 34:1007-1014, 2013.

46. Thorstensson, A, Grimby, G, and Karlsson, J. Force-velocity relations and fiber composition in human knee extensor muscles. *J Appl Physiol* 40:12-16, 1976.

47. Wilson, GJ, Walshe, AD, and Fisher, MR. The development of an isokinetic squat device: reliability and relationship to functional performance. *Eur J Appl Physiol Occup Physiol* 75:455-461, 1997.

48. Yamauchi, J, and Ishii, N. Relations between force-velocity characteristics of the knee-hip extension movement and vertical jump performance. *J Strength Cond Res* 21:703-709, 2007.

Chapter 14

1. Achten, J, and Jeukendrup, AE. Heart rate monitoring: applications and limitations. *Sports Med* 33:517-538, 2003.

2. Al-Ani, M, Munir, SM, White, M, Townend, J, and Coote, JH. Changes in RR variability before and after endurance training

measured by power spectral analysis and by the effect of isometric muscle contraction. *Eur J Appl Physiol Occup Physiol* 74:397-403, 1996.

3. Al Ghatrif, M, and Lindsay, J. A brief review: history to understand fundamentals of electrocardiography. *J Community Hosp Intern Med Perspect* 2:14383, 2012.

4. Aubert, AE, Seps, B, and Beckers, F. Heart rate variability in athletes. *Sports Med* 33:889-919, 2003.

5. Banister, EW. Modeling elite athletic performance. In *Physiological Testing of Elite Athletes.* Green, H, McDougal, J, and Wenger, H, eds. Champaign, IL: Human Kinetics, 403-424, 1991.

6. Billman, GE. Heart rate variability - a historical perspective. *Front Physiol* 2:86, 2011.

7. Borresen, J, and Lambert, MI. Changes in heart rate recovery in response to acute changes in training load. *Eur J Appl Physiol* 101:503-511, 2007.

8. Borresen, J, and Lambert, MI. The quantification of training load, the training response and the effect on performance. *Sports Med* 39:779-795, 2009.

9. Bouchard, CL, and Rankinen TU. Individual differences in response to regular physical activity. *Med Sci Sports Exerc* 33:S446-S451, 2001.

10. Brink, MS, Nederhof, E, Visscher, C, Schmikli, SL, and Lemmink, KA. Monitoring load, recovery, and performance in young elite soccer players. *J Strength Cond Res* 24:597-603, 2010.

11. Brink, MS, Visscher, C, Schmikli, SL, Nederhof, E, and Lemmink, KA. Is an elevated submaximal heart rate associated with psychomotor slowness in young elite soccer players? *Eur J Sport Sci* 13:207-214, 2013.

12. Brown, TE, Beightol, LA, Koh, J, and Eckberg, DL. Important influence of respiration on human RR interval power spectra is largely ignored. *J Appl Physiol* 75:2310-2317, 1993.

13. Buchheit, M. Monitoring training status with HR measures: do all roads lead to Rome? *Front Physiol* 5:1-19, 2014.

14. Buchheit, M, Simpson, MB, Al Haddad, H, Bourdon, PC, and Mendez-Villanueva, A. Monitoring changes in physical performance with heart rate measures in young soccer players. *Eur J Appl Physiol* 112:711-723, 2012.

15. Camm, AJ, Malik, M, Bigger, JT, Breithardt, G, Cerutti, S, Cohen, RJ, Coumel, P, Fallen, EL, Kennedy, HL, Kleiger, RE, and Lombardi, F. Heart rate variability: standards of measurement, physiological interpretation, and clinical use. *Eur Heart J* 17:354-381, 1996.

16. Carter, JB, Banister, EW, and Blaber, AP. Effect of endurance exercise on autonomic control of heart rate. *Sports Med* 3:33-46, 2003.

17. Charkoudian, N, Eisenach, JH, Joyner, MJ, Roberts, SK, and Wick, DE. Interactions of plasma osmolality with arterial and central venous pressures in control of sympathetic activity and heart rate in humans. *Am J Physiol Heart Circ Physiol* 289:H2456-H2460, 2005.

18. Chen, JL, Yeh, DP, Lee, JP, Chen, CY, Huang, CY, Lee, SD, Chen, CC, Kuo, TB, Kao, CL, and Kuo, CH. Parasympathetic nervous activity mirrors recovery status in weightlifting performance after training. *J Strength Cond Res* 25:1546-1552, 2011.

19. Coutts, AJ, Reaburn, P, Piva, TJ, and Rowsell, GJ. Monitoring for overreaching in rugby league players. *Eur J Appl Physiol* 99:313-324, 2007.

20. Daanen, HM, Lamberts, RP, Kallen, VL, Jin, A, and Van Meeteren, NU. A systematic review on heart-rate recovery to monitor changes in training status in athletes. *Int J Sport Physiol* 7:251-260, 2012.

21. Edwards, S. *The Heart Rate Monitor Book.* Sacramento, CA: Fleet Feet Press, 127, 1993.

22. Esco, MR, and Flatt, AA. Ultra-short-term heart rate variability indexes at rest and post-exercise in athletes: evaluating the agreement with accepted recommendations. *J Sports Sci Med* 13:535-541, 2014.

23. Esco, M, Flatt, A, and Nakamura, F. Agreement between a smartphone pulse sensor application and electrocardiography for determining lnRMSSD. *J Strength Cond Res* 31:380-385, 2017.

24. Fahmy, HMA. *Wireless Sensor Networks: Concepts, Applications, Experimentation and Analysis.* Singapore: Springer, 496, 2016.

25. Flatt, AA, and Esco, MR. Validity of the ithlete™ smart phone application for determining ultra-short-term heart rate variability. *J Hum Kinet.* 39:85-92, 2013.

26. Friel, J. *Total Heart Rate Training: Customize and Maximize Your Workout Using a Heart Rate Monitor.* Berkeley: Ulysses Press, 13, 2006.

27. Fukushima, H, Kawanaka, H, Bhuiyan, MS, and Oguri, K. Estimating heart rate using wrist-type Photoplethysmography and acceleration sensor while running. *Conf Proc IEEE Eng Med Biol Soc* 2012:2901-2904, 2012.

28. Ganzfried, S, and Sandholm, T. Game theory-based opponent modeling in large imperfect-information games. In *Proc of 10th Int. Conf. on Autonomous Agents and Multiagent Systems.* Taipei, Taiwan: International Foundation for Autonomous Agents and Multiagent Systems, 2533-2540, 2011.

29. Geib, RW, Swink, PJ, Vorel, AJ, Shepard, CS, Gurovich, AN, and Waite, GN. The bioengineering of changing lifestyle and wearable technology: a mini review. *Biomed Sci Instrum* 51:69-76, 2015.

30. Gillinov, AM, Etiwy, M, Gillinov, S, Wang, R, Blackburn, G, Phelan, D, Houghtaling, P, Javadikasgari, H, and Desai, MY. Variable accuracy of commercially available heart rate monitors. *J Am Coll Cardiol* 69:336, 2017.

31. Gomez, C, Oller, J, and Paradells, J. Overview and evaluation of Bluetooth low energy: an emerging low-power wireless technology. *Sensors* 12:11734-11753, 2012.

32. Hajar, R. The pulse from ancient to modern medicine: part 3. *Heart Views* 3:117-120, 2018.

33. Halson, SL. Monitoring training load to understand fatigue in athletes. *Sports Med* 44:139-147, 2014.

34. Hart, EC, Charkoudian, N, and Miller, VM. Sex, hormones, and neuroeffector mechanisms. *Acta Physiol* 203:155-165, 2011.

35. Heathers, JA. Smartphone-enabled pulse rate variability: an alternative methodology for the collection of heart rate variability in psychophysiological research. *Int J Psychophysiol* 89:297-304, 2013.

36. Hedelin, R, Kenttä, G, Wiklund, U, Bjerle, P, and Henriksson-Larsén, K, Short-term overtraining: effects on performance, circulatory responses, and heart rate variability. *Med Sci Sports Exerc* 32:1480-1484, 2000.

37. Herzig, D, Eser, P, Omlin, X, Riener, R, Wilhelm, M, and Achermann, P. Reproducibility of heart rate variability is parameter and sleep stage dependent. *Front Physiol* 8:1100, 2018.

38. Higgins, CB, Vatner, SF, and Braunwald, E. Parasympathetic control of the heart. *Pharmacol Rev* 25:119-155, 1973.

39. Hough, P, Glaister, M, and Pledger, A. The accuracy of wrist-

worn heart rate monitors across a range of exercise intensities. *J Phys Act Res* 2:112-116, 2017.

40. Iellamo, F, Legramante, JM, Massaro, M, Raimondi, G, and Galante, A. Effects of a residential exercise training on baroreflex sensitivity and heart rate variability in patients with coronary artery disease: a randomized, controlled study. *Circulation* 102:2588-2592, 2000.

41. Iellamo, F, Legramante, JM, Pigozzi, F, Spataro, A, Norbiato, G, Lucini, D, and Pagani, M. Conversion from vagal to sympathetic predominance with strenuous training in high-performance world class athletes. *Circulation* 105:2719-2724, 2002.

42. Iwasaki, KI, Zhang, R, Zuckerman, JH, and Levine, BD. Dose-response relationship of the cardiovascular adaptation to endurance training in healthy adults: how much training for what benefit? *J Appl Physiol* 95:1575-1583, 2003.

43. Jose, AD, Collison, D. The normal range and determinants of the intrinsic heart rate in man. *Cardiovasc Res* 4:160-167, 1970.

44. Karvonen, J, and Vuorimaa, T. Heart rate and exercise intensity during sports activities. *Sports Med* 5:303-311, 1988.

45. Lambert, MI, and Borresen, J. Measuring training load in sports. *Int J Sports Physiol Perform* 5:406-411, 2010.

46. Lamberts, RP, and Lambert, MI. Day-to-day variation in heart rate at different levels of submaximal exertion: implications for monitoring training. *J Strength Cond Res* 23:1005-1010, 2009.

47. Lamberts, R, Swart, J, Capostagno, B, Noakes, T, and Lambert, M. Heart rate recovery as a guide to monitor fatigue and predict changes in performance parameters. *Scand J Med Sci Sports* 20:449-57, 2009.

48. Landsberg, L, and Young, J. Effects of nutritional status on autonomic nervous system function. *Am J Clin Nutr* 35:1234-1240, 1982.

49. Leicht, AS, Allen, GD, and Hoey, AJ. Influence of intensive cycling training on heart rate variability during rest and exercise. *Can J Appl Physiol* 28:898-909, 2003.

49a. Lucia, A, Hoyos, J, Santalla, A, Earnest, C, and Chicharro, JL. Tour de France versus Vuelta a Espana: which is harder? *Med Sci Sports Exerc* 35:872-878, 2003.

50. Makivic, B, Nikić, MD, and Willis, M. Heart rate variability (HRV) as a tool for diagnostic and monitoring performance in sport and physical activities. *J. Exerc Physiol Online* 16:103-131, 2013.

51. Manzi, V, Castagna, C, Padua, E, Lombardo, M, D'Ottavio, S, Massaro, M, Volterrani, M, and Iellamo, F. Dose-response relationship of autonomic nervous system responses to individualized training impulse in marathon runners. *Am J Physiol Heart Circ Physiol* 296:H1733-H1740, 2009.

51a. Manzi, V, Iellamo, F, Impellizzeri, F, D'Ottavio, S, and Castagna, C. Relation between individualized training impulses and performance in distance runners. *Med Sci Sports Exerc* 41:2090-2096, 2009.

52. Michael, S, Jay, O, Halaki, M, Graham, K, and Davis, GM. Submaximal exercise intensity modulates acute post-exercise heart rate variability. *Eur J Appl Physiol* 116:697-706, 2016.

52a. Milanez, VF, and Pedro, RE. Application of different load quantification methods during a karate training session. *Rev Bras Med Esporte* 18:278-282, 2012.

53. Morgulev, E, Azar, OH, and Lidor, R. Sports analytics and the big-data era. *Int J Data Sci Anal* 5:213-222, 2018.

54. Nederhof, E, Zwerver, J, Brink, M, Meeusen, R, and Lemmink, K. Different diagnostic tools in nonfunctional overreaching. *Int J Sports Med* 29:590-597, 2008.

55. Nunan, D, Donovan, GAY, Jakovljevic, DG, Hodges, LD, Sandercock, GR, and Brodie, DA. Validity and reliability of short-term heart-rate variability from the Polar S810. *Med Sci Sports Exerc* 41:243-250, 2009.

56. Obrist, PA, Webb, RA, Sutterer, JR, and Howard, JL. The cardiac-somatic relationship: some reformulations. *Psychophysiology* 6:569-587, 1970.

57. Ostojic, SM, Stojanovic, MD, and Calleja-Gonzalez, J. Ultra short-term heart rate recovery after maximal exercise: relations to aerobic power in sportsmen. *Chin J Physiol* 54:105-110, 2011.

58. Parak, J, and Korhonen, I. Evaluation of wearable consumer heart rate monitors based on photoplethysmography. *Conf Proc IEEE Eng Med Biol Soc* 2014:3670-3673, 2014.

59. Pereira, LA, Flatt, AA, Ramirez-Campillo, R, Loturco, I, and Nakamura, FY. Assessing shortened field-based heart-rate-variability-data acquisition in team-sport athletes. *Int J Sport Physiol* 11:154-158, 2016.

60. Phan, D, Siong, LY, Pathirana, PN, and Seneviratne, A. Smartwatch: performance evaluation for long-term heart rate monitoring. *International Symposium on Bioelectronics and Bioinformatics (ISBB)* 144-147, 2015.

61. Pichot, V, Busso, T, Roche, F, Garet, M, Costes, F, Duverney, D, Lacour, JR, and Barthélémy, JC. Autonomic adaptations to intensive and overload training periods: a laboratory study. *Med Sci Sports Exerc* 34:1660-1666, 2002.

62. Pichot, V, Roche, F, Gaspoz, JM, Enjolras, F, Antoniadis, A, Minini, P, Costes, F, Busso, T, Lacour, JR, and Barthelemy, JC. Relation between heart rate variability and training load in middle-distance runners. *Med Sci Sports Exerc* 32:1729-1736, 2000.

63. Pinna, GD, Maestri, R, Torunski, A, Danilowicz-Szymanowicz, L, Szwoch, M, La Rovere, MT, and Raczak, G. Heart rate variability measures: a fresh look at reliability. *Clin Sci* 113:131-140, 2007.

64. Plews, DJ, Laursen, PB, Kilding, AE, and Buchheit, M. Heart rate variability in elite triathletes, is variation in variability the key to effective training? A case comparison. *Eur J Appl Physiol* 112:3729-3741, 2012.

65. Plews, DJ, Laursen, PB, Kilding, AE, and Buchheit, M. Training adaptation and heart rate variability in elite endurance athletes - opening the door to effective monitoring. *Sports Med* 43:773-781, 2013.

66. Plews, DJ, Laursen, PB, Kilding, AE, and Buchheit, M. Heart rate variability and training intensity distribution in elite rowers. *Int J Sports Physiol Perform* 9:1026-1032, 2014.

67. Plews, DJ, Laursen, PB, Le Meur, Y, Hausswirth, C, Kilding, AE, and Buchheit, M. Monitoring training with heart rate variability: how much compliance is needed for valid assessment? *Int J Sports Physiol Perform* 9:783-790, 2014.

68. Plews, DJ, Scott, B, Altini, M, Wood, M, Kilding, AE, and Laursen, PB. Comparison of heart-rate-variability recording with smartphone photoplethysmography, Polar H7 chest strap, and electrocardiography. *Int J Sports Physiol Perform* 12:1324-1328, 2017.

69. Robinson, BF, Epstein, SE, Beiser, DG, and Braunwald, E. Control of heart rate by the autonomic nervous system: studies in man on the interrelation between baroreceptor mechanisms and exercise. *Circ Res* 19:400-411, 1966.

70. Rousselle, JG, Blascovich, J, and Kelsey, RM. Cardiorespiratory response under combined psychological and exercise stress. *Int J Psychophysiol* 20:49-58, 1995.

71. Sandercock, GRH, and Brodie, DA. The use of heart rate variability measures to assess autonomic control during exercise. *Scand J Med Sci Sport* 16:302-313, 2006.

72. Schmitt, L, Regnard, J, Desmarets, M, Mauny, F, Mourot,

L, Fouillot, JP, Coulmy, N, and Millet, G. Fatigue shifts and scatters heart rate variability in elite endurance athletes. *PLoS One* 8:e71588, 2013.

72a. Seiler, KS, and Kjerland, GO. Quantifying training intensity distribution in elite endurance athletes: is there evidence for an "optimal" distribution? *Scand J Med Sci Sport* 16:49-56, 2006.

73. Seiler, S. What is best practice for training intensity and duration distribution in endurance athletes?. *Int J Sports Physiol Perform* 5:276-291, 2010.

74. Selye, H. The evolution of the stress concept: the originator of the concept traces its development from the discovery in 1936 of the alarm reaction to modern therapeutic applications of syntoxic and catatoxic hormones. *Am Scientist* 61:692-699, 1973.

75. Shin, K, Minamitani, H, Onishi, S, Yamazaki, H, and Lee, M. Autonomic differences between athletes and nonathletes: spectral analysis approach. *Med Sci Sports Exerc* 29:1482-90, 1997.

76. Spierer, DK, Rosen, Z, Litman, LL, and Fujii, K. Validation of photoplethysmography as a method to detect heart rate during rest and exercise. *J Med Eng Technol* 39:264-271, 2015.

76a. Stagno, KM, Thatcher, R, and Van Someren, KA. A modified TRIMP to quantify the in-season training load of team sport players. *J Sports Sci* 25:629-634, 2007.

77. Stanley, J, Peake, JM, and Buchheit, M. Cardiac parasympathetic reactivation following exercise: implications for training prescription. *Sports Med* 43:1259-1277, 2013.

78. Tortora, GJ, and Derrickson, BH. *Principles of Anatomy and Physiology.* Vol 1, 12th ed. Hoboken, NJ: John Wiley & Sons, 426, 2009.

79. Tran, Y, Wijesuriya, N, Tarvainen, M, Karjalainen, P, and Craig, A. The relationship between spectral changes in heart rate variability and fatigue. *J Psychophysiol* 23:143-151, 2009.

80. Vanrenterghem, J, Nedergaard, NJ, Robinson, MA, and Drust, B. Training load monitoring in team sports: a novel framework separating physiological and biomechanical load-adaptation pathways. *Sports Med* 47:2135-2142, 2017.

81. Vesterinen, V, Häkkinen, K, Hynynen, E, Mikkola, J, Hokka, L, and Nummela, A. Heart rate variability in prediction of individual adaptation to endurance training in recreational endurance runners. *Scand J Med Sci Sport* 23:171-180, 2013.

82. Wallace, LK, Slattery, KM, and Coutts, AJ. A comparison of methods for quantifying training load: relationships between modelled and actual training responses. *Eur J Appl Physiol* 114:11-20, 2014.

83. Weghorn, H. Usability and engineering aspects of competing RF technologies for communication with commercial sports sensors in ubiquitous applications - experimental comparison of power consumption and use cases for ANT+ and Bluetooth Low Energy sensor devices. In *Proceedings of the 3rd International Congress on Sport Sciences Research and Technology Support – Volume 1:icSPORTS.* Setúbal, Portugal, Science and Technology Publications, Lda, 263-270, 2015.

84. Weiler, DT, Villajuan, SO, Edkins, L, Cleary, S, and Saleem, JJ. Wearable heart rate monitor technology accuracy in research: a comparative study between PPG and ECG technology. *Proceedings of the Human Factors and Ergonomics Society Annual Meeting* 61:1292-1296, 2017.

85. Weipert, M, Kumar, M, Kreuzfeld, S, Arndt, D, Rieger, A, and Stoll, R. Comparison of three mobile devices for measuring R-R intervals and heart rate variability: Polar S810i, Sunnto t6 and an ambulatory ECG system. *Eur J Appl Physiol* 109:779-786, 2010.

86. Williams, S, Booton, T, Watson, M, Rowland, D, and Altini, M. Heart rate variability is a moderating factor in the workload-injury relationship of competitive CrossFit™ athletes. *J Sports Sci Med* 16:443-449, 2017.

87. Yang, XL, Liu, GZ, Tong, YH, Yan, H, Xu, Z, Chen, Q, Liu, X, Zhang, HH, Wang, HB, and Tan, SH. The history, hotspots, and trends of electrocardiogram. *J Geriatr Cardiol* 12:448-456, 2015.

Chapter 15

1. Aagaard, P. Spinal and supraspinal control of motor function during maximal eccentric muscle contraction: effects of resistance training. *J Sport Health Sci* 7:282-293, 2018.

2. Babiloni, C, Marzano, N, Iacoboni, M, Infarinato, F, Aschieri, P, Buffo, P, Cibelli, G, Soricelli, A, Eusebi, F, and Del Percio, C. Resting state cortical rhythms in athletes: a high-resolution EEG study. *Brain Res Bull* 81:149-156, 2010.

3. Behrens, M, Weippert, M, Wassermann, F, Bader, R, Bruhn, S, and Mau-Moeller, A. Neuromuscular function and fatigue resistance of the plantar flexors following short-term cycling endurance training. *Front Physiol* 6:145, 2015.

4. Budini, F, and Tilp, M. Changes in H-reflex amplitude to muscle stretch and lengthening in humans. *Rev Neurosci* 27:511-522, 2016.

5. Buhlmayer, L, Birrer, D, Rothlin, P, Faude, O, and Donath, L. Effects of mindfulness practice on performance-relevant parameters and performance outcomes in sports: a meta-analytical review. *Sports Med* 47:2309-2321, 2017.

6. Cantou, P, Platel, H, Desgranges, B, and Groussard, M. How motor, cognitive and musical expertise shapes the brain: focus on fMRI and EEG resting-state functional connectivity. *J Chem Neuroanat* 89:60-68, 2018.

7. Cheng, MY, Huang, CJ, Chang, YK, Koester, D, Schack, T, and Hung, TM. Sensorimotor rhythm neurofeedback enhances golf putting performance. *J Sport Exerc Psychol* 37:626-636, 2015.

8. Cheng, MY, Hung, CL, Huang, CJ, Chang, YK, Lo, LC, Shen, C, and Hung, TM. Expert-novice differences in SMR activity during dart throwing. *Biol Psychol* 110:212-218, 2015.

9. Cheng, MY, Wang, KP, Hung, CL, Tu, YL, Huang, CJ, Koester, D, Schack, T, and Hung, TM. Higher power of sensorimotor rhythm is associated with better performance in skilled air-pistol shooters. *Psychol Sport Exerc* 32:47-53, 2017.

10. Chuang, LY, Huang, CJ, and Hung, TM. The differences in frontal midline theta power between successful and unsuccessful basketball free throws of elite basketball players. *Int J Psychophysiol* 90:321-328, 2013.

11. Colyer, SL, and McGuigan, PM. Textile electrodes embedded in clothing: a practical alternative to traditional surface electromyography when assessing muscle excitation during functional movements. *J Sports Sci Med* 17:101-109, 2018.

12. Del Percio, C, Infarinato, F, Marzano, N, Iacoboni, M, Aschieri, P, Lizio, R, Soricelli, A, Limatola, C, Rossini, PM, and Babiloni, C. Reactivity of alpha rhythms to eyes opening is lower in athletes than non-athletes: a high-resolution EEG study. *Int J Psychophysiol* 82:240-247, 2011.

13. De Luca, CJ. The use of surface electromyography in biomechanics. *J Appl Biomech* 13:135-163, 1997.

14. De Luca, CJ, Kuznetsov, M, Gilmore, LD, and Roy, SH. Inter-electrode spacing of surface EMG sensors: reduction of crosstalk contamination during voluntary contractions. *J Biomech* 45:555-561, 2012.

15. Fabre, JB, Martin, V, Gondin, J, Cottin, F, and Grelot, L. Effect of playing surface properties on neuromuscular fatigue in tennis. *Med Sci Sports Exerc* 44:2182-2189, 2012.

16. Gorodnichev, RM, and Fomin, RN. Presynaptic inhibition of

spinal α motoneurons in humans adapted to different types of motor activity. *Hum Physiol* 33:215, 2007.

17. Grey, MJ, Pierce, CW, Milner, TE, and Sinkjaer, T. Soleus stretch reflex during cycling. *Motor Control* 5:36-49, 2001.

18. Jackson, AF, and Bolger, DJ. The neurophysiological bases of EEG and EEG measurement: a review for the rest of us. *Psychophysiology* 51:1061-1071, 2014.

19. Kao, SC, Huang, J, and Hung, M. Frontal midline theta is a specific indicator of optimal attentional engagement during skilled putting performance. *J Sport Exerc Psychol* 35:470-478, 2013.

20. Larsen, B, Voigt, M, and Grey, MJ. Changes in the soleus stretch reflex at different pedaling frequencies and crank loads during pedaling. *Motor Control* 10:265-279, 2006.

20a. Malmivuo, P, Malmivuo, J, and Plonsey R. Electroencephalography. In *Bioelectromagnetism: principles and applications of bioelectric and biomagnetic fields.* USA: Oxford University Press, 247-264, 1995.

21. Mantini, D, Perrucci, MG, Del Gratta, C, Romani, GL, and Corbetta, M. Electrophysiological signatures of resting state networks in the human brain. *Proc Natl Acad Sci U S A* 104:13170-13175, 2007.

21a. Motamedi-Fakhr, S, Moshrefi-Torbati, M, Hill, M, Hill, CM, and White, P R. Signal processing techniques applied to human sleep EEG signals—A review. *Biomedical Signal Processing and Control*, 10:21-33, 2014.

22. Palmieri, RM, Ingersoll, CD, and Hoffman, MA. The Hoffmann reflex: methodologic considerations and applications for use in sports medicine and athletic training research. *J Athl Train* 39:268-277, 2004.

23. Pearcey, GEP, Noble, SA, Munro, B, and Zehr, EP. Spinal cord excitability and sprint performance are enhanced by sensory stimulation during cycling. *Front Hum Neurosci* 11:612, 2017.

24. Perez, MA, Lundbye-Jensen, J, and Nielsen, JB. Task-specific depression of the soleus H-reflex after cocontraction training of antagonistic ankle muscles. *J Neurophysiol* 98:3677-3687, 2007.

25. Raichlen, DA, Bharadwaj, PK, Fitzhugh, MC, Haws, KA, Torre, GA, Trouard, TP, and Alexander, GE. Differences in resting state functional connectivity between young adult endurance athletes and healthy controls. *Front Hum Neurosci* 10:610, 2016.

26. Ramos-Campo, DJ, Martinez-Guardado, I, Rubio-Arias, JA, Freitas, TT, Othalawa, S, Andreu, L, Timon, R, and Alcaraz, PE. Muscle architecture and neuromuscular changes after high-resistance circuit training in hypoxia. *J Strength Cond Res,* 2019. [e-pub ahead of print].

27. Sala-Llonch, R, Pena-Gomez, C, Arenaza-Urquijo, EM, Vidal-Piñeiro, D, Bargallo, N, Junque, C, and Bartres-Faz, D. Brain connectivity during resting state and subsequent working memory task predicts behavioral performance. *Cortex* 48:1187-1196, 2012.

28. Scott-Hamilton, J, Schutte, NS, and Brown, RF. Effects of a mindfulness intervention on sports-anxiety, pessimism, and flow in competitive cyclists. *Appl Psychol Health Well Being* 8:85-103, 2016.

29. Srinivasan, R, Winter, WR, Ding, J, and Nunez, PL. EEG and MEG coherence: measures of functional connectivity at distinct spatial scales of neocortical dynamics. *J Neurosci Methods* 166:41-52, 2007.

30. Stevanovic, VB, Jelic, MB, Milanovic, SD, Filipovic, SR, Mikic, MJ, and Stojanovic, MDM. Sport-specific warm-up attenuates static stretching-induced negative effects on vertical jump but not neuromuscular excitability in basketball players. *J Sports Sci Med* 18:282-289, 2019.

31. Teplan, M. Fundamentals of EEG measurement. *Meas Sci Rev* 2:1-11, 2002.

32. Thompson, R, Kaufman, KA, De Petrillo, LA, Glass, CR, and Arnkoff, DB. One-year follow-up of mindful sport performance enhancement (MSPE) with archers, golfers, and runners. *J Clin Sport Psychol* 5:99-116, 2011.

33. Vila-Cha, C, Falla, D, Correia, MV, and Farina, D. Changes in H reflex and V wave following short-term endurance and strength training. *J Appl Physiol (1985)* 112:54-63, 2012.

34. Zehr, EP. Considerations for use of the Hoffmann reflex in exercise studies. *Eur J Appl Physiol* 86:455-468, 2002.

Chapter 16

1. Alghannam, AF, Gonzalez, JT, and Betts, JA. Restoration of muscle glycogen and functional capacity: role of post-exercise carbohydrate and protein co-ingestion. *Nutrients* 10:253, 2018.

2. Arratibel-Imaz, I, Calleja-Gonzalez, J, Emparanza, JI, Terrados, N, Mjaanes, JM, and Ostojic, SM. Lack of concordance amongst measurements of individual anaerobic threshold and maximal lactate steady state on a cycle ergometer. *Phys Sportsmed* 44:34-45, 2016.

3. Atkinson, G, and Nevill, AM. Statistical methods for assessing measurement error (reliability) in variables relevant to sports medicine. *Sports Med* 26:217-238, 1998.

4. Banfi, G, and Dolci, A. Free testosterone/cortisol ratio in soccer: usefulness of a categorization of values. *J Sports Med Phys Fitness* 46:611-616, 2006.

5. Barsotti, RJ. Measurement of ammonia in blood. *J Pediatr* 138:S11-S19, 2001.

6. Batterham, AM, and Hopkins, WG. Making meaningful inferences about magnitudes. *Int J Sport Physiol Perform* 1:50-57, 2006.

7. Baum, A, and Grunberg, N. Measurement of stress hormones. In *Measuring Stress: A Guide for Health and Social Scientists.* Cohen, S, Kessler, RC, and Gordon, LU, eds. New York: Oxford University Press, 175-192, 1997.

8. Beneke, R, Leithauser, RM, and Ochentel, O. Blood lactate diagnostics in exercise testing and training. *Int J Sports Physiol Perform* 6:8-24, 2011.

9. Bernard, C. *Leçons sur les phenomenes de la vie communs aux animaux et aux vegetaux.* Paris: Bailliere, 1878.

10. Bland, JM, and Altman, DG. Applying the right statistics: analyses of measurement studies. *Ultrasound Obstet Gynecol* 22:85-93, 2003.

11. Booth, FW, and Laye, MJ. The future: genes, physical activity and health. *Acta Physiol (Oxf)* 199:549-556, 2010.

12. Bouchard, C. Exercise genomics--a paradigm shift is needed: a commentary. *Br J Sports Med* 49:1492-1496, 2015.

13. Bouchard, C, Blair, SN, Church, TS, Earnest, CP, Hagberg, JM, Hakkinen, K, Jenkins, NT, Karavirta, L, Kraus, WE, Leon, AS, Rao, DC, Sarzynski, MA, Skinner, JS, Slentz, CA, and Rankinen, T. Adverse metabolic response to regular exercise: is it a rare or common occurrence? *PLoS One* 7:e37887, 2012.

14. Bouchard, C, and Rankinen, T. Individual differences in response to regular physical activity. *Med Sci Sports Exerc* 33:S446-S451, 2001.

15. Bouchard, C, Rankinen, T, and Timmons, JA. Genomics and genetics in the biology of adaptation to exercise. *Compr Physiol* 1:1603-1648, 2011.

16. Bourdon, PC, Cardinale, M, Murray, A, Gastin, P, Kellmann, M, Varley, MC, Gabbett, TJ, Coutts, AJ, Burgess, DJ, Gregson,

W, and Cable, NT. Monitoring athlete training loads: consensus statement. *Int J Sports Physiol Perform* 12:S2161-S2170, 2017.

17. Brancaccio, P, Lippi, G, and Maffulli, N. Biochemical markers of muscular damage. *Clin Chem Lab Med* 48:757-767, 2010.

18. Brandt, C, and Pedersen, BK. The role of exercise-induced myokines in muscle homeostasis and the defense against chronic diseases. *J Biomed Biotechnol* 2010:520258, 2010.

19. Buyse, L, Decroix, L, Timmermans, N, Barbe, K, Verrelst, R, and Meeusen, R. Improving the diagnosis of nonfunctional overreaching and overtraining syndrome. *Med Sci Sport Exerc,* 2019. [e-pub ahead of print].

20. Calleja-Gonzalez, J, Mielgo-Ayuso, J, Sampaio, J, Delextrat, A, Ostojic, SM, Marques-Jimenez, D, Arratibel, I, Sanchez-Urena, B, Dupont, G, Schelling, X, and Terrados, N. Brief ideas about evidence-based recovery in team sports. *J Exerc Rehabil* 14:545-550, 2018.

21. Campbell, JP, and Turner, JE. Debunking the myth of exercise-induced immune suppression: redefining the impact of exercise on immunological health across the lifespan. *Front Immunol* 9:648, 2018.

22. Cannon, WB. Organization for physiological homeostasis. *Physiol Rev* 9:399-431, 1929.

23. Cavero-Redondo, I, Peleteiro, B, Alvarez-Bueno, C, Artero, EG, Garrido-Miguel, M, and Martinez-Vizcaino, V. The effect of physical activity interventions on glycosylated haemoglobin (HbA1c) in non-diabetic populations: a systematic review and meta-analysis. *Sports Med* 48:1151-1164, 2018.

24. Cook, CE. Clinimetrics corner: the minimal clinically important change score (MCID): a necessary pretense. *J Man Manip Ther* 16:E82-E83, 2008.

25. Cooper, SJ. From Claude Bernard to Walter Cannon. Emergence of the concept of homeostasis. *Appetite* 51:419-427, 2008.

26. da Nobrega, AC. The subacute effects of exercise: concept, characteristics, and clinical implications. *Exerc Sport Sci Rev* 33:84-87, 2005.

27. Enoka, RM, and Duchateau, J. Translating fatigue to human performance. *Med Sci Sports Exerc* 48:2228-2238, 2016.

28. Fernandez-Garcia, B, Lucia, A, Hoyos, J, Chicharro, JL, Rodriguez-Alonso, M, Bandres, F, and Terrados, N. The response of sexual and stress hormones of male pro-cyclists during continuous intense competition. *Int J Sports Med* 23:555-560, 2002.

29. Fernandez-Sanjurjo, M, de Gonzalo-Calvo, D, Fernandez-Garcia, B, Diez-Robles, S, Martinez-Canal, A, Olmedillas, H, Davalos, A, and Iglesias-Gutierrez, E. Circulating microRNA as emerging biomarkers of exercise. *Exerc Sport Sci Rev* 46:160-171, 2018.

30. Finaud, J, Lac, G, and Filaire, E. Oxidative stress: relationship with exercise and training. *Sports Med* 36:327-358, 2006.

31. Finaud, J, Scislowski, V, Lac, G, Durand, D, Vidalin, H, Robert, A, and Filaire, E. Antioxidant status and oxidative stress in professional rugby players: evolution throughout a season. *Int J Sports Med* 27:87-93, 2006.

32. Finch, CF, and Marshall, SW. Let us stop throwing out the baby with the bathwater: towards better analysis of longitudinal injury data. *Br J Sports Med* 50:712-715, 2016.

33. Finsterer, J. Biomarkers of peripheral muscle fatigue during exercise. *BMC Musculoskelet Disord* 13:218-231, 2012.

34. Garlick, PJ. The role of leucine in the regulation of protein metabolism. *J Nutr* 135:1553S-1556S, 2005.

35. Ginsburg, GS, and Phillips, KA. Precision medicine: from science to value. *Health Aff (Millwood)* 37:694-701, 2018.

36. Goldberger, AL. Heartbeats, hormones, and health; is variability the spice of life? *Am J Respir Crit Care Med* 163:1289-1290, 2001.

37. Goldberger, AL, Amaral, LA, Hausdorff, JM, Ivanov, PC, Peng, CK, and Stanley, HE. Fractal dynamics in physiology: alterations with disease and aging. *Proc Natl Acad Sci U S A* 99:2466-2472, 2002.

38. Goodwin, ML, Harris, JE, Hernández, A, and Gladden, LB. Blood lactate measurements and analysis during exercise: a guide for clinicians. *J Diabetes Sci Technol* 1:558-569, 2007.

39. Halson, SL. Monitoring training load to understand fatigue in athletes. *Sports Med* 44 Suppl 2:S139-147, 2014.

40. Halson, SL, and Jeukendrup, AE. Does overtraining exist? An analysis of overreaching and overtraining research. *Sports Med* 34:967-981, 2004.

41. Hawkins, RC. Laboratory turnaround time. *Clin Biochem Rev* 28:179-194, 2007.

42. Hemingway, H, Croft, P, Perel, P, Hayden, JA, Abrams, K, Timmis, A, Briggs, A, Udumyan, R, Moons, KG, Steyerberg, EW, Roberts, I, Schroter, S, Altman, DG, and Riley, RD. Prognosis research strategy (PROGRESS) 1: a framework for researching clinical outcomes. *BMJ* 346:e5595, 2013.

43. Higgins, JP. Nonlinear systems in medicine. *Yale J Biol Med* 75:247-260, 2002.

44. Hristovski, R, Balague, N, Daskalovski, B, Zivkovic, V, Aleksovska-Velickovska, L, and Naumovski, M. Linear and nonlinear complex systems approach to sports. Explanatory differences and applications. *Res Phys Educ Sport Health* 1:25-31, 2012.

45. Iberall, AS, and McCulloch, WS. Homeokinesis - the organizing principle of complex living systems. *IFAC Proceedings Volumes* 2:39-50, 1968.

46. Julian, R, Meyer, T, Fullagar, HH, Skorski, S, Pfeiffer, M, Kellmann, M, Ferrauti, A, and Hecksteden, A. Individual patterns in blood-borne indicators of fatigue-trait or chance. *J Strength Cond Res* 31:608-619, 2017.

47. Karkazis, K, and Fishman, JR. Tracking U.S. Professional athletes: the ethics of biometric technologies. *Am J Bioeth* 17:45-60, 2017.

48. Knicker, AJ, Renshaw, I, Oldham, AR, and Cairns, SP. Interactive processes link the multiple symptoms of fatigue in sport competition. *Sports Med* 41:307-328, 2011.

49. Kreider, AC, Fry, R, and O'Toole, ML. *Overtraining in Sport.* Champaign, IL: Human Kinetics, 1998.

50. LabCorp. Introduction to Specimen Collection. 2019. www.labcorp.com/resource/introduction-to-specimen-collection. Accessed July 18, 2019.

51. Lambert, EV, St Clair Gibson, A, and Noakes, TD. Complex systems model of fatigue: integrative homoeostatic control of peripheral physiological systems during exercise in humans. *Br J Sports Med* 39:52-62, 2005.

52. Lee, EC, Fragala, MS, Kavouras, SA, Queen, RM, Pryor, JL, and Casa, DJ. Biomarkers in sports and exercise: tracking health, performance, and recovery in athletes. *J Strength Cond Res* 31:2920-2937, 2017.

53. Legaz-Arrese, A, Carranza-Garcia, LE, Serrano-Ostariz, E, Gonzalez-Rave, JM, and Terrados, N. The traditional maximal lactate steady state test versus the 5 x 2000 m test. *Int J Sports Med* 32:845-850, 2011.

54. MacKinnon, LT. Special feature for the Olympics: effects of exercise on the immune system: overtraining effects on immunity and performance in athletes. *Immunol Cell Biol* 78:502-509, 2000.

55. Meerson, FZ. Intensity of function of structures of the differentiated cell as a determinant of activity of its genetic apparatus. *Nature* 206:483-484, 1965.

56. Meeusen, R, Duclos, M, Foster, C, Fry, A, Gleeson, M, Nieman, D, Raglin, J, Rietjens, G, Steinacker, J, and Urhausen, A. Prevention, diagnosis, and treatment of the overtraining syndrome: joint consensus statement of the European College of Sport Science and the American College of Sports Medicine. *Med Sci Sports Exerc* 45:186-205, 2013.

57. Mendez-Villanueva, A, Fernandez-Fernandez, J, Bishop, D, Fernandez-Garcia, B, and Terrados, N. Activity patterns, blood lactate concentrations and ratings of perceived exertion during a professional singles tennis tournament. *Br J Sports Med* 41:296-300, 2007.

58. Mikulecky, DC. Complexity, communication between cells, and identifying the functional components of living systems: some observations. *Acta Biotheoretica* 44:179-208, 1996.

59. Minchella, PA, Chipungu, G, Kim, AA, Sarr, A, Ali, H, Mwenda, R, Nkengasong, JN, and Singer, D. Specimen origin, type and testing laboratory are linked to longer turnaround times for HIV viral load testing in Malawi. *PLoS One* 12:e0173009, 2017.

60. Modell, H, Cliff, W, Michael, J, McFarland, J, Wenderoth, MP, and Wright, A. A physiologist's view of homeostasis. *Adv Physiol Educ* 39:259-266, 2015.

61. Mujika, I, and Burke, LM. Nutrition in team sports. *Ann Nutr Metab* 57:26-35, 2010.

62. Osborne, B, and Cunningham, JL. Legal and ethical implications of athletes' biometric data collection in professional sport. *Marq Sports L Rev* 37, 2017.

63. Palacios, G, Pedrero-Chamizo, R, Palacios, N, Maroto-Sanchez, B, Aznar, S, and Gonzalez-Gross, M. Biomarkers of physical activity and exercise. *Nutr Hosp* 31(suppl 3):237-244, 2015.

64. Parker, L, McGuckin, TA, and Leicht, AS. Influence of exercise intensity on systemic oxidative stress and antioxidant capacity. *Clin Physiol Funct Imaging* 34:377-383, 2014.

65. Paulsen, G, Mikkelsen, UR, Raastad, T, and Peake, JM. Leucocytes, cytokines and satellite cells: what role do they play in muscle damage and regeneration following eccentric exercise? *Exerc Immunol Rev* 18:42-97, 2012.

66. Philippe, P, and Mansi, O. Nonlinearity in the epidemiology of complex health and disease processes. *Theor Med Bioeth* 19:591-607, 1998.

67. Pickering, C, and Kiely, J. Do non-responders to exercise exist-and if so, what should we do about them? *Sports Med (Auckland, NZ)* 49:1-7, 2019.

68. Pitsiladis, YP, Tanaka, M, Eynon, N, Bouchard, C, North, KN, Williams, AG, Collins, M, Moran, CN, Britton, SL, Fuku, N, Ashley, EA, Klissouras, V, Lucia, A, Ahmetov, II, de Geus, E, and Alsayrafi, M. Athlome Project Consortium: a concerted effort to discover genomic and other "omic" markers of athletic performance. *Physiol Genomics* 48:183-190, 2016.

69. Pitsiladis, Y, Wang, G, Wolfarth, B, Scott, R, Fuku, N, Mikami, E, He, Z, Fiuza-Luces, C, Eynon, N, and Lucia, A. Genomics of elite sporting performance: what little we know and necessary advances. *Br J Sports Med* 47:550-555, 2013.

70. Prior, RL, and Cao, G. In vivo total antioxidant capacity: comparison of different analytical methods. *Free Radic Biol Med* 27:1173-1181, 1999.

71. Rennie, MJ, Edwards, RH, Krywawych, S, Davies, CT, Halliday, D, Waterlow, JC, and Millward, DJ. Effect of exercise on protein turnover in man. *Clin Sci (Lond)* 61:627-639, 1981.

72. Rennie, MJ, and Tipton, KD. Protein and amino acid metabolism during and after exercise and the effects of nutrition. *Annu Rev Nutr* 20:457-483, 2000.

73. Rodríguez-Alonso, M, Fernández-García, B, Pérez-Landaluce, J, and Terrados, N. Blood lactate and heart rate during national and international women's basketball. *J Sports Med Phys Fitness* 43:432-436, 2003.

74. Rosenblueth, A, Wiener, N, and Bigelow, J. Behavior, purpose and teleology. *Philos Sci* 10:18-24, 1943.

75. Schelling, X, Calleja-Gonzalez, J, Torres-Ronda, L, and Terrados, N. Using testosterone and cortisol as biomarker for training individualization in elite basketball: a 4-year follow-up study. *J Strength Cond Res* 29:368-378, 2015.

76. Seshadri, DR, Li, RT, Voos, JE, Rowbottom, JR, Alfes, CM, Zorman, CA, and Drummond, CK. Wearable sensors for monitoring the internal and external workload of the athlete. *NPJ Digit Med* 2:71, 2019.

77. Simopoulos, AP. The importance of the ratio of omega-6/omega-3 essential fatty acids. *Biomed Pharmacother* 56:365-379, 2002.

78. Smith, LL. Cytokine hypothesis of overtraining: a physiological adaptation to excessive stress? *Med Sci Sports Exerc* 32:317-331, 2000.

79. Steinacker, JM, Lormes, W, Reissnecker, S, and Liu, Y. New aspects of the hormone and cytokine response to training. *Eur J Appl Physiol* 91:382-391, 2004.

80. Sterling, P, and Eyer, J. Allostasis: a new paradigm to explain arousal pathology. In *Handbook of Life Stress, Cognition and Health*. Fisher, S and Reason, J, eds. New York: John Wiley & Sons, 629, 1988.

81. Tainter, JA, Allen, TFH, Little, A, and Hoekstra, TW. Resource transitions and energy gain: contexts of organization. *Conserv Ecol* 7:4, 2003.

82. Terrados, N, Melichna, J, Sylven, C, and Jansson, E. Decrease in skeletal muscle myoglobin with intensive training in man. *Acta Physiol Scand* 128:651-652, 1986.

83. Theofilidis, G, Bogdanis, GC, Koutedakis, Y, and Karatzaferi, C. Monitoring exercise-induced muscle fatigue and adaptations: making sense of popular or emerging indices and biomarkers. *Sports (Basel)* 6:153, 2018.

84. Thomas, DT, Erdman, KA, and Burke, LM. American College of Sports Medicine joint position statement. Nutrition and athletic rerformance. *Med Sci Sports Exerc* 48:543-568, 2016.

85. Thorpe, RT, Atkinson, G, Drust, B, and Gregson, W. Monitoring fatigue status in elite team-sport athletes: implications for practice. *Int J Sports Physiol Perform* 12:S227-S234, 2017.

86. Timmons, JA. Variability in training-induced skeletal muscle adaptation. *J Appl Physiol (1985)* 110:846-853, 2011.

87. Torres-Ronda, L, and Schelling, X. Critical process for the implementation of technology in sport organizations. *Strength Cond J* 39:54-59, 2017.

88. Viru, A, and Viru, M. *Biochemical Monitoring of Sport Training*. Champaign, IL: Human Kinetics, 11-26, 2001.

89. Vlahovich, N, Fricker, PA, Brown, MA, and Hughes, D. Ethics of genetic testing and research in sport: a position statement from the Australian Institute of Sport. *Br J Sports Med* 51:5-11, 2017.

90. Walsh, NP, Gleeson, M, Shephard, RJ, Gleeson, M, Woods, JA, Bishop, NC, Fleshner, M, Green, C, Pedersen, BK, Hoffman-Goetz, L, Rogers, CJ, Northoff, H, Abbasi, A, and Simon, P. Position statement. Part one: Immune function and exercise. *Exerc Immunol Rev* 17:6-63, 2011.

91. Wang, D, DE Vito, G, Ditroilo, M, and Delahunt, E. Different effect of local and general fatigue on knee joint stiffness. *Med Sci Sports Exerc* 49:173-182, 2017.

92. Wang, K, Lee, I, Carlson, G, Hood, L, and Galasa, D. Systems biology and the discovery of diagnostic biomarkers. *Dis Markers* 28:199-207, 2010.

93. Webborn, N, Williams, A, McNamee, M, Bouchard, C, Pitsiladis, Y, Ahmetov, I, Ashley, E, Byrne, N, Camporesi, S, Collins, M, Dijkstra, P, Eynon, N, Fuku, N, Garton, FC, Hoppe, N, Holm, S, Kaye, J, Klissouras, V, Lucia, A, Maase, K, Moran, C, North, KN, Pigozzi, F, and Wang, G. Direct-to-consumer genetic testing for predicting sports performance and talent identification: consensus statement. *Br J Sports Med* 49:1486-1491, 2015.

94. Wyrwich, KW, Tierney, WM, and Wolinsky, FD. Further evidence supporting an SEM-based criterion for identifying meaningful intra-individual changes in health-related quality of life. *J Clin Epidemiol* 52:861-873, 1999.

Chapter 17

1. Abbiss, CR, Peiffer, JJ, Meeusen, R, and Skorski, S. Role of ratings of perceived exertion during self-paced exercise: what are we actually measuring? *Sports Med* 45:1235-1243, 2015.

2. Abbott, W, Brownlee, TE, Harper, LD, Naughton, RJ, and Clifford, T. The independent effects of match location, match result and the quality of opposition on subjective wellbeing in under 23 soccer players: a case study. *Res Sports Med* 26:262-275, 2018.

3. Adcock, R, and Collier, D. Measurement validity: a shared standard for qualitative and quantitative research. *Am Polit Sci Rev* 95:529-546, 2001.

4. Akenhead, R, and Nassis, GP. Training load and player monitoring in high-level football: current practice and perceptions. *Int J Sports Physiol Perform* 11:587-593, 2016.

5. Ary, D, Jacobs, LC, Sorensen, C, and Walker, D. *Introduction to Research in Education.* Boston: Cengage, 2019.

6. Baldwin, W. Information no one else knows: the value of self-report. In *The Science of Self-report: Implications for Research and Practice.* Stone, AA, Turkkan, JS, Bachrach, CA, Jobe, JB, Kurtzman, HS, and Cain, VS, eds. Mahwah, NJ; Lawrence Erlbaum Associates, 3-7, 2000.

7. Banister, EW. Modeling elite athletic performance. In *Physiological Testing of Elite Athletes.* 2nd ed. MacDougall JD, Wenger HA, and Green HJ, eds. Champaign, IL: Human Kinetics, 403-424, 1991.

8. Barça Innovation Hub. The influence of the perceived exertion rating on football training and competition. April 8, 2019. https://barcainnovationhub.com/influence-of-perceived-exertion-on-football-training-and-competition. Accessed January 4, 2020.

9. Bittencourt, N, Meeuwisse, WH, Mendonça, LD, Nettel-Aguirre, A, Ocarino, JM, and Fonseca, ST. Complex systems approach for sports injuries: moving from risk factor identification to injury pattern recognition—narrative review and new concept. *Br J Sports Med* 50:1309-1314, 2016.

10. Borg, G. Interindividual scaling and perception of muscular force. *Kungliga fysiografiska sällskapets i Lund förhandlingar* 12:117-125, 1961.

11. Borg, G. *Physical Performance and Perceived Exertion. Studia Psychologica Et Paedagogica, Series Altera, Investigationes XI.* Lund, Sweden: Gleerup, 1962.

12. Borg, G. Perceived exertion as an indicator of somatic stress. *Scand J Rehabil Med* 2:92-98, 1970.

13. Borg, G. Ratings of perceived exertion and heart rates during short-term cycle exercise and their use in a new cycling strength test. *Int J Sports Med* 3:153-158, 1982.

14. Borg, G. *An Introduction to Borg's RPE-Scale.* Ithaca, NY: Movement Publications, 1985.

15. Borg, G. *Borg's Perceived Exertion and Pain Scales.* Champaign, IL: Human Kinetics, 1998.

16. Borg, E. *On Perceived Exertion and its Measurement.* (Doctoral dissertation). Stockholm, Sweden: Stockholm University, 2007.

17. Borg, E. Placing verbal descriptors on a ratio scale. In *Fechner Day 2011: Proceedings of the Twenty-Seventh Annual Meeting of the International Society for Psychophysics.* Algom, D, Zakay, D, Chajut, E, Shaki, S, Mama, Y, and Shakuf, V, eds. Raanana, Israel: International Society for Psychophysics, 119-124, 2011.

18. Borg, E. Perception of blackness as a training material for the Borg centiMax scale. In *Fechner Day 2013: Proceedings of the 20th Annual Meeting of the International Society for Psychophysics.* Wackermann, J, Wittman, M, and Skrandies, eds. Freiburg, Germany, 98, 2013.

19. Borg, G, and Borg, E. *A General Psychophysical Scale of Blackness and Its Possibilities as a Test of Rating Behavior (Report No. 737).* Stockholm: Department of Psychology, Stockholm University, 1991.

20. Borg, G, and Borg, E. A new generation of scaling methods: level-anchored ratio scaling. *Psychologica* 28:15-45, 2001.

21. Borg, E, and Borg, G. A comparison of AME and CR100 for scaling perceived exertion. *Acta Psychol (Amst)* 109:157-175, 2002.

22. Borg, G, and Borg, E. *The Borg CR Scales® Folder.* Hasselby, Sweden: Borg Perception, 1-4, 2010.

23. Borg, E, and Kaijser, L. A comparison between three rating scales for perceived exertion and two different work tests. *Scand J Med Sci Sports* 6:57-69, 2006.

24. Borg, E, and Love, C. A demonstration of the Borg centiMax® Scale (CR100) for performance evaluation in diving. *Nord Psychol* 70:228-244, 2017.

25. Borresen, J, and Lambert, MI. The quantification of training load, the training response, and the effect on performance. *Sports Med* 39:779-795, 2009.

26. Bowling, A. Just one question: if one question works, why ask several? *J Epidemiol Community Health* 59:342-345, 2005.

27. Brink, MS, Frencken, WGP, Jordet, G, and Lemmink, KAPM. Coaches' and players' perceptions of training dose: not a perfect match. *Int J Sports Physiol Perform* 9:497-502, 2014.

28. Calvert, TW, Banister, EW, and Savage, MV. A systems model of the effects of training on physical performance. *IEEE Transactions on Systems, Man and Cybernetics* SMC-6:94-102, 1976.

29. Calvert, M, Kyte, D, Price, G, Valderas, JM, and Hjollund, NH. Maximising the impact of patient reported outcome assessment for patients and society. *BMJ* 364:k5267, 2019.

30. Chamari, K, Haddad, M, Wong, DP, Dellal, A, and Chaouachi, A. Injury rates in professional soccer players during Ramadan. *J Sports Sci* 30:S93-S102, 2012.

31. Chan, JT, and Mallett, CJ. The value of emotional intelligence for high performance coaching. *Int J Sports Sci Coach* 6:315-328, 2011.

32. Chen, MJ, Fan, X, and Moe, ST. Criterion-related validity of the Borg ratings of perceived exertion scale in healthy individuals: a meta-analysis. *J Sports Sci* 20:873-899, 2002.

33. Choi, PYL, and Salmon, P. Symptom changes across the menstrual cycle in competitive sportswomen, exercisers and sedentary women. *Br J Clin Psychol* 34:447-460, 1995.

34. Christen, J, Foster, C, Porcari, JP, and Mikat, RP. Temporal robustness of the session rating of perceived exertion. *Int J Sports Physiol Perform* 11:1088-1093, 2016.

35. Cohen, S, Kamarck, T, and Mermelstein R. A global measure of perceived stress. *J Health Soc Behav* 24:385-396, 1983.

36. Coquart, JBJ, Dufour, Y, Groslambert, A, Matran, R, and Garcin, M. Relationships between psychological factors, RPE and time limit estimated by teleoanticipation. *Sport Psychol* 26:359-374, 2012.

37. Coutts, AJ. In the age of technology, Occam's razor still applies. *Int J Sports Physiol Perform* 9:741, 2014.

38. Coutts, AJ, and Cormack, SJ. Monitoring the training response. In *High-Performance Training for Sports*. 1st ed. Joyce, D and Lewindon, D, eds. Champaign, IL: Human Kinetics, 71-84, 2014.

39. Coutts, AJ, Rampinini, E, Marcora, SM, Castagna, C, and Impellizzeri, FM. Heart rate and blood lactate correlates of perceived exertion during small-sided soccer games. *J Sci Med Sport* 12:79-84, 2009.

40. Crowcroft, S, McCleave, E, Slattery, K, and Coutts, AJ. Assessing the measurement sensitivity and diagnostic characteristics of athlete-monitoring tools in national swimmers. *Int J Sports Physiol Perform* 12:S295-S2100, 2016.

41. Cunanan, AJ, DeWeese, BH, Wagle, JP, Carroll, KM, Sausaman, R, Hornsby, WG, Haff, GG, Triplett, NT, Pierce, KC, and Stone, MH. The general adaptation syndrome: a foundation for the concept of periodization. *Sports Med* 48:787-797, 2018.

42. Cutsem, J, Marcora, S, Pauw, K, Bailey, S, Meeusen, R, and Roelands, B. The effects of mental fatigue on physical performance: a systematic review. *Sports Med* 47:1569-1588, 2017.

43. Day, ML, McGuigan, MR, Brice, G, and Foster, C. Monitoring exercise intensity during resistance training using the session RPE scale. *J Strength Cond Res* 18:353-358, 2004.

44. de Boer, AGEM, van Lanschot, JJB, Stalmeier, PFM, van Sandick, JW, Hulscher, JB, de Haes, JC, and Sprangers, MA. Is a single-item visual analogue scale as valid, reliable, and responsive as multi-item scales in measuring quality of life? *Qual Life Res* 13:311-320, 2004.

45. Del Giudice, M, Bonafiglia, JT, Islam, H, Preobrazenski, N, Amato, A, and Gurd, BJ. Investigating the reproducibility of maximal oxygen uptake responses to high-intensity interval training. *J Sci Med Sport* 23:94-99, 2020.

46. Derogatis, LR. *SCL-90: Administration, Scoring & Procedures Manual for the R (evised) Version and Other Instruments of the Psychopathology Rating Scale Series*. Baltimore: Johns Hopkins University School of Medicine, 1977.

47. de Vet, H, Terwee, CB, and Bouter, LM. Clinimetrics and psychometrics: two sides of the same coin. *J Clin Epidemiol* 56:1146-1147, 2003.

48. Diamantopoulos, A, Sarstedt, M, Fuchs, C, Wilczynski, P, and Kaiser, S. Guidelines for choosing between multi-item and single-item scales for construct measurement: a predictive validity perspective. *J Acad Mark Sci* 40:434-449, 2012.

49. Ekkekakis, P. Affect, mood, and emotions. In *Measurement in Sport and Exercise Psychology*. Tenenbaum, G, Eklund, R, and Kamata, A, eds. Champaign, IL: Human Kinetics, 321-332, 2012.

50. Fanchini, M, Ferraresi, I, Petruolo, A, Azzalin, A, Ghielmetti, R, Schena, F, and Impellizzeri, FM. Is a retrospective RPE appropriate in soccer? Response shift and recall bias. *Sci Med Football* 1:53-59, 2017.

51. Fanchini, M, Ghielmetti, R, Coutts, AJ, Schena, F, and Impellizzeri, FM. Effect of training-session intensity distribution on session rating of perceived exertion in soccer players. *Int J Sports Physiol Perform* 10:426-430, 2015.

52. Fechner, GT. Elemente Der Psychophysik. Vol 2 Vols. Leipzig: Breitkopf und Härtel, 1860.

53. Foster, C. Monitoring training in athletes with reference to overtraining syndrome. *Med Sci Sports Exerc* 30:1164-1168, 1998.

54. Foster, C, Florhaug, JA, Franklin, J, Gottschall, L, Hrovatin, LA, Parker, S, Doleshal, P, and Dodge, C. A new approach to monitoring exercise training. *J Strength Cond Res* 15:109-115, 2001.

55. Fox, JL, Stanton, R, Sargent, C, Wintour, S-A, and Scanlan, AT. The association between training load and performance in team sports: a systematic review. *Sports Med* 48:2743-2774, 2018.

56. Gabbett, TJ, and Domrow, N. Relationships between training load, injury, and fitness in sub-elite collision sport athletes. *J Sports Sci* 25:1507-1519, 2007.

57. Gathercole, R, Sporer, B, and Stellingwerff, T. Countermovement jump performance with increased training loads in elite female rugby athletes. *Int J Sports Med* 36:722-728, 2015.

58. Goldstein, EB. *Blackwell Handbook of Sensation and Perception*. Malden, MA: Blackwell Publishing Ltd, 2005.

59. Grove, JR, Main, LC, Partridge, K, Bishop, DJ, Russell, S, Shepherdson, A, and Ferguson, L. Training distress and performance readiness: laboratory and field validation of a brief self-report measure. *Scand J Med Sci Sports* 24:e483-e490, 2014.

60. Grove, JR, and Prapavessis, H. Preliminary evidence for the reliability and validity of an abbreviated Profile of Mood States. *Intl J Sport Psychol* 23:92-109, 1992.

61. Haddad, M, Stylianides, G, Djaoui, L, Dellal, A, and Chamari, K. Session-RPE method for training load monitoring: validity, ecological usefulness, and influencing factors. *Front Neurosci* 11:113-114, 2017.

62. Hall, EE, Ekkekakis, P, and Petruzzello, SJ. Is the relationship of RPE to psychological factors intensity-dependent? *Med Sci Sports Exerc* 37:1365-1373, 2005.

63. Halperin, I, and Emanuel, A. Rating of perceived effort: methodological concerns and future directions. *Sports Med* 50:679-687, 2019.

64. Hampson, DB, St Clair Gibson, A, Lambert, MI, and Noakes, TD. The influence of sensory cues on the perception of exertion during exercise and central regulation of exercise performance. *Sports Med* 31:935-952, 2001.

65. Hardy, CJ, and Rejeski, WJ. Not what, but how one feels: the measurement of affect during exercise. *J Sport Exerc Psychol* 11:304-317, 1989.

66. Herman, L, Foster, C, Maher, MA, Mikat, RP, and Porcari, JP. Validity and reliability of the session RPE method for monitoring exercise training intensity. *S Afr J Sports Med* 18:14-17, 2006.

67. Hiscock, DJ, Dawson, BT, and Peeling, P. Perceived exertion responses to changing resistance training programming variables. *J Strength Cond Res* 29:1564-1569, 2015.

68. Hitzschke, B, Holst, T, Ferrauti, A, Meyer, T, Pfeiffer, M, and Kellmann, M. Entwicklung des Akutmaßes zur Erfassung von Erholung und Beanspruchung im Sport. *Diagnostica* 62:212-226, 2016.

69. Hitzschke, B, Kölling, S, Ferrauti, A, Meyer, T, Pfeiffer, M, and Kellmann, M. Development of the short recovery and stress scale for sports (SRS). *Zeitschrift fur Sportpsychologie* 22:146-161, 2015.

70. Hooper, SL, and Mackinnon, LT. Monitoring overtraining in athletes. *Sports Med* 20:321-327, 1995.

71. Hopkins, WG. Quantification of training in competitive sports. *Sports Med* 12:161-183, 1991.

72. Hutchinson, JC, and Tenenbaum, G. Perceived effort—can it be considered gestalt? *Psychol Sport Exerc* 7:463-476, 2006.

73. Impellizzeri, FM, Borg, E, and Coutts, AJ. Intersubjective comparisons are possible with an accurate use of the Borg CR scales. *Int J Sports Physiol Perform* 6:2-7, 2011.

74. Impellizzeri, FM, and Marcora, SM. Test validation in sport physiology: lessons learned from clinimetrics. *Int J Sports Physiol Perform* 4:269-277, 2009.

75. Impellizzeri, FM, Marcora, SM, and Coutts, AJ. Internal and external training load: 15 years on. *Int J Sports Physiol Perform* 14:270-273, 2019.

76. Impellizzeri, FM, Rampinini, E, and Marcora, SM. Physiological assessment of aerobic training in soccer. *J Sports Sci* 23:583-592, 2005.

77. Jaspers, A, Brink, MS, Probst, SGM, Frencken, WGP, and Helsen, WF. Relationships between training load indicators and training outcomes in professional soccer. *Sports Med* 47:533-544, 2017.

78. Jones, HS, Williams, EL, Marchant, D, Sparks, A, Midgley, A, Bridge, C, and McNaughton, L. Distance-dependent association of affect with pacing strategy in cycling time trials. *Med Sci Sports Exerc* 47:825-832, 2015.

79. Kallus, W, and Kellmann, M. *The Recovery-Stress Questionnaires: User Manual*. Frankfurt, Germany: Pearson Assessment, 1-35, 2016.

80. Kellmann, M. Preventing overtraining in athletes in high-intensity sports and stress/recovery monitoring. *Scand J Med Sci Sports* 20:95-102, 2010.

81. Kellmann, M, and Günther, K-D. Changes in stress and recovery in elite rowers during preparation for the Olympic Games. *Med Sci Sports Exerc* 32:676-683, 2000.

82. Kellmann, M, Patrick, T, Botterill, C, and Wilson, CT. The recovery-cue and its use in applied settings: practical suggestions regarding assessment and monitoring of recovery. In *Enhancing Recovery: Preventing Underperformance in Athletes*. Kellmann, M, ed. Champaign, IL; Human Kinetics, 219-229, 2002.

83. Kiely, J. Periodization theory: confronting an inconvenient truth. Sports Med 48:753-764, 2017.

84. Kraft, JA, Green, JM, and Thompson, KR. Session ratings of perceived exertion responses during resistance training bouts equated for total work but differing in work rate. *J Strength Cond Res* 28:540-545, 2014.

85. Kraft, JA, Laurent, ML, Green, JM, Helm, J, Roberts, C, and Holt, S. Examination of coach and player perceptions of recovery and exertion. *J Strength Cond Res* 34:1383-1391, 2020.

86. Lacome, M, Carling, C, Hager, J-P, Dine, G, and Piscione, J. Workload, fatigue, and muscle damage in an under-20 rugby union team over an intensified international tournament. *Int J Sports Physiol Perform* 13:1059-1066, 2018.

87. Laurent, CM, Green, JM, Bishop, PA, Sjökvist, J, Schumacker, RE, Richardson, MT, and Curtner-Smith, M. A practical approach to monitoring recovery: development of a perceived recovery status scale. *J Strength Cond Res* 25:620-628, 2011.

88. Lea, J, Hulbert, S, O'Driscoll, J, Scales, J, and Wiles, J. Criterion-related validity of ratings of perceived exertion during resistance exercise in healthy participants: a meta-analysis. Presented at the 23rd Annual Congress of the European College of Sport Science, Dublin, Ireland; 2018.

89. Legros, P. Le surentraînement: Diagnostic des manifestations psychocomportementales précoces. *Sci Sports* 8:71-74, 1993.

90. Lochner, K. Affect, mood, and emotions. In *Successful Emotions*. Wiesbaden: Springer Fachmedien Wiesbaden, 43-67, 2016.

91. Lolli, L, Bahr, R, Weston, M, Whiteley, R, Tabben, M, Bonanno, D, Gregson, W, Chamari, K, Di Salvo, V, and van Dyk, N. No association between perceived exertion and session duration with hamstring injury occurrence in professional football. *Scand J Med Sci Sports* 30:523-530, 2019.

92. Los Arcos, A, Martínez-Santos, R, Yanci, J, Mendiguchia, J, and Mendez-Villanueva, A. Negative associations between perceived training load, volume and changes in physical fitness in professional soccer players. *J Sports Sci Med* 14:394-401, 2015.

93. Lundqvist, C, and Kenttä, G. Positive emotions are not simply the absence of the negative ones: development and validation of the emotional recovery questionnaire (EmRecQ). *Sport Psychol* 24:468-488, 2010.

94. Ma'ayan, A. Complex systems biology. J R Soc Interface 14:20170391-20170399, 2017.

95. Macpherson, TW, McLaren, SJ, Gregson, W, Lolli, L, Drust, B, and Weston, M. Using differential ratings of perceived exertion to assess agreement between coach and player perceptions of soccer training intensity: an exploratory investigation. *J Sports Sci* 37:2783-2788, 2019.

96. Main, L, and Grove, JR. A multi-component assessment model for monitoring training distress among athletes. *Eur J Sport Sci* 9:195-202, 2009.

97. Malcata, RM, Vandenbogaerde, TJ, and Hopkins, WG. Using athletes' world rankings to assess countries' performance. *Int J Sports Physiol Perform* 9:133-138, 2014.

98. Manzi, V, D'Ottavio, S, Impellizzeri, FM, Chaouachi, A, Chamari, K, and Castagna, C. Profile of weekly training load in elite male professional basketball players. *J Strength Cond Res* 24:1399-1406, 2010.

99. Marcora, SM. Do we really need a central governor to explain brain regulation of exercise performance? *Eur J Appl Physiol* 104:929-931, 2008.

100. Marcora, S. Counterpoint: afferent feedback from fatigued locomotor muscles is not an important determinant of endurance exercise performance. *J Appl Physiol* 108:454-456, 2010.

101. Marcora, SM. Effort: perception of. In *Encyclopedia of Perception*. Goldstein, EB, ed. Thousand Oaks, CA; Sage Publications, 380-383, 2010.

102. Marcora, SM, and Staiano, W. The limit to exercise tolerance in humans: mind over muscle? *Eur J Appl Physiol* 109:763-770, 2010.

103. Marcora, SM, Staiano, W, and Manning, V. Mental fatigue impairs physical performance in humans. *J Appl Physiol* 106:857-864, 2009.

104. Martens, R, Vealey, RS, Burton, D, Bump, LA, and Smith, DE. Development and validation of the competitive sports anxiety inventory 2. In *Competitive Anxiety in Sport*. Martens, R, Vealey, RS, and Burton, D, eds. Champaign, IL: Human Kinetics, 117-178, 1990.

105. Marx, RG, Bombardier, C, Hogg-Johnson, S, and Wright, JG.

Clinimetric and psychometric strategies for development of a health measurement scale. *J Clin Epidemiol* 52:105-111, 1999.

106. Mather, G. *Essentials of Sensation and Perception (Foundations of Psychology)*. New York: Routledge, 1-165, 2011.

107. McAuley, E, and Courneya, KS. Self-efficacy relationships with affective and exertion responses to exercise1. *J Appl Soc Psychol* 22:312-326, 1992.

108. McLaren, SJ, Macpherson, TW, Coutts, AJ, Hurst, C, Spears, IR, and Weston, M. The relationships between internal and external measures of training load and intensity in team sports: a meta-analysis. *Sports Med* 48:641-658, 2018.

109. McLaren, SJ, Smith, A, Spears, IR, and Weston, M. A detailed quantification of differential ratings of perceived exertion during team-sport training. *J Sci Med Sport* 20:290-295, 2017.

110. McLaren, SJ, Taylor, JM, Macpherson, TW, Spears, IR, and Weston, M. Systematic reductions in differential ratings of perceived exertion across a 2-wk repeated-sprint training intervention that improved soccer player's high-speed running abilities. *Int J Sports Physiol Perform*, 2020 [e-pub ahead of print].

111. McNair, P, Lorr, M, and Droppleman, L. *POMS Manual*. 2nd ed. San Diego, CA: Education and Industrial Testing Service, 1981.

112. Micklewright, D, Gibson, ASC, Gladwell, V, and Salman Al, A. Development and validity of the rating-of-fatigue scale. *Sports Med* 47:2375-2393, 2017.

113. Moalla, W, Fessi, MS, Farhat, F, Nouira, S, Wong, DP, and Dupont, G. Relationship between daily training load and psychometric status of professional soccer players. *Res Sports Med* 24:387-394, 2016.

114. Mokkink, LB, Prinsen, CAC, Bouter, LM, Vet, HCW de, and Terwee, CB. The COnsensus-based Standards for the selection of health Measurement INstruments (COSMIN) and how to select an outcome measurement instrument. *Braz J Phys Ther* 20:105-113, 2016.

115. Morgan, WP, Brown, DR, Raglin, JS, O'Connor, PJ, and Ellickson, KA. Psychological monitoring of overtraining and staleness. *Br J Sports Med* 21:107-114, 1987.

116. Morton, RH, Stannard, SR, and Kay, B. Low reproducibility of many lactate markers during incremental cycle exercise. *Br J Sports Med* 46:64-69, 2011.

117. Nassis, GP, and Gabbett, TJ. Is workload associated with injuries and performance in elite football? A call for action. *Br J Sports Med* 51:486-487, 2017.

118. Nassis, GP, Hertzog, M, and Brito, J. Workload assessment in soccer: an open-minded, critical thinking approach is needed. *J Strength Cond Res* 31:e77-e78, 2017.

119. Nederhof, E, Brink, MS, and Lemmink, KAPM. Reliability and validity of the Dutch recovery stress questionnaire for athletes. *Int J Sports Psychol* 39:301-311, 2008.

120. Nogueira, F, Miloski, B, Bara Filho, MG, and Lourenço, LM. Influência da presença ou da ausência de jogos nas percepções de fadiga de atletas profissionais de voleibol durante uma temporada competitiva. *Revista Portuguesa de Ciências do Desporto* 17:152-160, 2017.

121. Nunnally, J, and Bernstein, I. *Psychometric Theory*. 3rd ed. New York: McGraw-Hill, 1994.

122. Pageaux, B. The psychobiological model of endurance performance: an effort-based decision-making theory to explain self-paced endurance performance. *Sports Med* 44:1319-1320, 2014.

123. Pageaux, B. Perception of effort in exercise science: definition, measurement, and perspectives. *Eur J Sport Sci* 16:885-894, 2016.

124. Pender, NJ, Bar-Or, O, Wilk, B, and Mitchell, S. Self-efficacy and perceived exertion of girls during exercise. *Nurs Res* 51:86-91, 2002.

125. Pfeiffer, M. Modeling the relationship between training and performance-a comparison of two antagonistic concepts. *Int J Comput Sci* 7:13-32, 2008.

126. Prinsen, C, Vohra, S, Rose, MR, Boers, M, Tugwell, P, Clarke, P, Williamson, PR, and Terwee, CB. Guideline for selecting outcome measurement instruments for outcomes included in a Core Outcome Set. 2016. https://cosmin.nl/wp-content/uploads/COSMIN-guideline-selecting-outcome-measurement-COS.pdf. Accessed August 27, 2020.

127. Prinsen, CAC, Vohra, S, Rose, MR, Boers, M, Tugwell, P, Clarke, M, Williamson, PR, and Terwee, CB. How to select outcome measurement instruments for outcomes included in a "Core Outcome Set": a practical guideline. *Trials* 17:449, 2016.

128. Quarrie, KL, Raftery, M, Blackie, J, Cook, CJ, Fuller, CW, Gabbett, TJ, Gray, AJ, Gill, N, Hennessy, L, Kemp, S, and Lambert, M. Managing player load in professional rugby union: a review of current knowledge and practices. *Br J Sports Med* 51:421-427, 2017.

129. Raedeke, TD, and Smith, AL. Development and preliminary validation of an athlete burnout measure. *J Sport Exerc Psychol* 23:281-306, 2001.

130. Raglin, JS, and Morgan, WP. Development of a scale for use in monitoring training-induced distress in athletes. *Int J Sports Med* 15:84-88, 2008.

131. Rejeski, J. The perception of exertion: a social psychophysiological integration. *J Sport Psychol* 3:305-320, 1981.

132. Rejeski, J. Perceived exertion: an active or passive process. *J Sport Psychol* 7:371-378, 1985.

133. Robertson, S, Kremer, P, Aisbett, B, Tran, J, and Cerin, E. Consensus on measurement properties and feasibility of performance tests for the exercise and sport sciences: a Delphi study. *Sports Med Open* 3:2, 2017.

134. Robertson, RJ, and Noble, BJ. Perception of physical exertion: methods, mediators, and applications. *Exerc Sport Sci Rev* 25:407-452, 1997.

135. Robey, E, Dawson, BT, Halson, S, Gregson, W, Goodman, C, and Eastwood, P. Sleep quantity and quality in elite youth soccer players: a pilot study. *Eur J Sport Sci* 14:410-417, 2013.

136. Rushall, BS. A tool for measuring stress tolerance in elite athletes. *J Appl Sport Psychol* 2:51-66, 1990.

137. Saw, AE, Kellmann, M, Main, LC, and Gastin PB. Athlete self-report measures in research and practice: considerations for the discerning reader and fastidious practitioner. *Int J Sports Physiol Perform* 12:S2127-S2135, 2017.

138. Saw, AE, Main, LC, and Gastin, PB. Monitoring athletes through self-report: factors influencing implementation. *J Sports Sci Med* 14:137-146, 2015.

139. Saw, AE, Main, LC, and Gastin, PB. Monitoring the athlete training response: subjective self-reported measures trump commonly used objective measures: a systematic review. *Br J Sports Med* 50:281-291, 2016.

140. Scott, TJ, Black, CR, Quinn, J, and Coutts, AJ. Validity and reliability of the session-RPE method for quantifying training in Australian football: a comparison of the CR10 and CR100 scales. *J Strength Cond Res* 27:270-276, 2013.

141. Shacham, S. A shortened version of the Profile of Mood States. *J Pers Assess* 47:305-306, 2010.

142. Shiffman, S. Real-time self-report of momentary states in the natural environment: computerized ecological momentary

assessment. In *The Science of Self-Report Implications for Research and Practice.* Stone, AA, Turkkan, JS, Bachrach, CA, Jobe, JB, Kurtzman, HS, and Cain, VS, eds. Mahwah, NJ: Lawrence Erlbaum Associates, 227-296, 2000.

143. Sloan, JA, Aaronson, N, Cappelleri, JC, Fairclough, DL, Varricchio, C, Clinical Significance Consensus Meeting Group. Assessing the clinical significance of single items relative to summated scores. *Mayo Clin Proc* 77:479-487, 2002.

144. Smith, MR, Coutts, AJ, Merlini, M, Deprez, D, Lenoir, M, and Marcora, SM. Mental fatigue impairs soccer-specific physical and technical performance. *Med Sci Sports Exerc* 48:267-276, 2016.

145. Spielberger, CD. *The Preliminary Manual for the State-Trait Personality Inventory* [Unpublished Manual]. Tampa: University of South Florida, 1979.

146. Spielberger, CD, Gorsuch, RL, and Lushene, RE. *Manual for the State-Trait Anxiety Inventory.* Palo Alto, CA: Consulting Psychologists Press, 1970.

147. Starling, LT, and Lambert, MI. Monitoring rugby players for fitness and fatigue: what do coaches want? *Int J Sports Physiol Perform* 13:777-782, 2018.

148. Steele, J, Fisher, J, McKinnon, S, and McKinnon, P. Differentiation between perceived effort and discomfort during resistance training in older adults: reliability of trainee ratings of effort and discomfort, and reliability and validity of trainer ratings of trainee effort. *J Trainol* 6:1-8, 2016.

149. Streiner, DL, Norman, GR, and Cairney, J. *Health Measurement Scales.* 5th ed. Oxford, UK: Oxford University Press, 2014.

150. Taylor, K-L, Chapman, DW, Cronin, JB, Newton, MJ, and Gill, ND. Fatigue monitoring in high performance sport: a survey of current trends. *J Aust Strength Cond* 20:12-23, 2012.

151. Terry, PC, Lane, AM, and Fogarty, GJ. Construct validity of the Profile of Mood States–Adolescents for use with adults. *Psychol Sport Exerc* 4:125-139, 2003.

152. Terry, PC, Lane, AM, Lane, HJ, and Keohane, L. Development and validation of a mood measure for adolescents. *J Sports Sci* 17:861-872, 1999.

153. Terwee, CB, Bot, SDM, and de Boer, MR, Quality criteria were proposed for measurement properties of health status questionnaires. *J Clin Epidemiol* 60:34-42, 2007.

154. Terwee, CB, Prinsen, CA, Chiarotto, A, de Vet, HC, Bouter, LM, Alonso, J, Westerman, MJ, Patrick, DL, and Mokkink, LB. COSMIN methodology for assessing the content validity of PROMs. 2017. www.cosmin.nl/wp-content/uploads/COSMIN-methodology-for-content-validity-user-manual-v1.pdf. Accessed August 27, 2020.

155. Thorpe, RT, Atkinson, G, Drust, B, and Gregson, W. Monitoring fatigue status in elite team-sport athletes: implications for practice. *Int J Sports Physiol Perform* 12:S227-S234, 2017.

156. Turner, AN, Buttigieg, C, Marshall, G, Noto, A, Phillips, J, and Kilduff, L. Ecological validity of the session rating of perceived exertion for quantifying internal training load in fencing. *Int J Sports Physiol Perform* 12:124-128, 2016.

157. Uchida, MC, Teixeira, LFM, Godoi, VJ, Marchetti, PH, Conte, M, Coutts, AJ, and Bacurau, RF. Does the timing of measurement alter session-RPE in boxers? *J Sports Sci Med* 13:59-65, 2014.

158. Van Hooff, MLM, Geurts, SAE, Kompier, MAJ, and Taris, TW. "How fatigued do you currently feel?" Convergent and discriminant validity of a single-item fatigue measure. *J Occup Health* 49:224-234, 2007.

159. Vanrenterghem, J, Nedergaard, NJ, Robinson, MA, and Drust, B. Training load monitoring in team sports: a novel framework separating physiological and biomechanical load-adaptation pathways. *Sports Med* 47:2135-2142, 2017.

160. Viru, A, and Viru, M. Nature of training effects. In *Exercise and Sport Science.* Garrett, WE and Kirkendall, DT, eds. Philadelphia: Lippincott Williams & Wilkins, 67-96, 2000.

161. Wallace, LK, Slattery, KM, and Coutts, AJ. The ecological validity and application of the session-RPE method for quantifying training loads in swimming. *J Strength Cond Res* 23:33-38, 2009.

162. Wallace, LK, Slattery, KM, Impellizzeri, FM, and Coutts, AJ. Establishing the criterion validity and reliability of common methods for quantifying training load. *J Strength Cond Res* 28:2330-2337, 2014.

163. Weston, M. Training load monitoring in elite English soccer: a comparison of practices and perceptions between coaches and practitioners. *Sci Med Football* 2:216-224, 2018.

164. Weston, M, Siegler, J, Bahnert, A, McBrien, J, and Lovell, R. The application of differential ratings of perceived exertion to Australian Football League matches. *J Sci Med Sport* 18:704-708, 2015.

165. Wilson, M. *Constructing Measures.* Mahwah, NJ: Lawrence Erlbaum Associates, 2005.

Chapter 18

1. Albanese, D, Filosi, M, Visintainer, R, Riccadonna, S, Jurman, G, and Furlanello, C. Minerva and minepy: a C engine for the MINE suite and its R, Python and MATLAB wrappers. *Bioinformatics* 29:407-408, 2013.

2. Allen, MJ, and Yen, WM. *Introduction to Measurement Theory.* Long Grove, IL: Waveland Press, 2001.

3. Amrhein, V, Trafimow, D, and Greenland, S. Inferential statistics as descriptive statistics: there is no replication crisis if we don't expect replication. *Am Stat* 73:262-270, 2019.

4. Angrist, JD, and Pischke, JS. *Mastering 'Metrics: The Path From Cause To Effect.* Princeton, NJ: Princeton University Press, 2015.

5. Anvari, F, and Lakens, D. Using anchor-based methods to determine the smallest effect size of interest. *PsyArXiv Preprints*, 2019.

6. Barker, RJ, and Schofield, MR. Inference about magnitudes of effects. *Int J Sports Physiol Perform* 3:547-557, 2008.

7. Batterham, AM, and Hopkins, WG. Making meaningful inferences about magnitudes. *Int J Sports Physiol Perform* 1:50-57, 2006.

8. Borg, DN, Minett, GM, Stewart, IB, and Drovandi, CC. Bayesian methods might solve the problems with magnitude-based inference. *Med Sci Sports Exerc* 50:2609-2610, 2018.

9. Breiman, L. Statistical modeling: the two cultures. *Statist Sci* 16:199-215, 2001.

10. Buchheit, M, and Rabbani, A. The 30-15 intermittent fitness test versus the yo-yo intermittent recovery test level 1: relationship and sensitivity to training. *Int J Sports Physiol Perform* 9:522-524, 2014.

11. Caldwell, AR, and Cheuvront, SN. Basic statistical considerations for physiology: the journal *Temperature* toolbox. *Temperature* 6:181-210, 2019.

12. Carsey, T, and Harden, J. *Monte Carlo Simulation and Resampling Methods for Social Science.* Los Angeles: Sage Publications, 2013.

13. Cohen, J. *Statistical Power Analysis for the Behavioral Sciences.* 2nd ed. Hillsdale, NJ: Lawrence Erlbaum Associates, 1988.

14. Cumming, G. The new statistics: why and how. *Psychol Sci* 25:7-29, 2014.

15. Curran-Everett, D. Magnitude-based inference: good idea but flawed approach. *Med Sci Sports Exerc* 50:2164-2165, 2018.

16. Dienes, Z. *Understanding Psychology as a Science: An Introduction to Scientific and Statistical Inference.* New York: Red Globe Press, 2008.

17. Efron, B, and Hastie, T. *Computer Age Statistical Inference: Algorithms, Evidence, and Data Science.* New York: Cambridge University Press, 2016.

18. Friedman, J, Hastie, T, and Tibshirani, R. Regularization paths for generalized linear models via coordinate descent. *J Statist Softw* 33:1-22, 2010.

19. Gelman, A. Causality and statistical learning. *Am J Sociol* 117:955-966, 2011.

20. Gelman, A, and Hennig, C. Beyond subjective and objective in statistics. *J R Statist Soc A* 180:967-1033, 2017.

21. Hernán, MA. Does water kill? A call for less casual causal inferences. *Ann Epidemiol* 26:674-680, 2016.

22. Hernán, MA. Causal diagrams: draw your assumptions before your conclusions course. PH559x, 2017.

23. Hernán, MA. The C-word: scientific euphemisms do not improve causal inference from observational data. *Am J Public Health* 108:616-619, 2018.

24. Hernán, MA, and Cole, SR. Invited commentary: causal diagrams and measurement bias. *Am J Epidemiol* 170:959-962, 2009.

25. Hernán, MA, Hsu, J, and Healy, B. A second chance to get causal inference right: a classification of data science tasks. *CHANCE* 32:42-49, 2019.

26. Hernán, MA, and Robins, J. *Causal Inference.* Boca Raton FL: Chapman & Hall/CRC, 2010.

27. Hernán, MA, and Taubman, SL. Does obesity shorten life? The importance of well-defined interventions to answer causal questions. *Int J Obes (Lond)* 32:S8-S14, 2008.

28. Hopkins, W. Spreadsheets for analysis of validity and reliability. *Sportscience* 19:36-42, 2015.

29. Hopkins, WG. Measures of reliability in sports medicine and science. *Sports Med* 30:1-15, 2000.

30. Hopkins, WG. Bias in Bland-Altman but not regression validity analyses. *Sportscience* 8:42-47, 2004.

31. Hopkins, WG. How to interpret changes in an athletic performance test. *Sportscience* 8:1-7, 2004.

32. Hopkins, WG. A new view of statistics. 2006. www.sportsci.org/resource/stats/effectmag.html. Accessed August 27, 2020.

33. Hopkins, WG. Understanding statistics by using spreadsheets to generate and analyze samples. *Sportscience* 1; 11:23-27, 2007.

34. Hopkins, WG. A Socratic dialogue on comparison of measures. *Sportscience* 14:15-22, 2010.

35. Hopkins, WG. Individual responses made easy. *J Appl Physiol* 118:1444-1446, 2015.

36. Hopkins, WG, and Batterham, AM. The vindication of magnitude-based inference (draft 2). *Sportscience* 22:9-27, 2018.

37. Hopkins, WG, Marshall, SW, Batterham, AM, and Hanin, J. Progressive statistics for studies in sports medicine and exercise science. *Med Sci Sports Exerc* 41:3-13, 2009.

38. James, G, Witten, D, Hastie, T, and Tibshirani, R. *An Introduction to Statistical Learning: With Applications in R.* New York: Springer, 2017.

39. King, MT. A point of minimal important difference (MID): a critique of terminology and methods. *Expert Rev Pharmacoecon Outcomes Res* 11:171-184, 2011.

40. Kleinberg, S. *Why: A Guide to Finding and Using Causes.* Boston: O'Reilly Media, 2015.

41. Kruschke, JK, and Liddell, TM. Bayesian data analysis for newcomers. *Psychonomic Bull Rev* 25:155-177, 2018.

42. Kruschke, JK, and Liddell, TM. The Bayesian new statistics: hypothesis testing, estimation, meta-analysis, and power analysis from a Bayesian perspective. *Psychonomic Bull Rev* 25:178-206, 2018.

43. Kuhn, M, and Johnson, K. *Applied Predictive Modeling.* New York: Springer, 2018.

44. Kuhn, M, and Johnson, K. *Feature Engineering and Selection: A Practical Approach for Predictive Models.* Milton Park, Abington, UK: CRC Press LLC, 2019.

45. Lakens, D, Scheel, AM, and Isager, PM. Equivalence testing for psychological research: a tutorial. *Adv Methods Pract Psychol Sci* 1:259-269, 2018.

46. Lang, KM, Sweet, SJ, and Grandfield, EM. Getting beyond the null: statistical modeling as an alternative framework for inference in developmental science. *Res Hum Dev* 14:287-304, 2017.

47. Lederer, DJ, Bell, SC, Branson, RD, Chalmers, JD, Marshall, R, Maslove, DM, Ost, DE, Punjabi, NM, Schatz, M, Smyth, AR, and Stewart, W. Control of confounding and reporting of results in causal inference studies: guidance for authors from editors of respiratory, sleep, and critical care journals. *Ann Am Thorac Soc* 16:22-28, 2019.

48. McElreath, R. *Statistical Rethinking: A Bayesian Course with Examples in R and Stan.* Boca Raton, FL: Chapman & Hall/CRC, 2015.

49. McGraw, KO, and Wong, SP. A common language effect size statistic. *Psychol Bull* 111:361-365, 1992.

50. Miller, T. Explanation in artificial intelligence: Insights from the social sciences. *Artificial Intelligence* 267: 1-38, 2019.

51. Mitchell, SD. Integrative pluralism. *Biol Philos* 17:55-70, 2002.

52. Mitchell, S. *Unsimple Truths: Science, Complexity, and Policy.* Chicago: University of Chicago Press, 2012.

53. Molnar, C. *Interpretable Machine Learning.* Victoria, BC: Leanpub, 2018.

54. Molnar, C, Bischl, B, and Casalicchio, G. Iml: an R package for interpretable machine learning. *J Open Source Softw* 3:786, 2018.

55. Nevill, AM, Williams, AM, Boreham, C, Wallace, ES, Davison, GW, Abt, G, Lane, AM., and Winter, EM. Can we trust "magnitude-based inference"? *J Sports Sci* 36:2769-2770, 2018.

56. Novick, MR. The axioms and principal results of classical test theory. *J Math Psychol* 3:1-18, 1966.

57. Page, SE. *The Model Thinker: What You Need to Know to Make Data Work for You.* New York: Basic Books, 2018.

58. Pearl, J. Causal inference in statistics: an overview. *Stat Surv* 3:96-146, 2009.

59. Pearl, J. The seven tools of causal inference, with reflections on machine learning. *Commun ACM* 62:54-60, 2019.

60. Pearl, J, Glymour, M, and Jewell, NP. *Causal Inference in Statistics: A Primer.* Chichester, West Sussex: Wiley, 2016.

61. Pearl, J, and Mackenzie, D. *The Book of Why: The New Science of Cause and Effect.* New York: Basic Books, 2018.

62. Reshef, DN, Reshef, YA, Finucane, HK, Grossman, SR, McVean, G, Turnbaugh, PJ, Lander, ES, Mitzenmacher, M, and Sabeti, PC. Detecting novel associations in large data sets. *Science* 334:1518-1524, 2011.

63. Ribeiro, MT, Singh, S, and Guestrin, C. "Why should I trust

you?": explaining the predictions of any classifier. 2016. http://arxiv.org/abs/1602.04938. Accessed August 27, 2020.

64. Rohrer, JM. Thinking clearly about correlations and causation: graphical causal models for observational data. *Adv Methods and Pract Psychol Sci* 1:27-42, 2018.

65. Rousselet, GA, Pernet, CR, and Wilcox, RR. A practical introduction to the bootstrap: a versatile method to make inferences by using data-driven simulations [reproducibility package]. 2019. https://doi.org/10.17605/OSF.IO/8B4T5. Accessed August 27, 2020.

66. Sainani, KL. Clinical versus statistical significance. *PM R* 4:442-445, 2012.

67. Sainani, KL. The problem with "magnitude-based inference." *Med Sci Sports Exerc* 50:2166-2176, 2018.

68. Sainani, KL, Lohse, KR, Jones, PR, and Vickers, A. Magnitude-based inference is not Bayesian and is not a valid method of inference. *Scand J Med Sci Sports* 29:1428-1436, 2019.

69. Shmueli, G. To explain or to predict? *Stat Sci* 25:289-310, 2010.

70. Shrier, I, and Platt, RW. Reducing bias through directed acyclic graphs. *BMC Med Res Methodol* 8:70, 2008.

71. Swinton, PA, Hemingway, BS, Saunders, B, Gualano, B, and Dolan, E. A statistical framework to interpret individual response to intervention: paving the way for personalized nutrition and exercise prescription. *Front Nutr* 5:41, 2018.

72. Turner, A, Brazier, J, Bishop, C, Chavda, S, Cree, J, and Read, P. Data analysis for strength and conditioning coaches: using Excel to analyze reliability, differences, and relationships. *Strength Cond J* 37:76-83, 2015.

73. Weinberg, G, and McCann, L. *Super Thinking: The Big Book of Mental Models*. New York: Portfolio/Penguin, 2019.

74. Welsh, AH, and Knight, EJ. "Magnitude-based inference": a statistical review. *Med Sci Sports Exerc* 47:874-884, 2015.

75. Yarkoni, T, and Westfall, J. Choosing prediction over explanation in psychology: lessons from machine learning. *Perspect Psychol Sci* 12:1100-1122, 2017.

Chapter 19

1. Aasheim, C, Stavenes, H, Andersson, SH, Engbretsen, L, and Clarsen, B. Prevalence and burden of overuse injuries in elite junior handball. *BMJ Open Sport Exerc Med* 4:e000391, 2018.

2. Anderson, L, Triplett-McBride, T, Foster, C, Doberstein, S, and Brice, G. Impact of training patterns on incidence of illness and injury during a women's collegiate basketball season. *J Strength Cond Res* 17:734-738, 2003.

3. Bahr, R. Why screening tests to predict injury do not work—and probably never will…: a critical review. *Br J Sports Med* 50:776-780, 2016.

4. Bahr, MA, and Bahr, R. Jump frequency may contribute to risk of jumper's knee: a study of interindividual and sex differences in a total of 11 943 jumps video recorded during training and matches in young elite volleyball players. *Br J Sports Med* 48:1322-1326, 2014.

5. Bahr, R, Clarsen, B, and Ekstrand, J. Why we should focus on the burden of injuries and illnesses, not just their incidence. *Br J Sports Med* 52:1018-1021, 2018.

6. Bahr, R, and Holme, I. Risk factors for sports injuries — a methodological approach. *Br J Sports Med* 37:384-392, 2003.

7. Bahr, R, and Krosshaug, T. Understanding injury mechanisms: a key component of preventing injuries in sport. *Br J Sports Med* 39:324-329, 2005.

8. Banister, EW, and Calvert, TW. Planning for future performance: implications for long term training. *Can J Appl Sport Sci* 5:170-176, 1980.

9. Banister, E, Calvert, T, Savage, M, and Bach, T. A systems model of training for athletic performance. *Aust J Sports Med* 7:57-61, 1975.

10. Barboza, SD, Bolling, CS, Nauta, J, Mechelen, W van, and Verhagen, E. Acceptability and perceptions of end-users towards an online sports-health surveillance system. *BMJ Open Sport Exerc Med* 3:e000275, 2017.

11. Bertelsen, ML, Hulme, A, Petersen, J, Brund, RK, Sørensen, H, Finch, CF, Parner, ET, and Neilsen, RO. A framework for the etiology of running-related injuries. *Scand J Med Sci Sports* 27:1170-1180, 2017.

12. Bittencourt, NFN, Meeuwisse, WH, Mendonça, LD, Nettel-Aguirre, A, Ocarino, JM, and Fonseca, ST. Complex systems approach for sports injuries: moving from risk factor identification to injury pattern recognition—narrative review and new concept. *Br J Sports Med* 50:1309-1314, 2016.

13. Black, GM, Gabbett, TJ, Cole, MH, and Naughton, G. Monitoring workload in throwing-dominant sports: a systematic review. *Sports Med* 46:1503-1516, 2016.

14. Borresen, J, and Lambert, MI. Quantifying training load: a comparison of subjective and objective methods. *Int J Sports Physiol Perform* 3:16-30, 2008.

15. Bourdon, PC, Cardinale, M, Murray, A, Gastin, P, Kellmann, M, Varley, MC, Gabbett, TJ, Coutts, AJ, Burgess, DJ, Gregson, W, and Cable, NT. Monitoring athlete training loads: consensus statement. *Int J Sports Physiol Perform* 12:S2161-S2170, 2017.

16. Buchheit, M. Applying the acute:chronic workload ratio in elite football: worth the effort? *Br J Sports Med* 51:1325-1327, 2016.

17. Carey, DL, Blanch, P, Ong, K-L, Crossley, KM, Crow, J, and Morris, ME. Training loads and injury risk in Australian football—differing acute: chronic workload ratios influence match injury risk. *Br J Sports Med* 51:1215-1220, 2017.

18. Carey, DL, Crossley, KM, Whiteley, R, Mosler, A, Ong, KL, Crow, J, and Morris, ME. Modelling training loads and injuries: the dangers of discretization. *Med Sci Sports Exerc* 50:2267-2276, 2018.

19. Carey, DL, Ong, K, Whiteley, R, Crossley, KM, Crow, J, and Morris, ME. Predictive modelling of training loads and injury in Australian football. *Int J Comput Sci Sport* 17:49-66, 2018.

20. Colby, MJ, Dawson, B, Peeling, P, Heasman, J, Rogalski, B, Drew, MK, Stares, J, Zouhal, H, and Lester, L. Multivariate modelling of subjective and objective monitoring data improve the detection of non-contact injury risk in elite Australian footballers. *J Sci Med Sport* 20:1068-1074, 2017.

21. Collins, L. Analysis of longitudinal data: the integration of theoretical model, temporal design, and statistical model. *Ann Rev Psychol* 57:505-528, 2006.

22. Crutzen, R, and Peters, G-JY. Targeting next generations to change the common practice of underpowered research. *Front Psychol* 8:1184, 2017.

23. Drew, MK, Blanch, P, Purdam, C, and Gabbett, TJ. Yes, rolling averages are a good way to assess training load for injury prevention. Is there a better way? Probably, but we have not seen the evidence. *Br J Sports Med* 51:618-619, 2017.

24. Drew, MK, and Finch, CF. The relationship between training load and injury, illness and soreness: a systematic and literature review. *Sports Med* 45:861-863, 2016.

25. Drew, MK, Raysmith, BP, and Charlton, PC. Injuries impair the chance of successful performance by sportspeople: a systematic review. *Br J Sports Med* 51:1209-1214, 2017.

26. Dyk, N van, Made, AD van der, Timmins, RG, Opar, DA, and Tol, JL. There is strength in numbers for muscle injuries: it is time to establish an international collaborative registry. *Br J Sports Med* 52:1228-1229, 2018.

27. Eckard, TG, Padua, DA, Hearn, DW, Pexa, BS, and Frank, BS. The relationship between training load and injury in athletes: a systematic review. *Sports Med* 48:1929-1961, 2018.

28. Ekstrand, J. Keeping your top players on the pitch: the key to football medicine at a professional level. *Br J Sports Med* 47:723-724, 2013.

29. Ekstrand, J, Lundqvist, D, Davison, M, D'Hooghe, M, and Pensgaard, AM. Communication quality between the medical team and the head coach/manager is associated with injury burden and player availability in elite football clubs. *Br J Sports Med* 53:304-308, 2019.

30. Fanchini, M, Rampinini, E, Riggio, M, Coutts, AJ, Pecci, C, and McCall, A. Despite association, the acute:chronic work load ratio does not predict non-contact injury in elite footballers. *Sci Med Football* 2:108-114, 2018.

31. Foster, C, Rodriguez-Marroyo, JA, and de Koning, JJ. Monitoring training loads: the past, the present, and the future. *Int J Sports Physiol Perform* 12:S22-S28, 2017.

32. Fuller, C. Injury definitions. In *Sports Injury Research*. Verhagen, E and van Mechelen, W, eds. New York: Oxford University Press, 43-53, 2010.

33. Gabbett, TJ. Debunking the myths about training load, injury and performance: empirical evidence, hot topics and recommendations for practitioners. *Br J Sports Med* 54:58-66, 2018.

34. Gabbett, TJ, Nassis, GP, Oetter, E, Pretorius, J, Johnston, N, Medina, D, Rodas, G, Myslinski, T, Howells, D, Beard, A, and Ryan, A. The athlete monitoring cycle: a practical guide to interpreting and applying training monitoring data. *Br J Sports Med* 20:1451-1452, 2017.

35. Gupta, A, Wilkerson, GB, Sharda, R, and Colston, MA. Who is more injury-prone? Prediction and assessment of injury risk. *Decision Sci* 50:374-409, 2018.

36. Haddad, M, Stylianides, G, Djaoui, L, Dellal, A, and Chamari, K. Session-RPE method for training load monitoring: validity, ecological usefulness, and influencing factors. *Front Neurosci* 11:612, 2017.

37. Hägglund, M, Waldén, M, Magnusson, H, Kristenson, K, Bengtsson, H, and Ekstrand, J. Injuries affect team performance negatively in professional football: an 11-year follow-up of the UEFA Champions League injury study. *Br J Sports Med* 47:738-742, 2013.

38. Hickey, J, Shield, AJ, Williams, MD, and Opar, DA. The financial cost of hamstring strain injuries in the Australian Football League. *Br J Sports Med* 48:729-730, 2014.

39. Hoffman, DT, Dwyer, DB, Bowe, SJ, Clifton, P, and Gastin, PB. Is injury associated with team performance in elite Australian football? 20 years of player injury and team performance data that include measures of individual player value. *Br J Sports Med* 54:475-479, 2020.

40. Hulin, BT. The never-ending search for the perfect acute:chronic workload ratio: what role injury definition? *Br J Sports Med* 51:991-992, 2017.

41. Hulme, A, and Finch, CF. From monocausality to systems thinking: a complementary and alternative conceptual approach for better understanding the development and prevention of sports injury. *Inj Epidemiol* 2:31, 2015.

42. Hulme, A, Thompson, J, Nielsen, RO, Read, GJM, and Salmon, PM. Towards a complex systems approach in sports injury research: simulating running-related injury development with agent-based modelling. *Br J Sports Med* 53:560-569, 2019.

43. Jones, CM, Griffiths, PC, and Mellalieu, SD. Training load and fatigue marker associations with injury and illness: a systematic review of longitudinal studies. *Sports Med* 47:943-974, 2017.

44. Killen, NM, Gabbett, TJ, and Jenkins, DG. Training loads and incidence of injury during the preseason in professional rugby league players. *J Strength Cond Res* 24:2079-2084, 2010.

45. Lacome, M, Avrillon, S, Cholley, Y, Simpson, BM, Guilhem, G, and Buchheit, M. Hamstring eccentric strengthening program: does training volume matter? *Int J Sports Physiol Perform* 15:81-90, 2018.

46. Lacome, M, Simpson, B, Broad, N, and Buchheit, M. Monitoring players' readiness using predicted heart rate responses to football drills. *Int J Sports Physiol Perform* 1:13, 1273-1280, 2018.

47. Lolli, L, Batterham, AM, Hawkins, R, Kelly, DM, Strudwick, AJ, Thorpe, R, Gregson, W, and Atkinson, G. Mathematical coupling causes spurious correlation within the conventional acute-to-chronic workload ratio calculations. *Br J Sports Med* 53:921-922, 2017.

48. Lolli, L, Batterham, AM, Hawkins, R, Kelly, DM, Strudwick, AJ, Thorpe, RT, Gregson, W, and Atkinson, G. The acute-to-chronic workload ratio: an inaccurate scaling index for an unnecessary normalisation process? *Br J Sports Med* 53:1510-1512, 2018.

49. Lyman, S, Fleisig, GS, Waterbor, JW, Funkhouser, EM, Pulley, L, Andrews, JR, Osinski, ED, and Roseman, JM. Longitudinal study of elbow and shoulder pain in youth baseball pitchers. *Med Sci Sports Exerc* 33:1803-1810, 2001.

50. Malone, S, Roe, M, Doran, DA, Gabbett, TJ, and Collins, KD. Aerobic fitness and playing experience protect against spikes in workload: the role of the acute:chronic workload ratio on injury risk in elite Gaelic football. *Int J Sports Physiol Perform* 12:393-401, 2017.

51. Malone, S, Roe, M, Doran, DA, Gabbett, TJ, and Collins, K. High chronic training loads and exposure to bouts of maximal velocity running reduce injury risk in elite Gaelic football. *J Sci Med Sport* 20:250-254, 2016.

52. McCall, A, Fanchini, M, and Coutts, AJ. Prediction: the modern day sports science/medicine "quest for the holy grail." *Int J Sports Physiol Perform* 12:704-706, 2017.

53. Mechelen, W van, Hlobil, H, and Kemper, HC. Incidence, severity, aetiology and prevention of sports injuries. A review of concepts. *Sports Med* 14:82-99, 1992.

54. Meeuwisse, WH. Assessing causation in sport injury: a multifactorial model. *Clin J Sport Med* 4:166-170, 1994.

55. Meeuwisse, WH, Tyreman, H, Hagel, B, and Emery, C. A dynamic model of etiology in sport injury: the recursive nature of risk and causation. *Clin J Sport Med* 17: 215-219, 2007.

56. Menaspà, P. Are rolling averages a good way to assess training load for injury prevention? *Br J Sports Med* 51:618-619, 2017.

57. Menaspà, P. Building evidence with flawed data? The importance of analysing valid data. *Br J Sports Med* 51:1173, 2017.

58. Møller, M, Nielsen, RO, Attermann, J, Wedderkopp, N, Lind, M, Sørensen, H, and Myklebust, G. Handball load and shoulder injury rate: a 31-week cohort study of 679 elite youth handball players. *Br J Sports Med* 51:231-237, 2017.

59. Munafò, MR, Nosek, BA, Bishop, DVM, Button, KS, Chambers, CD, Sert, NP du, Simonsohn, U, Wagenmaker, E-J, Ware, JJ, and Loannidis, JPA. A manifesto for reproducible science. *Nat Hum Behav* 1:0021, 2017.

60. Murray, NB, Gabbett, TJ, and Townshend, AD. Relationship between pre-season training load and in-season availability in elite Australian football players. *Int J Sports Physiol Perform* 12:749-755, 2017.

61. Neupert, EC, Cotterill, ST, and Jobson, SA. Training monitoring

engagement: an evidence-based approach in elite sport. *Int J Sports Physiol Perform* 28:1-21, 2018.

62. Nielsen, RO, Bertelsen, ML, Møller, M, Hulme, A, Windt, J, Verhagen, E, Mansournia, MA, Casals, M, and Parner, ET. Training load and structure-specific load: applications for sport injury causality and data analyses. *Br J Sports Med* 52:1016-1017, 2017.

63. Nielsen, RO, Bertelsen, ML, Ramskov, D, Møller, M, Hulme, A, Theisen, D, Finch, CF, Fortington, LV, Mansournia, MA, and Parner, ET. Time-to-event analysis for sports injury research part 1: time-varying exposures. *Br J Sports Med* 53:61-68, 2019.

64. Nielsen, RO, Bertelsen, ML, Ramskov, D, Møller, M, Hulme, A, Theisen, D, Finch, CF, Fortington, LV, Mansournia, MA, and Parner, ET. Time-to-event analysis for sports injury research part 2: time-varying outcomes. *Br J Sports Med* 53:70-78, 2019.

65. Nielsen, RØ, Parner, ET, Nohr, EA, Sørensen, H, Lind, M, and Rasmussen, S. Excessive progression in weekly running distance and risk of running-related injuries: an association which varies according to type of injury. *J Orthop Sports Phys Ther* 44:739-747, 2014.

66. Olsen, SJ, Fleisig, GS, Dun, S, Loftice, J, and Andrews, JR. Risk factors for shoulder and elbow injuries in adolescent baseball pitchers. *Am J Sports Med* 34:905-912, 2006.

67. Opar, DA, Williams, MD, Timmins, RG, Hickey, J, Duhig, SJ, and Shield, AJ. Eccentric hamstring strength and hamstring injury risk in Australian footballers. *Med Sci Sports Exerc* 47:857-865, 2015.

68. Orchard, JW, James, T, Portus, M, Kountouris, A, and Dennis, R. Fast bowlers in cricket demonstrate up to 3- to 4-week delay between high workloads and increased risk of injury. *Am J Sports Med* 37:1186-1192, 2009.

69. Rasmussen, CH, Nielsen, RO, Juul, MS, and Rasmussen, S. Weekly running volume and risk of running-related injuries among marathon runners. *Int J Sports Phys Ther* 8:111-120, 2013.

70. Raysmith, BP, and Drew, MK. Performance success or failure is influenced by weeks lost to injury and illness in elite Australian track and field athletes: a 5-year prospective study. *J Sci Med Sport* 19:778-783, 2016.

71. Robertson, S, Bartlett, JD, and Gastin, PB. Red, amber, or green? Athlete monitoring in team sport: the need for decision-support systems. *Int J Sports Physiol Perform* 12:S273-S279, 2016.

72. Rossi, A, Pappalardo, L, Cintia, P, Iaia, FM, Fernàndez, J, and Medina, D. Effective injury forecasting in soccer with GPS training data and machine learning. *PLoS One* 13:e0201264, 2018.

73. Ruddy, JD, Cormack, SJ, Whiteley, R, Williams, MD, Timmins, RG, and Opar, DA. Modeling the risk of team sport injuries: a narrative review of different statistical approaches. *Front Physiol* 10:829, 2019.

74. Ruddy, JD, Pollard, CW, Timmins, RG, Williams, MD, Shield, AJ, and Opar, DA. Running exposure is associated with the risk of hamstring strain injury in elite Australian footballers. *Br J Sports Med* 52:919-928, 2018.

75. Sampson, JA, Fullagar, HHK, and Murray, A. Evidence is needed to determine if there is a better way to determine the acute:chronic workload. *Br J Sports Med* 51:621-622, 2017.

76. Sampson, JA, Murray, A, Williams, S, Halseth, T, Hanisch, J, Golden, G, and Fullagar, HHK. Injury risk-workload associations in NCAA American college football. *J Sci Med Sport* 21:1215-1220, 2018.

77. Sands, W, Cardinale, M, McNeal, J, Murray, S, Sole, C, Reed, J, Apostolopoulos, N, and Stone, M. Recommendations for

measurement and management of an elite athlete. *Sports (Basel)* 7:105, 2019.

78. Sands, WA, Kavanaugh, AA, Murray, SR, McNeal, JR, and Jemni, M. Modern techniques and technologies applied to training and performance monitoring. *Int J Sports Physiol Perform* 12:S263-S272, 2017.

79. Shaw, G, Lee-Barthel, A, Ross, ML, Wang, B, and Baar, K. Vitamin C–enriched gelatin supplementation before intermittent activity augments collagen synthesis. *Am J Clin Nutr* 105:136-143, 2017.

80. Shmueli, G. To explain or to predict? *Statist Sci* 25:289-310, 2010.

81. Shrier, I. Strategic assessment of risk and risk tolerance (StARRT) framework for return-to-play decision-making. *Br J Sports Med* 49:1311-1315, 2015.

82. Smith, DJ. A framework for understanding the training process leading to elite performance. *Sports Med* 33:1103-1126, 2003.

83. Soligard, T, Schwellnus, M, Alonso, J-M, Bahr, R, Clarsen, B, Dijkstra, HP, Gabbatt, T, Gleeson, M, Hagglund, M, Hutchinson, MR, van Rensburg, CJ, Khan, KM, Meeusen, R, Orchard, JW, Pluim, BM, Raferty, M, Budgett, R, and Engebretsen, L. How much is too much? (Part 1) International Olympic Committee consensus statement on load in sport and risk of injury. *Br J Sports Med* 50:1030-1041, 2016.

84. Thornton, HR, Delaney, JA, Duthie, GM, and Dascombe, BJ. Developing athlete monitoring systems in team-sports: data analysis and visualization. *Int J Sports Physiol Perform* 14:698-705, 2019.

85. Vanrenterghem, J, Nedergaard, NJ, Robinson, MA, and Drust, B. Training load monitoring in team sports: a novel framework separating physiological and biomechanical load-adaptation pathways. *Sports Med* 47:2135-2142, 2017.

86. Verhagen, E, and Gabbett, T. Load, capacity and health: critical pieces of the holistic performance puzzle. *Br J Sports Med* 53:5-6, 2019.

87. Walls, TA, Schafer, JL, eds. *Models for Intensive Longitudinal Data*. New York: Oxford University Press, 1-288, 2006.

88. Wang, C, Vargas, JT, Stokes, T, Steele, R, and Shrier, I. Analyzing activity and injury: lessons learned from the acute:chronic workload ratio." *Sports Medicine* 50: 1243–54, 2020.

89. Ward, P, Windt, J, and Kempton, T. Business intelligence: how sport scientists can support organisation decision making in professional sport. *Int J Sports Physiol Perform* 14:544-546, 2019.

90. Weaving, D, Dalton, NE, Black, C, Darrall-Jones, J, Phibbs, PJ, Gray, M, Jones, B, and Roe, GA. The same story or a unique novel? Within-participant principal-component analysis of measures of training load in professional rugby union skills training. *Int J Sports Physiol Perform* 13:1175-1181, 2018.

91. Williams, S, Trewartha, G, Cross, MJ, Kemp, SPT, and Stokes, KA. Monitoring what matters: a systematic process for selecting training load measures. *Int J Sports Physiol Perform* 12:S2101-S2106, 2017.

92. Williams, S, West, S, Cross, MJ, and Stokes, KA. Better way to determine the acute:chronic workload ratio? *Br J Sports Med* 51:209-210, 2017.

93. Windt, J, Ardern, CL, Gabbett, TJ, Khan, KM, Cook, CE, Sporer, BC, and Zumbo, BD. Getting the most out of intensive longitudinal data: a methodological review of workload–injury studies. *BMJ Open* 8:e022626, 2018.

94. Windt, J, and Gabbett, TJ. How do training and competition workloads relate to injury? The workload—injury aetiology model. *Br J Sports Med* 51:428-435, 2016.

95. Windt, J, and Gabbett, TJ. Is it all for naught? What does mathematical coupling mean for acute:chronic workload ratios? *Br J Sports Med* 53:988-990, 2019.

96. Windt, J, Gabbett, TJ, Ferris, D, and Khan, KM. Training load-injury paradox: is greater preseason participation associated with lower in-season injury risk in elite rugby league players? *Br J Sports Med* 51:645-650, 2017.

Chapter 20

1. Agrawal, R, Imieliński, T, and Swami, A. Mining association rules between sets of items in large databases. *Sigmod Record* 22:207-216, 1993.

2. Alpaydin, E. *Introduction to Machine Learning.* Cambridge, MA: MIT Press, 14, 2009.

3. Amigó, E, Gonzalo, J, Artiles, J, and Verdejo, F. A comparison of extrinsic clustering evaluation metrics based on formal constraints. *Inf Retr* 12:461-486, 2009.

3a. Anderson, C. The end of theory: the data deluge makes the scientific method obsolete. June 23, 2008. www.wired.com/2008/06/pb-theory/. Accessed March 8, 2020.

4. Andrienko, G, Andrienko, N, Budziak, G, Dykes, J, Fuchs, G, von Landesberger, T, and Weber, H. Visual analysis of pressure in football. *Data Min Knowl Disc* 31:1793-1839, 2017.

5. Ball, KA, and Best, RJ. Different centre of pressure patterns within the golf stroke I: cluster analysis. *J Sports Sci* 25:757-770, 2007.

6. Bartlett, JD, O'Connor, F, Pitchford, N, Torres-Ronda, L, and Robertson, SJ. Relationships between internal and external training load in team-sport athletes: evidence for an individualized approach. *Int J Sports Physiol Perform* 12:230-234, 2017.

7. Bate, L, Hutchinson, A, Underhill, J, and Maskrey, N. How clinical decisions are made. *Br J Clin Pharmacol* 74:614-620, 2012.

7a. Benioff, MR, and Lazowska, ED. Computational science: ensuring America's competitiveness. 2005. http://vis.cs.brown.edu/docs/pdf/Pitac-2005-CSE.pdf. Accessed March 8, 2020.

8. Bordes, A, Chopra, S, and Weston, J. Question answering with subgraph embeddings. 2014. https://arxiv.org/abs/1406.3676. Accessed August 5, 2019.

9. Bozdogan, H. Model selection and Akaike's information criterion (AIC): the general theory and its analytical extensions. *Psychometrika* 52:345-370, 1987.

10. Brefeld, U, Lasek, J, and Mair, S. Probabilistic movement models and zones of control. *Mach Learn* 108:127-147, 2019.

11. Browne, P, Morgan, S, Bahnisch, J, and Robertson, S. Discovering patterns of play in netball with network motifs and association rules. *Int J Comput Sci Sport* 18:64-79, 2019.

12. Calder, JM, and Durbach, IN. Decision support for evaluating player performance in rugby union. *Int J Sports Sci Coach* 10:21-37, 2015.

13. Chan, TC, and Singal, R. A Markov Decision Process-based handicap system for tennis. *J Quant Anal Sports* 12:179-188, 2016.

14. Cintia, P., Rinzivillo, S., and Pappalardo, L. *Machine Learning and Data Mining for Sports Analytics Workshop.* Porto, Portugal, September, 2015.

15. Croskerry, P. The theory and practice of clinical decision-making. *Can J Anaesth* 52:R1-R8, 2005.

16. Cun, Y Le, Bengio, Y, and Hinton, G. Deep learning. *Nature* 521:436-444, 2015.

17. Cust, EE, Sweeting, AJ, Ball, K, and Robertson, S. Machine and deep learning for sport-specific movement recognition: a systematic review of model development and performance. *J Sports Sci* 37:568-600, 2019.

18. Den Hartigh, RJ, Hill, Y, and Van Geert, PL. The development of talent in sports: a dynamic network approach. *Complexity* 1-13, 2018.

19. Dhar, V, and Chou, D. A comparison of nonlinear models for financial prediction. *IEEE Trans Neural Netw* 12:907-921, 2001.

20. Dietterich, T. Overfitting and undercomputing in machine learning. *ACM Comput Serv* 27:326-327, 1995.

21. Edelmann-Nusser, J, Hohmann, A, and Henneberg, B. Modeling and prediction of competitive performance in swimming upon neural networks. *Eur J Sport Sci* 2:1-10, 2002.

22. Fogel, DB, Chellapilla, K, and Angeline, PJ. Inductive reasoning and bounded rationality reconsidered. *IEEE Trans Evol Comput* 3:142-146, 1999.

23. Fong, S, Mohammed, O, Fiaidhi, J, Mohammed, S, and Kwoh, CK. Measuring similarity by prediction class between biomedical datasets via Fuzzy unordered rule induction. *Int J Bio Sci Bio Tech* 6:159-168, 2014.

24. Gama, J. Data stream mining: the bounded rationality. *Informatica* 37:21-25, 2013.

25. Garg, AX, Adhikari, NKJ, McDonald, H, Rosas-Arellano, MP, Devereaux, PJ, Beyene, J, and Haynes, RB. Effects of computerized clinical decision support systems on practitioner performance and patient outcomes: a systematic review. *JAMA* 293:1223-1238, 2005.

26. Gigerenzer, G, and Selten, R. *Bounded Rationality: The Adaptive Toolbox.* Cambridge, MA: MIT Press, 2002.

27. Gillet, N, Berjot, S, Vallerand, RJ, Amoura, S, and Rosnet, E. Examining the motivation-performance relationship in competitive sport: a cluster-analytic approach. *Int J Sport Psychol* 43:79-102, 2012.

28. Grove, WM, Zald, DH, Lebow, BS, Snitz, BE, and Nelson, C. Clinical versus mechanical prediction: a meta-analysis. *Psychol Assess* 12:19-30, 2000.

29. Hinton, G, Deng, L, Yu, D, Dahl, G, Mohamed, AR, Jaitly, N, Senior, A, Vanhoucke, V, Nguyen, P, Kingsbury, B, and Sainath, T. Deep neural networks for acoustic modeling in speech recognition. *IEEE Signal Process Mag* 29, 2012.

30. Hoch, SJ, and Schkade, DA. A psychological approach to decision support systems. *Manag Sci* 42:51-64, 1996.

31. Jaksch, T, Ortner, R, and Auer, P. Near-optimal regret bounds for reinforcement learning. *J Mach Learn Res* 11:1563-1600, 2010.

32. James, G, Witten, D, Hastie, T, and Tibshirani, R. *An Introduction to Statistical Learning.* New York: Springer, 2013.

33. Janssen, D, Schöllhorn, WI, Newell, KM, Jäger, JM, Rost, F, and Vehof, K. Diagnosing fatigue in gait patterns by support vector machines and self-organizing maps. *Hum Mov Sci* 30:966-975, 2011.

34. Jean, S, Cho, K, Memisevic, R, and Bengio, Y. On using very large target vocabulary for neural machine translation. 2007. https://arxiv.org/abs/1412.2007. Accessed August 5, 2019.

35. Kahneman, D. Maps of bounded rationality: psychology for behavioral economics. *Am Econ Rev* 93:1449-1475, 2003.

36. Kale, A, Nguyen, F, Kay, M, and Hullman, J. Hypothetical outcome lots help untrained observers judge trends in ambiguous data. *IEEE Trans Vis Comput Graph* 25:892-902, 2018.

37. Kawamoto, K, Houlihan, CA, Balas, EA, and Lobach, DF. Improving clinical practice using clinical decision support systems: a systematic review of trials to identify features critical to success. *BMJ* 330:765-772, 2005.

38. Kay, M, Kola, T, Hullman, JR, and Munson, SA. When (ish) is my bus?: user-centered visualizations of uncertainty in everyday, mobile predictive systems. In *Proc CHI Conf Hum Factor Comput Syst* 5092-5103, 2016.

39. Kearns, MJ. A bound on the error of cross validation using the approximation and estimation rates, with consequences for the training-test split. *Adv Neural Inf Process Syst* 183-189, 1996.

40. Kringle, EA, Knutson, EC, Engstrom, C, and Terhorst, L. Iterative processes: a review of semi-supervised machine learning in rehabilitation science. *Disabil Rehabil Assist Technol* 15:515-520, 2019.

41. Krizhevsky, A, Sutskever, I, and Hinton, GE. Imagenet classification with deep convolutional neural networks. In *Adv Neural Inf Process Syst* 1097-1105, 2012.

42. Lamb, P, and Croft, H. Visualizing rugby game styles using self-organizing maps. *IEEE Comput Graph Appl* 36:11-15, 2016.

43. Larkin, JH, and Simon, HA. Why a diagram is (sometimes) worth ten thousand words. *Cogn Sci* 11:65-100, 1987.

44. Lee, BK, Lessler, J, and Stuart, EA. Improving propensity score weighting using machine learning. *Stat Med* 29:337-346, 2010.

45. Liu, M, and Liu, H. Research on application of association rule mining in Chinese athletes' nutritional and biochemical indexes monitoring. *JDCTA* 6:174-180, 2012.

46. Liu, G, and Schulte, O. Deep reinforcement learning in ice hockey for context-aware player evaluation. 2018. https://arxiv.org/abs/1805.11088. Accessed August 5, 2019.

46a. Manyika, J, Chui, M, Brown, B, Bughin, J, Dobbs, R, Roxburgh, C, and Hung Byers, A. Big data: the next frontier for innovation, competition, and productivity. www.mckinsey.com/business-functions/mckinsey-digital/our-insights/big-data-the-next-frontier-for-innovation. Accessed March 8, 2020.

47. Maymin, PZ. The automated general manager: can an algorithmic system for drafts, trades, and free agency outperform human front offices? *J Glob Sport Manag* 2:234-249, 2017.

47a. Meehl, P. Clincal versus statistical prediction: A theoretical analysis and a review of the evidence. Minneapolis, MN, US. University of Minnesota Press. 1954.

48. Memmert, D, Lemmink, KA, and Sampaio, J. Current approaches to tactical performance analyses in soccer using position data. *Sports Med* 47:1-10, 2017.

49. Mingers, J. An empirical comparison of pruning methods for decision tree induction. *Mach Learn* 4:227-243, 1989.

50. Ofoghi, B, Zeleznikow, J, MacMahon, C, and Raab, M. Data mining in elite sports: a review and a framework. *Meas Phys Educ Exerc Sci* 17:171-186, 2013.

51. Pappalardo, L, Cintia, P, Pedreschi, D, Giannotti, F, and Barabasi, AL. Human perception of performance. 2017. https://arxiv.org/abs/1712.02224. Accessed August 5, 2019.

52. Pedersen, AV, Aksdal, IM, and Stalsberg, R. Scaling demands of soccer according to anthropometric and physiological sex differences: a fairer comparison of men's and women's soccer. *Front Psychol* 10:762, 2019.

53. Powrie, JK, Bassett, EE, Rosen, T, Jørgensen, JO, Napoli, R, Sacca, L, Christiansen, JS, Bengtsson, BA, Sönksen, PH, and GH-2000 Project Study Group. Detection of growth hormone abuse in sport. *Growth Horm IGF Res* 17:220-226, 2007

54. Prakash, CD, Patvardhan, C, and Lakshmi, CV. Team selection strategy in IPL 9 using Random Forests Algorithm. *Int J Comput Appl* 139:42-48, 2016.

55. Ramasubramanian, K, and Singh, A. *Machine Learning Using R.* New Delhi, India: Apress, 2017.

56. Rein, R, and Memmert, D. Big data and tactical analysis in elite soccer: future challenges and opportunities for sports science. *Springerplus* 5:1410, 2016.

57. Robertson, S, Back, N, and Bartlett, JD. Explaining match outcome in elite Australian rules football using team performance indicators. *J Sports Sci* 34:637-644, 2016.

58. Robertson, S, Bartlett, JD, and Gastin, PB. Red, amber, or green? Athlete monitoring in team sport: the need for decision-support systems. *Int J Sports Physiol Perform* 12:S273-S279, 2017.

59. Robertson, S, Gupta, R, and McIntosh, S. A method to assess the influence of individual player performance distribution on match outcome in team sports. *J Sports Sci* 34:1893-1900, 2016.

60. Robertson, S, and Joyce, D. Bounded rationality revisited: making sense of complexity in applied sport science. 2019. https://osf.io/preprints/sportrxiv/yh38j/. Accessed November 4, 2019.

61. Robertson, S, Spencer, B, Back, N, and Farrow, D. A rule induction framework for the determination of representative learning design in skilled performance. *J Sports Sci* 37:1280-1285, 2019.

62. Sampaio, J, McGarry, T, Calleja-González, J, Sáiz, SJ, i del Alcázar, XS, and Balciunas, M. Exploring game performance in the National Basketball Association using player tracking data. *PLoS One* 10:1-14, 2015.

63. Senanayake, SA, Malik, OA, Iskandar, PM, and Zaheer, D. A knowledge-based intelligent framework for anterior cruciate ligament rehabilitation monitoring. *Appl Soft Comput* 20:127-141, 2014.

64. Simon, HA. Rational choice and the structure of the environment. *Psych Rev* 63:129-138, 1956.

65. Spencer, B, Robertson, S, and Morgan, S. Modelling within-team relative phase couplings using position derivatives in Australian rules football. *Math Comput Model Dyn Syst* 23:372-383, 2017.

66. Sprague Jr, RH. A framework for the development of decision support systems. *MIS Q* 1-26, 1980.

67. Stöckl, M, and Morgan, S. Visualization and analysis of spatial characteristics of attacks in field hockey. *Int J Perform Anal Sport* 13:160-178, 2013.

68. Sutskever, I, Vinyals, O, and Le, QV. Sequence to sequence learning with neural networks. *Adv Neural Inf Process Syst* 3104-3112, 2014.

69. Taha, Z, Musa, RM, Majeed, AP, Alim, MM, and Abdullah, MR. The identification of high potential archers based on fitness and motor ability variables: a support vector machine approach. *Hum Mov Sci* 57:184-193, 2018.

70. Thornton, HR, Delaney, JA, Duthie, GM, Scott, BR, Chivers, WJ, Sanctuary, CE, and Dascombe, BJ. Predicting self-reported illness for professional team-sport athletes. *Int J Sports Physiol Perform* 11:543-550, 2016.

71. Wagenmakers, EJ, and Farrell, S. AIC model selection using Akaike weights. *Psychon Bull Rev* 11:192-196, 2004.

72. Weigelt, M, Ahlmeyer, T, Lex, H, and Schack, T. The cognitive representation of a throwing technique in judo experts–technological ways for individual skill diagnostics in high-performance sports. *Psych Sport Exerc* 12:231-235, 2011.

72a. Wing, J. Computational thinking benefits society. 2014. http://socialissues.cs.toronto.edu/2014/01/computational-thinking/. Accessed March 8, 2020.

73. Witten, IH, Frank, E, Hall, MA, and Pal, CJ. *Data Mining: Practical Machine Learning Tools and Techniques.* Cambridge, MA: Morgan Kaufmann, 5, 2016.

74. Wundersitz, DW, Josman, C, Gupta, R, Netto, KJ, Gastin, PB, and Robertson, S. Classification of team sport activities using a single wearable tracking device. *J Biomech* 48:3975-3981, 2015.

75. Zelič, I, Kononenko, I, Lavrač, N, and Vuga, V. Induction of decision trees and Bayesian classification applied to diagnosis of sport injuries. *J Med Syst* 21:429-444, 1997.

76. Zhang, D, Gatica-Perez, D, Bengio, S, and McCowan, I. Semi-supervised adapted HMMs for unusual event detection. In *IEEE Conf Comp Soc Comput Vis and Pattern Recognit* 1:611-618, 2005.

Chapter 21

1. Attneave, F. Some informational aspects of visual perception. *Psychol Rev* 61:183-193, 1954.

2. Bosch, T. Body composition in football players. *NSCA Coach* 4:50-56, 2019.

3. Bulger, RE. The responsible conduct of research, including responsible authorship and publication practices. In *Ethics for Life Scientists*, Korthals M and Bogers RJ, eds. Dordrecht, The Netherlands: Springer, 55-62, 2004.

4. Cavanagh, P. Visual cognition. *Vision Res* 51:1538-1551, 2011.

5. Dahlstrom, MF. Using narratives and storytelling to communicate science with nonexpert audiences. *Proc Natl Acad Sci U S A* 111:13614-13620, 2014.

6. Dengel, DR, Raymond, CJ, and Bosch, TB. Assessment of muscle mass. In *Body Composition: Health and Performance in Exercise and Sport.* Lukaski, HC, ed. Boca Raton, FL: CRC Press, 27-48, 2017.

7. Few, S. Visual perception and quantitative communication. In *Show Me the Numbers: Designing Tables and Graphs to Enlighten.* Oakland, CA: Analytics Press, 92-116, 2004.

8. Freytag, G. The construction of the drama. In *Technique of the Drama.* 2nd ed. Chicago: S.C. Griggs & Company, 104-209, 1896.

9. Griethe, H, and Schumann, H. Visualizing uncertainty for improved decision making. In *Proceedings of the 4th International Conference on Business Informatics Research, Skövde, Sweden, 3-4 October 2005.* Skövde, Sweden: University of Skövde, 1-11, 2005.

10. Healey, CG, Booth, KS, and Enns, JT. Harnessing preattentive processes for multivariate data visualization. In *Proceedings of Graphics Interface '93, Toronto, Canada, 19–21 May 1993.* Mississauga, Canada: Canadian Information Processing Society, 107-117, 1993.

11. Kay, M, Kola, T, Hullman, JR, and Munson, SA. When (ish) is my bus?: User-centered visualizations of uncertainty in everyday, mobile predictive systems. In *Proceedings of the 2016 CHI Conference on Human Factors in Computing Systems, San Jose, USA, 7–12 May 2016.* San Jose, CA: ACM, 5092-5103, 2016.

12. Kress, G, and Van Leeuwen, T. Colour as a semiotic mode: notes for a grammar of colour. *Vis Commun* 1:343-368, 2002.

13. Krzywinski, M, and Cairo, A. Storytelling. *Nat Methods* 10:687, 2013.

14. Lee, B, Riche, NH, Isenberg, P, and Carpendale, S. More than telling a story: transforming data into visually shared stories. *IEEE Comput Graph Appl* 35:84-90, 2015.

15. Padilla, LM, Creem-Regehr, SH, Hegarty, M, and Stefanucci, JK. Decision making with visualizations: a cognitive framework across disciplines. *Cogn Res Princ Implic* 3:29, 2018.

16. Perin, C, Vuillemot, R, Stolper, CD, Stasko, JT, Wood, J, and Carpendale, S. State of the art of sports data visualization. *Comput Graph Forum* 37:663-686, 2018.

17. Riveiro, M. Evaluation of uncertainty visualization techniques for information fusion. In *Proceedings of the 10th International Conference on Information Fusion, Québec, Canada, 9-12 July 2007.* Washington, DC: IEEE Computer Society, 1-8, 2007.

18. Riveiro, M, Helldin, T, Falkman, G, and Lebram, M. Effects of visualizing uncertainty on decision-making in a target identification scenario. *Comput Graph* 41:84-98, 2014.

19. Rosling, H, Rosling, O, and Rosling Rönnlund, A. The single perspective instinct. In *Factfulness.* London, UK: Sceptre, 185-203, 2018.

20. Skeels, M, Lee, B, Smith, G, and Robertson, GG. Revealing uncertainty for information visualization. *Inf Vis* 9:70-81, 2010.

21. Story, MF. The principles of universal design. In *Universal Design Handbook.* 2nd ed. Preiser, WFE and Smith, KH, eds. New York: McGraw-Hill, 4.3-4.12, 2011.

22. Story, MF, Mueller, JL, and Mace, RL. *The Universal Design File: Designing for People of All Ages and Abilities.* Raleigh, NC: North Carolina State University, 2-4, 1998.

23. Wagemans, J, Elder, JH, Kubovy, M, Palmer, SE, Peterson, MA, Singh M, and von der Heydt, R. A century of Gestalt psychology in visual perception: I. Perceptual grouping and figure-ground organization. *Psychol Bull* 138:1172-1217, 2012.

Chapter 22

1. Bompa, T, and Haff, GG. *Periodization: Theory and Methodology of Training.* 5th ed. Champaign, IL: Human Kinetics, 2009.

2. Brewer, C. Strength and conditioning in the elite sports environment. In *Routledge Handbook of Elite Sport Performance.* Collins, D, Cruickshank, A, and Jordet, G, eds. Milton Park, Abington, UK: Routledge, 85-98, 2019.

3. Cissik, J, Hedrick, A, and Barnes, M. Challenges applying the research on periodization. *Strength Cond J* 30:45-51, 2008.

4. Ham, DJ, Knez, WL, and Young, WB. A deterministic model of the vertical jump: implications for training. *J Strength Cond Res* 21:967-972, 2007.

5. Joyner, MJ, and Coyle, EF. Endurance exercise performance: the physiology of champions. *J Physiol* 586:35-44, 2008.

6. Oliver, GD, and Keeley, DW. Gluteal muscle group activation and its relationship with pelvis and torso kinematics in high school baseball pitchers. *J Strength Cond Res* 24:3015-3022, 2010.

7. Stone, MH, Stone, ME, and Sands, WA. *Principles and Practice of Resistance Training.* Champaign, IL: Human Kinetics, 2007.

8. Strudwick, T. Reshaping the future of sports science in football. *Football Medic and Scientist* 19:12-18, 2017.

Chapter 23

1. Argus, CK, Driller, MW, Ebert, TR, Martin, DT, and Halson, S. The effects of four different recovery strategies on repeat sprint cycling performance. *Int J Sports Physiol Perform* 8:542-548, 2013.

1a. Baird, MF, Graham, SM, Baker, JS, and Bickerstaff, GF. Creatine-kinase- and exercise-related muscle damage implications for muscle performance and recovery. *J Nutr Metab* 960363, 2012.

2. Banfi, G, Lombardi, G, Colombini, A, and Melegati, G. Whole-body cryotherapy in athletes. *Sports Med* 40:509-517, 2010.

3. Barnett, A. Using recovery modalities between training sessions in elite athletes. *Sports Med* 36:781-796, 2006.

4. Beaven, CM, Cook, C, Gray, D, Downes, P, Murphy, I, Drawer, S, Ingram, JR, Kilduff, LP, and Gill, N. Electrostimulation's

enhancement of recovery during a rugby preseason. *Int J Sports Physiol Perform* 8:92-98, 2013.

5. Behm, D. The effects and potential mechanisms of foam rolling on athletic performance. Presented at European Congress of Sport Science, MetropolisRhur, Germany, 7/7/17, 2017.

6. Bleakley, CM, Bieuzen, F, Davison, GW, and Costello, JT. Whole-body cryotherapy: empirical evidence and theoretical perspectives. *Open Access J Sports Med* 5:25-36, 2014.

6a. Bonnar, D, Bartel, K, Kakoschke, N and Lang, C. Sleep interventions designed to improve athletic performance and recovery: A systematic review of current approaches. *Sports medicine, 48*(3): 683-703, 2018.

7. Broatch, JR, Bishop, DJ, and Halson, S. Lower limb sports compression garments improve muscle blood flow and exercise performance during repeated-sprint cycling. *Int J Sports Physiol Perform* 13:882-890, 2018.

8. Brophy-Williams, N, Driller, MW, Kitic, CM, Fell, JW, and Halson, SL. Effect of compression socks worn between repeated maximal running bouts. *Int J Sports Physiol Perform* 12:621-627, 2017.

9. Brophy-Williams, N, Driller, MW, Shing, CM, Fell, JW, and Halson, SL. Confounding compression: the effects of posture, sizing and garment type on measured interface pressure in sports compression clothing. *J Sports Sci* 33:1403-1410, 2015.

10. Brown, F, Gissane, C, Howatson, G, van Someren, K, Pedlar, C, and Hill, J. Compression garments and recovery from exercise: a meta-analysis. *Sports Med* 47:2245-2267, 2017.

11. Caia, J, Kelly, VG, and Halson, SL. The role of sleep in maximising performance in elite athletes. In *Sport, Recovery and Performance*. Kellman, M and Beckman, J, eds. Abington, UK: Routledge, 151-167, 2017.

12. Costello, JT, Baker, PR, Minett, GM, Bieuzen, F, Stewart, IB, and Bleakley, C. Whole-body cryotherapy (extreme cold air exposure) for preventing and treating muscle soreness after exercise in adults. *Cochrane Database Syst Rev* 9:CD010789, 2015.

13. Ferguson, RA, Dodd, MJ, and Paley, VR. Neuromuscular electrical stimulation via the peroneal nerve is superior to graduated compression socks in reducing perceived muscle soreness following intense intermittent endurance exercise. *Eur J Appl Physiol* 114:2223-2232, 2014.

14. Halson, S. Does the time frame between exercise influence the effectiveness of hydrotherapy for recovery? *Int J Sports Physiol Perform* 6:147-159, 2011.

15. Halson, SL. Sleep in elite athletes and nutritional interventions to enhance sleep. *Sports Med* 44(suppl 1):S13-S23, 2014.

16. Heapy, AM, Hoffman, MD, Verhagen, HH, Thompson, SW, Dhamija, P, Sandford, FJ, and Cooper, MC. A randomized controlled trial of manual therapy and pneumatic compression for recovery from prolonged running - an extended study. *Res Sports Med* 26:354-364, 2018.

17. Hill, J, Howatson, G, van Someren, K, Leeder, J, and Pedlar, C. Compression garments and recovery from exercise-induced muscle damage: a meta-analysis. *Br J Sports Med* 48:1340-1346, 2014.

18. Ihsan, M, Watson, G, and Abbiss, CR. What are the physiological mechanisms for post-exercise cold water immersion in the recovery from prolonged endurance and intermittent exercise? *Sports Med* 46:1095-1109, 2016.

19. Institut National du Sport, Hausswirth, C, and Mujika, I. *Recovery for Performance in Sport*. Champaign, IL: Human Kinetics, 2013.

20. Juliff, LE, Halson, SL, and Peiffer, JJ. Understanding sleep disturbance in athletes prior to important competitions. *J Sci Med Sport* 18:13-18, 2015.

21. Killer, SC, Svendsen, IS, Jeukendrup, AE, and Gleeson, M. Evidence of disturbed sleep and mood state in well-trained athletes during short-term intensified training with and without a high carbohydrate nutritional intervention. *J Sports Sci* 35:1402-1410, 2017.

22. Kosar, AC, Candow, DG, and Putland, JT. Potential beneficial effects of whole-body vibration for muscle recovery after exercise. *J Strength Cond Res* 26:2907-2911, 2012.

23. Kraemer, WJ, Hooper, DR, Kupchak, BR, Saenz, C, Brown, LE, Vingren, JL, Luk, HY, DuPont, WH, Szivak, TK, Flanagan, SD, Caldwell, LK, Eklund, D, Lee, EC, Hakkinen, K, Volek, JS, Fleck, SJ, and Maresh, CM. The effects of a roundtrip trans-American jet travel on physiological stress, neuromuscular performance, and recovery. *J Appl Physiol (1985)* 121:438-448, 2016.

24. Lastella, M, Roach, GD, Halson, SL, Martin, DT, West, NP, and Sargent, C. The impact of a simulated grand tour on sleep, mood, and well-being of competitive cyclists. *J Sports Med Phys Fitness* 55:1555-1564, 2015.

25. Lastella, M, Roach, GD, Halson, SL, and Sargent, C. Sleep/wake behaviours of elite athletes from individual and team sports. *Eur J Sport Sci* 15:94-100, 2015.

26. Leeder, J, Glaister, M, Pizzoferro, K, Dawson, J, and Pedlar, C. Sleep duration and quality in elite athletes measured using wristwatch actigraphy. *J Sports Sci* 30:541-545, 2012.

26a. Leeder, J, Godfrey, M, Gibbon, D, Gaze, D, Davison, GW, Van Someren, KA, and Howatson, G. Cold water immersion improves recovery of sprint speed following a simulated tournament. *Eur J Sport Sci* 19:1166-1174, 2019.

27. Machado, AF, Almeida, AC, Micheletti, JK, Vanderlei, FM, Tribst, MF, Netto Junior, J, and Pastre, CM. Dosages of cold-water immersion post exercise on functional and clinical responses: a randomized controlled trial. *Scand J Med Sci Sports* 27:1356-1363, 2017.

28. Mujika, I, Halson, S, Burke, LM, Balague, G, and Farrow, D. An integrated, multifactorial approach to periodization for optimal performance in individual and team sports. *Int J Sports Physiol Perform* 13:538-561, 2018.

29. Overmayer, RG, and Driller, MW. Pneumatic compression fails to improve performance recovery in trained cyclists. *Int J Sports Physiol Perform* 13:490-495, 2018.

30. Pinar, S, Kaya, F, Bicer, B, Erzeybek, MS, and Cotuk, HB. Different recovery methods and muscle performance after exhausting exercise: comparison of the effects of electrical muscle stimulation and massage. *Biol Sport* 29:269-275, 2012.

31. Poppendieck, W, Wegmann, M, Ferrauti, A, Kellmann, M, Peiffer, M, and Meyer, T. Massage and performance recovery: a meta-analytical review. *Sports Med* 46:183-205, 2016.

32. Pournot, H, Tindel, J, Testa, R, Mathevon, L, and Lapole, T. The acute effects of local vibration as a recovery modality from exercise-induced increased muscle stiffness. *J Sci Med Sport* 15:142-147, 2016.

33. Rabita, G, and Delextrat, A. Stretching. In *Recovery for Performance in Sport*. Hausswirth, C and Mujika, I, eds. Champaign, IL: Human Kinetics, 55-70, 2013.

34. Roberts, LA, Raastad, T, Markworth, JF, Figueiredo, VC, Egner, IM, Shield, A, Cameron-Smith, D, Coombes, JS, and Peake, JM. Post-exercise cold water immersion attenuates acute anabolic signalling and long-term adaptations in muscle to strength training. *J Physiol* 593:4285-4301, 2015.

34a. Russell, S, Jenkins, D, Smith, M, Halson, S and Kelly, V. The application of mental fatigue research to elite team sport performance: New perspectives. *Journal of science and medicine in sport*, 22(6):723-728, 2019.

35. Sands, WA, McNeal, JR, Murray, SR, Ramsey, MW, Sato, K, Mizuguchi, S, and Stone, MH. Stretching and its effects on recovery. *Strength Cond J* 35:30-36, 2013.

36. Sargent, C, Halson, S, and Roach, GD. Sleep or swim? Early-morning training severely restricts the amount of sleep obtained by elite swimmers. *Eur J Sport Sci* 14(suppl 1):S310-S315, 2014.

37. Sargent, C, and Roach, GD. Sleep duration is reduced in elite athletes following night-time competition. *Chronobiol Int* 33:667-670, 2016.

38. Stephens, JM, Halson, S, Miller, J, Slater, GJ, and Askew, CD. Cold-water immersion for athletic recovery: one size does not fit all. *Int J Sports Physiol Perform* 12:2-9, 2017.

39. Stephens, JM, Sharpe, K, Gore, C, Miller, J, Slater, GJ, Versey, N, Peiffer, J, Duffield, R, Minett, GM, Crampton, D, Dunne, A, Askew, CD, and Halson, SL. Core temperature responses to cold-water immersion recovery: a pooled-data analysis. *Int J Sports Physiol Perform* 13:917-925, 2018.

40. Vaile, J, Halson, S, and Graham, S. Recovery review - science vs practice. *J Aust Strength Cond* 2(suppl 2):5-21, 2010.

40a. Vaile, J, Halson, S, Gill, N, and Dawson, B. Effect of hydrotherapy on the signs and symptoms of delayed onset muscle soreness. *European journal of applied physiology* 102:447-455, 2008.

41. Van Hooren, B, and Peake, JM. Do we need a cool-down after exercise? A narrative review of the psychophysiological effects and the effects on performance, injuries and the long-term adaptive response. *Sports Med* 48:1575-1595, 2018.

42. Versey, N, Halson, S, and Dawson, B. Effect of contrast water therapy duration on recovery of cycling performance: a dose-response study. *Eur J Appl Physiol* 111:37-46, 2011.

43. Versey, N, Halson, S, and Dawson, B. Effect of contrast water therapy duration on recovery of running performance. *Int J Sports Physiol Perform* 7:130-140, 2012.

44. Versey, NG, Halson, SL, and Dawson, BT. Water immersion recovery for athletes: effect on exercise performance and practical recommendations. *Sports Med* 43:1101-1130, 2013.

45. Webb, NP. The use of post game recovery modalities following team contact sport: a review. *J Aust Strength Cond* 21:70-79, 2013.

46. Wiewelhove, T, Doweling, A, Schneider, C, Hottenrott, L, Meyer, T, Kellmann, M, Pfeiffer, M, and Ferrauti, A. A meta-analysis of the effects of foam rolling on performance and recovery. *Front Physiol* 10:376, 2019.

47. Winke, M, and Williamson, S. Comparison of a pnumatic compression device to a compression garment during recovery from DOMS. *Int J Exerc Sci* 11:375-383, 2018.

Chapter 24

1. Ackerman, KE, Cano Sokoloff, N, De Nardo Maffazioli, G, Clarke, HM, Lee, H, and Misra, M. Fractures in relation to menstrual status and bone parameters in young athletes. *Med Sci Sports Exerc* 47:1577-1586, 2015.

2. Adams, JD, Capitan-Jimenez, C, Huggins, RA, Casa, DJ, Mauromoustakos, A, and Kavouras, SA. Urine reagent strips are inaccurate for assessing hypohydration: a brief report. *Clin J Sport Med* 29:506-508, 2019.

3. American College of Sports Medicine, Sawka, MN, Burke, LM, Eichner, ER, Maughan, RJ, Montain, SJ, and Stachenfeld, NS. American College of Sports Medicine position stand. Exercise and fluid replacement. *Med Sci Sports Exerc* 39:377-390, 2007.

4. Belval, LN, Hosokawa, Y, Casa, DJ, Adams, WM, Armstrong, LE, Baker, LB, Burke, L, Cheuvront, S, Chiampas, G, Gonzalez-Alonso, J, Huggins, RA, Kavouras, SA, Lee, EC, McDermott, BP, Miller, K, Schlader, Z, Sims, S, Stearns, RL, Troyanos, C, and Wingo, J. Practical hydration solutions for sports. *Nutrients* 11:1550, 2019.

5. Bennell, KL, Malcolm, SA, Thomas, SA, Ebeling, PR, McCrory, PR, Wark, JD, and Brukner, PD. Risk factors for stress fractures in female track-and-field athletes: a retrospective analysis. *Clin J Sports Med* 5:229-235, 1995.

6. Burke, LM. Re-examining high-fat diets for sports performance: did we call the "nail in the coffin" too soon? *Sports Med* 45(suppl 1):S33-S49, 2015.

7. Burke, LM, and Hawley, JA. Swifter, higher, stronger: what's on the menu? *Science* 362:781-787, 2018.

8. Burke, LM, Hawley, JA, Jeukendrup, A, Morton, JP, Stellingwerff, T, and Maughan, RJ. Toward a common understanding of diet-exercise strategies to manipulate fuel availability for training and competition preparation in endurance sport. *Int J Sport Nutr Exerc Metab* 28:451-463, 2018.

9. Burke, LM, Lundy, B, Fahrenholtz, IL, and Melin, AK. Pitfalls of conducting and interpreting estimates of energy availability in free-living athletes. *Int J Sport Nutr Exerc Metab* 28:350-363, 2018.

10. Burke, LM, and Maughan, RJ. The Governor has a sweet tooth - mouth sensing of nutrients to enhance sports performance. *Eur J Sport Sci* 15:29-40, 2015.

11. Burke, LM, Ross, ML, Garvican-Lewis, LA, Welvaert, M, Heikura, IA, Forbes, SG, Mirtschin, JG, Cato, LE, Strobel, N, Sharma, AP, and Hawley, JA. Low carbohydrate, high fat diet impairs exercise economy and negates the performance benefit from intensified training in elite race walkers. *J Physiol* 595:2785-2807, 2017.

12. Carr, AJ, Hopkins, WG, and Gore, CJ. Effects of acute alkalosis and acidosis on performance: a meta-analysis. *Sports Med* 41:801-814, 2011.

13. Casa, DJ, Cheuvront, SN, Galloway, SD, and Shirreffs, SM. Fluid needs for training, competition, and recovery in track-and-field athletes. *Int J Sport Nutr Exerc Metab* 29:175-180, 2019.

14. Chambers, ES, Bridge, MW, and Jones, DA. Carbohydrate sensing in the human mouth: effects on exercise performance and brain activity. *J Physiol* 587:1779-1794, 2009.

15. Cheuvront, SN, and Kenefick, RW. Dehydration: physiology, assessment, and performance effects. *Compr Physiol* 4:257-285, 2014.

16. Costa, RJS, Miall, A, Khoo, A, Rauch, C, Snipe, R, Camoes-Costa, V, and Gibson, P. Gut-training: the impact of two weeks repetitive gut-challenge during exercise on gastrointestinal status, glucose availability, fuel kinetics, and running performance. *Appl Physiol Nutr Metab* 42:547-557, 2017.

17. Coyle, EF, Coggan, AR, Hemmert, MK, and Ivy, JL. Muscle glycogen utilisation during prolonged strenuous exercise when fed carbohydrate. *J Appl Physiol* 61:165-172, 1986.

18. Deakin, V. Iron depletion in athletes. In *Clinical Sports Nutrition*. Burke, L and Deakin, V, eds. Sydney: McGraw-Hill, 263-312, 2006.

19. Geyer, H, Parr, MK, Reinhart, U, Schrader, Y, Mareck, U, and Schanzer, W. Analysis of non-hormonal nutritional supplements for anabolic-androgenic steroids - results of an international study. *Int J Sports Med* 25:124-129, 2004.

20. Goulet, EDB. Comment on drinking strategies: planned drinking versus drinking to thirst. *Sports Med* 49:631-633, 2018.

21. Havemann, L, West, S, Goedecke, JH, McDonald, IA, St-Clair Gibson, A, Noakes, TD, and Lambert, EV. Fat adaptation followed by carbohydrate-loading compromises high-intensity sprint performance. *J Appl Physiol* 100:194-202, 2006.

22. Hawley, JA, Schabort, EJ, Noakes, TD, and Dennis, SC. Carbohydrate-loading and exercise performance: an update. *Sports Med* 24:73-81, 1997.

23. Hew-Butler, T, Loi, V, Pani, A, and Rosner, MH. Exercise-associated hyponatremia: 2017 update. *Front Med* 4:21, 2017.

24. Impey, SG, Hearris, MA, Hammond, KM, Bartlett, JD, Louis, J, Close, GL, and Morton, JP. Fuel for the work required: a theoretical framework for carbohydrate periodization and the glycogen threshold hypothesis. *Sports Med* 48:1031-1048, 2018.

25. Jeukendrup, AE. Training the gut for athletes. *Sports Med* 47:101-110, 2017.

26. Kenefick, RW. Drinking strategies: planned drinking versus drinking to thirst. *Sports Med* 48:31-37, 2018.

27. Kenefick, RW. Author's reply to Goulet: Comment on drinking strategies: planned drinking versus drinking to thirst. *Sports Med* 49:635-636, 2019.

28. Kerr, D, Khan, K, and Bennell, K. Bone, exercise, and nutrition In *Clinical Sports Nutrition.* 5th ed. Burke, L and Deakin, V, eds. Sydney: McGraw-Hill, 234-265, 2015.

29. Koehler, K, Hoerner, NR, Gibbs, JC, Zinner, C, Braun, H, De Souza, MJ, and Schaenzer, W. Low energy availability in exercising men is associated with reduced leptin and insulin but not with changes in other metabolic hormones. *J Sports Sci* 34:1921-1929, 2016.

30. Kreider, RB, Kalman, DS, Antonio, J, Ziegenfuss, TN, Wildman, R, Collins, R, Candow, DG, Kleiner, SM, Almada, AL, and Lopez, HL. International Society of Sports Nutrition position stand: safety and efficacy of creatine supplementation in exercise, sport, and medicine. *J Int Soc Sports Nutr* 14:18, 2017.

31. Larson-Meyer, DE, and Willis, KS. Vitamin D and athletes. *Curr Sports Med Rep* 9:220-226, 2010.

32. Larson-Meyer, DE, Woolf, K, and Burke, L. Assessment of nutrient status in athletes and the need for supplementation. *Int J Sport Nutr Exerc Metab* 28:139-158, 2018.

33. Lieberman, JL, De Souza, MJ, Wagstaff, DA, and Williams, NI. Menstrual disruption with exercise is not linked to an energy availability threshold. *Med Sci Sports Exerc* 50:551-561, 2018.

34. Logan-Sprenger, HM, Palmer, MS, and Spriet, LL. Estimated fluid and sodium balance and drink preferences in elite male junior players during an ice hockey game. *Appl Physiol Nutr Metab* 36:145-152, 2011.

35. Loucks, AB, *Energy Balance and Energy Availability.* In Maughan, R.J. (ed). *Encyclopedia of Sports Medicine: Sports Nutrition,* London: John Wiley & Sons, 72-87, 2014.

36. Loucks, AB, Kiens, B, and Wright, HH. Energy availability in athletes. *J Sports Sci* 29(suppl 1):S7-S15, 2011.

37. Marquet, LA, Brisswalter, J, Louis, J, Tiollier, E, Burke, LM, Hawley, JA, and Hausswirth, C. Enhanced endurance performance by periodization of carbohydrate intake: "Sleep Low" strategy. *Med Sci Sports Exerc* 48:663-672, 2016.

38. Maughan, RJ, Burke, LM, Dvorak, J, Larson-Meyer, DE, Peeling, P, Phillips, SM, Rawson, ES, Walsh, NP, Garthe, I, Geyer, H, Meeusen, R, van Loon, LJC, Shirreffs, SM, Spriet, LL, Stuart, M, Vernec, A, Currell, K, Ali, VM, Budgett, RG, Ljungqvist, A, Mountjoy, M, Pitsiladis, YP, Soligard, T, Erdener, U, and Engebretsen, L. IOC consensus statement: dietary supplements and the high-performance athlete. *Br J Sports Med* 52:439-455, 2018.

39. Maughan, RJ, and Gleeson, M. *The Biochemical Basis of Sports Performance.* London: Oxford University Press, 2010.

40. McDermott, BP, Anderson, SA, Armstrong, LE, Casa, DJ, Cheuvront, SN, Cooper, L, Kenney, WL, O'Connor, FG, and Roberts, WO. National Athletic Trainers' Association position statement: fluid replacement for the physically active. *J Athl Train* 52:877-895, 2017.

41. Melin, AK, Heikura, IA, Tenforde, A, and Mountjoy, M. Energy availability in athletics: health, performance, and physique. *Int J Sport Nutr Exerc Metab* 29:152-164, 2019.

42. Mountjoy, M, Sundgot-Borgen, J, Burke, L, Ackerman, KE, Blauwet, C, Constantini, M, Lebrun, C, Lundy, B, Melin, A, Meyer, N, Sherman, R, Tenforde, AS, Torstveit, MK, and Budgett, R. International Olympic Committee (IOC) consensus statement on relative energy deficiency in sport (RED-S): 2018 update. *Int J Sport Nutr Exerc Metab* 28:316-331, 2018.

43. Nattiv, A, Loucks, AB, Manore, MM, Sanborn, CF, Sundgot-Borgen, J, and Warren, MP. American College of Sports Medicine position stand. The female athlete triad. *Med Sci Sports Exerc* 39:1867-1882, 2007.

43a. Otten, JJ, Hellwig, JP, and Meyers, LD, eds. *Dietary Reference Intakes: The Essential Guide to Nutrient Requirements.* Washington, DC: National Academies Press, 2006.

44. Owens, DJ, Allison, R, and Close, GL. Vitamin D and the athlete: current perspectives and new challenges. *Sports Med* 48:3-16, 2018.

45. Phinney, SD, Bistrian, BR, Evans, WJ, Gervino, E, and Blackburn, GL. The human metabolic response to chronic ketosis without caloric restriction: preservation of submaximal exercise capability with reduced carbohydrate oxidation. *Metabolism* 32:769-776, 1983.

46. Savoie, FA, Kenefick, RW, Ely, BR, Cheuvront, SN, and Goulet, ED. Effect of hypohydration on muscle endurance, strength, anaerobic power and capacity and vertical jumping ability: a meta-analysis. *Sports Med* 45:1207-1227, 2015.

47. Sim, M, Garvican-Lewis, LA, Cox, GR, Govus, A, McKay, AKA, Stellingwerff, T, and Peeling, P. Iron considerations for the athlete: a narrative review. *Eur J Appl Physiol* 119:1463-1478, 2019.

48. Spriet, LL. New insights into the interaction of carbohydrate and fat metabolism during exercise. *Sports Med* 44(suppl 1):87-96, 2014.

49. Stellingwerff, T, and Cox, GR. Systematic review: carbohydrate supplementation on exercise performance or capacity of varying durations. *Appl Physiol Nutr Metab* 39:998-1011, 2014.

50. Stellingwerff, T, Spriet, LL, Watt, MJ, Kimber, NE, Hargreaves, M, Hawley, JA, and Burke, LM. Decreased PDH activation and glycogenolysis during exercise following fat adaptation with carbohydrate restoration. *Am J Physiol Endocrinol Metab* 290:E380-E388, 2006.

51. Tenforde, AS, Barrack, MT, Nattiv, A, and Fredericson, M. Parallels with the female athlete triad in male athletes. *Sports Med* 46:171-182, 2016.

52. Thomas, DT, Erdman, KA, and Burke, LM. American College of Sports Medicine joint position statement. Nutrition and athletic performance. *Med Sci Sports Exerc* 48:543-568, 2016.

53. Trexler, ET, Smith-Ryan, AE, Stout, JR, Hoffman, JR, Wilborn, CD, Sale, C, Kreider, RB, Jager, R, Earnest, CP, Bannock, L, Campbell, B, Kalman, D, Ziegenfuss, TN, and Antonio, J. International Society of Sports Nutrition position stand: beta-alanine. *J Int Soc Sports Nutr* 12:30, 2015.

54. United States Anti-Doping Agency. Supplement 411. www.usada.org/athletes/substances/supplement-411/. Accessed August 27, 2020.

55. Vanheest, JL, Rodgers, CD, Mahoney, CE, and De Souza, MJ. Ovarian suppression impairs sport performance in junior elite female swimmers. *Med Sci Sports Exerc* 46:156-166, 2014.

56. Volek, JS, Noakes, T, and Phinney, SD. Rethinking fat as a fuel for endurance exercise. *Eur J Sport Sci* 15:13-20, 2015.

57. Walsh, NP. Nutrition and athlete immune health: new perspectives on an old paradigm. *Sports Med* 49(suppl 2):153-168, 2019.

58. Walsh, NP, Gleeson, M, Pyne, DB, Nieman, DC, Dhabhar, FS, Shephard, RJ, Oliver, SJ, Bermon, S, and Kajeniene, A. Position statement. Part two: Maintaining immune health. *Exerc Immunol Rev* 17:64-103, 2011.

59. Webster, CC, Swart, J, Noakes, TD, and Smith, JA. A carbohydrate ingestion intervention in an elite athlete who follows a LCHF diet. *Int J Sports Physiol Perform* 13:957-960, 2018.

60. Windsor, R. July 15, 2016. "This is what it took to fuel Chris Froome and Team Sky through the Tour de France." Cycling Weekly, Accessed August 27, 2020. www.cyclingweekly.com/news/racing/tour-de-france/took-fuel-chris-froome-team-sky-tour-de-france-265684.

61. Witard, OC, Garthe, I, and Phillips, SM. Dietary protein for training adaptation and body composition manipulation in track and field athletes. *Int J Sport Nutr Exerc Metab* 29:165-174, 2019.

62. Wittbrodt, MT, and Millard-Stafford, M. Dehydration impairs cognitive performance: a meta-analysis. *Med Sci Sports Exerc* 50:2360-2368, 2018.

Chapter 25

1. Adams, WM, Hosokawa, Y, and Casa, DJ. Body-cooling paradigm in sport: maximizing safety and performance during competition. *J Sport Rehabil* 25:382-394, 2016.

2. Adams, JD, Kavouras, SA, Robillard, JI, Bardis, CN, Johnson, EC, Ganio, MS, McDermott BP, and White MA. Fluid balance of adolescent swimmers during training. *J Strength Cond Res* 30:621-625, 2016.

3. Alhadad, SB, Tan, PMS, and Lee, JKW. Efficacy of heat mitigation strategies on core temperature and endurance exercise: a meta-analysis. *Front Physiol* 10:71, 2019.

4. Al Haddad, H, Laursen, PB, Chollet, D, Lemaitre, F, Ahmaidi, S, and Buchheit, M. Effect of cold or thermoneutral water immersion on post-exercise heart rate recovery and heart rate variability indices. *Auton Neurosci* 156:111-116, 2010.

5. Armstrong, LE. *Exertional Heat Illnesses*. Champaign, IL: Human Kinetics, 2003.

6. Armstrong, LE. Hydration assessment techniques. *Nutr Rev* 63:S40-S54, 2005.

7. Armstrong, LE. Assessing hydration status: the elusive gold standard. *J Am Coll Nutr* 26:575S-584S, 2007.

8. Armstrong, LE, and Casa, DJ. Methods to evaluate electrolyte and water turnover of athletes. *Athl Train Sports Health Care* 1:169-179, 2009.

9. Armstrong, LE, and Maresh, CM. The induction and decay of heat acclimatisation in trained athletes. *Sports Med* 12:302-312, 1991.

10. Armstrong, LE, Maresh, CM, Castellani, JW, Bergeron, MF, Kenefick, RW, LaGasse, KE, and Riebe, D. Urinary indices of hydration status. *Int J Sport Nutr* 4:265-279, 1994.

11. Armstrong, LE, Millard-Stafford, M, Moran, DS, Pyne, SW, and Roberts, WO. American College of Sports Medicine position stand. Exertional heat illness during training and competition. *Med Sci Sports Exerc* 39:556-572, 2007.

12. Arnaoutis, G, Kavouras, SA, Kotsis, YP, Tsekouras, YE, Makrillos, M, and Bardis, CN. Ad libitum fluid intake does not prevent dehydration in suboptimally hydrated young soccer players during a training session of a summer camp. *Int J Sport Nutr Exerc Metab* 23:245-251, 2013.

13. Baker, LB, Dougherty, KA, Chow, M, and Kenney, WL. Progressive dehydration causes a progressive decline in basketball skill performance. *Med Sci Sports Exerc* 39:1114-1123, 2007.

14. Baker, LB, Stofan, JR, Hamilton, AA, and Horswill, CA. Comparison of regional patch collection vs. whole body washdown for measuring sweat sodium and potassium loss during exercise. *J Appl Physiol* 107:887-895, 2009.

15. Baker, LB, Stofan, JR, Lukaski, HC, and Horswill, CA. Exercise-induced trace mineral element concentration in regional versus whole-body wash-down sweat. *Int J Sport Nutr Exerc Metab* 21:233-239, 2011.

16. Bardis, CN, Kavouras, SA, Arnaoutis, G, Panagiotakos, DB, and Sidossis, LS. Mild dehydration and cycling performance during 5-kilometer hill climbing. *J Athl Train* 48:741-747, 2013.

17. Benjamin, CL, Sekiguchi, Y, Fry, LA, and Casa, DJ. Performance changes following heat acclimation and the factors that influence these changes: meta-analysis and meta-regression. *Front Physiol* 10:1448, 2019.

18. Binkley, HM, Beckett, J, Casa, DJ, Kleiner, DM, and Plummer, PE. National Athletic Trainers' Association position statement: exertional heat illnesses. *J Athl Train* 37:329-343, 2002.

19. Bolster, DR, Trappe, SW, Short, KR, Scheffield-Moore, M, Parcell, AC, Schulze, KM, and Costill DL. l. Effects of precooling on thermoregulation during subsequent exercise. *Med Sci Sports Exerc* 31:251-257, 1999.

20. Bongers, CCWG, Hopman, MTE, and Eijsvogels, TMH. Cooling interventions for athletes: an overview of effectiveness, physiological mechanisms, and practical considerations. *Temperature (Austin)* 4:60-78, 2017.

21. Bottin, JH, Lemetais, G, Poupin, M, Jimenez, L, and Perrier, ET. Equivalence of afternoon spot and 24-h urinary hydration biomarkers in free-living healthy adults. *Eur J Clin Nutr* 70:904-907, 2016.

22. Breen, E, Tang, K, Olfert, M, Knapp, A, and Wagner, P. Skeletal muscle capillarity during hypoxia: VEGF and its activation. *High Alt Med Biol* 9:158-166, 2008.

23. Buchheit, M, Racinais, S, Bilsborough, J, Hocking, J, Mendez-Villanueva, A, Bourdon, PC, Voss, S, Livingston, S, Christian, R, Périard, J, Cordy, J, and Coutts, AJ. Adding heat to the live-high train-low altitude model: a practical insight from professional football. *Br J Sports Med* 47(suppl 1):i59-i69, 2013.

24. Budd, GM. Wet-bulb globe temperature (WBGT)—its history and its limitations. *J Sci Med Sport* 11:20-32, 2008.

25. Casa, DJ, Becker, SM, Ganio, MS, Brown, CM, Yeargin, SW, Roti, MW, Siegler, J, Blowers, JA, Glaviano, NR, Huggins, RA, Armstrong, LE, and Maresh, CM. Validity of devices that assess body temperature during outdoor exercise in the heat. *J Athl Train* 42:333-342, 2007.

26. Casadio, JR, Kilding, AE, Cotter, JD, and Laursen, PB. From lab to real world: heat acclimation considerations for elite athletes. *Sports Med* 47:1467-1476, 2017.

27. Cheuvront, SN, Carter, R, Montain, SJ, and Sawka, MN. Daily body mass variability and stability in active men undergoing exercise-heat stress. *Int J Sport Nutr Exerc Metab* 14:532-540, 2004.

28. Cheuvront, SN, and Haymes, EM. Thermoregulation and marathon running: biological and environmental influences. *Sports Med* 31:743-762, 2001.

29. Cheuvront, SN, and Kenefick, RW. Am I drinking enough? Yes, no, and maybe. *J Am Coll Nutr* 35:185-192, 2016.

30. Daanen, HAM, Jonkman, AG, Layden, JD, Linnane, DM, and Weller, AS. Optimising the acquisition and retention of heat acclimation. *Int J Sports Med* 32:822-828, 2011.

31. Daanen, HAM, Racinais, S, and Périard, JD. Heat acclimation decay and re-induction: a systematic review and meta-analysis. *Sports Med* 48:409-430, 2018.

32. Dixon, PG, Kraemer, WJ, Volek, JS, Howard, RL, Gomez, AL, Comstock, BA, Dunn-Lewis, C, Fragala, MS, Hooper, DR, Häkkinen, K, and Maresh, CM. The impact of cold-water immersion on power production in the vertical jump and the benefits of a dynamic exercise warm-up. *J Strength Cond Res* 24:3313-3317, 2010.

33. Duffield, R, Coutts, A, and Quinn, J. Core temperature responses and match running performance during intermittent-sprint exercise competition in warm conditions. *J Strength Cond Res* 23:1238-1244, 2009.

34. Dupuy, O, Douzi, W, Theurot, D, Bosquet, L, and Dugué, B. An evidence-based approach for choosing post-exercise recovery techniques to reduce markers of muscle damage, soreness, fatigue, and inflammation: a systematic review with meta-analysis. *Front Physiol* 9:403, 2018.

35. Figaro, MK, and Mack, GW. Regulation of fluid intake in dehydrated humans: role of oropharyngeal stimulation. *Am J Physiol* 272:R1740-R1746, 1997.

36. Flaherty, G, O'Connor, R, and Johnston, N. Altitude training for elite endurance athletes: a review for the travel medicine practitioner. *Travel Med Infect Dis* 14:200-211, 2016.

37. Garrett, AT, Creasy, R, Rehrer, NJ, Patterson, MJ, and Cotter, JD. Effectiveness of short-term heat acclimation for highly trained athletes. *Eur J Appl Physiol* 112:1827-1837, 2012.

38. Garrett, AT, Goosens, NG, Rehrer, NG, Patterson, MJ, and Cotter, JD. Induction and decay of short-term heat acclimation. *Eur J Appl Physiol* 107:659, 2009.

39. Gibson, OR, Dennis, A, Parfitt, T, Taylor, L, Watt, PW, and Maxwell, NS. Extracellular Hsp72 concentration relates to a minimum endogenous criteria during acute exercise-heat exposure. *Cell Stress Chaperones* 19:389-400, 2014.

40. Girard, O, Brocherie, F, and Millet, GP. Effects of altitude/hypoxia on single- and multiple-sprint performance: a comprehensive review. *Sports Med* 47:1931-1949, 2017.

41. Jacobs, RA, Lundby, A-KM, Fenk, S, Gehrig, S, Siebenmann, C, Flück, D, Kirk, N, Hilty, MP, and Lundby, C. Twenty-eight days of exposure to 3454 m increases mitochondrial volume density in human skeletal muscle. *J Physiol (Lond)* 594:1151-1166, 2016.

42. Judelson, DA, Maresh, CM, Anderson, JM, Armstrong, LE, Casa, DJ, Kraemer, WJ, and Volek JS. Hydration and muscular performance: does fluid balance affect strength, power and high-intensity endurance? *Sports Med* 37:907-921, 2007.

43. Kavouras, SA. Assessing hydration status. *Curr Opin Clin Nutr Metab Care* 5:519-524, 2002.

44. Kavouras, SA, Johnson, EC, Bougatsas, D, Arnaoutis, G, Panagiotakos, DB, Perrier, E, and Klein A. Validation of a urine color scale for assessment of urine osmolality in healthy children. *Eur J Nutr* 55:907-915, 2016.

45. Keiser, S, Flück, D, Hüppin, F, Stravs, A, Hilty, MP, and Lundby, C. Heat training increases exercise capacity in hot but not in temperate conditions: a mechanistic counter-balanced cross-over study. *Am J Physiol Heart Circ Physiol* 309:H750-H761, 2015.

46. Kenefick, RW. Author's reply to Valenzuela et al.: Comment on "drinking strategies: planned drinking versus drinking to thirst." *Sports Med* 48:2215-2217, 2018.

47. Kenefick, RW. Drinking strategies: planned drinking versus drinking to thirst. *Sports Med* 48:31-37, 2018.

48. Kerr, ZY, Register-Mihalik, JK, Pryor, RR, Hosokawa, Y, Scarneo, SE, and Casa, DJ. Compliance with the National Athletic Trainers' Association Inter-Association Task Force preseason heat-acclimatization guidelines in high school football. *J Athl Train* 54:749-757, 2019.

49. Korey Stringer Institute. Wet Bulb Globe Temperature Monitoring. https://ksi.uconn.edu/prevention/wet-bulb-globe-temperature-monitoring/. Accessed August 27. 2020.

50. Lorenzo, S, Halliwill, JR, Sawka, MN, and Minson, CT. Heat acclimation improves exercise performance. *J Appl Physiol (1985)* 109:1140-1147, 2010.

51. Lynch, GP, Périard, JD, Pluim, BM, Brotherhood, JR, and Jay, O. Optimal cooling strategies for players in Australian Tennis Open conditions. *J Sci Med Sport* 21: 232-237, 2018.

52. McDermott, BP, Anderson, SA, Armstrong, LE, Casa, DJ, Cheuvront, SN, Cooper, L, Kenney, WL, O'Connor, FG, and Roberts, WO. National Athletic Trainers' Association position statement: fluid replacement for the physically active. *J Athl Train* 52:877-895, 2017.

53. McDermott, BP, Casa, DJ, Ganio, MS, Lopez, RM, Yeargin, SW, Armstrong, LE, and Maresh, CM. Acute whole-body cooling for exercise-induced hyperthermia: a systematic review. *J Athl Train* 44:84-93, 2009.

54. McKenzie, AL, Muñoz, CX, and Armstrong, LE. Accuracy of urine color to detect equal to or greater than 2% body mass loss in men. *J Athl Train* 50:1306-1309, 2015.

55. Millet, GP, Roels, B, Schmitt, L, Woorons, X, and Richalet, JP. Combining hypoxic methods for peak performance. *Sports Med* 40:1-25, 2010.

56. Morris, JG, Nevill, ME, Lakomy, HKA, Nicholas, C, and Williams, C. Effect of a hot environment on performance of prolonged, intermittent, high-intensity shuttle running. *J Sports Sci* 16:677-686, 1998.

57. Mounier, R, Pedersen, BK, and Plomgaard, P. Muscle-specific expression of hypoxia-inducible factor in human skeletal muscle. *Exp Physiol* 95:899-907, 2010.

58. Nassis, GP. Effect of altitude on football performance: analysis of the 2010 FIFA World Cup data. *J Strength Cond Res* 27:703-707, 2013.

59. Nuccio, RP, Barnes, KA, Carter, JM, and Baker, LB. Fluid balance in team sport athletes and the effect of hypohydration on cognitive, technical, and physical performance. *Sports Med* 47:1951-1982, 2017.

60. Nybo, L, and González-Alonso, J. Critical core temperature: a hypothesis too simplistic to explain hyperthermia-induced fatigue. *Scand J Med Sci Sports* 25:4-5, 2015.

61. Pandolf, KB, Burse, RL, and Goldman, RF. Role of physical fitness in heat acclimatisation, decay and reinduction. *Ergonomics* 20:399-408, 1977.

62. Périard, JD, Racinais, S, and Sawka, MN. Adaptations and mechanisms of human heat acclimation: applications for competitive athletes and sports. *Scand J Med Sci Sports* 25(suppl 1):20-38, 2015.

63. Périard, JD, Travers, GJS, Racinais, S, and Sawka, MN. Cardiovascular adaptations supporting human exercise-heat acclimation. *Auton Neurosci* 196:52-62, 2016.

64. Pryor, JL, Johnson, EC, Roberts, WO, and Pryor, RR. Application of evidence-based recommendations for heat acclimation: individual and team sport perspectives. *Temperature (Austin)* 6:37-49, 2019.

65. Pryor, JL, Pryor, RR, Vandermark, LW, Adams, EL, VanScoy, RM, Casa, DJ, Armstrong, LE, Lee, EC, DiStefano, LJ, Anderson, JM, and Maresh, CM. Intermittent exercise-heat exposures and intense physical activity sustain heat acclimation adaptations. *J Sci Med Sport* 22:117-122, 2019.

66. Racinais, S, Alonso, J-M, Coutts, AJ, Flouris, AD, Girard, O, González-Alonso, J, Hausswirth, C, Jay, O, Lee, JK, Mitchell, N, Nassis, GP, Nybo, L, Pluim, BM, Roelands, B, Sawka, MN, Wingo, J, and Périard, JD. Consensus recommendations on training and competing in the heat. *Sports Med* 45:925-938, 2015.

67. Racinais, S, Cocking, S, and Périard, JD. Sports and environmental temperature: from warming-up to heating-up. *Temperature (Austin)* 4:227-257, 2017.

68. Robbins, PA. Role of the peripheral chemoreflex in the early stages of ventilatory acclimatization to altitude. *Respir Physiol Neurobiol* 158:237-242, 2007.

69. Rusko, HK, Tikkanen, HO, and Peltonen, JE. Altitude and endurance training. *J Sports Sci* 22:928-944, 2004.

70. Saunders, PU, Pyne, DB, and Gore, CJ. Endurance training at altitude. *High Alt Med Biol* 10:135-148, 2009.

71. Sawka, MN, Burke, LM, Eichner, ER, Maughan, RJ, Montain, SJ, and Stachenfeld, NS. American College of Sports Medicine position stand. Exercise and fluid replacement. *Med Sci Sports Exerc* 39:377-390, 2007.

72. Sawka, MN, Leon, LR, Montain, SJ, and Sonna, LA. Integrated physiological mechanisms of exercise performance, adaptation, and maladaptation to heat stress. *Compr Physiol* 1:1883-1928, 2011.

73. Sawka, MN, Pandolf, KB, Avellini, BA, and Shapiro, Y. Does heat acclimation lower the rate of metabolism elicited by muscular exercise? *Aviat Space Environ Med* 54:27-31, 1983.

74. Schoene, RB. Limits of human lung function at high altitude. *J Exp Biol* 204:3121-3127, 2001.

75. Shirreffs, SM, Armstrong, LE, and Cheuvront, SN. Fluid and electrolyte needs for preparation and recovery from training and competition. *J Sports Sci* 22:57-63, 2004.

76. Shirreffs, SM, and Maughan, RJ. Urine osmolality and conductivity as indices of hydration status in athletes in the heat. *Med Sci Sports Exerc* 30:1598-1602, 1998.

77. Sunderland, C, Morris, JG, and Nevill, ME. A heat acclimation protocol for team sports. *Br J Sports Med* 42:327-333, 2008.

78. Tyler, CJ, Reeve, T, Hodges, GJ, and Cheung, SS. The effects of heat adaptation on physiology, perception and exercise performance in the heat: a meta-analysis. *Sports Med* 46:1699-1724, 2016.

79. Wilber, RL. Current trends in altitude training. *Sports Med* 31:249-265, 2001.

80. Willmott, AGB, Hayes, M, James, CA, Dekerle, J, Gibson, OR, and Maxwell, NS. Once- and twice-daily heat acclimation confer similar heat adaptations, inflammatory responses and exercise tolerance improvements. *Physiol Rep* 6:e13936, 2018.

81. Young, AJ, Sawka, MN, Levine, L, Cadarette, BS, and Pandolf, KB. Skeletal muscle metabolism during exercise is influenced by heat acclimation. *J Appl Physiol* 59:1929-1935, 1985.

82. Zoll, J, Ponsot, E, Dufour, S, Doutreleau, S, Ventura-Clapier, R, Vogt, M, Hoppeler, H, Richard, R, and Flück, M. Exercise training in normobaric hypoxia in endurance runners. III. Muscular adjustments of selected gene transcripts. *J Appl Physiol* 100:1258-1266, 2006.

Chapter 26

1. Ashinoff, BK, and Abu-Akel, A. Hyperfocus: the forgotten frontier of attention. *Psychol Res* 20:1-9, 2019.

2. Baggetta, P, and Alexander, PA. Conceptualization and operationalization of executive function. *Mind Brain Educ* 10:10-33, 2016.

3. Baumeister, J, Reinecke, K, Liesen, H, and Weiss, M. Cortical activity of skilled performance in a complex sports related motor task. *Eur J Appl Physiol* 104:625-631, 2008.

4. Bender, AM, Van Dongen, HPA, and Samuels, CH. Sleep quality and chronotype differences between elite athletes and non-athlete controls. *Clocks Sleep* 1:3-12, 2018.

5. Berka, C, Behneman, A, Kintz, N, Johnson, R, and Raphael, G. Accelerating training using interactive neuro-educational technologies: applications to archery, golf, and rifle marksmanship. *J Int Soc Sports Nutr* 1:87-104, 2010.

6. Bertram, CP, Guadagnoli, MA, Greggain, J, and Pauls, A. The effect of blocked versus random warm-up on performance in skilled golfers. Proceedings from the 2016 World Scientific Congress of Golf, 7, 2016.

7. Bertram, CP, Guadagnoli, MA, and Marteniuk, RG. The stages of learning and implications for optimized learning environments. In *Routledge International Handbook of Golf Science*. New York: Routledge, 119-128, 2017.

8. Biederman, J, and Spencer, T. Attention-deficit/hyperactivity disorder (ADHD) as a noradrenergic disorder. *Biol Psychiatry* 46:1234-1242, 1999.

9. Bjork, EL, and Bjork, RA. Making things hard on yourself, but in a good way: creating desirable difficulties to enhance learning. In *Psychology and the Real World: Essays Illustrating Fundamental Contributions to Society*. Gernsbacher, MA, Pew, RW, Hough, LM, and Pomerantz, JR, eds. World Publishers, 59-64, 2011.

10. Boecker, H, Sprenger, T, Spilker, ME, Henriksen, G, Koppenhoefer, M, Wagner, KJ, and Tolle, TR. The runner's high: opioidergic mechanisms in the human brain. *Cereb Cortex* 18:2523-2531, 2008.

11. Boksem, MAS, and Tops, M. Mental fatigue: costs and benefits. *Brain Res Rev* 59:125-139, 2008.

12. Brownsberger, J, Edwards, A, Crowther, R, and Cottrell, D. Impact of mental fatigue on self-paced exercise. *Int J Sports Med* 34:1029-1036, 2013.

13. Cahn, BR, and Polich, J. Meditation states and traits: EEG, ERP, and neuroimaging studies. *Psychol Bull* 132:180-211, 2006.

14. Caldwell, JA, Hall, KK, and Erickson, BS. EEG data collected from helicopter pilots in flight are sufficiently sensitive to detect increased fatigue from sleep deprivation. *Int J Aviat Psychol* 12:19-32, 2002.

15. Caseras, X, Mataix-Cols, D, Giampietro, V, Rimes, KA, Brammer, M, Zelaya, F, Chalder, T, and Godfrey, EL. Probing the working memory system in chronic fatigue syndrome: a functional magnetic resonance imaging study using the n-back task. *Psychosom Med* 68:947-955, 2006.

16. Chiviacowsky, S, Wulf, G, and Wally, R. An external focus of attention enhances balance learning in older adults. *Gait Posture* 32:572-575, 2010.

17. Cook, DB, O'Connor, PJ, Lange, G, and Steffener, J. Functional neuroimaging correlates of mental fatigue induced by cognition among chronic fatigue syndrome patients and controls. *Neuroimage* 36:108-122, 2007.

18. Csíkszentmihályi, M. *Beyond Boredom and Anxiety*. San Francisco: Jossey-Bass, 1975.

19. Csíkszentmihályi, M. The flow experience and its significance for human psychology. In *Optimal Experience: Psychological Studies of Flow in Consciousness*. Csíkszentmihályi, M and Csíkszentmihályi, IS, eds. Cambridge, England: Cambridge University Press, 15-35, 1988.

20. Csíkszentmihályi, M. *Flow: The Psychology of Optimal Experience.* New York: HarperPerennial, 1990.

21. Csíkszentmihályi, M. *The Evolving Self: A Psychology for the Third Millennium.* New York: Harper-Collins, 1993.

22. Deloitte. Workplace Burnout Survey. March 14, 2018. www2. deloitte.com/us/en/pages/about-deloitte/articles/burnout-survey.html. Accessed November 23, 2019.

23. de Manzano, Ö, Cervenka, S. Jucaite, A, Hellenäs, O, Farde, L, and Ullén, F. Individual differences in the proneness to have flow experiences are linked to dopamine D2-receptor availability in the dorsal striatum. *Neuroimage* 67:1-6, 2013.

24. Dietrich, A. Functional neuroanatomy of altered states of consciousness: the transient hypofrontality hypothesis. *Consciousness Cogn* 12:231-256, *2003.*

25. Dietrich, A. Neurocognitive mechanisms underlying the experience of flow. *Consciousness Cogn* 13:746-761, *2004.*

26. Dietrich, A. Transient hypofrontality as a mechanism for the psychological effects of exercise. *Psychiatry Res* 145:79-83, 2006.

27. Dietrich, A, and McDaniel, WF. Endocannabinoids and exercise. *Br J Sports Med* 38:536-541, *2004.*

28. Egner, T, and Gruzelier, JH. Ecological validity of neurofeedback: modulation of slow wave EEG enhances musical performance. *Neuroreport* 14:1221-1224, 2003.

29. Farb, NAS, Segal, ZV, Mayberg, H, Bean, J, McKeon, D, Fatima, Z, and Anderson, AK. Attending to the present: mindfulness meditation reveals distinct neural modes of self-reference. *Soc Cogn Affect Neurosci* 2:313-322, 2007.

30. Farrow, D, and Robertson, S. Development of a skill acquisition periodisation framework for high-performance sport. *Sports Med* 47:1043-1054, 2017.

31. Ferreri, L, Mas-Herrero, E, Zatorre, RJ, Ripollés, P, Gomez-Andres, A, Alicart, H, and Rodriguez-Fornells, A. Dopamine modulates the reward experiences elicited by music. *Proc Natl Acad Sci U S A* 116:3793-3798, *2019.*

32. Fitts, PM, and Posner, MI. *Human Performance.* Belmont, CA: Brooks/Cole, 1967.

33. Fong, CJ, Zaleski, DJ, and Leach, JK. The challenge–skill balance and antecedents of flow: a meta-analytic investigation. *J Positive Psychol* 10:425-446, *2015.*

34. Fullagar, CJ, and Kelloway, EK. Flow at work: an experience sampling approach. *J Occup Organ Psychol* 82:595-615, 2009.

35. Fuss, J, Steinle, J, Bindila, L, Auer, MK, Kirchherr, H, Lutz, B, and Gass, P. A runner's high depends on cannabinoid receptors in mice. *Proc Natl Acad Sci U S A* 112:13105-13108, *2015.*

36. García-Pérez, MA. Forced-choice staircases with fixed step sizes: asymptotic and small-sample properties. *Vision Res* 38:1861-1881, 1998.

37. Garfield, CA, and Bennett, HZ. *Peak Performance: Mental Training Techniques of the World's Greatest Athletes.* New York: Warner Books, 1989.

38. Genovesio, A, Tsujimoto, S, and Wise, SP. Feature- and order-based timing representations in the frontal cortex. *Neuron* 63:254-266, 2009.

39. Gerber, M, Best, S, Meerstetter, F, Walter, M, Ludyga, S, Brand, S, Binachi, R, Madigan, DJ, Isoard-Gautheur, S, and Gustafsson, H. Effects of stress and mental toughness on burnout and depressive symptoms: a prospective study with young elite athletes. *J Sci Med Sport* 21:1200-1205, 2018.

40. Goldfarb, AH, and Jamurtas, AZ. β-Endorphin response to exercise. *Sports Med* 24:8-16, 1997.

41. Gruber, MJ, Gelman, BD, and Ranganath, C. States of curiosity modulate hippocampus-dependent learning via the dopaminergic circuit. *Neuron* 84:486-496, 2015.

42. Guadagnoli, MA, and Bertram, CP. Optimizing practice for performance under pressure. *Int J Golf Sci* 3:119-127, 2014.

43. Guadagnoli, MA, and Lee, TD. Challenge point: a framework for conceptualizing the effects of various practice conditions in motor learning. *J Mot Behav* 36:212-224, 2004.

44. Gyurkovics, M, Kotyuk, E, Katonai, ER, Horvath, EZ, Vereczkei, A, and Szekely, A. Individual differences in flow proneness are linked to a dopamine D2 receptor gene variant. *Conscious Cogn* 42:1-8, 2016.

45. Hamari, J, and Koivisto, J. Measuring flow in gamification: Dispositional Flow Scale-2. *Comput Hum Behav* 40:133-143, 2014.

46. Harris, DJ, Vine, SJ, and Wilson, MR. Neurocognitive mechanisms of the flow state. *Prog Brain Res* 234:221-243, 2017.

47. Harung, HS, Travis, F, Pensgaard, AM, Boes, R, Cook-Greuter, S, and Daley, K. Higher psycho-physiological refinement in world-class Norwegian athletes: brain measures of performance capacity. *Scand J Med Sci Sports* 21:32-41, *2011.*

48. Hatfield, BD, Haufler, AJ, Hung, T-M, and Spalding, TW. Electroencephalographic studies of skilled psychomotor performance. *J Clin Neurophysiol* 21:144-156, 2004.

49. Ishikura, T. Reduced relative frequency of knowledge of results without visual feedback in learning a golf-putting task. *Percept Mot Skills* 106:225-233, 2008.

50. Jackson, SA, and Eklund, RC. Assessing flow in physical activity: The Flow State Scale–2 and Dispositional Flow Scale–2. *J Sport Exerc Psychol* 24:133-150, *2002.*

51. Jackson, SA, and Marsh, HW. Development and validation of a scale to measure optimal experience: The Flow State Scale. *J Sport Exerc Psychol* 18:17-35, 1996.

52. Jackson, SA, Thomas, PR, Marsh, HW, and Smethurst, CJ. Psychological links with optimal performance: understanding the flow experience. *J Sci Med Sport* 2:418, 1999. http://dx.doi. org/10.1016/s1440-2440(99)80029-2

53. Jin, S-A. Toward integrative models of flow: effects of performance, skill, challenge, playfulness, and presence on flow in video games. *J Broadcast Electron Media* 56:169-186, *2012.*

54. Johnson, JA, Keiser, HN, Skarin, EM, and Ross, SR. The dispositional flow scale–2 as a measure of autotelic personality: an examination of criterion-related validity. *J Pers Assess* 96:465-470, *2014.*

55. Kamiński, J, Brzezicka, A, Gola, M, and Wróbel, A. Beta band oscillations engagement in human alertness process. *Int J Psychophysiol* 85:125-128, *2012.*

56. Katahira, K, Yamazaki, Y, Yamaoka, C, Ozaki, H, Nakagawa, S, and Nagata, N. EEG correlates of the flow state: a combination of increased frontal theta and moderate frontocentral alpha rhythm in the mental arithmetic task. *Front Psychol* 9:300, 2018.

57. Keller, J, and Bless, H. Flow and regulatory compatibility: an experimental approach to the flow model of intrinsic motivation. *Pers Soc Psychol Bull* 34:196-209, 2008.

58. Knöpfli, B, Calvert, R, Bar-Or, O, Villiger, B, and Von Duvillard, SP. Competition performance and basal nocturnal catecholamine excretion in cross-country skiers. *Med Sci Sports Exerc* 33:1228-1232, *2001.*

59. Lal, SKL, and Craig, A. Driver fatigue: electroencephalography and psychological assessment. *Psychophysiology* 39:313-321, 2002.

60. Langner, R, Steinborn, MB, Chatterjee, A, Sturm, W, and Willmes, K. Mental fatigue and temporal preparation in simple reaction-time performance. *Acta Psychologica* 133:64-72, 2010.

61. Lee, Y-J, Kim, H-G, Cheon, E-J, Kim, K, Choi, J-H, Kim, J-Y, Kim, J-M, and Koo, B-H. The analysis of electroencephalography changes before and after a single neurofeedback alpha/theta training session in university students. *Appl Psychophysiol Biofeedback* 44:173-184, 2019.

62. Limb, CJ, and Braun, AR. Neural substrates of spontaneous musical performance: an FMRI study of jazz improvisation. *PLoS One* 3:e1679, 2008.

63. Lin, C-HJ, Yang, H-C, Knowlton, BJ, Wu, AD, Iacoboni, M, Ye, Y-L, Huang, SL, and Chiang, M-C. Contextual interference enhances motor learning through increased resting brain connectivity during memory consolidation. *Neuroimage* 181:1-15, 2018.

64. Liu, S, Chow, HM, Xu, Y, Erkkinen, MG, Swett, KE, Eagle, MW, Rizik-Baer, DA, and Braun, AR. Neural correlates of lyrical improvisation: an fMRI study of freestyle rap. *Sci Rep* 2:834, 2012.

65. Lohse, KR, and Sherwood, DE. Defining the focus of attention: effects of attention on perceived exertion and fatigue. *Front Psychol* 2:332, 2011.

66. Longe, O, Maratos, FA, Gilbert, P, Evans, G, Volker, F, Rockliff, H, and Rippon, G. Having a word with yourself: neural correlates of self-criticism and self-reassurance. *Neuroimage* 49:1849-1856, 2010.

67. Lorist, MM, Boksem, MAS, and Ridderinkhof, KR. Impaired cognitive control and reduced cingulate activity during mental fatigue. *Brain Res Cogn Brain Res* 24:199-205, 2005.

68. Lou, JS, Kearns, G, Oken, B, Sexton, G, and Nutt, J. Exacerbated physical fatigue and mental fatigue in Parkinson's disease. *Mov Disord* 16:190-196, 2001.

69. Lustenberger, C, Boyle, MR, Foulser, AA, Mellin, JM, and Fröhlich, F. Functional role of frontal alpha oscillations in creativity. *Cortex* 67:74-82, 2015.

70. Mahler, SV, Smith, KS, and Berridge, KC. Endocannabinoid hedonic hotspot for sensory pleasure: anandamide in nucleus accumbens shell enhances "liking" of a sweet reward. *Neuropsychopharmacology* 32:2267-2278, 2007.

71. Marcora, SM, Staiano, W, and Manning, V. Mental fatigue impairs physical performance in humans. *J Appl Physiol* 106:857-864, 2009.

72. Marin, MM, and Bhattacharya, J. Getting into the musical zone: trait emotional intelligence and amount of practice predict flow in pianists. *Front Psychol* 4:853, 2013.

73. Maslow, AH. *Religions, Values, and Peak Experiences*. Columbus, OH: Ohio State University Press, 1964.

74. Morgan, JD, and Coutts, RA. Measuring peak experience in recreational surfing. *J Sport Behav* 39:202-217, 2016.

75. Nakamura, J, and Csikszentmihalyi, M. Flow theory and research. In *The Oxford Handbook of Positive Psychology*. Oxford: Oxford University Press, 195-206, 2009.

76. Nakashima, K, and Sato, H. The effects of various mental tasks on appearance of frontal midline theta activity in EEG. *J Hum Ergol (Tokyo)* 21:201-206, 1992.

77. Natarajan, K, Acharya, UR, Alias, F, Tiboleng, T, and Puthusserypady, SK. Nonlinear analysis of EEG signals at different mental states. *Biomed Eng Online* 3:7, 2004.

78. Navarro Gil, M, Escolano Marco C, Montero-Marín, J, Minguez Zafra, J, Shonin, E, and García Campayo, J. Efficacy of neurofeedback on the increase of mindfulness-related capacities in healthy individuals: a controlled trial. *Mindfulness* 9:303-311, 2018.

79. *Nietzsche, F. The Will to Power*. Kaufmann, W, trans. New York: Hollingdale, 1968.

80. Okogbaa, OG, Shell, RL, and Filipusic, D. On the investigation of the neurophysiological correlates of knowledge worker mental fatigue using the EEG signal. *Appl Ergon* 25:355-365, 1994.

81. Panisch, LS, and Hai, AH. The effectiveness of using neurofeedback in the treatment of post-traumatic stress disorder: a systematic review. *Trauma Violence Abuse* 21:541-550, 2020.

82. Pauls, AL, Bertram, CP, and Guadagnoli, MA. Is technology the saviour or the downfall of modern golf instruction? In *Routledge International Handbook of Golf Science*. New York: Routledge, 79-87, 2017.

83. Peifer, C, Schulz, A, Schächinger, H, Baumann, N, and Antoni, CH. The relation of flow-experience and physiological arousal under stress—Can u shape it? *J Exp Soc Psychol* 53:62-69, 2014.

84. Perkins-Ceccato, N, Passmore, SR, and Lee, TD. Effects of focus of attention depend on golfers' skill. *J Sports Sci* 21:593-600, 2003.

85. Philip, P, and Akerstedt, T. Transport and industrial safety, how are they affected by sleepiness and sleep restriction? *Sleep Med Rev* 10:347-356, 2006.

86. Pliszka, SR, McCracken, JT, and Maas, JW. Catecholamines in attention-deficit hyperactivity disorder: current perspectives. *J Am Acad Child Adolesc Psychiatry* 35:264-272, 1996.

87. Ravizza, K. Peak experiences in sport. *J Humanist Psychol* 17:35-40, 1977.

88. Ravizza, K. Qualities of the peak experience in sport. In *Psychological Foundations of Sport*, (JM Silva and RS Weinberg Eds.). Human Kinetics Publishers, Champaign, IL, 452-461, 1984.

89. Raymond, J, Sajid, I, Parkinson, LA, and Gruzelier, JH. Biofeedback and dance performance: a preliminary investigation. *Appl Psychophysiol Biofeedback* 30:64-73, 2005.

90. Reardon, CL, Hainline, B, Aron, CM, Baron, D, Baum, AL, Bindra, A, Budgett, R, Campriani, N, Castaldelli-Maia, JM, Currie, A, Derevensky, JL, Glick, ID, Gorczynski, P, Gouttebarge, V, Grandner, MA, Han, DH, McDuf, D, Mountjoy, M, Polat, A, Purcell, R, Putukian, M, Rice, S, Sills, A, Stull, T, Swartz, L, Zhu, LJ, and Engebretsen, L. Mental health in elite athletes: International Olympic Committee consensus statement (2019). *Br J Sports Med* 53:667-699, 2019.

91. Russell, S, Jenkins, D, Rynne, S, Halson, SL, and Kelly, V. What is mental fatigue in elite sport? Perceptions from athletes and staff. *Eur J Sport Sci* 10:1367-1376, 2019.

92. Salehzadeh Niksirat, K, Park, K, Silpasuwanchai, C, Wang, Z, and Ren, X. The relationship between flow proneness in everyday life and variations in the volume of gray matter in the dopaminergic system: a cross-sectional study. *Pers Individ Dif* 141:25-30, 2019.

93. Schacter, DL. EEG theta waves and psychological phenomena: a review and analysis. *Biol Psychol* 5:47-82, 1977.

94. Shereena, EA, Gupta, RK, Bennett, CN, Sagar, KJV, and Rajeswaran, J. EEG neurofeedback training in children with attention deficit/hyperactivity disorder: a cognitive and behavioral outcome study. *Clin EEG Neurosci* 50:242-255, 2019.

95. Singer, K. The effect of neurofeedback on performance anxiety in dancers. *J Dance Med Sci* 8:78-81, 2004.

96. Smith, MR, Coutts, AJ, Merlini, M, Deprez, D, Lenoir, M, and Marcora, SM. Mental fatigue impairs soccer-specific physical and technical performance. *Med Sci Sports Exerc* 48:267-276, 2016.

97. Smith, ME, McEvoy, LK, and Gevins, A. Neurophysiological indices of strategy development and skill acquisition. *Brain Res Cogn Brain Res* 7:389-404, 1999.

98. Smith, MR, Zeuwts, L, Lenoir, M, Hens, N, De Jong, LMS, and Coutts, AJ. Mental fatigue impairs soccer-specific decision-making skill. *J Sports Sci* 34:1297-1304, 2016.

99. Soderstrom, NC, and Bjork, RA. Learning versus performance: an integrative review. *Perspect Psychol Sci* 10:176-199, 2015.

100. Sparling, PB, Giuffrida, A, Piomelli, D, Rosskopf, L, and Dietrich, A. Exercise activates the endocannabinoid system. *Neuroreport* 14:2209-2211, 2003.

101. Swann, C, Keegan, RJ, Piggott, D, and Crust, L. A systematic review of the experience, occurrence, and controllability of flow states in elite sport. *Psychol Sport Exerc* 13:807-819, 2012.

102. Tenenbaum, G, Fogarty, GJ, and Jackson, SA. The flow experience: a Rasch analysis of Jackson's Flow State Scale. *J Outcome Meas* 3:278-294, 1999.

103. Ullén, F, de Manzano, Ö, Theorell, T, and Harmat, L. The physiology of effortless attention: correlates of state flow and flow proneness. In *Effortless Attention: A New Perspective in the Cognitive Science of Attention and Action*. Bruya, B, ed. Cambridge, MA: MIT Press, 205, 2010.

104. Van Cutsem, J, Marcora, S, De Pauw, K, Bailey, S, Meeusen, R, and Roelands, B. The effects of mental fatigue on physical performance: a systematic review. *Sports Med* 47:1569-1588, 2017.

105. van der Linden, D, Massar, SAA, Schellekens, AFA, Ellenbroek, BA, and Verkes, R-J. Disrupted sensorimotor gating due to mental fatigue: preliminary evidence. *Int J Psychophysiol* 62:168-174, 2006.

106. Williams, TD, Tolusso, DV, Fedewa, MV, and Esco, MR. Comparison of periodized and non-periodized resistance training on maximal strength: a meta-analysis. *Sports Med* 10:2083-2100, 2017.

107. Wilson, RC, Shenhav, A, Straccia, M, and Cohen, JD. The eighty five percent rule for optimal learning. *Nat Commun* 10:1-9, 2019.

108. Wrigley, WJ, and Emmerson, SB. The experience of the flow state in live music performance. *Psychol Music* 41:292-305, 2013.

109. Wulf, G. Attentional focus and motor learning: a review of 15 years. *Int Rev Sport Exerc Psychol* 6:77-104, 2013.

110. Wulf, G, Dufek, JS, Lozano, L, and Pettigrew, C. Increased jump height and reduced EMG activity with an external focus. *Hum Mov Sci* 29:440-448, 2010.

111. Wulf, G, McNevin, N, and Shea, CH. The automaticity of complex motor skill learning as a function of attentional focus. *Q J Exp Psychol A* 54:1143-1154, 2001.

112. Xing, B, Li, Y-C, and Gao, W-J. Norepinephrine versus dopamine and their interaction in modulating synaptic function in the prefrontal cortex. *Brain Res* 1641:217-233, 2016.

113. Yoshida, I, Hirao, K, and Kobayashi, R. The effect on subjective quality of life of occupational therapy based on adjusting the challenge–skill balance: a randomized controlled trial. *Clin Rehabil* 33:1732-1746, 2019.

114. Zhang, H, Watrous, AJ, Patel, A, and Jacobs, J. Theta and alpha oscillations are traveling waves in the human neocortex. *Neuron* 98:1269-1281.e4, 2018.

115. Zhang, X, Zhao, X, Du, H, and Rong, J. A study on the effects of fatigue driving and drunk driving on drivers' physical characteristics. *Traffic Inj Prev* 15:801-808, 2014.

Chapter 27

1. Barker, AT, Jalinous, R, and Freeston, IL. Non-invasive magnetic stimulation of human motor cortex. *Lancet* 1:1106-1107, 1985.

2. Baumeister, J, Reinecke, K, Liesen, H, and Weiss, M. Cortical activity of skilled performance in a complex sports related motor task. *Eur J Appl Physiol* 104:625, 2008.

3. Berthelot, G, Sedeaud, A, Marck, A, Antero-Jacquemin, J, Schipman, J, Sauliere, G, Marc, A, Desgorces, FD, and Toussaint, JF. Has athletic performance reached its peak? *Sports Med* 45:1263-1271, 2015.

4. Brandt, R, Bevilacqua, GG, and Andrade, A. Perceived sleep quality, mood states, and their relationship with performance among Brazilian elite athletes during a competitive period. *J Strength Cond Res* 31:1033-1039, 2017.

5. Brownsberger, J, Edwards, A, Crowther, R, and Cottrell, D. Impact of mental fatigue on self-paced exercise. *Int J Sports Med* 34:1029-1036, 2013.

6. Cantone, M, Lanza, G, Vinciguerra, L, Puglisi, V, Ricceri, R, Fisicaro, F, Vagli, C, Bella, R, Ferri, R, Pennisi, G, and Di Lazzaro, V. Age, height, and sex on motor evoked potentials: translational data from a large Italian cohort in a clinical environment. *Front Hum Neurosci* 13:185, 2019.

7. Carroll, TJ, Taylor, JL, and Gandevia, SC. Recovery of central and peripheral neuromuscular fatigue after exercise. *J Appl Physiol* 122:1068-1076, 2016.

8. Chang, KH, Lu, FJ, Chyi, T, Hsu, YW, Chan, SW, and Wang, ET. Examining the stress-burnout relationship: the mediating role of negative thoughts. *PeerJ* 5:e4181, 2017.

9. Cheng, MY, Huang, CJ, Chang, YK, Koester, D, Schack, T, and Hung, TM. Sensorimotor rhythm neurofeedback enhances golf putting performance. *J Sport Exerc Psychol* 37:626-636, 2015.

10. Cheng, MY, Hung, CL, Huang, CJ, Chang, YK, Lo, LC, Shen, C, and Hung, TM. Expert-novice differences in SMR activity during dart throwing. *Biol Psychol* 110:212-218, 2015.

11. Cheng, MY, Wang, KP, Hung, CL, Tu, YL, Huang, CJ, Koester, D, Schack, S, and Hung, TM. Higher power of sensorimotor rhythm is associated with better performance in skilled air-pistol shooters. *Psychol Sport Exerc* 32:47-53, 2017.

12. Cosman, JD, Lowe, KA, Zinke, W, Woodman, GF, and Schall, JD. Prefrontal control of visual distraction. *Curr Biol* 28:414-420, 2018.

13. Davenne, D. Sleep of athletes–problems and possible solutions. *Biol Rhythm Res* 40:45-52, 2009.

14. De Beaumont, L, Mongeon, D, Tremblay, S, Messier, J, Prince, F, Leclerc, S, Lassonde, M, and Théoret, H. Persistent motor system abnormalities in formerly concussed athletes. *J Athl Train* 46:234-240, 2011.

15. Dietrich, A. Neurocognitive mechanisms underlying the experience of flow. *Conscious Cogn* 13:746-761, 2004.

16. Draganski, B, Gaser, C, Busch, V, Schuierer, G, Bogdahn, U, and May, A. Neuroplasticity: changes in grey matter induced by training. *Nature* 427:311, 2004.

17. Farzan, F, Barr, MS, Hoppenbrouwers, SS, Fitzgerald, PB, Chen, R, Pascual-Leone, A, and Daskalakis, ZJ. The EEG correlates of the TMS-induced EMG silent period in humans. *Neuroimage* 83:120-134, 2013.

18. Gómez-Pinilla, F. Brain foods: the effects of nutrients on brain function. *Nat Rev Neurosci* 9:568, 2008.

19. Groppa, S, Oliviero, A, Eisen, A, Quartarone, A, Cohen, LG, Mall, V, Kaelin-Lang, A, Mima, T, Rossi, S, Thickbroom, GW, Rossini, PM, Ziemann, U, Valls-Sole, J, and Siebner, HR. A practical guide to diagnostic transcranial magnetic stimulation: report of an IFCN committee. *Clin Neurophysiol* 123:858-882, 2012.

20. Jackson, SA, and Marsh, HW. Development and validation of a scale to measure optimal experience: the flow state scale. *J Sport Exerc Psychol* 18:17-35, 1996.

21. Klomjai, W, Katz, R, and Lackmy-Vallée, A. Basic principles of transcranial magnetic stimulation (TMS) and repetitive TMS (rTMS). *Ann Phys Rehabil Med* 58:208-213, 2015.

22. Lefaucheur, JP, Andre-Obadia, N, Antal, A, Ayache, SS, Baeken, C, Benninger, DH, Cantello, RM, Cincotta, M, de Carvalho, M, De Ridder, D, Devanne, H, Di Lazzaro, V, Filipovic, SR, Hummel, FC, Jaaskelainen, SK, Kimiskidis, VK, Koch, G, Langguth, B, Nyffeler, T, Oliviero, A, Padberg, F, Poulet, E, Rossi, S, Rossini, PM, Rothwell, JC, Schonfeldt-Lecuona, C, Siebner, HR, Slotema, CW, Stagg, CJ, Valls-Sole, J, Ziemann, U, Paulus, W, and Garcia-Larrea, L. Evidence-based guidelines on the therapeutic use of repetitive transcranial magnetic stimulation (rTMS). *Clin Neurophysiol* 125:2150-2206, 2014.

23. Lobo, V, Patil, A, Phatak, A, and Chandra, N. Free radicals, antioxidants, and functional foods: impact on human health. *Pharmacogn Rev* 4:118, 2010.

24. Lorist, MM, Bezdan, E, ten Caat, M, Span, MM, Roerdink, JB, and Maurits, NM. The influence of mental fatigue and motivation on neural network dynamics; an EEG coherence study. *Brain Res* 1270:95-106, 2009.

25. Lotze, M, and Halsband, U. Motor imagery. *J Physiol Paris* 99:386-395, 2006.

26. Mann, DT, Williams, AM, Ward, P, and Janelle, CM. Perceptual-cognitive expertise in sport: a meta-analysis. *J Sport Exerc Psychol* 29:457-478, 2007.

27. Martinez-Valdes, E, Farina, D, Negro, F, Del Vecchio, A, and Falla, D. Early motor unit conduction velocity changes to HIIT versus continuous training. *Med Sci Sports Exerc* 50:2339-2350, 2018.

28. McEwen, BS, Nasca, C, and Gray, JD. Stress effects on neuronal structure: hippocampus, amygdala, and prefrontal cortex. *Neuropsychopharmacology* 41:3, 2016.

29. McKay, WB, Stokic, DS, Sherwood, AM, Vrbova, G, and Dimitrijevic, MR. Effect of fatiguing maximal voluntary contraction on excitatory and inhibitory responses elicited by transcranial magnetic motor cortex stimulation. *Muscle Nerve* 19:1017-1024, 1996.

30. Miller, BT, and Clapp, WC. From vision to decision: the role of visual attention in elite sports performance. *Eye Contact Lens* 37:131-139, 2011.

31. Moscatelli, F, Messina, G, Valenzano, A, Petito, A, Triggiani, AI, Messina, A, Monda, V, Viggiano, A, De Luca, V, Capranica, L, and Monda, M. Differences in corticospinal system activity and reaction response between karate athletes and non-athletes. *Neurol Sci* 37:1947-1953, 2016.

32. Nakata, H, Yoshie, M, Miura, A, and Kudo, K. Characteristics of the athletes' brain: evidence from neurophysiology and neuroimaging. *Brain Res Rev* 62:197-211, 2010.

33. Oliveira, MF, Zelt, JT, Jones, JH, Hirai, DM, O'Donnell, DE, Verges, S, and Neder, JA. Does impaired O_2 delivery during exercise accentuate central and peripheral fatigue in patients with coexistent COPD-CHF? *Front Physiol* 5:514, 2015.

34. Park, JL, Fairweather, MM, and Donaldson, DI. Making the case for mobile cognition: EEG and sports performance. *Neurosci Biobehav Rev* 52:117-130, 2015.

35. Pascual-Leone, A, Amedi, A, Fregni, F, and Merabet, LB. The plastic human brain cortex. *Annu Rev Neurosci* 28:377-401, 2005.

36. Rossi, S, Hallett, M, Rossini, PM, Pascual-Leone, A, and Safety of TMS Consensus Group. Safety, ethical considerations, and application guidelines for the use of transcranial magnetic stimulation in clinical practice and research. *Clin Neurophysiol* 120:2008-2039, 2009.

37. Rossini, PM, Burke, D, Chen, R, Cohen, LG, Daskalakis, Z, Di Iorio, R, Di Lazzaro, V, Ferreri, F, Fitzgerald, PB, George, MS, Hallett, M, Lefaucheur, JP, Langguth, B, Matsumoto, H, Miniussi, C, Nitsche, MA, Pascual-Leone, A, Paulus, W, Rossi, S, Rothwell, JC, Siebner, HR, Ugawa, Y, Walsh, V, and Ziemann, U. Non-invasive electrical and magnetic stimulation of the brain, spinal cord, roots and peripheral nerves: basic principles and procedures for routine clinical and research application. An updated report from an I.F.C.N. Committee. *Clin Neurophysiol* 126:1071-1107, 2015.

38. Ruffino, C, Papaxanthis, C, and Lebon, F. Neural plasticity during motor learning with motor imagery practice: review and perspectives. *Neuroscience* 341:61-78, 2017.

39. Sáenz-Moncaleano, C, Basevitch, I, and Tenenbaum, G. Gaze behaviors during serve returns in tennis: a comparison between intermediate-and high-skill players. *J Sport Exerc Psychol* 40:49-59, 2018.

40. Stangor, C, and Walinga, J. The neuron is the building block of the nervous system. In *Introduction to Psychology - 1st Canadian Edition.* PressBooks, 2014.

41. Stickgold, R, and Walker, MP. Sleep-dependent memory consolidation and reconsolidation. *Sleep Med* 8:331-343, 2007.

42. Taubert, M, Lohmann, G, Margulies, DS, Villringer, A, and Ragert, P. Long-term effects of motor training on resting-state networks and underlying brain structure. *Neuroimage* 57:1492-1498, 2011.

43. Taylor, JL, Butler, JE, Allen, GM, and Gandevia, SC. Changes in motor cortical excitability during human muscle fatigue. *J Physiol* 490:519-528, 1996.

44. Watson, AM. Sleep and athletic performance. *Curr Sports Med Rep* 16:413-418, 2017.

45. Yavari, A, Javadi, M, Mirmiran, P, and Bahadoran, Z. Exercise-induced oxidative stress and dietary antioxidants. *Asian J Sports Med* 6:e34898, 2015.

46. Zarzycki, R, Morton, SM, Charalambous, CC, Marmon, A, and Snyder-Mackler, L. Corticospinal and intracortical excitability differ between athletes early after ACLR and matched controls. *J Orthop Res* 36:2941-2948, 2018.

Chapter 28

1. Abdollahipour, R, Palomo Nieto, M, Psotta, R, and Wulf, G. External focus of attention and autonomy support have additive benefits for motor performance in children. *Psychol Sport Exerc* 32:17-24, 2017.

2. Ávila, LTG, Chiviacowsky, S, Wulf, G, and Lewthwaite, R. Positive social-comparative feedback enhances motor learning in children. *Psychol Sport Exerc* 13:849-853, 2012.

3. Chiviacowsky, S, and Wulf, G. Feedback after good trials enhances learning. *Res Q Exerc Sport* 78:40-47, 2007.

4. Chiviacowsky, S, Wulf, G, Lewthwaite, R, and Campos, T. Motor learning benefits of self-controlled practice in persons with Parkinson's disease. *Gait Posture* 35:601-605, 2012.

5. Clark, SE, and Ste-Marie, DM. The impact of self-as-a-model interventions on children's self-regulation of learning and swimming performance. *J Sports Sci* 25:577-586, 2007.

6. Chua, L-K, Wulf, G, and Lewthwaite, R. Onward and upward: optimizing motor performance. *Hum Mov Sci* 60:107-114, 2018.

7. Freudenheim, AM, Wulf, G, Madureira, F, and Corrêa, UC. An external focus of attention results in greater swimming speed. *Int J Sports Sci Coach* 5:533-542, 2010.

8. Guss-West, C, and Wulf, G. Attentional focus in classical ballet: a survey of professional dancers. *J Dance Med Sci* 20:23-29, 2016.

9. Halperin, I, Chapman, DT, Martin, DT, Lewthwaite, R, and Wulf, G. Choices enhance punching performance of competitive kickboxers. *Psychol Res* 81:1051-1058, 2017.

10. Hooyman, A, Wulf, and Lewthwaite, R. Impacts of autonomy-supportive versus controlling instructional language on motor learning. *Hum Mov Sci* 36:190-198, 2014.

11. Hutchinson, JC, Sherman, T, Martinovic, N, and Tenenbaum, G. The effect of manipulated self-efficacy on perceived and sustained effort. *J Appl Sport Psychol* 20:457-472, 2008.

12. Iwatsuki, T, Abdollahipour, R, Psotta, R, Lewthwaite, R, and Wulf, G. Autonomy facilitates repeated maximum force productions. *Hum Mov Sci* 55:264-268, 2017.

13. Iwatsuki, T, Navalta, J, and Wulf, G. Autonomy enhances running efficiency. *J Sports Sci* 37:685-691, 2013.

14. Iwatsuki, T, Shih, HT, Abdollahipour, R, and Wulf, G. More bang for the buck: autonomy support increases muscular efficiency. *Psychol Res* 37: 685-691, 2019..

15. Janelle, CM, Barba, DA, Frehlich, SG, Tennant, LK, and Cauraugh, JH. Maximizing performance effectiveness through videotape replay and a self-controlled learning environment. *Res Q Exerc Sport* 68:269-279, 1997.

16. Kuhn, YA, Keller, M, Ruffieux, J, and Taube, W. Adopting an external focus of attention alters intracortical inhibition within the primary motor cortex. *Acta Physiologica* 220:289-299, 2017.

17. Lewthwaite, R, Chiviacowsky, S, Drews, R, and Wulf, G. Choose to move: the motivational impact of autonomy support on motor learning. *Psychon Bull Rev* 22:1383-1388, 2015.

18. Lewthwaite, R, and Wulf, G. Social-comparative feedback affects motor skill learning. *Q J Exp Psychol* 63:738-749, 2010.

19. Lewthwaite, R, and Wulf, G. Motor learning through a motivational lens. In *Skill Acquisition in Sport: Research, Theory & Practice.* 2nd ed. Hodges, NJ and Williams, AM, eds.. London: Routledge, 173-191, 2012.

20. Lohse, KR, and Sherwood, DE. Defining the focus of attention: effects of attention on perceived exertion and fatigue. *Front Psychol* 2:232, 2011.

21. Lohse, KR, Sherwood, DE, and Healy, AF. How changing the focus of attention affects performance, kinematics, and electromyography in dart throwing. *Hum Mov Sci* 29:542-555, 2010.

22. Lohse, KR, Sherwood, DE, and Healy, AF. Neuromuscular effects of shifting the focus of attention in a simple force production task. *J Mot Behav* 43:173-184, 2011.

23. Marchant, DC, Greig, M, Bullough, J, and Hitchen, D. Instructions to adopt an external focus enhance muscular endurance. *Res Q Exerc Sport* 82:466-473, 2011.

24. Marchant, D.C., Greig, M., and Scott, C. Attentional focusing strategies influence bicep EMG during isokinetic biceps curls. *Athletic Insight* 10(2): 11, 2008.

25. Marchant, DC, Greig, M, and Scott, C. Attentional focusing instructions influence force production and muscular activity during isokinetic elbow flexions. *J Strength Cond Res* 23:2358-2366, 2009.

26. McKay, B, Wulf, G, Lewthwaite, R, and Nordin, A. The self: your own worst enemy? A test of the self-invoking trigger hypothesis. *Q J Exp Psychol* 68:1910-1919, 2015.

27. Milton, J, Solodkin, A, Hluštík, P, and Small, SL. The mind of expert motor performance is cool and focused. *Neuroimage* 35:804-813, 2007.

28. Montes, J, Wulf, G, and Navalta, JW. Maximal aerobic capacity can be increased by enhancing performers' expectancies. *J Sports Med Phys Fitness* 58:744-749, 2018.

29. Montoya, ER, Bos, PA, Terburg, D, Rosenberger, LA, and van Honk, J. Cortisol administration induces global down-regulation of the brain's reward circuitry. *Psychoneuroendocrinology* 47:31-42, 2014.

30. Murayama, K, Izuma, K, Aoki, R, and Matsumoto, K. "Your choice" motivates you in the brain: the emergence of autonomy neuroscience. In *Recent Developments in Neuroscience Research on Human Motivation.* Kim, S, Reeve, J, and Bong, M, eds. Bingley, UK: Emerald Group Publishing, 95-125, 2016.

31. Palmer, K, Chiviacowsky, S, and Wulf, G. Enhanced expectancies facilitate golf putting. *Psychol Sport Exerc* 22:229-232, 2016.

32. Pascua, LAM, Wulf, G, and Lewthwaite, R. Additive benefits of external focus and enhanced performance expectancy for motor learning. *J Sports Sci* 33:58-66, 2015.

33. Porter, JM, Anton, PM, and Wu, WFW. Increasing the distance of an external focus of attention enhances standing long jump performance. *J Strength Cond Res* 26:2389-2393, 2012.

34. Porter, JM, Nolan, RP, Ostrowski, EJ, and Wulf, G. Directing attention externally enhances agility performance: a qualitative and quantitative analysis of the efficacy of using verbal instructions to focus attention. *Front Psychol* 1:216, 2010.

35. Porter, JM, Ostrowski, EJ, Nolan, RP, and Wu, WFW. Standing long-jump performance is enhanced when using an external focus of attention. *J Strength Cond Res* 24:1746-1750, 2010.

36. Porter, JM, Wu, WFW, Crossley, RM, and Knopp, SW. Adopting an external focus of attention improves sprinting performance in low-skilled sprinters. *J Strength Cond Res* 29:947-953, 2015.

37. Porter, JM, Wu, WFW, and Partridge, JA. Focus of attention and verbal instructions: strategies of elite track and field coaches and athletes. *Sport Sci Rev* 19:199-211, 2010.

38. Post, PG, Fairbrother, JT, and Barros, JAC. Self-controlled amount of practice benefits learning of a motor skill. *Res Q Exerc Sport* 82:474-481, 2011.

39. Reeve, J, and Tseng, CM. Cortisol reactivity to a teacher's motivating style: the biology of being controlled versus supporting autonomy. *Motivation Emotion* 35:63-74, 2011.

40. Rosenqvist, O, and Skans, ON. Confidence enhanced performance?—the causal effects of success on future performance in professional golf tournaments. *J Econ Behav Organ* 117:281-295, 2015.

41. Saemi, E, Porter, JM, Ghotbi-Varzaneh, A, Zarghami, M, and Maleki, F. Knowledge of results after relatively good trials enhances self-efficacy and motor learning. *Psychol Sport Exerc* 13:378-382, 2012.

42. Schmidt, RA, Lee, TD, Winstein, CJ, Wulf, G, and Zelaznik, HN. *Motor Control and Learning.* 6th ed. Champaign, IL: Human Kinetics, 2019.

43. Schücker, L, Hagemann, N, Strauss, B, and Völker, K. The effect of attentional focus on running economy. *J Sport Sci* 12:1242-1248, 2009.

44. Schultz, W. Updating dopamine reward signals. *Curr Opin Neurobiol* 23:229-238, 2013.

45. Stoate, I, and Wulf, G. Does the attentional focus adopted by swimmers affect their performance? *Int J Sport Sci Coach* 6:99-108, 2011.

46. Stoate, I, Wulf, G, and Lewthwaite, R. Enhanced expectancies improve movement efficiency in runners. *J Sports Sci* 30:815-823, 2012.

47. Trempe, M, Sabourin, M, and Proteau, L. Success modulates consolidation of a visuomotor adaptation task. *J Exp Psychol Learn Mem Cogn* 38:52-60, 2012.

48. Vance, J, Wulf, G, Töllner, T, McNevin, NH, and Mercer, J. EMG activity as a function of the performer's focus of attention. *J Mot Behav* 36:450-459, 2004.

49. Wu, WFW, Porter, JM, and Brown, LE. Effect of attentional focus strategies on peak force and performance in the standing long jump. *J Strength Cond Res* 26:1226-1231, 2012.

50. Wulf, G. Attentional focus and motor learning: a review of 15 years. *Int Rev Sport Exerc Psychol* 6:77-104, 2013.

51. Wulf, G, and Adams, N. Small choices can enhance balance learning. *Hum Mov Sci* 38:235-240, 2014.

52. Wulf, G, Chiviacowsky, S, and Cardozo, P. Additive benefits of autonomy support and enhanced expectancies for motor learning. *Hum Mov Sci* 37:12-20, 2014.

53. Wulf, G, Chiviacowsky, S, and Drews, R. External focus and autonomy support: two important factors in motor learning have additive benefits. *Hum Mov Sci* 40:176-184, 2015.

54. Wulf, G, Chiviacowsky, S, and Lewthwaite, R. Normative feedback effects on learning a timing task. *Res Q Exerc Sport* 81:425-431, 2010.

55. Wulf, G, Chiviacowsky, S, and Lewthwaite, R. Altering mindset can enhance motor learning in older adults. *Psychol Aging* 27:14-21, 2012.

56. Wulf, G, and Dufek, JS. Increased jump height with an external attentional focus is due to augmented force production. *J Mot Behav* 41:401-409, 2009.

57. Wulf, G, Dufek, JS, Lozano, L, and Pettigrew, C. Increased jump height and reduced EMG activity with an external focus of attention. *Hum Mov Sci* 29:440-448, 2010.

58. Wulf, G, Freitas, HE, and Tandy, RD. Choosing to exercise more: small choices can increase exercise engagement. *Psychol Sport Exerc* 15:268-271, 2014.

59. Wulf, G, Höß, M, and Prinz, W. Instructions for motor learning: differential effects of internal versus external focus of attention. *J Mot Behav* 30:169-179, 1998.

60. Wulf, G, and Lewthwaite, R. Optimizing Performance Through Intrinsic Motivation and Attention for Learning: the OPTIMAL theory of motor learning. *Psychon Bull Rev* 23:1382-1414, 2016.

61. Wulf, G, Lewthwaite, R, Cardozo, P, and Chiviacowsky, S. Triple play: additive contributions of enhanced expectancies, autonomy support, and external attentional focus to motor learning. *Q J Exp Psychol* 71:824-834, 2018.

62. Wulf, G, McNevin, NH, and Shea, CH. The automaticity of complex motor skill learning as a function of attentional focus. *Q J Exp Psychol* 54A:1143-1154, 2001.

63. Wulf, G, Zachry, T, Granados, C, and Dufek, JS. Increases in jump-and-reach height through an external focus of attention. *Int J Sports Sci Coach* 2:275-284, 2007.

64. Yu, C, Rouse, PC, Veldhuijzen, J, Van Zanten, JCS, Metsios, GS, Ntoumanis, N, Kitas, JD, and Duda, JL. Motivation-related predictors of physical activity engagement and vitality in rheumatoid arthritis patients. *Health Psychol Open* 2:2055102915600359, 2015.

65. Zachry, T, Wulf, G, Mercer, J, and Bezodis, N. Increased movement accuracy and reduced EMG activity as the result of adopting an external focus of attention. *Brain Res Bull* 67:304-309, 2005.

66. Zarghami, M, Saemi, E, and Fathi, I. External focus of attention enhances discus throwing performance. *Kinesiology* 44:47-51, 2012.

67. Ziv, G, Ochayon, M, and Lidor, R. Enhanced or diminished expectancies in golf putting—which actually affects performance? *Psychol Sport Exerc* 40:82-86, 2019.

Chapter 29

1. Ardern, CL, Glasgow, P, Schneiders, A, Witvrouw, E, Clarsen, B, Cools, A, Gojanovic, B, Griffin, S, Khan, KM, Moksnes, H, Mutch, SA, Phillips, N, Reurink, G, Sadler, R, Silbernagel, KG, Thorborg, K, Wangensteen, A, Wilk, KE, and Bizzini, M. Consensus statement on return to sport from the First World Congress in Sports Physical Therapy, Bern. *Br J Sports Med* 50:853-864, 2016.

2. Baker, CE, Moore-Lotridge, SN, Hysong, AA, Posey, SL, Robinette, JP, Blum, DM, Benvenuti, MA, Cole, HA, Egawa, S, Okawa, A, Saito, M, McCarthy, JR, Nyman, JS, Yuasa, M, and Schoenecker, JG. Bone fracture acute phase response—a unifying theory of fracture repair: clinical and scientific implications. *Clin Rev Bone Miner Metab* 16:142-158, 2018.

3. Blanch, P, and Gabbett, TJ. Has the athlete trained enough to return to play safely? The acute:chronic workload ratio permits clinicians to quantify a player's risk of subsequent injury. *Br J Sports Med* 50:471-475, 2016.

4. Bleakley, C, McDonough, S, and MacAuley, D. The use of ice in the treatment of acute soft-tissue injury: a systematic review of randomized controlled trials. *Am J Sports Med* 32:251-261, 2004.

5. Bryant, AE, Aldape, MJ, Bayer, CR, Katahira, EJ, Bond, L, Nicora, CD, Fillmore, TL, Clauss, TR, Metz, TO, Webb-Robertson, BJ, and Stevens, DL. Effects of delayed NSAID administration after experimental eccentric contraction injury: a cellular and proteomics study. *PLoS One* 12:e0172486, 2017.

6. Caine, D, DiFiori, J, and Maffulli, N. Physeal injuries in children's and youth sports: reasons for concern? *Br J Sports Med* 40:749-760, 2006.

7. Cohen, P. Long Bone Fracture. *BMJ Best Practice*. March 2020. www.bestpractice.bmj.com/topics/en-us/386. Accessed August 28, 2020.

8. Coleman, N. General fracture considerations. *Curr Sports Med Rep* 17:175-176, 2018.

9. Cook, JL, and Purdam, CR. Is tendon pathology a continuum? A pathology model to explain the clinical presentation of load-induced tendinopathy. *Br J Sports Med* 43:409-416, 2009.

10. Ekeland, A, Engebretsen, L, Fenstad, AM, and Heir, S. Similar risk of ACL graft revision for alpine skiers, football and handball players: the graft revision rate is influenced by age and graft choice. *Br J Sports Med* 54:33-37, 2020.

11. Flachsmann, R, Broom, ND, Hardy, AE, and Moltschaniwskyj, G. Why is the adolescent joint particularly susceptible to osteochondral shear fracture? *Clin Orthop Relat Res* 212-221, 2000.

12. Fleming, BC, Hulstyn, MJ, Oksendahl, HL, and Fadale, PD. Ligament injury, reconstruction and osteoarthritis. *Curr Opin Orthop* 16:354-362, 2005.

13. Frank, CB. Ligament structure, physiology and function. *J Musculoskelet Neuronal Interact* 4:199-201, 2004.

14. Frizziero, A, Vittadini, F, Gasparre, G, and Masiero, S. Impact of estrogen deficiency and aging on tendon: concise review. *Muscles Ligaments Tendons J* 4:324-328, 2014.

15. Galiuto, L. The use of cryotherapy in acute sports injuries. *Ann Sports Medicine Res* 3:1060, 2016.

16. Hauser, R, and Dolan, E. Ligament injury and healing: an overview of current clinical concepts. *J Prolother* 3:836-846, 2011.

17. Hickey, JT, Timmins, RG, Maniar, N, Williams, MD, and Opar, DA. Criteria for progressing rehabilitation and determining return-to-play clearance following hamstring strain injury: a systematic review. *Sports Med* 47:1375-1387, 2017.

18. Jarvinen, TA, Jarvinen, TL, Kaariainen, M, Kalimo, H, and Jarvinen, M. Muscle injuries: biology and treatment. *Am J Sports Med* 33:745-764, 2005.

19. Khan, KM, Cook, JL, Taunton, JE, and Bonar, F. Overuse tendinosis, not tendinitis part 1: a new paradigm for a difficult clinical problem. *Phys Sportsmed* 28:38-48, 2000.

20. Macdonald, B, McAleer, S, Kelly, S, Chakraverty, R, Johnston, M, and Pollock, N. Hamstring rehabilitation in elite track and field athletes: applying the British Athletics Muscle Injury Classification in clinical practice. *Br J Sports Med* 53:1464-1473, 2019.

21. Magnusson, SP, Langberg, H, and Kjaer, M. The pathogenesis of tendinopathy: balancing the response to loading. *Nat Rev Rheumatol* 6:262-268, 2010.

22. Mountjoy, M, Sundgot-Borgen, JK, Burke, LM, Ackerman, KE, Blauwet, C, Constantini, N, Lebrun, C, Lundy, B, Melin, AK, Meyer, NL, Sherman, RT, Tenforde, AS, Klungland, Torstveit, M, and Budgett, R. IOC consensus statement on relative energy deficiency in sport (RED-S): 2018 update. *Br J Sports Med* 52:687-697, 2018.

23. Mueller-Wohlfahrt, HW, Haensel, L, Mithoefer, K, Ekstrand, J, English, B, McNally, S, Orchard, J, van Dijk, CN, Kerkhoffs, GM, Schamasch, P, Blottner, D, Swaerd, L, Goedhart, E, and Ueblacker, P. Terminology and classification of muscle injuries in sport: the Munich consensus statement. *Br J Sports Med* 47:342-350, 2013.

24. Muller, SA, Todorov, A, Heisterbach, PE, Martin, I, and Majewski, M. Tendon healing: an overview of physiology, biology, and pathology of tendon healing and systematic review of state of the art in tendon bioengineering. *Knee Surg Sports Traumatol Arthrosc* 23:2097-2105, 2015.

25. Nork, SE. Initial fracture management and results. *J Orthop Trauma* 19:S7-S10, 2005.

26. Panics, G, Tallay, A, Pavlik, A, and Berkes, I. Effect of proprioception training on knee joint position sense in female team handball players. *Br J Sports Med* 42:472-476, 2008.

27. Perron, AD, Brady, WJ, and Keats, TA. Principles of stress fracture management. The whys and hows of an increasingly common injury. *Postgrad Med* 110:115-124, 2001.

28. Pollock, N, James, SL, Lee, JC, and Chakraverty, R. British athletics muscle injury classification: a new grading system. *Br J Sports Med* 48:1347-1351, 2014.

29. Scott, A, Backman, LJ, and Speed, C. Tendinopathy: update on pathophysiology. *J Orthop Sports Phys Ther* 45:833-841, 2015.

30. Sharma, P, and Maffulli, N. Biology of tendon injury: healing, modeling and remodeling. *J Musculoskelet Neuronal Interact* 6:181-190, 2006.

31. Sherry, MA, and Best, TM. A comparison of 2 rehabilitation programs in the treatment of acute hamstring strains. *J Orthop Sports Phys Ther* 34:116-125, 2004.

32. Shrier, I. Strategic Assessment of Risk and Risk Tolerance (StARRT) framework for return-to-play decision-making. *Br J Sports Med* 49:1311-1315, 2015.

33. Stares, J, Dawson, B, Peeling, P, Drew, M, Heasman, J, Rogalski, B, and Colby, M. How much is enough in rehabilitation? High running workloads following lower limb muscle injury delay return to play but protect against subsequent injury. *J Sci Med Sport* 21:1019-1024, 2018.

34. Wajswlner, H, and Nimphius, S. Bone injuries. In *Sports Injury Prevention and Rehabilitation*. Oxford: Routledge, 2016.

35. Warren, P, Gabbe, BJ, Schneider-Kolsky, M, and Bennell, KL. Clinical predictors of time to return to competition and of recurrence following hamstring strain in elite Australian footballers. *Br J Sports Med* 44:415-419, 2010.

Chapter 30

1. Arnold, B, and Schilling, B. *Evidence-Based Practice in Sport and Exercise: A Guide to Using Research.* Philadelphia: F.A. Davis Company, 2-19, 2016.

2. Bell, L. Patterns of interaction in multidisciplinary child protection teams in New Jersey. *Child Abuse Neglect* 2:65-80, 2001.

3. Corning, P. The re-emergence of "emergence": a venerable concept in search of a theory. *Complexity* 7:18-30, 2002.

4. Coutts, A. Challenges in developing evidence-based practice in high-performance sport. *Int J Sport Physiol Perform* 12:717-718, 2017.

5. Dijkstra, H, Pollock, N, Chakraverty, R, and Alonso, J. Managing the health of the elite athlete: a new integrated performance health management and coaching model. *Br J Sports Med* 48:523-531, 2014.

6. Faulkner, G, Taylor, A, Ferrence, R, Munro, S, and Selby, P. Exercise science and the development of evidence-based practice: a "better practices" framework. *Eur J Sport Sci* 6:117-126, 2006.

7. Gambrill, E. *Critical Thinking in Clinical Practice: Improving the Quality of Judgments and Decisions.* Hoboken, NJ: John Wiley & Sons, 3-28, 2005.

8. Goldstein, J. Emergence as a construct: history and issues. *Emergence* 1:49-72, 1999.

9. Kelledy, L, and Lyons, B. Circular causality in family systems theory. In *Encyclopedia of Couple and Family Therapy*. Lebow, J, Chambers, A, and Breunlin, D, eds. Cham, Switzerland: Springer, 1-4, 2019.

10. Koskie, J, and Freeze, R. A critique of multidisciplinary teaming: problems and possibilities. *Dev Disabil Bull* 28:1-17, 2000.

11. Lilienfeld, S, Lynn, S, and Lohr, J. Science and pseudoscience in clinical psychology: initial thoughts, reflections, and considerations. In *Science and Pseudoscience in Clinical Psychology.* Lilienfeld, S, Lynn, S, and Lohr, J, eds. New York: Guilford Press, 1-14, 2003.

12. Moore, Z. Critical thinking and the evidence-based practice of sport psychology. *J Clin Sport Psychol* 1:9-22, 2007.

13. Moreau, W, and Nabhan, D. Organizational and multidisciplinary work in Olympic high performance centers in USA. *Rev Med Clin Condes* 23:337-342, 2012.

14. Norris, S, and Smith, D. Planning, periodization, and sequencing training and competition: the rationale for a competently planned, optimally executed training and competition program, supported by a multidisciplinary team. In *Enhancing Recovery: Preventing Underperformance in Athletes*. Kellmann, M, ed. Champaign, IL: Human Kinetics, 121-161. 2002.

15. Popper, K. *Conjectures and Refutations: The Growth of Scientific Lnowledge.* London: Routledge & Kegan Paul, 1972.

16. Reid, C, Stewart, E, and Thorne, G. Multidisciplinary sport science teams in elite sport: comprehensive servicing or conflict and confusion? *Sport Psychol* 18:204-217, 2004.

17. Riedy, C. Holocracy – a social technology for purpose-ful organization. 2013. https://medium.com/@chrisjriedy/holocracy-a-social-technology-for-purposeful-organisation-14347a6f3453#:~:text=Holacracy%20is%20a%20real%2Dworld,distributed%20(Holacracy.org). Accessed August 27, 2020.

18. Robertson, B.J. Holacracy: A complete system for agile organizational governance and steering. *Agile Project Management Executive Report* 7(7):1-21, 2006.

19. Robertson, B. Organization at the leading edge: introducing holacracy. *Integral Leadership Rev* 7, 2007.

20. Roncaglia, I. A practitioner's perspective of multidisciplinary teams: analysis of potential barriers and key factors for success. *Psychol Thought* 9:15-23, 2016.

21. Smith, J. and Smolianov, P. The high performance management model: From Olympic and professional to university sport in the United States. *Sports Journal* 21:1-12, 2016.

22. Stember, M. Advancing the social sciences through the interdisciplinary enterprise. *Soc Sci J* 28:1-14, 1991.

23. Tucker, R, and Collins, M. What makes champions? A review of the relative contribution of genes and training to sporting success. *Br J Sports Med* 46:555-561, 2012.

24. Turner, A, Bishop, C, Cree, J, Carr, P, McCann, A, Bartholomew, B, and Halsted, L. Building a high-performance model for sport: a human development-centered approach. *Strength Cond J* 41:100-107, 2019.

25. van de Kamp, P. Holacracy - a radical approach to organizational design. In *Elements of the Software Development Process - Influences on Project Success and Failure*. Dekkers, H, Leeuwis, W, and Plantevin, I, eds. Amsterdam: University of Amsterdam, 13-26, 2014.

26. Zeigler, E. Professional preparation and discipline specialiation in Canadian PE and kinesiology. *J Phys Ed Rec Dance* 61:40-44, 1990.

Chapter 31

1. Barton, C. The current sports medicine journal model is outdated and ineffective. *Aspetar Sports Med J* 7:58-63, 2017.

2. Björk, BO, and Solomon, D. The publishing delay in scholarly peer-reviewed journals. *J Informetr* 7:914-923, 2013.

3. Buchheit, M. Houston, we still have a problem. *Int J Sports Physiol Perform* 12:1111-1114, 2017.

4. Buchheit, M. Want to see my report, coach? *Aspetar Sports Med J* 6:36-43, 2017.

5. Burke, LM. Communicating sports science in the age of the Twittersphere. *Int J Sport Nutr Metab* 27:1-5, 2017.

6. Côté, J, and Darling, E. Scientists on Twitter: preaching to the choir or singing from the rooftops? *Facets* 3:682694, 2018.

7. Dunleavy, P. How to write a blogpost from your journal article in eleven easy steps. January 2016. https://blogs.lse.ac.uk/impactofsocialsciences/2016/01/25/how-to-write-a-blogpost-from-your-journal-article. Accessed August 27, 2020.

8. Grand, A, Wilkinson, C, Bultitude, K, and Winfield, AFT.

Open science: a new "trust technology"? *Sci Commun* 34:679-689, 2012.

9. Impellizzeri, F. Social media in sport science and medicine: with great power comes great responsibility. *Int J Sport Physiol Perform* 13:253-254, 2018.

10. Jones, B, Till, K, Emmonds, S, Hendricks, S, Mackreth, P, Darrall-Jones, J, Roe, G, McGeechan, SI, Mayhew, R, Hunwicks, R, and Potts, N. Accessing off-field brains in sport: an applied research model to develop practice. *Br J Sports Med* 53:791-793, 2019.

11. Le Meur, Y, and Torres, L. 10 Challenges facing today's applied sport scientist. *Sport Perform Sci Rep* 57:v1, 2019.

12. Lemyre, F, Trudel, P, and Durand-Bush, N. How youth sport coaches learn to coach. *Sport Psychol* 21:191-209, 2007.

13. Malone, JJ, Harper, LD, Jones, B, Perry, J, Barnes, C, and Towlson, C. Perspectives of applied collaborative sport science research within professional team sports. *Eur J Sport Sci* 19:147-155, 2019.

14. Martindale, R, and Nash, C. Sport science relevance and application: perceptions of UK coaches. *J Sports Sci* 31:807-819, 2013.

15. Morris, ZS, Wooding, S, and Grant, J. The answer is 17 years, what is the question: understanding time lags in translational research. *J R Soc Med* 104:510-520, 2011.

16. Niyazov, Y, Vogel, C, Price, R, Lund, B, Judd, D, Akil, A, Mortonson, M, Schwartzman, J, and Shron, M. Open access meets discoverability: citations to articles posted to academia.edu. *PLoS One* 11:e0148257, 2016.

17. Norris, M. *The Citation Advantage of Open Access Articles.* Loughborough, UK: Loughborough University, 2018.

18. Purdam, K, and Zhu, Y. Social media, science communication, and academic super users in the UK. *First Monday (Chicago)* 11:1-18, 2017.

19. Stoszkowski, J, and Collins, D. Sources, topics, and use of knowledge by coaches. *J Sport Sci* 34:1-9, 2015.

20. Thornton, HR, Delaney, JA, Duthie, GM, and Dascombe, BJ. Developing athlete monitoring systems in team sports: data analysis and visualization *Int J Sport Physiol Perform* 1;14:698-705, 2019.

21. Vargas-Tonsing, TM. Coaches' preferences for continuing coaching education. *Int J Sports Sci Coach* 2:25-35, 2007.

22. Wright, T, Trudel, P, and Culver, D. Learning how to coach: the different learning situations reported by youth ice hockey coaches. *Phys Educ Sport Pedagogy* 12:127-144, 2007.

INDEX

Note: The italicized *f* and *t* following page numbers refer to figures and tables, respectively.

ABOUT THE EDITORS

Duncan N. French, PhD, is the vice president of performance at the Ultimate Fighting Championship (UFC) Performance Institute and has more than 20 years of experience working with elite professional and Olympic athletes. Prior to joining the UFC, French was the director of performance sciences at the University of Notre Dame and a technical lead for strength and conditioning at the English Institute of Sport.

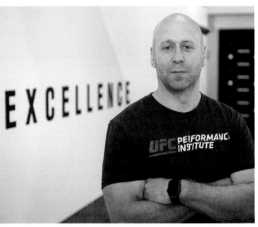

© Chris Unger/Zuffa LLC

French has worked three Olympic cycles as the national lead for strength and conditioning to Great Britain's basketball and, more recently, taekwondo Olympic programs. He earned his PhD from the University of Connecticut in 2004 and has authored or coauthored over 60 peer-reviewed scientific manuscripts. He is a fully accredited strength and conditioning coach with the United Kingdom Strength and Conditioning Association (UKSCA), Australian Strength and Conditioning Association (ASCA), and the National Strength and Conditioning Association (NSCA). French is a former chairman of the UKSCA and received an honorary fellowship in 2014 for his services to the strength and conditioning industry. French holds academic honorary fellowships with Australia Catholic University in Melbourne Australia and Edith Cowan University in Perth, Australia.

Lorena Torres Ronda, PhD, has extensive experience as a high-performance specialist in professional and Olympic sports. She has served as the performance director for the Philadelphia 76ers (NBA), the sport scientist and research and development coordinator for the San Antonio Spurs (NBA), and the sport scientist and strength and conditioning coach for the F.C. Barcelona basketball team and the Spanish national swimming team. Additionally, she has been a part of the NBA scientific committee.

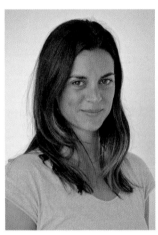

Torres Ronda is currently an adjunct fellow at the Institute for Health and Sport (iHeS) at Victoria University in Melbourne, Australia. She holds a PhD in sport science, is a strength and conditioning coach, and has a wide educational and research background spanning five different universities across the globe, with specializations in sport performance and sport science. In addition to leadership and high-performance culture, her focus centers on athletic performance, sport science, technology and innovation, data analysis and visualization (decision support systems), training and competition monitoring, load management, advanced recovery, and sports nutrition.

Torres Ronda has authored or coauthored more than 50 peer-reviewed scientific papers on athletic performance topics. She is passionate about merging science with practical applications.

CONTRIBUTORS

Courteney L. Benjamin, PhD, CSCS
  Samford University, USA

Chris P. Bertram, PhD
  University of the Fraser Valley, Canada

Tyler A. Bosch, PhD
  Red Bull Athlete Performance Center, USA

Clive Brewer, BSc (Hons), MSc, CSCS
  Columbus Crew SC, USA

Martin Buchheit, PhD
  HIIT Science, France
  Kitman Labs, France

Louise M. Burke, PhD
  Australia Catholic University, Australia

Julio Calleja-González, PhD
  University of the Basque Country, Spain

Marco Cardinale, PhD
  Aspetar Orthopaedic and Sports Medicine
  Hospital, Qatar

David Carey, PhD
  La Trobe University, Australia

Douglas J. Casa, PhD, CSCS
  University of Connecticut, USA

Jo Clubb, MSc
  Buffalo Bills, USA

Daniel Cohen, PhD
  Mindeporte (Colombian Ministry of Sport),
  Columbia

Cassandra C. Collins, BS
  Streaming Foods, Brazil

Stuart Cormack, PhD
  Australia Catholic University, Australia

Aaron J. Coutts, PhD
  University of Technology Sydney, Australia

Roman N. Fomin, PhD
  UFC Performance Institute, USA

Duncan N. French, PhD, CSCS,*D
  UFC Performance Institute, USA

Tim Gabbett, BHSc (Hons), PhD
  Gabbett Performance Solutions, Australia

G. Gregory Haff, PhD, CSCS,*D, FNSCA
  Edith Cowan University, Australia

Shona L. Halson, PhD
  Australia Catholic University, Australia

Franco M. Impellizzeri, PhD
  University of Technology Sydney, Australia

Joel Jamieson
  8WeeksOut, USA

Mladen Jovanović, MS
  University of Belgrade, Serbia

David Joyce, BPhty (Hons), MPhty (Sports), MSc
  The Performance Union, Australia

Cory Kennedy, MSc, CSCS
  Chicago Cubs Baseball Club, USA

Enda King, PhD
  Sports Surgery Clinic, Ireland

William J. Kraemer, PhD, CSCS,*D, FNSCA
  The Ohio State University, USA

Paul Laursen, PhD
  HIIT Science, Canada

Yann Le Meur, PhD
  YLMSportScience, France

Ric Lovell, PhD
  Western Sydney University, Australia

Mike McGuigan, PhD, CSCS,*D
  Auckland University of Technology, New Zealand

Shaun J. McLaren, PhD
  Durham University, UK

Jean-Benoît Morin, PhD
  University Jean Monnet Saint-Etienne, France

Andrew M. Murray, PhD, CSCS
  NBA, USA

Darcy Norman, PT
  Kitman Labs, USA
  US Men's National Soccer Team, USA

Eric S. Rawson, PhD, CSCS, NSCA-CPT
  Messiah University, USA

Chris Richter, PhD
  Sports Surgery Clinic, Germany

Sam Robertson, PhD
  Victoria University, Australia

Kay Robinson, BSc (Hons)
  GWS Giants Football Club, Australia

Pierre Samozino, PhD
University Savoie Mont Blanc, France

Xavier Schelling i del Alcázar, PhD, CSCS
Victoria University, USA

Yasuki Sekiguchi, PhD, CSCS
University of Connecticut, USA

Jessica M. Stephens, PhD
Australian Capital Territory Academy of Sport,
Australia

Michael H. Stone, PhD, CSCS, FNSCA
East Tennessee State University, USA

Nicolás Terrados, MD, PhD
Regional Unit of Sports Medicine and Health
Research Institute of the Principality of Asturias,
Spain

Lorena Torres Ronda, PhD
Victoria University, USA

Jacqueline Tran, PhD
High Performance Sport New Zealand, New
Zealand

Matthew C. Varley, PhD
La Trobe University, Australia

Johann Windt, PhD, CSCS
Vancouver Whitecaps FC, Canada

Nick Winkelman, PhD, CSCS, NSCA-CPT
Irish Rugby Football Union, Ireland

Gabriele Wulf, PhD
University of Nevada–Las Vegas, USA

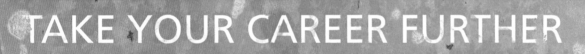
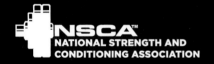
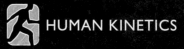